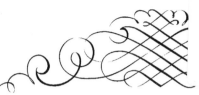

ISBN 978-1-330-58638-9
PIBN 10036850

1 MONTH OF
FREE
READING

at

www.ForgottenBooks.com

By purchasing this book you are eligible for one month membership to ForgottenBooks.com, giving you unlimited access to our entire collection of over 1,000,000 titles via our web site and mobile apps.

To claim your free month visit:

www.forgottenbooks.com/free36850

English
Français
Deutsche
Italiano
Español
Português

www.forgottenbooks.com

Mythology Photography **Fiction**
Fishing Christianity **Art** Cooking
Essays Buddhism Freemasonry
Medicine **Biology** Music **Ancient
Egypt** Evolution Carpentry Physics
Dance Geology **Mathematics** Fitness
Shakespeare **Folklore** Yoga Marketing
Confidence Immortality Biographies
Poetry **Psychology** Witchcraft
Electronics Chemistry History **Law**
Accounting **Philosophy** Anthropology
Alchemy Drama Quantum Mechanics
Atheism Sexual Health **Ancient History**
Entrepreneurship Languages Sport
Paleontology Needlework Islam
Metaphysics Investment Archaeology
Parenting Statistics Criminology
Motivational

A TREATISE

ON

THE SURGICAL DISEASES OF THE EYE.

A TREATISE

ON THE

SURGICAL DISEASES OF THE EYE.

BY

H. HAYNES WALTON,

FELLOW OF THE ROYAL COLLEGE OF SURGEONS IN ENGLAND;
SURGEON TO THE CENTRAL LONDON OPHTHALMIC HOSPITAL, AND
TO ST MARY'S HOSPITAL, PADDINGTON;
TEACHER OF THE SURGICAL OPERATIONS IN ST MARY'S MEDICAL SCHOOL.

SECOND EDITION.

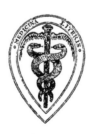

LONDON:
JOHN CHURCHILL, NEW BURLINGTON STREET.

MDCCCLXI.

LONDON :
REED AND PARDON, PRINTERS,
PATERNOSTER ROW.

TO

SAMUEL BROWNE, ESQ.,

LICENTIATE OF KING'S AND QUEEN'S COLLEGE OF PHYSICIANS IN IRELAND,
M.R.C.S., SURGEON R.N.,

SURGEON TO THE GENERAL HOSPITAL, BELFAST, AND TO THE
OPHTHALMIC INSTITUTION,

A ZEALOUS TEACHER OF OPHTHALMIC SURGERY, AND A SUCCESSFUL PRACTITIONER,

This Work is inscribed,

AS A HIGH MARK OF ESTEEM FOR HIS PROFESSIONAL ATTAINMENTS AND HIS
MORAL WORTH,

BY

THE AUTHOR.

PREFACE TO THE FIRST EDITION.

As an untried writer, I cannot be otherwise than anxious for the success of this work. I have spared no pains in my attempt to make it of practical value, and I have laid under contribution all the literature that has come within my reach or my knowledge, whether English or Foreign, on the subject of Ophthalmic Pathology and Surgery. I have given at length my own personal experience. It remains for me to particularize some of those to whom I feel myself especially indebted.

First of all I mention the venerable Dr. John Richard Farre, who, in conjunction with Mr. John Cunningham Saunders, established the first public Institution in this Kingdom for the treatment of Ophthalmic Diseases.

To this great Physician, full of years and of honour, I am indebted for the advice to study Ophthalmic Medicine and Surgery, and by him I was introduced as a pupil into this department of Science.

Having had the good fortune to be both pupil and, for a short period, Acting House-Surgeon of the Ophthalmic Institution, under the superintendence of Mr. Tyrrell, Mr. Scott, and Mr. Dalrymple, I must record my admiration of the zeal, the practical skill, and the advanced science which characterised the practice of those illustrious men, whose premature death is a loss as well to the Public as to the Medical Profession. To Mr. Lawrence also, eminent alike as a scholar and as a surgeon, I am under deep obligations for the knowledge which I gained on Ophthalmic subjects, while acting under him as Dresser and House-Surgeon.

To Dr. Mackenzie, of Glasgow, I am much indebted, and have compared my own observations with his valuable experience, as detailed in his excellent work on the diseases of the eye.

No one who is at all acquainted with Ophthalmic Surgery is ignorant of the immense value of the profoundly scientific and eminently practical researches of Dr. Jacob, of Dublin : his writings I have studied with care.

To Mr. Wilde, of Dublin, I must also pay my tribute of thanks and admiration ; and no less to my friend Mr. Browne, of Belfast, who has greatly assisted me by many important suggestions.

My colleague, Mr. Taylor, has rendered me most important assistance by working with me, and taking many of the sketches that adorn this volume.

I am under obligations to others whom I name not in detail, that I may escape the charge of parading the catalogue of my kind friends. To all and each, I tender my warm and respectful thanks.

The Illustrations, one hundred and sixty-nine in number, by the Messrs. Bagg, will doubtless fully sustain the high character which these Artists have acquired.

H. HAYNES WALTON.

69, Brook Street, Hanover Square.
December 31*st*, 1852.

PREFACE TO THE SECOND EDITION.

This is a New Edition in the fullest sense of the word.

The history of Ophthalmic Surgery, consisting of forty-six pages, has been omitted.

Chapters II., VI., X., XXVI., XXVII., are entirely new.

Chapters I., XIV., XVI., XXII., have been re-written.

The remaining chapters have been either recast, or thoroughly revised in every page. I would allude particularly to the IV., V., XIII., XXIII., and XXV., as being those most changed.

Several new wood-cuts have been introduced.

All of the many reviews of the last edition were most satisfactory. Some of them were by the highest Ophthalmic authorities in England, Scotland, and Ireland. That by the father of British Ophthalmology, Dr. Mackenzie, of Glasgow, in the "British and Foreign Medico-Chirurgical Review," and to which he appended his name, was the most elaborate, extended, and valuable. I have availed myself of the many remarks and suggestions it contains.

There have been several reprints of the work.

From friends I have received numerous hints and more or less assistance; for all of which I am grateful. But I must particularize among them, my colleagues Mr. R. Taylor and Mr. E. Hulme, the former of whom has besides overlooked the proof sheets with his characteristic kindness and carefulness.

Mr. G. H. Davis, a former pupil of St. Mary's Hospital, and a late House-Surgeon, has rendered me much help with the Index, which is very copious.

H. HAYNES WALTON.

69, BROOK STREET, HANOVER SQUARE, W.
July 1st, 1861.

CONTENTS.

A TREATISE

ON THE

SURGICAL DISEASES OF THE EYE.

CHAPTER I.

THE USE OF CHLOROFORM IN OPHTHALMIC SURGERY.

IMPORTANCE OF AN EXPERIENCED CHLOROFORMIST — EFFECTS AT DIFFERENT PERIODS OF LIFE—CONTRA-INDICATIONS—TESTS—PREPARATION OF PATIENT — QUANTITY REQUIRED TO PRODUCE STUPOR — MODE OF INHALATION — EXCEPTIONS TO EMPLOYMENT.

THE benefit of chloroform happily extends to ophthalmic surgery. It is scarcely possible to overrate the value of a discovery which tranquillizes the mind of the patient by banishing the anticipation of pain, deadens the sensibility, and prevents the reality of suffering; while to the operator it brings the inestimable advantage of quieting the struggles of children or of irresolute adults, which are so apt to frustrate all the care, foresight, and dexterity that the most assiduous application to practical surgery can command.

I shall give a short sketch of the method of dealing with this wonderful agent. Does it not deserve a notice? Is it not as important as any subject in the volume, and does it not require to be taught? Students should have instruction in all that concerns this anæsthetic.

No one who has at all looked into the matter can, I think, doubt that nearly all the deaths under chloroform have been due to carelessness, often to extreme neglect. What surgeon is there, much engaged in his profession, who has not witnessed narrow escapes? I am sure that I have saved several lives by

B

timely interference, by stopping the inhalation, or adopting resuscitating measures. Therefore, whenever it is practicable, I stipulate for the services of a proficient chloroformist; for when the administration is undertaken by a chance person, or, as more frequently happens, by the general medical attendant of the patient, I almost always have to be the chloroformist and the operator too, so little is the process generally understood, although attention to a few rules, with some opportunities of actual practice, will enable most men to officiate with safety. I say most men, because the physical incapabilities of some wholly unfit them to see with composure the convulsions and struggles that might arise, or tedious and bloody dissections, as in the removal of orbital tumours, or to exercise the necessary judgment and perseverance not unfrequently required with those persons who are less easily affected.

That some individuals are better subjects for chloroform than others is a fact. Young persons and children take it easier and with less unpleasant effect, and with less risk, than the aged. Very old persons should not be chloroformed for any slight matter, and never without due representation to themselves or their friends of the increased danger arising from their time of life. I should certainly not give it to a patient who had any disease of the heart, or chronic organic disease of the brain; and assuredly with very great reluctance to one with an intermitting pulse. Embarrassed pulmonary circulation is a condition in which it should not be given without much consideration. Disease of the lungs, however, as in phthisis, does not contra-indicate it. Attention was drawn to this by Mr. Wells, who, by the special and dying request of a nobleman whom he attended during the ravages of phthisis, brought before the Medico-Chirurgical Society of London the important fact of the relief derived from it in that malady. The extreme violence of the cough, and the very oppressive dyspnœa, uncontrolled by the usual remedies, suggested the trial of chloroform. The inhalation was successful; every repetition of it equally so; and during the remaining seven months of the patient's life great alleviation of suffering, without any discoverable ill effects, was obtained by its frequent employment. Several years ago I attended a phthisical patient, who would not allow a bandage to be removed from his diseased leg without first deadening his sensibility by the influence of chloroform. This was repeated about three times a week for nearly three months. The distressing cough was always allayed for many hours after inhalation.

Great care should be taken to procure pure chloroform; and generally the most sure way of doing this, and certainly the readiest, is to purchase only at an establishment that can be depended on. Once, and once only, have I been disappointed in so doing. The chloroform was just about to be used by myself, when I quickly detected the escape of hydrochloric acid vapour from the bottle. At once I made the fact known to the manufacturer, who called on me to explain the cause—an error in distillation, that certainly should have been avoided. The following hints, therefore, may be useful. The formula is $C^2 H Cl^3$. Its specific gravity was fixed at 1·480 by Liebig, but it is constantly produced at 1·496 by Soubeiran. Dr. Simpson gives it as 1·500. It is frequently empirically prepared by persons who know nothing of its composition, and it is seldom that an absolutely pure sample can be obtained. In different specimens there have been discovered alcohol, chlorine, hydrochloric acid, and hydrochloric ether, compounds of methyle, besides water and fixed substances. Chloroform may be depended on that has a sp. gr. of 1·480; a higher density is to be preferred, and it should stand the following tests. When poured on the hand, it should evaporate entirely, without leaving any odour. It should not give any reaction with red or blue litmus paper or nitrate of silver. When shaken with twice its weight of distilled water, and allowed to stand two or three hours in a graduated tube, it should not sensibly diminish in bulk. When placed in contact with concentrated sulphuric acid, the acid should not become blackened. If it will stand this examination, it may be safely relied on. It should be kept in a well-stopped bottle, and from the influence of the light.

The stomach should be empty previous to inhalation, a precaution secured by enjoining a strict fast for four or five hours. A loaded stomach is sure to occasion violent vomiting; and besides the annoyance and filth that this occasions, there is risked the likelihood of interruption to the operation, the prolonging of the whole proceeding, and consequently the more unpleasant after-results. I have frequently witnessed, in consequence of the stomach being full, a degree of depression like that caused by severe sea-sickness, so intense, that it has been deemed prudent not to continue the inhalation. There is often nausea when the stomach contains nothing, but the retching, when it occurs, is generally of short duration, and much depression is uncommon.

I think it of much importance that the patient should loosen any tight article of dress ; indeed, that his chest and abdomen be wholly unrestricted in their movements; and in the case of females, the stays should be loosened. In this unrestrained state, when respiration is easier, the desired effect is quicker accomplished, insensibility sooner passes away, and there is no hindrance to artificial respiration, or any other measure for resuscitation, should circumstances demand it.

While I do not sometimes hesitate myself to administer the chloroform with a handkerchief, or on a bit of lint—a wasteful method,—I am sure that, for general use, and, above all, for prolonged inhalations, a graduated inhaler is more safe, and especially because a small quantity can be given at a time, under all circumstances, including struggles or resistance, with a proper supply of air. Much fallacy prevails respecting the quantity actually taken. I find this so well considered by my friend Dr. Druitt, in the eighth edition of his "Surgeon's Vade Mecum," in the masterly and comprehensive chapter on the means of producing insensibility to pain, that I quote it:—"In speaking of the dose of chloroform, it must be remembered that it is not the mere quantity inhaled, without reference to time, but the quantity present in the blood in a given time, which is to be regarded. Patients may be kept under its influence a long time, and thus may inhale a large quantity with safety ; but even a small quantity too rapidly inhaled, and sufficiently diluted

with air, may be dangerous. When we hear the dose of chloroform estimated by drachms, and are told of a patient who con-
sumed thirty-two ounces in twenty-four hours, we must not
forget that it is the actual quantity present in a given time in
the blood, and its effects on the sensibility and respiration, that
are to be the real guides as to the safety or danger of the quantity administered, and not the mere quantity by measure that is
evaporated. Dr. Snow calculated that about twelve minims of
chloroform circulating in the blood of an adult produce the
second degree of narcotism; eighteen minims the degree in
which operations are performed ; a little more than thirty suffice
to arrest respiration, and thirty-six or thirty-seven to stop the
action of the heart. These numbers refer to the quantity
actually circulating in the blood at a given time. It is necessary, also, to bear in mind, that when a patient is inhaling air
highly charged with chloroform, the narcotic effects continue to
increase, as Dr. Snow pointed out, for twenty seconds after the
inhalation is discontinued, owing to the absorption of the vapour
remaining in the lungs. But it seems very certain that much
less is requisite for producing full insensibility in some persons
than in others."

The administration should be effected as gently as possible,
and with perfect stillness in the room. It matters not how much
chloroform is put into the inhaler, if the stop-cocks or valves are
so arranged—and they should be—that the chloroformist can at
will regulate the quantity he wishes the patient to take, and on
this chiefly the safety of the process depends. Proceed very
slowly, and allow but a very small quantity of vapour to enter
the lungs at once. In proportion as it is given quickly, so is the
danger to life.

The chloroformist should attend to his special duty, and that
only : he should keep his finger on the pulse, and his eye on the
breathing. "There should be," continues Dr. Druitt, "no
hurry in the first stage of the process, because complete insensibility to pain, and absence of involuntary movement and
wincing, are more safely obtained after the vapour has had time
to permeate all the capillaries and benumb all the peripheral

nerves. Dr. Snow makes the most valuable observation,—that
insensibility to pain cannot be obtained in a *very rapid* manner
without a dangerous degree of narcotism of the nervous centres.
The inhalation should occupy at least from four to seven minutes
before the third degree of narcotism is established, and then it
will usually be another minute more before the surgeon should
begin. The loud talking or violence of the intoxication stage is
no cause of alarm—quite the reverse : it shows that the vapour
has not produced a dangerous effect, and that a slight increase is
necessary to produce the next degree."

The time to commence an operation is the moment voluntary
motion is suspended, and the proof of this is the loss of the
sensibility of the conjunctiva ; for, as long as there remains
sensibility in that membrane, there will be contraction of the
eyelids, when the globe of the eye is touched. After the full
influence has been produced, the chloroform should be still more
diluted, as much less of it will suffice to keep up the effect, and
it will be wise to take the inhaler away from the face from time
to time. There are two common errors in the use of chloroform,—the one on the part of the chloroformist in not getting a
sufficient effect, and the other on the part of the surgeon in
commencing the operation too soon. Operations are often
indeed finished, at the time when they ought to be commenced.

Now, as regards the use of chloroform in the special department of ophthalmic surgery, most unquestionably, in infancy, it
does afford very great assistance ; for, without it, resistance on
the part of the little patient is certain. The very diminutiveness of the organ, whereby there is much less room for the use
of the fingers and for instruments, together with the great
delicacy of the parts, demand the utmost exposure of the surface
of the eyeball, with the greatest steadiness. In former years,
the operation for congenital cataract was frequently postponed,
because these desiderata could not be commanded ; and I believe
that occasionally in the present day their acquisition is considered impossible, and an operation delayed, to the great detriment of the patient. I strongly suspect that the reason why
the posterior operation for " solution " of cataract has been so

frequently but wrongly advised in infancy is, because of the much greater nicety required to perform the anterior. Without the effect of chloroform, to retract the palpebræ, to introduce the needle, and to employ it in a proper manner, not dividing the capsule too extensively, nor moving it too freely in the lens, lest dislocation should occur, without touching the iris, or using injurious force, is no easy matter, or, at least, it may not be easy. True it is, that the modern spring-eyelid retractor, of silver wire or steel, removes some of the difficulty, but only a part; for the task of securing the child, as well as other obstacles, still remain.

Again, from what I hear, · and indeed I may say, from what I see, it would appear that, before the use of anæsthetics, the operation for congenital cataract was not unfrequently left unfinished. The capsule which blocked up the pupil was not always removed; and the operation, in any given case, was more often and injuriously repeated, not merely from the erroneous idea that then existed, and unfortunately still does exist to some extent, about the necessary repetition of them, but also on account of the difficulty that frequently prevented the surgeon from carrying out his previous intentions.

With children, and young persons in general, even when an operation is painless, there is an expectation of something worse than what is actually felt, and generally a deficiency of resolution that renders it impossible for them to be sufficiently quiet without violent resistance, or the employment of mechanical restraint; and failures and mishaps are more commonly due than could be supposed, to the unsteadiness of the eye. If I had noted down all the instances that I have witnessed of foiled endeavours, they would form a large page in my note-book.

An infant that has lost its pupil from purulent ophthalmia, or any other cause, is not now doomed to darkness till the adult period, or, at least, need not be, as in past years. We can operate on the smallest eye, and the consent of the patient is not necessary.

The public are becoming alive to the disadvantages of holding down children. A lady called on me recently, to make an arrangement for an operation on her child's eye, and at once asked if I used chloroform in such cases. I answered that I did, and, requesting her reason for the question, she said, " I have just left the house of Mr. ——, who has declined to employ it; he declared that, by rolling up my child in a table-cloth, and the aid of two strong assistants, he could manage her, or the most unruly young lady. I told him that her timidity and highly nervous susceptibility made me dread the effect of such an ordeal on her mind."

It is curious to read in the work of the talented and ingenious Mr. Wardrop, of the mechanical contrivances he resorted to, in order to quiet the resistance of a blind and deaf boy. Persons have been bled till they fainted, to obtain a passive state.

I now pass to those operations on the adult eye in which we may receive considerable assistance from insensibility. It is evident that here there should be a distinction between such cases as require chloroform merely because of lack of moral courage, and those in which it is of positive advantage under any condition; as in the one, we may leave the choice to the patient, or we may object; in the other, it is our duty to recommend it. It is a fact that, with the fullest consent and greatest determination on the part of a person, indeed with a resolution that could endure a limb to be severed from the body without a groan or a cry, and with every desire to assist the operator, anæsthetic sleep may be advantageous. The majority of operations for artificial pupil, especially where the proceeding is complicated, and requires the use of more than one, or the re-introduction of the same instrument, falls under the latter category. An eye, for the most part, that requires this aid, is much damaged, and the vitreous humour is too frequently disorganized; so that there is needed the greatest steadiness of the eyeball, with long continuance of a given position, and an absence of much pressure. Now, the movements of the eyeball may be quite involuntary, and the eyelids will twitch, in spite of the most resolute will. But not the least disadvantage of consciousness is the compression that the straight and oblique muscles can and do exercise in such operations. When acting violently, they exert considerable influence; and the effect of such an agency, at such a time, is always hazardous, in several ways. Again, in many operations of general surgery, the sooner the manipulation ends, and the instruments are out of the body, the more certain is the result: this is doubly true of the eye. These remarks may be said to apply, in the main, when the eyeball is to be opened for the extraction of any body, be it capsule, animalcule, or any particle driven into it from without, and decided difficulty or intricacy is apprehended.

Surgeons do not generally adopt my plan of closing the eyelids, after the operation for " extraction," with straps of plaster; but, when chloroform has been used, the practice is imperative, or the vitreous humour will be lost if vomiting should ensue. The same holds good in any case when the cornea has been extensively incised. Except in a diseased and very fluid state of the vitreous humour, it is effectual.

Timidity, and the accompanying restlessness of a patient, may render it impossible to operate successfully. I have seen this over and over, even under the hands of operators who have not been surpassed in this kingdom for self-possession and brilliancy in execution. On each occasion, the eye was either lost or much damaged, from the unavoidable results of operating against the patient's resistance. Here chloroform removes all difficulty. I cannot give a case more to the point than the following. A man sixty-five years of age, with hard cataracts, was brought up to the operating-room at the Central London Ophthalmic Hospital, for extraction to be performed on one of his eyes; but so great was his agitation, that he could not be induced to keep quiet enough to allow his eye to be sufficiently opened for the operation. He almost fainted when ascending the stairs, and required to be lifted by the porter. All this was from sheer mental emotion, for he was neither feeble nor infirm. As there was no probability of his ever having self-command enough, I determined to give him chloroform. It was decided, however, not to do it on that day—for he had recently taken food,—but on the following, when his stomach was empty. I operated while he was insensible, easily and successfully. This was on a Friday. On the Saturday, delirium tremens set in, and continued with violence, the head being tossed freely about, till the Monday, when it began to yield to remedies. On the Wednesday he had recovered. With the exception of a few hours, when the delirium first came on, the eyes were kept closed by plasters ; a nurse was, however, constantly at his side, to prevent him from tearing them off again. Eleven days after the operation, the eye was found, contrary to all expectation, to be proceeding well, the corneal section having united, there being no prolapse of the iris, and the pupil being quite circular. He did not at any time complain of pain. His sight was restored.

There are physical peculiarities of the eye which impede the operation for extraction of cataract, and which may be surmounted by the aid of chloroform. They are mainly those that present impediments to exposing and steadying the eyeball sufficiently to enable the cornea to be divided in an ample manner, such as a sunken eye, a narrow palpebral aperture, unusual prominence of the orbital ridge. In any of these states, more pressure with the fingers is generally required than the eye will bear. During stupor the eyelids can be more widely extended, and the eyeball fixed with a lightness of touch that would, on account of the peculiarities, be insufficient during sensibility ; there being, in fact, all the difference between involuntary resistance, however slight, and absolute quiet. Beyond this chloroform does not assist us here. When a patient has tolerable fortitude, at all events, whatever be his mental emotion, so long as he remains master of his will, and can direct his eye to the position desired, and there are no impediments to exposing his eyeball to the required extent, I would rather that he retain his senses during the operation ; for then, I believe that the crystalline lens is better started from its position, that it escapes much more readily, that the pupil is more quickly restored to its natural state, and the iris less liable to prolapse after the terrible stretching it has received. Even without this, is it not far better to save an aged person, if only from all the formality and distress of an inhalation? Is it not better to see a patient rise and walk to his bed or couch, rational and thankful, than for him to be removed, half-conscious, sick and miserable, requiring careful and anxious attention, both on account of the constitutional effects of the chloroform, and the injury he might inflict on his eye? Although a patient might not vomit or even retch after the inhalation of chloroform, he might remain twelve or twenty-four hours in a squeamish state, with but little appetite for food; and this might be more injurious than vomiting, for it is of the greatest importance, especially late in life, that nutrition should be well maintained. I have several times calmed the fears of elderly persons on whom I was about to perform extraction, and dissuaded them from an inhalation, and in every instance I have been thanked for my advice. I have been asked repeatedly, even by patients, if the anæsthetic sleep does not give confidence to the operator, and enable the operation to be the better done. I can only say that if, in any given instance, this is likely to be true, the timid surgeon had better avail himself of every admissible assistance that is likely to restore sight to his patient.

As it is after the meridian of life, and often in the very aged, that extraction is needed, we should be careful not to use chloroform needlessly. In the early period of our existence, the risk of a fatal termination is exceedingly small. Not so, however, in the old and enfeebled, in whom the heart is so often diseased by being degenerated,—a state which the most rigid scrutiny during life may fail to detect. Disease of the heart, however, has not been always found in those who have been killed by chloroform. The operation is unattended with acute pain when well executed. We should not, therefore, use such an agent as a matter of routine, but withhold it when it may be dispensed with; and whenever we employ it, exercise the most searching scrutiny as to its admissibility. We should not lightly place an aged person in a state so closely resembling apoplexy that it would be quite impossible, at the moment, for any one to point out the difference.

I cannot close this subject without a slight tribute of respect to the late Dr. Snow. Among those who have devoted themselves to the extension of our knowledge of the precautions under which chloroform should be employed, his name stands pre-eminent. His extensive researches, and his numerous and scientific experiments, were conducted with a degree of accuracy hardly to be surpassed; and the results have been so important as to place the medical profession and the public under the greatest obligations to him. To operate when the patient had been narcotised by one so conversant with all the peculiarities of its action on the human body, was to obtain an advantage heretofore unknown in surgery. I refer with pleasure to his communications in the "Medical Gazette," during the period from 1847 to 1850; to No. 180 of the "Edinburgh Journal of Medicine" for April, 1847; and to the "Medical Times" for August 31st, 1850; and lastly, to his posthumous work "On Chloroform and other Anæsthetics: their Action and Administration," edited by his friend Dr. Richardson.

CHAPTER II.

THERE is no novelty in the local application of water in a continuous stream, as a remedial agent, by the douche; yet one very seldom sees the appliance in use. Why such a valuable means of treating disease—for valuable it has been proved to be—is not more commonly resorted to, can only be accounted for, I imagine, on the supposition that there is general lack of knowledge on the subject. Among the men of reputation who have pointed out the advantages of the douche, Mr. James, of Exeter, one of the bright ornaments of our profession, stands prominent. Those who have had the advantage of attending his hospital practice could not fail to be struck with the benefit of it under his supervision. He told me that private individuals were in the habit of resorting to the hospital to be douched. They repaired to the bath-room, put on the waterproof dress, according to the part to be acted on, whether arm or leg, and having received the application, paid the hospital a certain fee.

I believe in the efficacy of an eye-douche: I believe it to be a valuable addition to our ophthalmic therapeutics. It is several years since I have been prescribing it, especially for those of my patients who are old enough to manage it.

In acute, and particularly in chronic inflammatory affections of the eyeball, or of the eyelids, its directly sensitive effects are soothing and sedative. The temperature must be regulated by the sensations of the user, for, after all that theory may suggest on this head, his discretion is, I think, the best criterion. To this is added, in purulent ophthalmia, a real and effectual method of cleansing the eye.

It is not less valuable as a means of applying cold to the overworked and fatigued eye.

It is a ready and efficient manner of soothing the eye after some operations.

It may be useful in washing away extraneous substances.

FIG. 1.

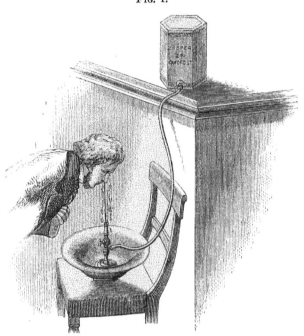

The figure shows the one I recommend and the manner of using it.

It was made at my suggestion, by Mr. W. Cooper, of 26, Oxford-street, who has bestowed pains on its construction. It consists of a metal box, capable of holding about six pints of water, and can be suspended, or rested on a bracket. To this is attached an elastic tube, terminated by a pedestal stop-cock, that will stand easily in a basin. As there are no valves, the apparatus is so much the less likely to get out of order.

The full quantity of the water may be taken at once. The frequency of the application must of course depend on the circumstances of individual cases and the effect. One need not be afraid of repetition, as it can hardly be abused.

I do not like to enter more into detail, and so risk tiring my reader. Any surgeon who gives the system a trial will soon become acquainted with all necessary details.

Every ophthalmic institution should have a douche, with a continuous supply of water, and so arranged that warm water may be used. For the poor man I extemporize a douche with a pail or a pan for the reservoir, a bit of small gas-tubing bent in a syphon, and a simple stop-cock with one jet, all of which can be got for a shilling or two.

There are several hand-douches at present before the public. They are very extensively advertised. I need not particularize them.

CHAPTER III.

IT is easy to comprehend the extent of influence exerted over the success of a surgical operation by the perfection or imperfection of the instrument with which it is performed; and if this be the case in surgery at large, it is more particularly true in ophthalmic operations.

To lessen the defects of an instrument is tantamount to an improvement in the branch of surgery to which it belongs. Simplicity and due adaptation to the purpose intended are the qualities which a surgeon who operates on the eye should endeavour to acquire for his implements. The improvement of those in our day contrasts advantageously with the coarseness of form and inferiority of workmanship in times past. For these reasons alone I should deem it proper to notice the subject; but, further, I take this view of the matter—that in treating of any department of operative surgery, an opportunity for communicating practical instruction is lost when hints and observations on the instruments concerned are omitted.

The plan proposed is, to introduce the several instruments with the subjects requiring their use, and to describe them apart from the operations, as it possesses the advantage of securing a fuller attention for them than if they were spoken of digressively: while the subsequent details of the operations themselves, being uninterrupted, will then most readily command attention. Some few, of general use, will be given at the end of the chapter.

As each instrument will be illustrated by an engraving which will convey the most exact ideas of it, those points only which deserve especial attention, or which the figure less prominently sets forth, will be dwelt on in the description. The instruments that are introduced are those I am actually in the habit of using, and which appear to me to be the most appropriate to each operation, and the most convenient for the several purposes which they are intended to fulfil.

With ophthalmic instruments, lightness is an element of the highest importance. The lighter they are, the greater is the delicacy with which they can be applied. With light instruments the resistance to be overcome is better appreciated, as well as the amount of force required for that purpose. The blades should not be of greater size than the use intended requires: but in a far greater degree the same property is attained by exchanging the ivory handle so generally adopted, notwithstanding the nicer appearance, for one of light wood. In all other respects the minimum of the dimensions compatible with the kind of instrument should be made the rule. In successive years, as I have required to renew my instruments, I have gradually had their size reduced; and the effect has been to adapt them better to the several operations. Besides remedying the clumsiness and awkwardness which attach to those of greater bulk, in several instances positive evils, arising from inordinate size, have been avoided.

To all small instruments, such as cataract knives, cataract needles, and the like, I prefer round handles; for, when of this form, they can be held with more ease and freedom, while stiffness and constraint are overcome, and a more individual independent control is thus given to the fingers. I am also of opinion that the handles should be smooth and not crosscut. There can be no other reason why the handle of a surgical instrument should be roughened, and thereby rendered unpleasant to the touch, as well as less suitable for delicate use, than that surgeons, having been careless about the subject, have permitted the instrument-maker to indulge his fancy, merely to give an air of finish to his workmanship. I believe it to be true—and if so, it is a fact of much significance—that there is no other manual art in which rough-handled instruments are used.

All instruments designed to puncture the cornea should have such a form, from the gradual increase of thickness from the point, as to act on the principle of a stopper in the aperture that is made : the effect of this is to retain the aqueous humour as long as possible, so that the natural prominence of the cornea is for a time preserved, and the subsequent steps of the operation are facilitated. The gradual augmentation of size sufficient for this purpose, while at the same time a proper stiffness of point is preserved, need not, in cataract needles, exceed at the largest part from 1-36th to 1-40th of an inch.

Sharpness of point, and keenness of edge, are of paramount importance; and these qualities of a perfect instrument should

FIG. 2.

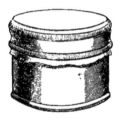

be carefully sought after, and ascertained by delicate processes. To test the point, the best criterion I know is the little drum made of the cuticle stripped from the softest kid skin, and stretched over a metallic cylinder, of which the above figure is a representation. A less perfect method is, to stretch the cuticle across the fingers. In either case, if the point be in order, little more than the weight of the instrument should cause it insensibly to penetrate the tissue. If, on the contrary, the point be dull, it requires to be forced through ; if otherwise defective by being turned or broken, in addition to the force required to make it penetrate, a sharp cracking sound is emitted. In consequence of the natural pores in the cuticle, several punctures should be made, to insure the passage of the point of the instrument through an unbroken space.

The edge should be tried on the palm of the hand where the cuticle is thinnest; for instance, on the ball of the thumb. And I cannot express myself more concisely than by saying, that with a slight drawing motion it should at once enter, or bite, as instrument-makers say.

Properly tempered instruments may always be secured by dealing at some highly respectable London shop, such as that of Messrs. Weiss, or Whicker and Blaise, where each, from the largest to the smallest, is separately hardened, and individually tempered, and where the extent of sale is such as to enable the maker to maintain in constant employment a workman whose sole occupation it is to manufacture delicate instruments of this class; for by such exclusive attention alone can the highest perfection be reached.

It is necessary, also, that scissors be inspected. Their efficiency depends not only on the blades being properly sharpened, but also on their being lightly made and securely riveted. The simplest, and, at the same time, the surest test, is to close the blades gently, and without any lateral pressure, on a very thin piece of wetted paper. If properly made, they will readily divide it; if not, they will close over it without cutting.

I cannot refrain from adding a remark on sponges. It is hardly conceivable that the success of an operation can, in any degree, be dependent on the mere purity of a sponge; yet I have the strongest reason to suspect that the partial or even the entire failure of the process of adhesion after incisions has depended on the transmission of particles of sand from the sponges to the edges of wounds. The impossibility of buying a new sponge that is not loaded with earthy particles is well known. To remove these, time is requisite; washing, necessary as it is, cannot at once cleanse them. The best method of procuring them free of grit is, to employ the best sponges of the shops for common domestic purposes for several months, taking care that on frequent occasions, when dry, they are beaten for some time.

c 2

FIG. 3.

SCALPEL.

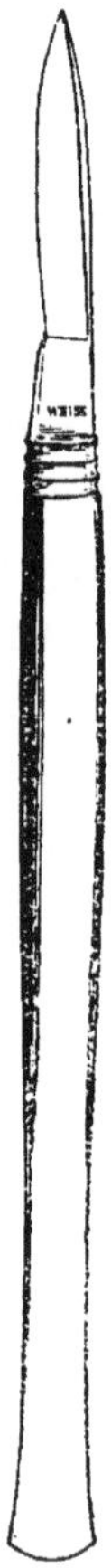

An instrument in such general use, and so well known, would have been passed over in silence, were it not that the kind here advocated is reduced considerably below the size of scalpels in general. The ordinary ones are decidedly too large for all dissecting operations on a small scale, especially such as those on the eyelids, where precision and neatness are imperatively demanded; and those for the removal of tumours about the eye and its appendages, particularly when encroaching upon, or actually lying within the orbit. The point is placed centrally, and this position, while it allows of a requisite amount of curve, renders it better adapted for minute dissection than when it is in a line with the back of the blade; and in a central point there may be the union of the greatest fineness with the greatest strength. In nearly all operations with the scalpel, it is the point of the blade that is principally available, and to its properties the value of the knife is chiefly due. The breadth of the handle is of some consequence; for if carried beyond a certain extent, it is not readily fingered. I also recommend that the parts to which the points of the fingers are applied should be rounded. The length may be what fancy suggests, unless, as is the case with myself, the instrument be held in a particular manner, as a common table-knife is held, my fingers being placed near the blade,—a method which demands shortness of handle. This mode of holding it I adopt for almost all purposes, finding that it combines the greatest freedom of motion with the greatest power, and the lightest touch.

FORCEPS.

The proper length is such as allows them to rest on the hand between the thumb and the finger, when held in the ordinary manner. Any length beyond this is useless, and

increases their weight. The blades should be
slightly bowed, well hardened, and of a substance, in thickness rather than in breadth, that
will not allow them to slip on each other; or
bend under any force of pressure that can be
required during their use, for were
their extremities to gape, which they
surely would if the centres of the
blades were weak, they must cease to
be effectual. The spring should not
be made stronger than sufficient to
sustain their weight. Round points
are, I think, superior to any other
form. The holding, or interior surfaces of the extremities, should be
raised, and obliquely cut for at least a quarter
of an inch, the serratures being large, and
exactly fitting. This roughness is quite compatible with an accuracy of edge adapted for
minute purposes.

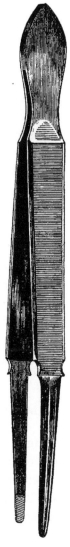

FIG. 4.

FIG. 5.

It is frequently required to use tenaculum
forceps in operations about the ocular appendages, for the ordinary ones do not lay hold
with sufficient firmness. The lesser figure,
representing merely the points, shows the
direction the teeth should have. When so
placed, they seize very readily, although they
cannot retain their grasp quite so securely as
when made to meet at a right angle. In order
to be effectual, their blades should be stout
enough to enable sufficient pressure to be made at the points.
When shut without an intervening substance, the teeth necessarily cross. A catch-spring, like that usually added to tenaculum forceps, and originally introduced for Amussat's treatment of bleeding arteries by torsion, is not only useless for
dissection, but a decided impediment.

EYELID-RETRACTOR.

Of the many single instruments in use for the FIG. 6.
purpose of retracting the eyelids, whether to procure
an examination of the eye, or to facilitate the performance of operations, I give the preference to this,
which is designed to be passed within the eyelid, and
which is of full size for an adult. For infants and
children a smaller one is necessary. Its length and
lightness are such as to enable it to be applied with
delicacy, and to be maintained in the desired position
without the exercise of force. The bent portion
deserves attention. It should not be longer or more
obtuse than is sufficient to secure and confine the
edge of the eyelid, otherwise its action might be
detrimental; because if the sinus or sulcus of the
eyelid were reached, a resistance would be immediately encountered, which would not only prevent
the eyelid from being properly raised, but be a
source of pain, owing to the dragging and violence
then requisite to effect any degree of retraction.

DOUBLE WIRE EYELID-RETRACTOR.

This might be called the operator's assistant, as it
quite supersedes the fingers of an assistant in nearly
all the operations that need efficient retraction of the
eyelids. It is more generally useful than any instrument in the ophthalmic case. It is rather less effective when used without chloroform, because the involuntary
muscular action of the orbicularis palpebrarum overcomes
much of the spring force. It is well to have two sizes:
one as in fig. 7—applicable for most purposes, and a smaller for
children. The manner of application can hardly be mistaken.
The spiral or spring part, the outer end, is to be on the temporal
side of the eye, while the retracting portions, at the ends of the
blades, are to be inserted under the eyelids.

FIG. 7.

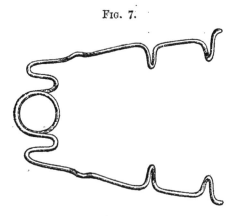

Another (fig. 8) is constructed for the spring part to pass over the nose, so that the outside of the eye shall be left free for any necessary use of instruments.

FIG. 8.

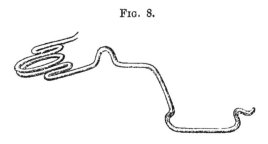

SUTURE NEEDLES.

That the stitching of wounds is very often the most painful part of an operation is a fact early impressed upon the student of surgery. Without doubt, much of the suffering is too frequently to be attributed to the imperfection of the needle. Good surgical needles are rarely to be met with, merely because their manufacture is in general neglected, and they are not rendered hard enough to bear proper sharpening. The point, or cutting part, should be large enough to make a channel through which the shaft can glide with ease, or at least pass without force sufficient to stretch or tear the skin. These requisites seem to be fully united in the well-formed glover's needle, which has three edges, of which this is an illustration. The stoutness should be proportionate to the thread which is required, by

FIG. 9.

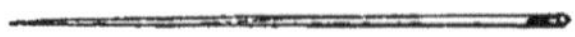

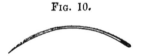

which standard the size of a needle should invariably be regulated. The length is a matter of convenience. Where circumstances admit of choice, I always prefer the straight form, because a straight needle enters more readily, and is more easily guided than a curved one.

A different body is desirable for a bent needle. The front, or concave part, should be quite flat from side to side, and the posterior, or convex side, oval across. If both are oval, the edges cannot be made thin enough, consistently with smallness and strength. This pattern illustrates the description.

FIG. 10.

The figures represent the size of those I employ. Besides there being no advantage derivable from shorter ones, there is a positive disadvantage attached to lesser length, arising from difficulty in use. A variety of porte-aiguilles have been invented to obviate this, all of which may be dispensed with, so far as my experience goes, by employing a proper needle.

CURVED SCISSORS.

The slight bend in the blades of these scissors renders them very useful on many occasions, and the ophthalmic case is scarcely perfect without them. The points should be of a certain width, and not too delicate, in order to ensure proper strength.

Messrs. Weiss have registered two kinds of joints for

scissors, and other double-bladed instruments of the same class. The one is called the lever joint, the rivet being placed at the side in an angular projection; by which it is said that greater power is given, and the mode of cutting is rather improved, and a substance is less likely to slip from between the blades. The other, which I highly approve of, is a sort of lock-joint, a screw not being used, and the advantage of which is, that the blades do not become loose, but ever keep their degree of tightness, and the instrument can be the more readily used with either hand, and easily unlocked for the purpose of being cleaned.

Fig. 11.

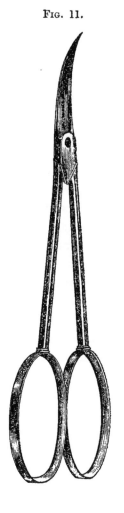

I have seen scalpel edges recommended for scissors that are intended, like these, to be used for cutting the living tissues. Such are impracticable. At the same time, the blades should be made as thin as is consistent with efficient use, for there is a great difference in the practical effect, between those of ordinary make and those so prepared.

I would suggest that scissors are not sharpened sufficiently often. I frequently see them employed when they are long past service.

CHAPTER IV.

BURNS AND SCALDS—ECCHYMOSIS—BLOWS, AND THEIR RESULTS—WOUNDS—
CHEMICAL INJURIES.

BURNS AND SCALDS.

THE surface of the eye is liable to be injured by heated liquids, by explosions of gas, of gunpowder, and other inflammable compounds, and by glowing or molten metal projected with violence. Yet it enjoys wonderful immunity from ordinary burns and scalds, which more or less overspread or involve the face and head, by virtue of the involuntary closing of the eyelids, and the instinctive tendency to maintain them shut. It would be a waste of time to attempt to describe the several conditions that are met with from these accidents, varying, as they do, from simple redness, to charring or calcination. The conjunctiva often suffers when other parts escape, and, with but a very insignificant lesion, may be much swollen and inflamed. There can be no mistake about the nature of these injuries, and the treatment is comprehended in a few simple rules.

Tepid bathing with the eye-douche or syringe is the first general measure, not only to soothe, but to remove any extraneous material. After this, diligent search should be made, to ascertain if anything has intruded. When the cornea or the conjunctiva has been abraded, more comfort is imparted by the application of olive oil than anything else I know of.

Not the least important of all—and it is important in proportion to the extent of the damage, especially when the cornea is hurt—is to keep the eyelids closed. By this we exclude the air, ensure moisture and warmth, and maintain the parts in quietude. Anodyne applications, and a strict daily attention to cleanliness, are among the necessaries. The eyelids should not be allowed to get gummed together, that there may be a free exit to any discharges; and this is most certainly best accomplished by cutting off the cilia, and keeping the edges greased. I do not think that further topical treatment is available. I suspect that stimulating and astringent ointments and lotions, of all kinds, are injurious, by increasing irritation. If the vitality of a part have been destroyed, or a wound inflicted, a definite process of repair must be passed through, which, I think, cannot in general be better assisted or directed than by the means mentioned.

Bodily rest and attention to constitutional symptoms are too often overlooked, and neglect of them might bring the penalty of prolonged suppuration, or inflammatory action of the entire eyeball.

What is to be most feared when the accident is severe, next to the loss of sight, is contraction and adhesion of the eyelids to each other, or to the eyeball; inevitable conditions accordingly as the conjunctiva is lost, or the angles of the eyelids injured. Cicatrization cannot be effected without it; and the quicker this is brought about, the less will be the defect. The prudent course is, I believe, to endeavour to reduce the healing process to the shortest limit, and afterwards to attend to the adhesions.

The slight injury that particles of melted metal generally inflict is a matter of marvel. I might fill pages with the wonderful escapes that are recorded, the greater number of which relate to the entrance of lead that had moulded itself to the surfaces of the eyeball and to the eyelids, thereby showing that it had entered the eye in a fluid state. The theory suggested to account for this is, the protection afforded by the evaporation of the fluid on the eye.

In the last occurrence of the kind that I saw, many of the cilia of both the eyelids were soldered together with a lump of solder, and the eye could not be opened till they were cut off. The edges of the eyelids were severely singed.

The following remarkable accident from molten iron is recorded in the " Ophthalmic Hospital Reports," page 217. A very healthy man was employed in an iron-foundry. While at work, some of the molten metal at a white heat had been spirted into his left eye. It struck the eyeball over the lower edge of the cornea and the adjacent part of the sclerotic coat. One of his fellow-labourers removed the metal with some difficulty after it had solidified on account of its adhering firmly to the charred tissues. It had in cooling been accurately moulded to the surface of the eyeball and to the edge of the lower eyelid. The affected parts of the cornea and sclerotica, which included the greater part of the thickness of each, sloughed off, as also did some of the palpebral mucous membrane. The eyeball itself, however, did not inflame. In the healing of the scar, the pupil was drawn downwards by puckering of the iris at its attached margin, but union was retained. Some adhesions between the eyeball and the lower eyelid resulted, but they did not constitute any material deformity, nor occasion much inconvenience.

Burns and scalds of the eyelids are generally followed by very distressing contraction, from the thinness and looseness of the skin, and the mobility of the tarsi. Paramount attention is therefore required, to prevent or to lessen the suppurative stage. Of all applications that I have myself tried and seen used, none are equal to nicely-dressed cotton-wool ; it is soft, light, and cleanly. It should not be applied in a lump, but put on in minute bits, and pressed with a probe so as to make it smooth and uniform. Where there is merely an abraded surface, from loss of cuticle, it excludes the air, and soaks up any superfluous secretion. If suppuration should exist, it absorbs the superabundant fluid, while enough is left for the purpose of sufficient moisture. With it the sore does not grow flabby and indolent, requiring stimulants, as so frequently happens with water-dressing, and the granulations are kept in a condition that precludes the necessity for escharotics. I have frequently seen ordinary ulcers that had resisted other applications heal under this, the simplest of all means. The changing of the material is readily effected. Any portion adhering to the sound skin must be wetted, and that over the raw surface will always readily separate when surcharged with moisture. Should a mild astringent ointment seem requisite, the Pharmacopœia supplies many to choose from.

No method of treatment that is known will prevent subsequent contraction, if the true skin, the cutis vera, be much damaged or destroyed; and all that can then be done towards lessening the deformity is to endeavour to shorten the period of suppuration, or, in other words, to promote healing as quickly as possible.

The special indication arises, if the edges of the eyelids be involved, to prevent their edges from uniting; and this may be with certainty fulfilled, if their corners have escaped injury.

What is to be done when grains of powder, or the residue of powder, enter the skin of the eyelids? I have never seen a person sufficiently early after the accident to warrant any attempt at removal. A great authority, Dr. Mackenzie, advises the particles to be very carefully picked out with a cataract needle,—an operation, as he remarks, that may take hours to accomplish. He adds that we should not trust to the application of a poultice, which is recommended with the view of dissolving and bringing away the powder.

I think that any determination of "picking," or not interfering, should be decided by the amount of powder that had entered: if much, I should leave it alone; if slight, I should probably do my best to remove it, and especially if there were grains sticking superficially in the cornea or the conjunctiva. I doubt whether but a small portion of any individual particle can actually be removed from the latter structure without excision of a part of it, and this would be unjustifiable.

I have lately seen a recommendation, in a French journal, to apply violently stimulating lotions to the surface directly after the burn: strong solutions of corrosive sublimate, for instance, for days together. This produces a violent eczema, by which epidermic scabs are raised, and the gunpowder also, more or less, with them.

Which of the two, the remedy or the disease, is the worse, is a question that must occur to the mind of the reader !

ECCHYMOSIS.

The ready production of ecchymosis about the eye is, of course, owing to the superficial position of the bones of the orbit, and the contusion that the skin therefore receives from a slight blow; while the considerable tumefaction which is so common after any blow, is due to another peculiarity of the orbital region—the looseness of the skin.

I question whether any means, except gentle friction, can hasten the natural process of absorption. The employment by pugilists of briony root and ·Solomon's seal, scraped and made with bread into a poultice, or of rosemary and arnica infusions, has induced medical men to recommend these applications. The tincture of arnica and water is the present popular remedy for all bruises.

But it is not, I suspect, a fact that the prize-fighters can disperse these results of their savage encounters; and I believe they last in them as long as in other people: but as their accustomed personal exhibitions after fights are at night, and by gas-light, most of the colour, especially the lighter hues, are invisible, and hence the popular assumption of the potency of their remedies. If it be true that in them the extravasation is quickly dispelled, it is more probably owing to their youth, and to the perfection of the nutrient and absorbent processes which exist in their high bodily condition.

There does not appear to be satisfactory evidence that depressing the temperature of the surface by frigorific mixtures hastens absorption; and, theoretically speaking, I should rather expect it to retard Nature in her operation.

There are, however, degrees of ecchymosis some of which demand treatment, and neglect might be followed by injury to the eyelid. The extravasation may be increasing; the infra or supra-orbital vessels, or other arterial twigs, may continue to ooze, and recourse must be had to pressure, or cold, or the heart's action reduced by the loss of blood, or by a smart purge, and, above all, perfect rest.

When the extravasation is considerable, the probability of suppuration is to be borne in mind, and the state of the system must be looked after, and all febrile threatenings attended to. Neither incisions nor punctures should be made, with the intention of turning out coagula; for suppuration would be almost certain to follow. The knife should be withheld, unless there is suppuration or erysipelatous inflammation, or sloughing is impending or has commenced. Leeches on the injured part are worse than useless; they do not imbibe coagulated blood, while they add to the local injury. The feelings of the patient must sometimes guide us in the choice of local applications: when the extravasation is considerable, there may be pain, which possibly will be relieved only by warm opiate lotions.

Ecchymosis of the conjunctiva, as every one knows, is produced by very slight causes, such as the most trivial blow, a cough, or a sneeze. Indeed, it is not uncommon without the slightest trace of its origin. It is very persistent, but need not excite the smallest anxiety. Even with tumefaction from extravasated blood beneath, it is not to be dreaded. I fancy that I have seen every variety of this from accidents, and after operations; and I never have deemed it prudent in the worst examples of mere swelling to make incisions, nor have I ever regretted non-interference. I have seen the disadvantages of incision. I have known operators expect to give exit to blood, when of course they discovered it was coagulum they had exposed, and all that could escape was a small amount of serum.

My rule is to trust to Nature, and do nothing except there be pain, or heat, or any discomfort, or other conditions, when I treat the existing symptoms according to the general rules of surgery, or therapeutically, using cold, or warmth, or opiates, as may seem necessary; but I deprecate any routine of stimulants or astringents. I am often told "that patients will have something;" and my answer is, "Well, if they must be so amused, pray let them have a lotion weak enough to be harmless; but let us not lose sight of the distinction between usefulness and amusement."

BLOWS.

A blow on the eyeball, from a grain of shot, or a cork, or the lash of a whip, may considerably injure or annihilate vision, with but slight, perhaps without any trace of mechanical violence. Fortunately it is seldom, as compared with the number of accidents, that vision is at once and completely destroyed, even when the lesion is extensive.

Beer records an instance of a man having lost his sight from a person who, being behind him, suddenly covered his eyes with his hands, using at the same time some pressure. Yet loss, or impairment of sight from a blow, is rarely ultimately unaccompanied with some external symptoms of degeneration or change of some part of the eye. Ordinarily the pupil is dilated, and sometimes to such an extent as to give rise to the supposition that the iris has been totally destroyed. This is attributed to shock of the ciliary system, meaning particularly the ciliary muscle, and the ciliary nerves, which really explains nothing. The iris is likely to lose its colour and to become tremulous, shaking with every movement of the eye, while the vitreous body will probably become dissolved, a condition indicated by the eyeball feeling soft. Either may be the beginning of change which ends in entire atrophy.

As an example of a severe case, I may mention that of a young woman, who was struck in the eye, but not violently, by the corner of a baker's tray; inflammation soon followed, for which no particular treatment was adopted. Some months afterwards, when I was applied to, I found the iris discoloured, and partly adherent to an opaque capsule; the lens nearly or entirely absorbed, the eyeball soft, and not the slightest perception of light remained. Another circumstance connected with the case is worth noting. A band of lymph united the capsule to the cornea, to admit of which the capsule must have been at some time in contact with the cornea, and the connecting medium must have been gradually elongated, in proportion as the lens was absorbed.

The lesser injuries are more frequently met with, and it requires considerable judgment not to be deceived by a patient's exaggerated expressions, nor to be misguided by mere conjunctival redness, ecchymosis, or chemosis; for, so long as the sight is not impaired, the cornea is clear, and the iris is bright, all will end well. But there may be an exception as to the iris. The change in colour may be apparent, and not real, being due only to a serous state of the aqueous humour. For example, after the operation for squint, the conjunctiva became chemosed, and the iris seemed changed from a light auburn to a rusty hue. Vision was unaffected. A natural condition of parts was soon restored. A week after the extraction of a cataract—and a more successful case was never seen—a light-blue iris presented a bright-russet tinge, and the colour was deepest at the lowest part; this also became natural.

Yet the worst effects as regards sight may result from a blow on the eyebrow, without the eyeball having been touched. I have known a stroke on the temple from a stick, although not followed by a bruise, nearly destroy vision in the contiguous eye. An engineer was striking a bar of iron with a sledge-hammer, a piece of the metal broke off, was projected against his face, and fractured his nasal bones. I saw him three days after the accident; the conjunctiva of the left eye was slightly ecchymosed, and the pupil greatly dilated, and vision was extinct.

Within a short period, the prevailing theory referred defective sight from a blow on the eyeball, or its vicinity, unattended by acute inflammatory action of the eye, to concussion of the retina; even more, it attributed also to the same cause many of the physical changes that I have alluded to. When the blow, or the pressure, was thought to be insufficient alone for the concussion, spasmodic action of the orbital muscles was blamed, false analogy of spasmodic muscular power in other parts of the system was adduced in confirmation, and the very large cushion

D

of fat in the orbit on which the eyeball rests, and specially provided for to prevent such an occurrence, quite ignored.

When wounds about the circumference of the orbit were followed by blindness, the nutrition of the eye was supposed to be damaged through lesion of some ophthalmic division of the fifth nerve ramifying on the face. One wonders how the idea could have originated. It appears to me to be confounded with injury of the nerve-trunk, when it enters the orbit. The literature of the subject is extensive, and strange opinions are expressed therein. Dr. Mackenzie has entered fully into it, and combats many of the theories put forth to explain the mode in which the inference is conveyed. He commits himself to this explanation:

" In all such cases I should suspect that injury of the branches of the fifth nerve, having communicated irritation to the nervous centres, a reflex disease, probably inflammatory, was propagated from them to the optic nerve, and to the other nerves concerned in the function of vision. Such considerations would lead us, in cases of suspected injury of the branches of the fifth nerve, not only to enjoin rest, but to treat the patient antiphlogistically, and to administer calomel with opium, in doses sufficient to affect the system."

In the great mass of such cases we have now a demonstrative explanation. For the last twelve months I have submitted to a careful ophthalmoscopic examination the accidents of this class that I have had to treat. In all I have found marked physical changes, the effect of violence, that could be pointed to as the direct disturber of sight; or, internal inflammatory action of the eye produced by the injury. So far, then, as my recent investigation goes, the *rationale* of the impairment of the sense is mainly to be found in actual and perceptible alterations in the interior of the eye, sometimes accompanied with external symptoms, sometimes not. But this must be known to all inquiring ophthalmologists. Among the physical changes I have met with are, detachments of the retina and laceration of it posteriorly, extravasation of blood, especially in the vitreous humour, dislocation of the crystalline lens backwards.

I will illustrate some of the direct effects of violence. A workman, in middle age, was severely struck on his forehead, just over the left eyebrow, six years ago, and quickly lost all useful sight. He could not exactly say how quickly it went, as his memory did not serve him; but it was an immediate consequence, for, when the swelling of the eyebrow and the ecchymosis had passed away, the eye was useless. It would be difficult to name any method of treatment that had not been tried, for the man had been to some of the general hospitals in London, and to several of the special ones. He could not read type of any size, but only just count his fingers when they were held up against the light. There was now no objective symptom whatever, and therefore it was impossible, from a mere external survey of the eye, to say what was at fault. Detachment of the retina was at once discernible, in a cloudy whiteness at the fundus of the eye, instead of the natural red colour of the choroid. The optic disc could not be seen, nor any parts in detail; instead, there appeared the uneven white cloud, with a few vessels, not very definite, in irregular arrangement. Here was, of course, an irremediable injury, probably from an early period; and far better would it have been for the patient, and more for the credit of Surgery, had this been earlier made out.

Of inflammatory action consequent on a blow I shall give two examples. A lad applied at the hospital because he saw imperfectly with his right eye. He could only count his fingers. He had visited several ophthalmic institutions, and had been submitted to divers kinds of treatment. Sixteen months before he had been struck on the eye with a dead pigeon, and it became merely blood-shot; pain ensued, and vision was soon lost. I examined him, to determine whether there was any external sign of injury, and whether also I could, by a concentrated light on the pupil, get any indication of deep-seated alteration. Not the slightest defect could be observed. Atropine was then used, and with the ophthalmoscope minute black specks on the surface of the capsule of the lens showed that, during the inflammation which followed the injury, and of which the patient declared he knew nothing, the posterior part of the iris had been in contact with it. But a greater change was yet to be observed. In the turbid vitreous humour hung shreds, or threads, which, from their arrangement, appeared to be of an inflammatory origin. The optic disc could not be seen. The choroid coat had undergone much pathological change. The external evidence of inflammatory action was slight, and, except so far as the loss of sight was a symptom—of course a marked one—there was nothing to arouse suspicion of the great mischief going on in the eyeball.

A boy was struck on the eye with a stick, and brought to the hospital a week afterwards, having in the mean time been bled and blistered because of the pain that ensued. The eyelids were swollen, from the enormous blister on the temple, causing much effusion around. The surface of the eyeball was a little injected, but the pupil dilated under atropine—no slight evidence of the absence of much inflammatory action in it. The lens was clear, but the vitreous humour was turbid, and the state of the retina could not be made out satisfactorily in consequence. The choroid seemed spotted, as if from the removal of the choroidal pigment. There was scarcely any vision, and as all evidence went to show that the eye was perfect before the accident, the conclusion was, that the changes which were seen were the result of the injuries, and were all effected in a very short space of time, and that with but little, if any, external evidence of what was passing within.

Very lately the question of damage to vision through injury to the orbital branches of the fifth nerve was legally brought before me. I was engaged, on behalf of the London and North-Western Railway Company, to attend a trial at Guildhall, in which they appeared as defendants, to resist an exorbitant demand for damages by the plaintiff, a watch-finisher in a small business, who alleged that the slight superficial wound which he received in the integuments of the eyebrow incapacitated him from using the peculiar eyeglass employed by the trade.

Mr. Skelding, one of the surgeons to the Company, Mr. Skey, and Mr. Lawrence were also for the defendants.

There could be no doubt that there was some loss of sensation, or impaired sensation of a very limited portion of the scalp ; that some of the branches of the supra-orbital nerve had been injured. One of the plaintiff's witnesses stated there was a probability of impairment of sight as an ultimate consequence, although the eyeball was at the time in perfect integrity. This produced a great impression on the jury. The Chief Baron questioned the witness on the point; and when, in answer, he was told that the archives of surgery bore such records, he commented on the worthlessness of many things that are recorded. He asked whether witness had ever met with such an example in his own practice, and was answered in the negative. But still the jury had received what I thought to be a wrong bias, and I did my best to remove it, and so did Mr. Skey; and I believe that we were successful, from the small damages allowed—much less in amount than the Company had offered. In my evidence, I gave concisely the views which I have expressed :—that mere injury to the nerve-branch on the head can have no effect on the function of the retina; that loss of sight, when associated with such lesion, is due to coincident injury of the eyeball; that in the case in question, as nearly a year had elapsed since the accident, and the plaintiff's eyesight was unimpaired, the eyeball must have escaped unhurt, and there was not a shadow of a chance of untoward consequences in that direction.

The method by which the watchmaker's glass is kept to the eye was fully discussed; and as I had previously studied the subject in reference to the trial, and had consulted many watchmakers and others, I was prepared to give an opinion. The plaintiff declared that he held it by muscular power, and in attempting to do this, pain and uneasiness ensued. I learnt, by experiment, that the glass may be so adapted to the eye by a purely mechanical process, and there held for an adequate time. This is done by pressing the lower part of the rim against the integuments of the lower eyelid, depressing them a little, and then locking the upper part under the edge of the orbit. I found that I could do this readily on either side of the face, and have perfect command of the glass as an optical instrument. This is doubtless the correct way of using it, and that employed by most workmen. But, strange to tell, there are numbers of mechanics who do not know this fact, and by muscular power only, keep the instrument in position, thereby producing much fatigue, to say nothing about limiting the application of the appliance. Besides, they are obliged to use the one eye always because only one eye is tutored; a decided and obvious disadvantage, as regards the function of vision, to say nothing of other drawbacks that occur in the details of workmanship.

Although pain is a common consequence of a blow on the eye, except it be accompanied by some disturbance of vision, a favourable prognosis may be given. But an unfavourable view should always be taken when, with or without pain, the sight is not restored in whole or in part for some hours after the stroke.

I think that I have said enough to direct attention to the general character of these accidents, and to put the student in the proper road of inquiry, and not less to show the necessity for examining each case with the ophthalmoscope. To prevent repetition, all that I have to say on this instrument, which has opened a new era in our diagnosis, and given a better guide to our practice, is given in a separate chapter at the end of the work.

I have avoided expanding my subject to a tiresome length, or attempting to exhaust it; neither have I multiplied cases, because I have, I think, produced enough for the sake of example, and more could not strengthen my statements. There are several physiological and pathological questions that I might open, but as these would be speculative rather than practical, I forbear.

Patients will not, I find, readily submit to an appropriate régime, except there be some very visible external injury, and the practitioner must be firm in enforcing his rules and his regulations.

When impaired vision at once follows an injury, unaccompanied by external lesion, I prescribe quiet for a few days; unstimulating and, except contra-indicated, rather low diet; cold to the eye, either by the douche, or a thin rag—for with one fold there is more evaporation,—dipped out of cold water and frequently changed. The French system of irrigation may be carried out. This consists in allowing the water to drop on the eye from a syphon of threads, or other material, connected with a reservoir above. The more elaborate apparatus is made of cistern, tube, and stop-cock. Should pain supervene, I generally give an aperient; besides this, I employ opiates, at first locally, and afterwards, if necessary, internally. The watery extract of opium, reduced to a proper consistence, and rubbed on the brow or the temple, or applied as a plaster, with an adhesive margin, is a good topical application; and so also is the Ung. opii. For the internal administration, I prefer small doses, often given, to a large prostrating quantity, because the narcotism is better, and there is less or no unpleasant consequences. I take cognizance of any general febrile state, and use those remedies that seem to me to be most appropriate.

No other treatment can be employed more likely to prevent further effusion of blood, or of any secretion, should these be poured out, or to hasten their absorption; nor is there any more effectual way of stopping the development of inflammatory action.

When there is more extensive disease—that is, when there is swelling of the eyelids, especially the upper one, pain, or flashes, scalding tears, accompanied by a hard pulse, acute disturbance of the digestive organs; and feverishness, or restlessness, or want of sleep, supervene,—we may be sure that very great disturbance exists, and that the integrity of the eye is threatened. There is now inflammation of the eyeball. It must ever be remembered that a given amount of injury to any part of the body is, as a rule, followed by a certain amount of action, and that the eye can scarcely receive a severe and rudely-inflicted hurt without marked local and general disturbance, the contrary being the exception. A reparative stage is set up, or attempted, a curative influence which we cannot stop, and that we interfere with legitimately only when we soothe and endeavour to keep it within certain bounds. If we attempt by heroic measures to inflict what has been called a " wrench " on the system, and suddenly to shut out all natural attempts, we shall fail, and besides, damage the patient.

I enter now on the treatment of inflammation of the eyeball, and with a desire to be concise, I cannot recognise the varieties and complications which arise in actual practice, and demand the best energies and most watchful care to detect, and much judgment to encounter. It is only the general rules that can be dwelt on. But it will be impossible to embody in a few words all that need be said here on this very important topic, especially as the subject will not be entertained again, but reference merely made to it, as occasion may demand.

Dr. Jacob has published a valuable volume on inflammation of the eyeball, which contains more original matter and sound practical precepts than any other work that I have read. He uses the term inflammation of the eyeball in a very wide sense—that in which I shall use it, and advances an opinion to which I fully subscribe—that a discoloured iris and a red sclerotica are not evidences of inflammation of the iris alone, but of the whole eyeball. He further asserts what I consider to be true,—that the attempt to describe inflammation as isolated or confined to particular structures, has not by any means proved serviceable ; for we find in practice that these distinctions vanish, and we discover only a progressive inflammation of the whole organ, though it may have been in the commencement more conspicuous in some particular tissues. I believe that the only exception to this rule will be found in acute idiopathic inflammation of the retina, a disease of very rare occurrence. Supplied by the arteria centralis retinæ, this membrane was long supposed to have no direct vascular connexion with other portions of the eyeball, until Professor Van Der Kolk succeeded in demonstrating a series of very minute vessels proceeding from the corona ciliaris, and connecting the retina and hyaloid membrane with the other tissues. This anatomical fact explains how retinitis, arising in the back part of the eye, has no tendency to involve the rest of the organ ; whereas, when it occurs in the vicinity of the corona ciliaris—as most always happens in traumatic cases—the inflammation becomes general. This point has been fully discussed and explained by my colleague, Mr. Taylor, in a paper in the " Medical Times and Gazette" for June 5th, 1852. Heretofore, inflammation of the eyeball has been considered to be that stage of disease which is followed by suppuration.

General blood-letting is frequently necessary, and is particularly applicable at the commencement of acute inflammation. It is especially indicated when there is rapidly-declining vision, together with congestion or effusion in the posterior part of the eye, which is rendered probable by the bulging of the lens and iris towards the cornea, even though there should be little external evidence of inflammation. It must, however, be borne in mind that extravasation of blood will throw the lens forward. Local bleeding will commonly be sufficient, and is often the only remedy to which the pain, that may be very distressing, will yield. Still no precise rule can be given as to whether the bleeding should be general or local; the practitioner must be guided by the individual peculiarities of each case. The necessity of moderation cannot be too energetically urged, for blood-letting has been truly called a spoliative remedy of the first class; and it should ever be remembered that depression is tolerably sure to follow the excitement of the acute inflammatory stage. The quantity should be regulated by the local symptoms, and the age and general condition of the patient; otherwise, destructive, rather than conservative effects may result. Disease cannot be bled out of the eye, as some writers seem to think. At the same time, when local bleeding is indicated, a decided effect must be obtained by the cupping-glass or by leeches. It is seldom that a leech or two will suffice, except during the earlier periods of life.

Dr. Jacob well observes, that the destructive consequences of inflammation are not proportioned to the acuteness of the attack, whether from accident or otherwise, but are frequently seen in a very remarkable degree where the inflammatory action is languid—a fact not less common in ophthalmic than in general surgery, although, unfortunately, not generally recognised.

Another excellent remark from his experience is, that patients are generally not seen until after the vessels have become permanently enlarged, and the inflammatory condition has been firmly established; then it is that the propriety of bleeding comes to be questionable. Again, the redness or increased vascularity may be but a consequence of inflammatory action, which has ceased or been subdued. As a rule, he says that bleeding should only be resorted to at the very commencement of an attack, when a hope may be entertained that by weakening the heart's action, and reducing the distension of the capillaries, the disorganizing process of inflammation may be prevented; and most assuredly to delay it until that stage arrives in which there is diminution in quantity, or deterioration in quality of the circulating fluid, would rather retard than promote the cure. This trustworthy observer, however, does not hesitate, in the progress of a case, to repeat the bleeding, if acute symptoms should return; a practice I myself would recommend.

But loss of blood may not control the disease; and opacity or suppuration of the cornea, or the effusion of pus into the anterior chamber, or discoloration of the iris and contraction of the pupil, with more or less adhesion to the lens, may declare still more plainly that the entire eyeball is implicated. Suppose, too, that these symptoms of advanced inflammation have set in without blood-letting having been admissible; or that the patient is seen for the first time in this state. Mercury, which is unfortunately as much abused in ophthalmic as in other affections, but which possesses powerful influence in checking inflammation of the eyeball, and in removing some of its products, must then be resorted to. It must not be lauded as a specific; for disease may continue to increase, even although the system be fully under its influence. A very marked influence will generally, although not invariably, follow its administration. Discrimination and judgment are as much called for in giving mercury as in blood-letting; and on this point I must again refer to Dr. Jacob's experience. After showing the impropriety of treating all injuries of the eye by antiphlogistics, pointing out that the destructive processes of inflammation are in many cases disproportionate to the injury sustained, and that a scratch or puncture of the cornea often causes destruction of the whole eye, while an extensive wound, with laceration and contusion, will sometimes be repaired without extension of inflammation to the rest of the organ, he lays down the important rule, that traumatic inflammation, so far from being invariably of the same type, is especially liable to be modified by the existing diathesis, and that it will be intense and rapid, or languid and chronic, according to the condition of the patient. He farther asserts, that it will assume the rheumatic, scrofulous, or even syphilitic character in patients who are suffering from those affections. These are important principles, and should form the key to our treatment. Here, then, a wide field is open for the exercise of practical skill. In some cases of great urgency, with strong constitutional powers, it is allowable, and even requisite, to give mercury till its effect on the mouth tells that the drug has entered the circulation; in others it must be but sparingly administered, and its influence assisted by the simultaneous support of the system by tonics; or it may be necessary to combine it with other medicines, or altogether to suspend its exhibition.

In my own practice, I am in the habit of using mercury in very small quantities, and almost always prescribe the Hydrargyrum cum cretâ, in doses of two, two and a half, or three grains, combining it with opium, hyoscyamus, or conium, as the bowels may require, and repeating it according to the urgency of the case; but never more frequently than four times in the twenty-four hours, and rarely so often. While this form is equal in potency to any other preparation of mercury, it is more under control, and it will be comparatively seldom that active salivation is quickly or unexpectedly developed,—no small advantage in debilitated constitutions. Salivation is certainly the poisonous influence of mercury; and I believe that the highest curative effect is to be obtained short of that state. At the same time, if a disease does not yield, and its violence be not lessening under its use, I should give the mercury till the mouth was in some degree affected, to ensure that the system was fully under its influence.

The potency and the manageableness of this form of the drug cannot be imagined by those who have not used it; and to those who are disposed to give it a trial,' I would recommend that they should select cases of syphilitic iritis to commence with; for then its effects can be readily watched, and the results appreciated; and in them, moreover, the fact may be learned that the disease will readily cease without the mouth being made sore.

I was requested to meet, in a case of syphilitic iritis, a well-known London surgeon, who uses very large doses of mercury in his syphilitic practice. The disease was far advanced, and the pupil contracted and irregular, the iris discoloured, the cornea hazy; in fact, all the symptoms of inflammation of the eyeball were present, and vision nearly extinct. The patient was sixty years of age, fat and feeble. I ordered him the chalk and mercury with hyoscyamus, in two grain doses each, three times a day, which this surgeon considered to be worse than useless. Five days after this, I saw the patient with Mr. Austin, of Rotherhithe, the regular family surgeon, who had been present at the consultation, and we found that the mouth was ‾sore, and the iritis yielding. The quantity of mercury was now lessened, and its administration so regulated that salivation was kept under; iodide of potass was ordered, and when I again saw him, at the end of a fortnight, the iris had quite recovered, the pupil acted well and dilated fully, a little redness of the sclerotica and of the conjunctiva alone remaining, and vision being nearly perfect. Here no blood was lost; indeed, it was necessary to support the patient with good diet. I am certain that relapses are very much less frequent under this cautious use of the mineral, than when it is lavishly administered.

I take it for granted that in these days of superior medical education it is sufficient to give a hint about properly maintaining the vital force, and thus sustaining and assisting power and action. Inflammation, as Dr. Markham truly says, in writing about pericarditis—and his words are equally valuable, although I am chiefly alluding to traumatic disease of the eyeball—" inflammation is a sign of weakness, not of strength; that in every inflammation where exudation has taken place, there is a process of absorption and reparation to be gone through, if the parts are to regain their integrity, and that for the furtherance of this process, vital force is absolutely necessary." Sinking, or weakness of the vital powers, therefore, he carefully anticipated in all inflammations. He continues to show that light and easily digested nourishment, milk, and weak broths, should be assiduously administered during the earliest periods of the inflammation, and stimuli when the acute period has ceased, and the process of absorption has commenced, or whenever the signs of enfeebled circulation begin to show themselves.

Modern science teaches, too, that much is to be gained by well-selected tonics; that quinine and mercury, and the use of preparations of iron, while we bleed locally, are not incompatible.

There is an excellent paper that bears forcibly on this subject, published in the 23rd volume of the "Medico-Chirurgical Transactions," by the late Mr. Dalrymple, on the rapid organization of lymph in cachexia. The author commences by stating that it is of high importance in a physiological, as well as a practical point of view, to ascertain whether effusion of the organizable materials of the blood become vitalized by the production of new vessels more readily and sooner in cachexia than in robust states of the constitution.

The conclusion he arrived at is, that in those who are enfeebled and depressed, effusions from the capillary vessels are more speedily and completely organized, with vessels capable of being permeated by minute injections, than in the more vigorous and plethoric, in whom inflammation is more acute in the outset, and passes through more speedy and determined stages. The greater tendency to the effusion and organization of fibrine on the surface of the iris in syphilitic cases, than in those of idiopathic iritis, is noticed; and the remark is made, that there will be no difficulty in admitting that the specific cases occur, at least, in London, in far greater proportion, in enfeebled constitutions and in those debilitated by excess and irregular habits, or the maladministration of mercury for the primary disease. A well-marked case of syphilitic iritis, peculiarly valuable and very worthy of perusal, is given in support of this view, and further most interesting evidence is adduced of the rapid organization of lymph in other instances of disease where life has been nearly extinct.

I have expatiated and endeavoured to be impressive, only on those agents which, although so valuable, are very likely to be abused in ophthalmic disease. I think it quite unnecessary to speak of remedies applicable to febrile and other disordered states of the system, incidental to acute ophthalmitis.

The artificial dilatation of the pupil should be effected whenever there is a tendency of the iris to adhere to the capsule of the lens, for the pupillary margin is very close to the capsule; indeed, it is almost certain, that in the earlier years of life they are in actual contact, and at no healthy period can there be any but the slightest space intervening between them. In inflammation of the eyeball, the iris and the capsule of the lens will adhere unless the pupillary edge be drawn outwards and towards the circumference of the lens, where the surfaces are necessarily separated. I rarely use the extract of belladonna around the lids, according to general custom, for it is a filthy application which soon dries and becomes inert. The sulphate of atropia, in the proportion of one or two grains to an ounce of water, a drop or two applied three times a day, on the conjunctiva of the outer part of the lower lid, will act as a sedative, and produce all the effects of dilatation. The atropia may be also applied to the lids, in an ointment composed of a grain to a drachm of lard or of glycerine, or belladonna lotion may be employed. With the use of this drug, when disease is disappearing, the pupil will often appear irregular; the result of some parts of the iris being more advanced to a healthy state than the others. The parts, however, which remain inactive are generally supposed to be adherent, and their yielding to the atropia is regarded as an indication of the adhesion giving way. I do not deny that this ever takes place, but I believe the rupture to be of rare occurrence,—rarer than generally stated, and rather attribute its supposed frequency to the causes now assigned.

The extent of dilatation of the pupil will generally be in

proportion to the integrity of the iris; and if its texture be much infiltrated, dilatation cannot be obtained. The use, however, of the atropia should not be regulated by the appearance of the iris ; for it may be influential when not expected, and in all instances of inflammation of the eyeball it should be employed. See what indication we may get from it. Directly that the iris begins to act, there is positive evidence of the disease passing away, and we reduce our remedies accordingly: when it acts fully, we may put aside all active measures. About half a dozen times in the course of my practice, I have seen the atropine irritate the conjunctiva and produce soreness of the cuticle. In each instance I ascertained that several grains of the drug had been used to half an ounce of water, and that the solution was therefore much too strong.

The evacuation of the aqueous humour has been proposed in inflammation of the eyeball ; it was practised a long while ago by Mr. Wardrop, and the manner in which he spoke of its advantages and the force of his authority, caused it to be for a time extensively adopted in most inflammatory affections of the eye; and reported cases of its utility in the purulent ophthalmia of infants, in gonorrhœal ophthalmia, inflammation of the cornea, ulceration of the cornea, abscess in the anterior chamber, iritis, and general inflammation of the eyeball, are very numerous. The theory is, to lessen or remove tension of the globe by the withdrawal of the humour, so as to admit of reparative action taking place; the same good effects being produced, whether the tension of the eyeball be lessened by diminution in the size and number of blood-vessels, or by the discharge of the aqueous humour. With reference to any danger arising from the diseased state of the eye, Mr. Wardrop remarks, that in those cases where the practice of evacuating the humour is judiciously had recourse to, although the operation may create some temporary irritation, yet its good effects will become immediately perceptible, and in most cases will be permanent; that considerable improvement in vision, particularly in those cases where there is a cloudiness in the anterior chamber, will take place ; that the sense of fulness of the eyeball, and pain in the eye and in the head, will cease; that in some cases a very remarkable change in the size of the inflamed vessels will occur; and that where the discharge of the aqueous humour has been found beneficial, it is not even necessary to suppose that its natural quantity is increased. I must not omit to state that Mr. Wardrop does not recommend it as a sole remedy, but as a powerful auxiliary in some, and in others, as a sure and perhaps the only means of preventing the total destruction of the vision. The paper entitled "The Effects of evacuating the Aqueous Humour in Inflammation of the Eyes, and in some Diseases of the Cornea," to which I allude, is in the fourth volume of the "Medico-Chirurgical Transactions."

I believe that this evacuation is seldom practised in the present day, and that for many years it has been discontinued. Mr. Lawrence writes forcibly against it, prefacing his objections with the statement that he has tried it in some instances, but with so little benefit that he has not been induced to persist in the practice : and that he has been the less inclined to do so in severe inflammations, because the ordinary antiphlogistic treatment enables us to control them. Dr. Jacob thinks that it is a measure that should be resorted to. Mr. Tyrrell was strongly in its favour, in some cases, and in connexion with local and general means. He practised it in inflammation of the aqueous membrane, not only when the size of the chambers was manifestly augmented, but when the globe felt very tense and tender, and there was much ophthalmia or sclerotitis; and he testified that he had several times known the operation produce not only immediate relief of suffering, but a very rapid subsidence of disease. The result of his observations induced him to advise that all the humour should not be allowed to escape, in which case the iris is pressed against the cornea, and severe suffering continues till these parts are again separated ; and when a repetition of the process is called for, from a recurrence of symptoms, he considered it proper to choose a fresh place in the cornea for the introduction of the instrument. We now know that there is no such thing as an aqueous membrane. Diseases of the cornea and of the iris were described by Mr. Tyrrell, as well as other authors, and included under the term "inflammation of the aqueous membrane, or aquo-capsulitis."

I must give my own experience of this remedy. I have not practised it when the cornea has been much inflamed, or contained pus between its layers, lest the mischief should be aggravated. I have often adopted it in sub-acute inflammation of the eyeball, attended with much pain : relief has frequently followed. The more I practise it, the more I approve of it. It may be regarded as a remedy temporarily eclipsed, and likely to be again employed. I shall give it a more extended trial. This is the method of operating.

Should chloroform not be used, considerable difficulty will be found in exposing and steadying the globe of the eye ; when the patient is insensible, the operation is very simple. The humour should be let out with the point of a cataract or an iris-knife. The operator stands behind the patient, who may be sitting or lying down, and proceeds as if about to operate for cataract, by raising the eyelid with the forefinger, fixing the globe with the point of that and of the middle finger, while an assistant depresses the lower eyelid. The incision should be near the margin of the cornea. Common care will save the iris from injury, and the lens will be spared if the point of the instrument be kept forwards. I find greater safety by making the cut laterally as soon as I have penetrated, than by thrusting. I have several times employed, with much readiness and operative effect, a broad needle, with a slit or perforation near the point, through which the aqueous humour escapes as soon as the cornea is fairly penetrated. The instrument-maker calls it a fenestrated needle. The humour is never thoroughly evacuated except the incision be ample, and withal it will be more effectually done if the eyeball be gently pressed on after being incised.

Pus may accumulate in the anterior chamber, from abscess of the iris, from ulceration at the back of the cornea, or from inflammation of the lining membrane. It would be imprudent as a rule to attempt its evacuation; for it is always absorbed if inflammation is arrested ; and opening the cornea in that stage of inflammation would, I fear, be followed by increased and

E

perhaps destructive inflammation of the eye. I find in my case-book an example of hypopium, headed "Rapid effusion and absorption of the pus." The anterior chamber was a third filled, and in ninety-six hours every particle was removed—purgation and counter-irritation behind the ears being the remedies. The presence of the pus does not seem to be injurious, when it occupies but a part of the chamber. I have never seen it rise to the level of the pupil without general suppuration of the globe. I have, however, been told by a surgeon in large ophthalmic practice, that he has seen the whole of the iris hidden by it, and that ultimately it was removed by absorption, and tolerable sight was regained.

Tapping the chamber, to evacuate serum, the presence of which is indicated by the colour of the fluid, is, I believe, a beneficial measure, if used with discretion. I do not recommend it except to relieve a symptom.

Pus may accumulate, too, in the texture of the cornea, and the proposal to evacuate it has been much censured. I have never practised it, nor seen it done; but in future I shall try it. My reasons will be found in the remarks on corneal wounds. Mr. Tyrrell approved of it when the abscess was extensive and the pain severe, with a distressing sensation of tension. But he recommended it in these cases rather with the view of relieving suffering than of hastening the cure, for he says that the matter is rarely so fluid as to escape by a small aperture; and the larger portion of it appears to be absorbed. The general opinion is, that the pus is infiltrated or diffused in the corneal tissue; but Dr. Jacob says that more frequently it is lodged in a distinct cavity, and recommends that if the accumulation be large, it should be opened, cautioning the operator to be prepared for prolapsus of the iris, and reminding him that such an occurrence should not be attributed to this act, as the operation, if done at the right time, often prevents the mischief; and when it does not prevent prolapse, renders it less injurious. An iris-knife would be the best instrument for performing the operation.

The unfortunate occurrence of suppuration of the contents of the eyeball can scarcely be mistaken. The symptoms are, great

constitutional disturbance, with fever and, perhaps, rigors, redness, and sometimes enormous swelling of the lids, especially the
upper; effusion of pus into the texture of the cornea, or into the
chambers of the eye; chemosis, and, above all, agonizing pain in
the eye, with throbbing in the orbit and in the temple. This
suffering lasts till the eye perishes, by the giving way of the
cornea and the escape of pus, and often of the disorganized lens
and some of the altered vitreous humour, when immediate relief
follows. But the period of the patient's suffering should always
be shortened by a free opening in the cornea, calculated to
give timely exit to the pus. This advanced stage of inflammation of the eyeball is generally treated by authors as a distinct
affection among the many subdivisions of ophthalmic inflammation. An eye cannot be saved after suppuration has commenced; indeed, when inflammation has arrived at that height
in which suppuration quickly follows, the organ is already
destroyed; and when it has actually suppurated, it is positively
cruel to bleed and purge a patient nearly to death, or to
involve him in all the horrors of a salivation, when there is
not any chance of benefit.

Anodyne fomentations, and fomentations of all kinds, to
assuage suffering, and to relieve engorged capillaries, are not,
I think, enough adopted. There is no more effectual way of
applying them than with a hollow sponge. All medicaments in
this form, and all opiates intended to act endermically, should
be used with the eyelids closed. The temperature must be
regulated by the patient's feelings.

The advantage of counter-irritation behind the ears or on the
temple has been questioned by some practical men; and the
supposed process of metastasis, which it is employed to imitate,
is now boldly denied, and, I think, successfully controverted. I
have not been able to satisfy myself of the supposed general
efficacy of blisters in ophthalmic diseases; and although I may
use them to give a patient every chance of benefit, I restrict
their employment to cases not complicated with fever and constitutional suffering. It is the fashion, at present, in this
metropolis, to prescribe blisters not larger than half an inch in

diameter; and these are said to be equally potent with the largest.

Effusion of blood in the eye is not unfrequent after a blow, and must then always be due to the mechanical lesion of some part, although the breach may not be apparent. The danger of its presence is in proportion to the quantity effused in the posterior parts. I have never adopted the practice which has been recommended by some continental surgeons, of evacuating it by opening the cornea, even when both aqueous chambers have seemed to be quite full of it; and I have never been disappointed in seeing it absorbed. A man, fifty-two years old, walking in the street on a Saturday night, was struck on his eye by a stone, and lost his sight; and on Sunday he was brought to me. The chambers of the eye were so discoloured with blood, that neither the iris nor pupil was visible. Cold lotion and a cathartic were ordered, and alcoholic drinks proscribed. On Tuesday evening the pupil was visible, the aqueous fluid still turbid, and a clot of blood was at the bottom of the anterior chamber. Sight was returning. On Thursday, at noon, the chambers were clear, and a very minute light-coloured clot was noticed lying across the capsule of the lens. The iris was thrown forward nearly in contact with the cornea, a state which was attributed to effusion of blood posteriorly. Just a fortnight later the eye had completely recovered the injury; the anterior chamber was restored, and vision had returned.

The removal of the blood may be rapid; in twenty-four hours a small quantity has disappeared, yet weeks may be required for the accomplishment of the same process, if coagulation ensues. Thus Mr. Bowman has pointed out in his lectures on the parts concerned in the operations on the eye, the very marked difference in the time required for the absorption, when the blood is effused into chambers occupied by serum, the consequence of pre-existing disease. He watched a clot during six months under these circumstances before it lost its shape or characteristic hue, and it was undergoing very slow absorption at the end of twelve months. Opportunities of noticing this interesting phenomenon are often afforded when an artificial pupil is made, or when the iris is wounded after any operation, or when, during the operation for extraction, blood from the wounded conjunctiva gets under the cornea. I have seen it removed as rapidly as when there has been no rupture of the eyeball, and therefore no escape of the aqueous humour. Effusion in the vitreous humour is very slowly removed, and may remain, as we now know, for months, and even years.

The careful management of the patient's apartment, as regards ventilation, temperature, and light, must not escape attention. It may be remarked, with regard to the light, that the room should not be made absolutely dark, not only because it would be useless, but domestic arrangements would thereby be interfered with, and much discomfort entailed on the attendants. Light judiciously admitted, and subdued, is the thing needed. In connexion with this subject, I strongly advise the perusal of "Notes on Nursing," by Florence Nightingale.

The patient's position in bed is not an unimportant particular. I have often found raising the shoulders and head add to his comfort; and allowing the easier return of blood, I imagine, must also exercise a curative effect.

BLOWS ON THE EYEBALL, ATTENDED WITH RUPTURE, LACERATION, AND DISTURBANCE OF THE CONTAINED PARTS.

Blows on the globe of the eye may cause rupture of its coats, or the separation, or dislocation, of some of its internal parts. Bursting is no uncommon occurrence; and when the sclerotica suffers, the superior portion, or the internal, between the cornea and a line concentric to the attachment of one of the recti muscles, generally gives way. I have seen but one exception, when the rupture was on the outer side. It has been suggested, in explanation, that the sclerotica tears at a point nearly opposite to that which is struck; the blows which reach the eyeball being, for the most part, on its lower or its outer side, the upper edge of the orbit and the nose protecting it in these positions. The vitreous humour may escape in greater or lesser quantity, and accompanying this may be prolapse of the retina and the choroid. With so much damage the organ is very often destroyed. I have seen profuse hæmorrhage in a few cases.

Loosening of the lens, or, more commonly, displacement of it, is another effect of blows on the eye and on the head. Dislocation of it forwards is that most usual ; and it may be either alone or in its capsule. If it be thrown against the back of the iris, and do not become opaque, the nature of the accident might be temporarily overlooked.

The lens may get fixed in the pupil, but rarely for any length of time, since it either falls against the iris, or, what is more likely, into the anterior chamber.

Pain is the usual concomitant of any form of this accident. It may exist with little or no inflammatory action. Sometimes it is of an intensely neuralgic character—portending destruction of vision, not only in the eye, but about the orbit and head. Acute inflammation mostly supervenes, and the organ is destroyed. I have, in a few cases, seen low inflammatory action, with little or no pain, equally fatal. In all cases the dislocated body must be extracted, if possible ; but if this be impracticable, it should be reclined.

But the lens may lie in the anterior chamber without any untoward symptoms ; and, most assuredly, if no irritation were set up, I should leave it alone, and trust to absorption. Even with slight local disturbance, in a patient under forty years of age, I should not interfere. Above forty, when the fibres increase in density, and absorption of them cannot quickly occur, I should make the earliest symptoms of irritation the signal for action.

A dislocated lens and capsule should be removed from the chamber at once ; that is, as soon as we have assurance that the capsule is present, for months and years may pass away before absorption occurs ; and even were it to be effected before the eye has been destroyed, the capsule might prove a source of much irritation, and, perhaps, become the seat of calcareous deposit. Mr. Lawrence mentions the particulars of a patient who occasionally visited the London Ophthalmic Infirmary, with the lens surrounded by its capsule in the anterior chamber, where it had been for twenty-eight years. The general state of the eye is not given.

But the capsule may not get opaque: and how is its presence to be detected? I answer this by an extract from a review of the last edition of this work, in the "British and Foreign Medico-Chirurgical Review," by Dr. Mackenzie. He says, "Weeks, months, and, I suspect, years, may pass before any decided opacity shows itself in the lens or capsule, provided the latter enclosing the former has been separated from its connexions, without any aperture by which the entrance of the aqueous humour is permitted. In such a case, the lens shows itself in the anterior chamber like a drop of water, of different specific gravity from the rest of the aqueous humour, and its margin seems surrounded by a narrow gilt ring of a splendid yellow colour! In this state he had extracted the lens and capsule before they exhibited the least opacity, although they had been dislocated for weeks."

I may mention incidentally the particulars of a case of spontaneous dislocation of the lens and its capsule into the anterior chamber, in which the eye was lost by the irritation produced. An overgrown girl of thirteen was brought to me about three years ago, with staphyloma completely around and close to the cornea, enlargement with semi-opacity of the cornea, much pain, extinction of vision, and general redness of the eyeball. While endeavouring to ascertain the cause of all this, an opaque capsule enclosing the lens passed forward into the anterior chamber. I now learnt that for some months this opaque body had been observed to pass from one chamber of the eye to the other. It was at once apparent that all the morbid action was produced by the dislocated part. As the other eye was suffering from supposed sympathetic implication, it was examined carefully, and its lens and capsule, quite opaque, were seen reclining backwards in the vitreous humour, but yet retaining a slight attachment to the lower portion of the suspensory ligament .The necessary operation on the right eye, that of "extraction," was followed by a cessation of all irritation. The parents of the girl would not allow the other eye to be touched.

Mr. Henry Howard relates, in one of the periodicals, an instance of spontaneous dislocation of lens into the anterior chamber of the eye being productive of cerebral derangement. A female, aged thirty, suffered from pain and inflammation in her left eye for nearly seven months, during the latter three of which, headaches, attended with vomiting, were so severe as to deprive her of her senses. Mr. Howard found the whole eyeball inflamed, and the lens, with a small quantity of lymph, lying in the anterior chamber. Extraction was performed. From that time the vomiting ceased, and the head symptoms gradually subsided, and were quite lost after forty-eight hours. The lens must have been contained in its capsule, and I am inclined to think that it escaped from its position so enclosed, and not, as Mr. Howard supposes, without it, in consequence of destruction of the capsule by inflammation. It is likely enough that there was softening and giving way of the suspensory ligament.

Many instances of spontaneous dislocation, some in young people, and which are, of course, always associated with morbid changes in the eye, are recorded by the late Mr. Dalrymple and others.

Sometimes a blow produces a rent in the sclerotica, while the conjunctiva remains intact, or but slightly torn, and the crystalline lens is forced out of the eye, and rests between these in close proximity to the cornea, constituting what is called " external dislocation of the lens." With this the iris is more or less paralysed or torn, and a portion, I believe, always carried out with the lens. Much blood is effused within the eyeball; yet vision may not be lost. The removal of the lens is the proper course. The simple process of raising the conjunctiva, snipping it, and removing the body, is easily effected. It has been suggested not to interfere till a fortnight after the accident, that an opportunity may be afforded for the healing of the sclerotica; and that a simple rupture thereby may not be converted into a compound one, and the chances of recovery perhaps materially diminished. Certainly this would not be advisable if the pressure of the lens was productive of pain or irritation. In two cases I tried the method, but I conferred no benefit on my patients. In one, a young adult female, at the end of a fortnight the lens had become decomposed, and now was revealed the cause of the undue irritation, which before was unaccountable. In the other, there was continual pain. Henceforth, I shall do that which appears to me more consonant with sound surgery, viz., to get rid of the extraneous body as soon as is practicable; in fact, to apply here the rule regarding the removal of extraneous matters from other parts of the body.

Here is another example of the change that the crystalline lens undergoes when allowed to remain dislocated. The case illustrates also other points that bear on my subject. An elderly man presented himself with a violent contusion of the right eye, that had been received during a drunken brawl some days before. So great was the degree of swelling and ecchymosis of the palpebræ and of the conjunctiva, that I could not discover the actual state of the organ, or give any definite prognosis. I feared, however, that the eyeball was ruptured, because, from the glimpse that could be obtained of the centre of the cornea, it was evident that the chambers of the eye contained blood. There was considerable pain, but no constitutional disturbance.

Rest, the local use of colds and opiates, constituted the treatment.

At my next visit to the hospital I was enabled, by the reduction of the tumefaction, to discover that there was a rupture at the inner part of the eyeball, at about the junction of the cornea and the sclerotica. Blood still filled the chambers. There was nothing, however, so far remarkable,—nothing but the ordinary course of events when the eye receives a certain amount of violence.

I did not discover for some days later, till the chemosis had greatly abated and the redness of the eye had much reduced, the presence of the crystalline lens on the outside of the eyeball, just posterior to the rupture, between the sclerotica and the conjunctiva. I could not, of course, see the lens; but discerning a tumour in that position, in connexion with the pupil drawn to the side, and the other objective symptoms, I naturally concluded that, in all probability, the lens was located there. At once I snipped the conjunctiva and removed the displaced body; but I·did not remove all of it, or, at least, take it away entire, for there was but a small part of it unchanged, apparently the nucleus,—the rest had broken down by decomposition into a gruel-like material. The selerotica beneath was much indented, puckered, and of an unhealthy aspect. This was just fourteen days from the accident.

The iris is apt to suffer from blows on the eye, to be torn, and even to be more or less separated from the ciliary attachment. I have several times witnessed partial detachment, so that a second pupil was formed, and I have seen a few instances of splitting from the pupil to the circumference, with partial detachment of the flaps. It may be torn away from corresponding parts of the circumference, leaving a central strap without any trace of pupil. I am indebted to my friend Mr. Browne, of the Belfast Ophthalmic Institution, for the following remarkable illustration. A sharp chip of metal wounded the cornea and the iris, and produced extravasation of blood in the chambers of the eye;

FIG. 12.

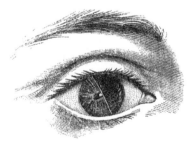

and when absorption had cleared the aqueous fluid, the eye exhibited nearly half the muscular fibres of the iris torn away from the uvea, and rolled up, as the above sketch shows.

These peculiar effects of violence, unattended as they may be with destruction of sight, are very remarkable. They remind us of other instances of most delicate results produced by violence. It would be useless to multiply examples, of which I could produce many from my case-book; enough has been cited to give the general characters of these accidents, and which, unfortunately, so far as the mere mechanical lesion is concerned, do not come within the scope of treatment. The edges of a rent will retract, and a partially detached iris will remain separated.

There is a form of injury that has only been lately properly accounted for,—I mean the apparent loss of a part or the whole of the iris after a blow. When entirely absent, it has been supposed that it might have escaped through any existing rupture of the eyeball, or wound,—a very unlikely thing when the breach has been small, and an impossibility when the cornea and the sclerotica have remained entire; and complete disappearance may be consequent on mere concussion. Mr. Solomon, who has long had his attention drawn to this state of things, has given a short and interesting communication on the subject, to the "British Medical Journal" for the 14th of April, 1860.

He alludes to these two conditions which must have been noticed by all men engaged in ophthalmic practice :—that if the iris be lacerated in its transverse diameter in two or three places, the whole of the segment included in the injury will, in the course of a few days, atrophy and cease to be apparent, although the aqueous humour shall be pellucid; and that if the ciliary nerves be divided by wounds, so much of the iris as the nerves supply will collapse, and the pupil extend to the rim of the cornea.

He continues,—"Or if in the extraction of a cataract, the vitreous body becomes dislocated in the front of the iris, and is allowed to remain there without interference (I do not know how we are to interfere with safety to the eye), that part of the iris which is in proximity with the corneal section atrophies, disappears, and, in time, loses its characteristic structure, being converted into a fibrous band." Moreover, dissection has proved

that the greater part of the iris may escape an external examination, and yet be found within the eyeball. Then follows this
valuable notice in connexion with the above, from the "Archiv
für Ophthalmologie," vol. i., part ii., page 119, by Von Ammon,
who gives the details of an examination after death, of an eye
in which the major part of the iris was rendered invisible by
the concussion from a musket, which was loaded with water
instead of lead, and discharged into the mouth, by a young
soldier who had determined on committing suicide. The only
visible portion of iris in the right eye was a crescentic fragment
towards the external side. The point where this portion disappeared was neither torn nor abruptly folded inwards, but
disappeared without its being possible to discern what had
become of it ; dissection showed that the upper, inner, and lower
borders of the iris were pushed back. The vitreous body was
displaced ; the lens, with its capsule, touched the upper border
of the middle of the superior ciliary processes; whilst the inferior
border was found near the centre of the abnormally large pupil.
The lens and vitreous body had displaced the iris. When the
lens and vitreous body were removed under water, the iris slowly
returned to its position.

Ammon's report is very long, and made up of the usual
German detail. It gives a most elaborate and tiresome description of the inspection of the two shattered eyeballs.

Now, while I recognise, I hope sufficiently, the immense
power of natural reparative action, and the danger of thwarting
or interfering with it, I am no less sure that much is either lost
or gained according as there is no treatment, or as judicious
means are used. Fortunately, there is no call for the exercise of
critical knowledge or of accurate diagnosis; nor is an intimate
acquaintance with ophthalmology needed. Nothing more is
wanted than attention to the first principles of surgery.

I emphatically caution my reader not to let any extent of
injury short of actual collapse destroy hope of being able to
restore an eye to some degree of usefulness. I beg him to take
my word for it, that many a golden opportunity is lost simply
because in the first instance a case has been thought hopeless.

To strengthen my assurance, I would add that physical repair and degrees of functional restoration are now and then almost incredible, and even surprise those practically well versed in surgical diseases of the eye. In the earlier years of my practice I published several of these wonderful recoveries in the weekly periodicals.

It must not be expected that perfection can be recovered after much mechanical lesion, including the loss of the lens; but I need not stop to show that an eye with even imperfect sight still possesses relative and absolute value.

If the direct inflammatory effects of an injury are quickly got over, the chances of the other eye ever suffering from irritation are immensely lessened. If inflammation lingers, many of the tunics are involved, pathological changes ensue, and the other eye is threatened.

Adaptation, as nearly as may be, of divided parts—slight sustaining pressure—local and general rest—are the things indicated, and the objects to be accomplished. When I see a patient sufficiently soon after an injury, I make no further examination than is needed to ascertain its nature, to be assured of the line of action required, and to be able to form a tolerable prognosis. Taking care to remove, by washing or otherwise, all extraneous substances, I close the eyelids, and keep them shut by one or two strips of court-plaster, which fulfils the first two indications —adaptation and slight sustaining pressure, with the great addition of excluding the atmosphere. When the accident is severe, I enjoin rest of body and disuse of the other eye. The quicker the union of the wound, the more certainly is the desired object gained, the more perfect the result, and the less the suffering.

It is positively hurtful to apply stimulating lotions; soothing, and not irritation, is needed. Swelling of the conjunctiva— chemosis, as it is called—is the inevitable result of an injury, and readily passes away. Sometimes it may be well to incise it. The frequent use of cold water, or a cold lotion applied with a rag sufficiently thin to allow of evaporation, is most advantageous; and if much pain exist, the addition of some preparations of opium will generally afford relief. Now and then warm applications are more grateful, so that the use of either must often be discretional.

I resort now more frequently to the internal use of opium, to produce sleep and to relieve pain, than formerly ; but for a prolonged or continuous effect, give it in very small quantities, and repeat the dose often : so that although in the end as much might be prescribed, a far better result is obtained. This affects the patient's system sufficiently, and keeps it so influenced, without that knock-down, prostrating result so likely to follow the large dose. Cases are met with in which nothing but the local abstraction of blood will give ease.

I learned, in the operations for the extraction of cataract and that for artificial pupil, how much is to be gained by not opening the eye for at least a week after it has been incised. That knowledge I apply here, and I find it advantageous to keep the eye plastered even longer. I am wholly unaware of a single object that is to be gained by an early inspection, or one from day to day, as has been advocated by some surgeons. If matters are doing well, it is not needed ; and if any untoward events supervene, their existence is always manifested in appearances of the upper eyelid ; and then it is, more than at any other period, that opening the eye is likely to be hurtful. I prefer that the patient should always of his own accord, and after the tarsal margins have been duly cleansed, open the eye. The act is then devoid of suffering. The application of the surgeon's fingers is very apt, where there has been much lesion, to produce pain, and that often of long duration.

But what is to be done when the iris is more or less prolapsed through the cornea, or perhaps through the sclerotica ? The latter state is the more common. Most assuredly, as a rule, the less that is done the better. But very seldom indeed can it be necessary to interfere. I have a few times thought it prudent, from the amount of the prolapse, from the large bit that was hanging out, to reduce the flap with a pair of scissors, and so to lessen or prevent irritation ; but I repeat, that in general nothing of the kind is needed. By a natural and a safe process, whatever is superfluous and not wanted in the progress of plugging and cicatrization is removed. The application of nitrate of silver cannot be beneficial. I know that it destroys primary cicatrization, and, besides, increases inflammatory action by irritating the eye; so that it is doubly hurtful. I say this after much investigation of the subject and a thorough conviction. In ulceration of the cornea the iris often protrudes in a bladder-like form, being pressed forwards by the aqueous humour; it is then often advantageous to puncture the protrusion and produce collapse. I have not, so far as I remember, met with a parallel example from an injury.

Constitutional treatment must not be neglected, and all measures likely to prevent or to reduce acute or chronic inflammatory action must be attended to; but all that need be said has been already expressed in this chapter in the treatment of inflammation of the eyeball.

I conclude this portion of the chapter by noticing a principle which, as yet, writers on ophthalmic surgery have not recognised. When it is clearly ascertained, however early, that a wounded eye is decidedly lost, and that the secondary action, which is tolerably sure to be suppurative, is attended with pain and constitutional disturbance, a portion of the eyeball should be removed—a mere incision will not answer,—or excision, after Bonnet's plan, adopted. Possessing such means for safe and instantaneous relief, and by which, besides, the greatest protection is afforded to the other eye from sympathetic ophthalmitis, we ought not to allow a continuation of suffering and prostration which no other treatment will check, and which ceases only after certain consecutive morbid changes in the lost organ.

WOUNDS OF THE CORNEA.

Abrasion of the corneal surface, whereby the epithelium is scraped, is, mechanically speaking, the slightest of corneal wounds, and generally of little import; but it may produce inflammation of the eyeball. I have had long and troublesome cases caused by infants scratching their mothers' eyes. A drop of oil is a comforting application to the recent accident. In severe instances the eye should be kept closed till the epithelium has been restored, cold applied, and the progress closely watched. For the treatment of any acute symptoms that may arise, I refer to what I have already written on inflammation of the eyeball.

Although I have spoken of suppuration in the cornea as an effect of general inflammatory action of the eye, and one of the later consequences of such disturbance, I entertain it again as a direct effect of injury.

Suppuration in the cornea, as the consequence of a scratch, or a blow, or impactment of a foreign body, is always perilous. It may appear very quickly, and at first with but little, generally with none or very little inflammatory implication of the rest of the tunics. But whatever be the accompanying symptoms, the eye will hardly escape much damage through destruction of the corneal texture. For some years I have pointed out the damage and the intractable character of the disease to all who have attended my practice. The slightest deposit of pus—a mere speck—should be regarded with the gravest prognosis. Over and over again, when I have quickly detected the earliest commencement, I have hoped by equally early measures to arrest the disorganizing action; but the increase has continued steadily, and the greater part, or whole of the cornea has been involved, and a dense white cicatrix has been the result, or staphyloma, or the entire eyeball has suppurated. It would serve no useful purpose to describe minutely the pathological appearances. I have tried myself, and seen tried, the antiphlogistic plan, including mercury, and with such bad results, that I have ceased to employ it. I have faith in the opposite, or tonic system, and this in accordance with common sense, and modern therapeutics, as the sufferers are generally enfeebled and badly cared-for persons, or those who have passed the meridian of life. Moreover, be the age or the system whatever it may, when the suppuration begins, prostration soon sets in. But, besides giving with discretion and judgment, and not overdoing it, such sustaining stimuli—I do not mean alcoholic drinks, or tonics that seem most appropriate or admissible,—I enjoin absolute rest and the avoidance of all mental labour. The bed is certainly the best place. It is not irksome, for, indeed, the attendant feebleness makes it desirable. Soothing applications are the only useful local ones. This then, so far as I know, with full recognition and attention to any deranged general state of health, will give the best results. Any portion of the cornea that can be saved, may be available in case of need for an artificial pupil. I have never tried Dr. Jacob's method, already given, of evacuating the pus.

WOUNDS OF THE CORNEA, WITH PROLAPSE OF THE IRIS.

Wounds of the cornea, accompanied by prolapse of the iris, are common, scarcely a month passing without some presenting themselves among my Ophthalmic Hospital patients. But the time for any benefit has generally passed before the surgeon is consulted. Children are very liable to them, from being allowed to play with sharp-pointed instruments.

The cornea is rarely ever accidentally divided without a part of the iris escaping; indeed, it is forced out and wedged in the aperture: and hence the general impossibility of spontaneous retraction, and the almost equal impossibility of forcing it back through the same aperture without unjustifiable and destructive violence. In the great majority of cases, the injury causes the lens and capsule to lose their transparency, and the opacity may commence in a few hours, or not be manifested for days, weeks, or even months.

The effect on the pupil is always marked; I have seen that aperture quite lost, from the greater part of the iris prolapsing at the margin of the cornea, through a wound inflicted by a bit of glass, and carrying with it the pupillary edge, the re-mainder of the iris being tightly stretched across the chambers. Yet it is seldom with a lateral wound that any part of the edge is involved.

With a central wound a very slight prolapse may destroy the pupil; and the worst class of cases is where there is a considerable rent, as in fig. 13, the anterior chamber destroyed, and the iris in contact with the cornea.

F

Although ordinary attempts at reduction are not always, I believe, necessarily fruitless—for I could mention authenticated examples to the contrary—yet success must be regarded as a

FIG. 13.

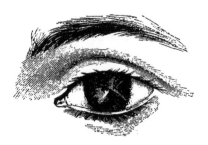

rare exception ; it is only with slight prolapse that it can ever be attained, and then at a very early period,—that is, while the accident is quite recent, and before cicatrization or repair has set in. A trustworthy observer, Roser, found in portions of prolapsed iris examined from two to six days after the accident, a layer of false membrane which was easily separated. This, of course, incorporates itself with the edges of the cornea, as happens in the formation of a partial staphyloma of the part. It is the tightness with which the iris is held in the wound that forms the difficulty. In one of the operations for artificial pupil, in which the iris is. purposely prolapsed, failure may ensue from the spontaneous return of the part; and this is so very likely to happen that the judicious surgeon guards against it by cutting off the greater portion that has been withdrawn. The only difference between the accidental and the surgical production of the prolapse—but it is the all-important difference—is in the relative proportions between the aperture and the mass of iris embraced.

Some surgical authorities say that in no slight case of prolapse which is seen quickly, or even a few days after the accident, should one abstain from attempts at reduction; and the readiest, and therefore first method, should be to rub the cornea gently through the medium of the upper eyelid for a few seconds, to push back. the iris, and then suddenly to expose the eye to a bright light, and to repeat this several times in succession, taking care that the sound eye is shaded while the friction is employed, and simultaneously exposed to the light with the injured one. I have never myself thus succeeded, neither has Dr. Mackenzie nor Mr. Lawrence; the plan has been recommended, no doubt, on the fact that an immediate prolapse, after the operation of extraction of a cataract, may sometimes be so reduced : but the cases are not analogous, as a moment's reflection must show.

I must tell the inexperienced in these matters, that the iris cannot be pushed back even when there is a large wound in the cornea, as we can thrust a bit of rag into a cavity; for whether the aqueous humour be present, or has been discharged, the action of the several orbital muscles, and the natural elasticity of the coats of the eye, maintain a tolerably close adaptation between the containing and the contained parts, and that in reality no cavity exists; so that, after all, the chief benefit must be looked for in those cases in which the iris is so little incarcerated that its action is not quite destroyed. Then with belladonna, or, what is better, the sulphate of atropia, the object may be attained, and I do not restrict its use to prolapse of the pupillary edge, as has been recommended, but employ it also when the circumference of the iris has been forced out; for dilatation of the pupil cannot be produced without traction being exerted on that part of the iris which is strangulated, be the hernia where it may; and, with the greatest attainable degree of artificial dilatation, the edge of the pupil is much within the circumference of the cornea. I may repeat what I said on the use of atropine in general, that its fullest influence is to be got by a drop of a strong solution applied to the conjunctiva. I saw a young gentleman, H. H. W., in less than a quarter of an hour after he had wounded the outer part of one of his corneæ with a scalpel. A portion of the iris was just embraced by the lips of the wound, to which the pupil was pulled, but did not protrude. A drop or two of a solution of a grain of atropine to two drachms of water, was at once used in the manner directed, and in three quarters of an hour the pupil was well dilated and perfectly round, showing that the iris was quite extricated. The dilatation was kept up for several days, till the wound was healed. A small scar on the cornea is the only trace of the accident.

It fortunately happens at times that, although the cornea is much divided, the iris merely rests against, and blocks up the wound, but does not prolapse. Within an hour after the accident, I saw a boy whose cornea was split vertically in the entire diameter, by something thrown at him. The iris did not prolapse, but merely rested on the wound. His mother would not allow any treatment, and brought him to the hospital no more.

But I do not see why, under favourable circumstances, a small prolapse may not be so acted on by instrumental means, and partially returned, or at least so influenced or released, as to enable the iris to be affected by atropine. It must be remembered that many manœuvres on the eye that could not formerly be done, except at a great risk, are, since the introduction of chloroform, easily and efficiently executed. I am not sure that it would always be impracticable to enlarge the corneal wound, although I fully admit that it would require the most delicate surgery, and that its performance is next to impossible, unless the patient be chloroformed.

Dr. Mackenzie thinks, that could the little bag of iris that protrudes be emptied of its aqueous humour, it would often return immediately into its place. Puncturing it would do this, but then a false pupil might be made. The method that he · recommends is, instantly after dropping a solution of atropine into both eyes, to bring the patient under the influence of chloroform, and with a small curette to press on the little bag of iris, so as to empty it of its contents. The curette should enter through the wound, carrying the bit of prolapsed iris before it.

The very general, but highly injurious system of touching a prolapsed iris with nitrate of silver, has been sufficiently noticed; but I may mention that the subject is again brought forward in the chapter on Cataract, when I speak of the treatment of prolapse after an operation. So, also, about cutting a bit of it off; this has been commented on, and is again spoken of in the same place.

The rules that I have already laid down for the local and general treatment of rupture or laceration of the eyeball, are no less applicable here. I need add but one suggestion. It is, not to be impatient for results, and neither to over-treat, nor too readily to despair. After the regular nutrition of a part has been interfered with and interrupted, a very long time must elapse before repair can be well established. Time, therefore, is the most important element in these circumstances.

WOUNDS OF THE EYELIDS, OF THE SURROUNDING INTEGUMENTS, AND OF THE CONJUNCTIVA.

These are, for the most part, detrimental from disarrangement attending the mal-approximation of their edges, and by which there may ensue trichiasis, entropium, ectropium, with more or less injurious exposure of the eyeball, accompanied with displacement of the punctum lacrymale, or from paralysis of the upper eyelid—ptosis. The most careful adaptation of the divided surfaces is, therefore, of the first importance. Plaster must not always be depended on, and should be used alone only in very superficial injuries. With deep, or extensive division of parts, sutures are absolutely needed. When, from loss of surface, the use of the needle is contra-indicated from the nature of the wound, and water-dressing, or even a poultice, is necessary, the process of cicatrization is materially assisted by drawing together and supporting the contiguous surfaces by plaster, or bandage and compress. I have often thereby effected much, in lessening deformity and shortening the period of cure.

Care should be taken that extraneous bodies are removed. Particles of grit will be best extricated by a stream of water from a strong syringe.

Whether it may be advisable to pare off or remove any torn or jagged edges and adapt the surfaces, must depend on the discretion of the surgeon, and the period at which the patient is seen; for, if more than a few hours have elapsed, and the suppuration stage has commenced, adhesion is impossible, and any interference of this kind will make matters worse. All operative proceedings must be then delayed till every trace of inflammatory action has ended.

A cook fell on the brass arm that suspended a bottle-jack over the fire-place, and tore the lower eyelid away from the corner of the eye, without injuring the canaliculus, in the manner shown in this sketch.

FIG. 14.

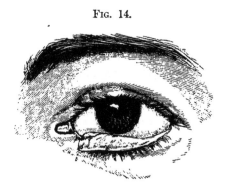

She did not apply at the Ophthalmic Hospital till the wound had been healed. I pared its edges and brought them together by suture, and, keeping the eyelid rather pulled up by semi-circular strips of plaster passed from the root of the nose to the temple for eight days, accomplished perfect restoration.

I have treated several like instances of injury to the inner part of the lower eyelid, which it would be useless to particularize, each of course requiring special little individual matters of attention that would be tedious to detail. The only point I think worthy of mention relates to the displacement or division of the canaliculus; but, to avoid repetition, I shall not do more in this place than refer my reader to the chapter on the affections of the Puncta, the Canaliculi, and the Lacrymal duct, in which all that relates to them is discussed. I may say, however, in passing, that the common recommendation to introduce a bristle or a bit of wire to maintain an aperture when this conduit is torn, is not a very practical one, and it would not prevent subsequent contraction.

I will give an example of injury to the outer portion of the eyelid. A naval officer, in a drunken brawl, by which he lost his eye and his commission, was pelted by a messmate with a broken decanter. The eyeball and the lower eyelid were cut across. I saw him six months after the accident. The outer portion of the eyelid was considerably everted, while the inner was adherent to the eyeball. The deformity induced him to wear a green patch to conceal the eye. By a rather free dissection, I brought the displaced bit in contact with that which was adherent to the eyeball. After the eyelashes—which I had cut off previous to my operation—had grown, so little trace was there of any injury that it was scarcely noticeable to a casual observer.

The upper eyelid is less seldom injured than the lower. An injury to the levator palpebræ muscle is often followed by ptosis, which is sometimes permanent.

A young brewer tore the upper eyelid, close to the orbit, very severely, against a gas-burner, and the integuments hung about in a manner which left me little hope of preventing much deformity, and ptosis seemed tolerably sure. With the exercise of some ingenuity in trimming and adapting the edges, I got a very satisfactory position of parts. The sequel was gratifying; for when all inflammatory action had passed away, the eyelid could be raised a little. A few months afterwards complete power of elevation returned, and there was little mark of what had happened.

Whenever the entire thickness of the eyelid is divided, the sutures should be carried through all the textures. I have had little experience as yet with the fine metallic suture, but from what I have seen, I believe it to be especially applicable to cases like this, in which accurate position is of so much consequence, and, from the dense nature of the textures, so difficult to be maintained by ordinary stitches.

Wounds of the integuments about the edge of the orbit, resulting from blows, partake of the character of incised wounds, and should be treated by suture; if primary union does not follow, the after result is none the worse for the attempt.

Broad and unsightly cicatrices may sometimes be advantageously dissected out, and a palpable disfiguration exchanged for a scar very much less disfiguring, or scarcely noticeable.

A rupture of some portion of the lacrymal duct above the bony canal in which it lies, is one of the accidents incidental to injury in this region, and, as far as I know, produces but temporary inconvenience. Charles Porter, a young man, received a slight scratch on the inner corner of one eye in a scuffle; he thought no more of it till the evening, when he blew his nose, and felt a puff of air in the corner of the eyelids. Rather amused by the novel sensation, he continued to inflate his nostrils, till he found that his eyes were nearly closed, and his face much swollen. When he came to Mr. Taylor, at the Central London Ophthalmic Hospital, two days after the accident, his eyelids were almost closed, and the swelling had extended down to the cheek as far as the under edge of the jaw; the air could easily be pressed in different directions, conveying a fine crepitating sensation to the finger. He soon got well without any treatment. Another case came under Mr. Taylor's notice, where a rupture of the sac followed the act of blowing the nose; and a third, caused by a slight blow from the branch of a tree: both these cases speedily recovered without special treatment. If the supply of air to the cellular tissue do not soon cease, pressure should be applied over the site of injury, for the cure consists in healing the breach through which the air passes.

Laceration of the tube within the bony canal, from fracture of the bone, is the more severe accident, and it may be advisable to maintain the aperture by a style, or occasionally to pass a probe.

In surgical operations about the eyelid, the incisions should be planned with reference to the least deformity; and where there is necessarily much loss of texture, some allowance may

frequently be made for after improvement by plastic operation;
the likelihood also of ptosis from injury to the levator palpebræ
should be remembered.

A surgeon may be compelled to remove parts of the eyelids,
or even to perform their entire amputation, after the bite of
rabid animals. The experiments of Youatt go far to show that
the nitrate of silver and sulphuric acid have power in neu-
tralising or destroying the poison; yet it is not considered
safe to trust to them alone. Bites about the face, or indeed
any uncovered part of the body, are the more serious from the
free contact of the dangerous saliva; and with this greater
chance of the morbid development, no well-assured method of
treatment should be neglected.

An intelligent and healthy lad, eight years old, was brought
to St. Bartholomew's Hospital, when I was house-surgeon, by
an elder sister, in consequence of injuries received from having
been knocked down by a strange dog while at play with his
schoolfellows. On the upper lid of the right eye was an abrasion
about three-quarters of an inch long, and half an inch broad,
and all the information that could be collected was, that the dog
leaped at him and knocked him down. As one knee bore the
evidence of a fall, and the face was covered with mud, the eyelid
was supposed to have suffered from the same cause. Some
simple dressing was applied, and I sent directions to the mother
to make inquiries about the dog. Just two months after, the
poor lad reappeared at the hospital with hydrophobia, and died
the next day. At the inquest a question was raised as to the
neglect of removing the eyelid; but I was able to prove that
the probability of danger was pointed out to the sister, and it
appeared that the mother had learned a day or two after that
the dog was killed as rabid, but was persuaded by a neighbour
not to let me know. To have resorted to such a severe measure
as the removal of an eyelid without any evidence that the part
had been bitten, would have been as culpable as to neglect it,
had I been in the possession of all the facts.

Wounds of the conjunctiva are of little consequence. The
operation for squinting has fully established the fact, that an

unfavourable result is not to be feared from extensive division of
this membrane, opening of the cellular sheath of the eyeball, and
exposure of the sclerotica. Prior to this operation, if a person
had received a wound of the conjunctiva, which was followed by
an equal amount of inflammation and swelling, the rigour of
strict antiphlogistic measures, and long confinement to a dark
room, would have been thought requisite. Sutures are not
required in slight injuries, although where the membrane is
much or irregularly torn, and more or less detached, a considerable portion that would otherwise perish may, I believe, be saved
by them. But more than this, the healing process is thereby
materially facilitated, and deformity may often be prevented.
In one instance I applied several, and obtained ready union. I
shall show, in the operation for squint, that the conjunctiva
unites as readily as skin, and that the threads do not produce
any irritation. I apply them at the very margin of the wound,
and allow them to come away of themselves—a process generally
accomplished in three days. I have used no smaller needle than
that which is figured among the instruments; but it may be
necessary to employ one very much more bent, and shorter.

Chemosis, or swelling of the conjunctiva and of the sub-
conjunctival cellular tissue from serous effusion, is a common
sequence of injury to any of the ocular appendages, and is very
likely to excite alarm, but is innocuous. Existing with a copious
purulent discharge, in which case the effusion is supposed to be
of a fibrinous nature—a state that is considered in the chapter
on Gonorrhœal Ophthalmia,—danger is at hand. The extent
need never create alarm; the brightness of the cornea, and the
integrity of sight, may be taken as certain assurances of the
absence of any danger. I have seen the cornea nearly covered
by it, from a blow on the eyebrow, and the swelling entirely
disappeared in a few days without treatment. I have never
used any remedy besides a cold lotion. Different forms may be
assumed according to the extent or position of the swelling, but
these are of no particular importance. I have observed very
extensive chemosis, with protrusion from between the lids, and
yet neither eyelid was everted, but the lower was so tightly

pressed against the eyeball that I could not depress it. This peculiarity was evidently from the conjunctiva of the lower palpebral sinus alone being affected. A blow on the eye had produced the mischief.

CHEMICAL INJURIES.

Strong chemical agents applied to the eye very rapidly exert their influence, but all reasonable effort should always be made to limit their action by the removal, as far as it may be, of the substance or any part of it which may not have exhausted its power, by washing and by neutralisation.

The free use of water should be the first treatment. But even when quickly resorted to, the time is passed for much saving benefit to be conferred, and especially if the cornea have been touched. Of course, the effect is chiefly in removing or diluting any excess of the destructive agent that may yet be about the eye. But this must not paralyse our efforts, and science must be resorted to, if only as a forlorn hope; for when not of actual service, a patient is none the less satisfied to find that all has been done and tried within the range of our power, practically and theoretically.

For an injury with an acid, an alkaline solution should be employed, and the bicarbonate of potass answers well.

When a strong alkali has entered the eye, we find in acetic acid a good re-agent. A drachm of the acidum aceticum of the London Pharmacopœia, to seven drachms of water, is the proper formula. A less proportion of the acid cannot be depended on, and for free use a greater quantity would render it too pungent to be borne. Vinegar may be used when at hand.

When lime or mortar enters the eye, the same diligent washing is demanded, and in addition the entire conjunctiva should be searched to discover any adherent bits, which should be picked off. The sinuses of the eyelids must be well inspected, and, in deep-set eyes, where this is not so readily effected, a camel's hair, or better still, a sable brush moistened with gum, should be swept along them. It is a rule, never to be departed from, that in all injuries of the eye from the introduction of extraneous bodies, the entire extent of the conjunctiva must be examined for any fragments that may remain adherent, or impacted; and the search will be imperfect unless the eyelids are everted, and their recesses well surveyed. Water is but a poor solvent for lime, and cold water takes up more than hot: a pint at 32° dissolves 13·25 grains; at 60°, 11·6; and at 212°, 6·7; and because of this it has been imagined that there is great scope for the exercise of practical chemistry, and from the specious recommendations that are published, the unwary student may be excused for supposing that the eye might be held harmless from any such injuries.

The true state of the case is, that this alkaline earth spoils the epithelium very quickly, always too quickly for us to stop certain effects; yet perhaps there is more opportunity to lessen the degree or intensity of action, than with most other escharotics. An acid lotion, as above recommended, should be tried. Modern chemistry teaches that a more effectual way is to employ a solution of sugar, and to apply the acid afterwards. Dissolve one part of sugar in one part of hot water, dilute with an equal bulk of cold water, so as to have a solution lukewarm, and apply it freely to the eye.

With the lime as lime, the sugar will in great part unite to form saccharate of lime; but with carbonate of lime, which is sure to be present, and will be quickly increased by exposure to air and moisture, no combination will be formed. It is therefore better to wash the eye subsequently with dilute acetic acid, which will dissolve out the lime in form of acetate of lime.

This is, so far as I know, the sum of all that can be done in these distressing injuries. I am aware that other reagents have been recommended, but some on such purely hypothetical grounds, and others so obviously inapplicable, that I shall not speak of them.

A few drops of glycerine as a local application will afford comfort. Unlike oil, it mingles freely with the water of the tears, and forms a protecting medium against the action of the air.

I think it unnecessary to continue further with the subject. However interesting it might be theoretically to suggest antidotes to affect the many substances that may touch the surface of the eye, for the circumstances of actual practice it is useless. Enough has been said, I hope, to establish the value of washing the eye at once, thoroughly, and not to waste useful time in seeking for remedies that can rarely ever be serviceable. If, for instance, particles of nitrate of silver were the offending material, it would be far more prudent instantaneously to resort to the water nearest at hand, than to delay succour till salt and water could be procured. First wash in every instance, and then seek for chemical aid if there be even a probability of assistance from it.

The effects of chemical injuries demand some notice.. We are most familiar with those that arise from lime in some form or combination. Weak mortar, although freely applied to the surface of the eye, may produce no worse effect than slightly whitening the conjunctiva, and giving a thin cloudiness to the cornea, from which there may be complete recovery. A stronger compound will have a greater effect, with more or less permanent result on the cornea; yet an opacity that seemed indelible and dense enough to render the eye almost useless, may be cleared enough to afford useful vision. When very strong mortar, lime, or worst of all, unslacked lime, enters the eye, the conjunctiva is entirely and rapidly acted on, and so is the epithelium on the cornea, as also the true corneal tissue, and the worst effects ensue. A person quickly appreciates the spoiling of the cornea by the loss of vision, but he cannot have any idea of the distressing results that are to ensue when the conjunctiva alone has been severely acted on; he should therefore be forewarned. The whitening and the swelling, and the absence of much pain, are not threatening symptoms, and even the separation of the decomposed part gives little or no indication of what must follow. There is an insidiousness about the process that deceives. The strong acids and alkalies char, or at once produce a sensible and apparent destructive change. It is only when the part injured by lime has been separated, and cicatrization is rather far advanced, that the inevitable contraction becomes apparent. Inevitable I say; for wherever there is destruction of the conjunctiva from this cause, or indeed by any escharotic, there must follow a cor-

responding amount of contraction, and of adhesion of the eyelids
to each other, or to the eyeball.

Having done all that mechanical and chemical skill places
within our reach, the after treatment must next occupy our
attention, and we should exercise great watchfulness to assist
the reparative efforts of nature. Total rest of the eye, with hot
or cold narcotic lotions, opium ointment, sedatives internally—
in short, anything that gives relief—is indicated. The use of
very cold, or iced water, for a limited period, I have found
to be very grateful, though occasionally objected to from mere
prejudice.

In the severer injuries, when the destroyed parts have been
cast off, granulations appear, and contractions begin to show
themselves, the common practice is to endeavour to destroy this
surface with caustics and escharotics. Even the probe is
brought into requisition, and the approximated edges are
rudely torn asunder.

I have seen all these most diligently used, and I am sure
that the practice is highly injurious. It irritates, inflames,
increases suppuration, prolongs the healing, augments the
damage, and produces greater contractions.

I suspect that most of the error that exists on this head is
perpetuated, because surgeons do not see their cases sufficiently
long—that is, to the end—but lose sight of them soon after they
have separated, by caustic or otherwise, contracting surfaces;
and think that the conclusion is as they desire.

There is no more production of new material than is required
for cicatrization and the drawing together of the surrounding
parts, the mass of which disappears in time, so that the breach
is mainly closed by a mechanical process. I am sure that actual
adhesion of granulating surfaces, when there is a continuous
ulcer, is rare—more so than is imagined,—and that the contractions are mistaken for it. The occurrence of adhesion would
be far more favourable for after-treatment by operation, and, if
this be true, should be encouraged. But I make the remark
suggestively, and to stimulate inquiry.

I say, then, use all means, and ensure speedy repair; for the less the wound is irritated, the shorter will be the suppurative stage, the quicker will be the healing, the less the contraction, and, necessarily, the fewer the bands and the bridles, and the greater chance will be thereby afforded for rectifying the deformity by practical surgery. The only exception to this rule is that rare condition in which the opposite sides of the palpebral and ocular conjunctiva have been damaged, while an intermediate portion of the membrane—the sinus, as it is called—remains intact, and adhesion is likely to ensue in an isthmus-like form. Persevering attempts must be made by daily dressing and guarding the surfaces with goldbeaters' skin and ointment, keeping the eyelid retracted, or by any ingenious plan to ensure the individual healing of each. If the glass guard, in shape like an artificial eye, with a hole in the centre, which has been so much recommended of late to be worn to prevent contractions, be at all admissible, it is here, although I think that the object may be obtained in a less objectionable way; for several persons who have used them for other purposes, and in vain, have complained of much pain and distress; but when one application fails, another must be tried.

While wishing to be most emphatic on abuse of treatment, I am not unaware of the timely advantage of a mild stimulant, or astringent, carefully and neatly applied to an indolent or unhealthy ulcer; and the only drugs contra-indicated are lead and nitrate of silver. When the cornea is ulcerated, or excoriated, lead lotions are inadmissible, on account of the deposit of insoluble sulphate and chloride. The most careful preparation with distilled water does not free it from this objection, because the saline matter in the tears will produce a precipitate. I have picked off the deposit many times.

I thoroughly believe that more harm has been inflicted by nitrate of silver in ophthalmic diseases and injuries than benefit conferred. Thousands and thousands of eyes have been destroyed by its injudicious use, by its caustic and irritating effects. It is the cause of a large number of men being invalided from the public services, and it produces a class of miserables, who spend their days in seeking relief from place to place. This salt, when resorted to as an astringent, should be employed of a less strength than produces pain. If one grain to the ounce of water is too strong, I use less. But I must leave this, and speak about the staining effect, which I desire to notice here.

In proportion to the strength of the nitrate of silver lotion is the danger of the conjunctiva becoming stained, and the time it is used has its influence in the probability of this unpleasant effect; yet a weak lotion, not long applied, may discolour. I have seen it happen in a fortnight's use, with only one daily application. I suspect that there is far greater likelihood of the nitrate being changed to the insoluble chloride, and ultimately to the oxide, and, as it is likely also, to the metallic state, during the repair of lesions about the conjunctiva. At all events, let caution be observed, and I have said enough to induce the point to be regarded.

I am not aware that a very decided stain can be removed by chemical action, but I know that it may be reduced by the application of hyposulphite of soda, as strong as the eye can bear it, beginning with eight or ten grains to an ounce of water, and applied with an eye-glass. I have never attempted to act on a slight stain.

Acute inflammation of the eyeball may ensue after any of these injuries, and at any stage of repair : for this, ample instructions have already been given.

CHAPTER V.

FIG. 15.

INSTRUMENTS FOR REMOVING FOREIGN BODIES FROM THE SURFACE OF THE CORNEA.

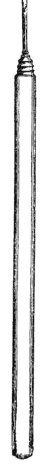

THE miniature gouge here figured is the twentieth part of an inch broad. It is hollowed or scooped, round at its extremity, bevelled, and sharp.

FOREIGN BODIES ON THE SURFACE OF THE EYE.

The intrusion of bodies in the eye is of very common occurrence, and the effects vary according to their size, their shape, and the manner in which they impinge.

An almost microscopic particle of matter may adhere, slightly irritate the eye, be readily dislodged by the movements of the eyelids, and washed away by the tears, or, perhaps, removed by the fingers from the cornea of the eye; or a body may be projected with great violence, become impacted in any part of the eye, and destroy it, either at once or, ultimately, from secondary causes.

I am sure that it is wholly unnecessary to describe minutely the symptoms of a patient thus injured; the thing is self-evident. The sensation, the irritability of the eye, with the flow of tears, and the almost impossibility of opening it, all point to the fact.

The excretory lacrymal channels must frequently convey away minute substances; for whatever is below the diameter of the punctum may be so carried away, if its length do not interfere. Hence the popular impression that blowing the nose will remove such things. One of my late colleagues at the St. Pancras Royal General Dispensary suffered from irritation of his eye that was to him inexplicable. Three days before he applied to me, while sitting in his drawing-room, he felt a very sharp pricking in the eye ; but neither could he discern the cause, nor could another surgeon succeed in discovering it. The semilunar fold of the conjunctiva was swollen and very red, and the entire conjunctiva inflamed ; while the end of a hair, protruding just sufficiently to allow of being laid hold of with a pair of forceps, was visible from the upper punctum. This was easily drawn out : it was half an inch in length, and evidently a portion of his own hair that had been hanging about his person, after the recent process of hair-cutting.

When a substance is lodged within the eyelids, the patient may be able to define its exact seat—a matter of some moment ; but when he cannot, and a survey of all the exposed parts of the eye fails to detect it, the eyelids should be retracted, and a greater surface of the globe of the eye exposed, the entire cornea, and some of the sclerotica beyond it, rendered visible. Should that not suffice to reveal it, the interior of the eyelids must be searched—the under by depressing it, and pulling it from the eyeball, which should be directed upwards ; the upper by reversing it, that is, turning it inside out—which may be easily done by holding some of the central cilia and the edge of the corresponding portion of the tarsus, drawing the eyelid down and away from the eyeball, resting a probe or any small instrument above the cartilage, and then folding the tarsus upwards and backwards over it. The retroversion may be adroitly effected with the forefinger and thumb. Nineteen times in twenty, the object sought will be found about midway on the tarsus, and rather near the edge. Yet, with all this, a small extraneous substance may still remain concealed, as the recess of the upper eyelid has not yet been exposed; and to unfold or open it to view, a narrow spatula, or paper-knife, or something of this kind, is required. When the object is perceived, its detachment is generally easy. But a minute particle may still escape observation in this situation, especially by artificial light; for the peculiarity of this recess may prevent perfect and satisfactory exposure. A jet of tepid water thrown up from a syringe with a bent pipe, projected with sufficient force, should be employed whenever, in such a case, there is reason to suppose that anything remains. Some surgeons use, as an instrument of search, a camel-hair brush; or what is better, as it is stiffer, one of sable, that has been oiled.

There are occasions when, from the multitude of the particles, the syringe cannot be dispensed with. A lad had both eyes filled with cement-powder. It was necessary to use the syringe for a long while, the eyelids being all the time held apart, before the material could be removed.

The less sensitiveness of the oculo-palpebral fold of conjunctiva of the upper eyelid—the sinus, as it is more frequently called—is the reason why the presence of a body may not be felt, or suspected, till suppuration or inflammation ensues, or a fungus sprouts out; or why it may produce so little annoyance, or even cause symptoms that may be referred to other causes. I examined the eye of a private patient, as I thought, carefully, but without discovering the cause of the slight annoyance which she felt. I saw her several days afterwards, and was requested to take another survey, as she was tolerably certain that something was present. A more thorough search discovered a fragment of window glass in the sinus, so large as to make it a wonder that its presence had not been most intolerable. Mr. Lawrence removed a bit of twig, from the bough of a tree, that had been under the eyelid for several weeks without the patient being aware of its having entered the eye. He gives another example, of a gentleman who consulted him on account of uneasiness in his eyes, into one of which a small insect had flown a few weeks before, although the patient was not disposed to attribute all his sufferings to that circumstance. Within the under lid was found one of the elytra (the wing cover) of a minute species of beetle, and within the upper, the corresponding one.

A gentleman consulted Dr. Jacob on account of a fungus growth resembling a polypus projecting from beneath the upper eyelid. The Doctor seized it with a pair of forceps, to extirpate it, and found it firm and resisting. He examined further, and discovered a bit of a rush, three quarters of an inch long, within it. The gentleman then recollected that, about a year before, he had a fall from his horse while hunting, and for several days felt as if something had got into his eye, but as the sensation went off he thought no more of it.

The first time I saw a fungus proceeding from this cause I was deceived for a time, because I had no knowledge on the subject, and I was unassisted in my diagnosis by any information from my patient, the morbid growth alone having attracted his attention.

In the Ophthalmic Hospital Reports, vol. i., p. 35, is recorded a case in which a husk remained under the eyelid for two months, and produced, by its irritation, a warty-looking growth, and besides, a fibrinous exudation that had become moulded by the movements of the eyelid. Ptosis was produced.

I will conclude these examples, which have been sufficiently numerous, by the following from Monteath's translation of Weller's "Manual of the Diseases of the Human Eye," quoted by Dr. Mackenzie. A young girl had a soft red fungus growing out of her eye, as large as a filbert; it was of some weeks' standing, and was attributed to a hurt inflicted by a straw striking the eye. The fungus originated in the conjunctiva, where it is reflected from the lower eyelid to the eyeball. It was cut away, but in three weeks was as large as ever. It was again removed; a bit of straw, half an inch in length, was observed and extracted; the cure was complete in a few days. A man consulted Dr. Monteath on account of an inflamed state of his eye, induced by a fall, five months before, among some bushes, in descending a steep mountain. He felt at the moment that some part of the eye was wounded; and, although he had applied a great variety of remedies, it had, from that period, remained in a tender state. On everting the upper eyelid, a fungous state of the conjunctiva was discovered very high up, and a probe gave assurance that something was there. It was seized with a pair of forceps, and, when extracted, proved to be a portion of twig from a bush, three-fourths of an inch in length, and nearly as thick as a crow-quill. This substance had remained in the upper fold of the conjunctiva for five months, and had got into that situation without wounding the eye.

I have always observed, as the effect of substances long lying under the eyelid, inflammation of the conjunctiva—more or less chronic or acute. The conjunctival papillæ enlarge, there is muco-purulent or purulent discharge, and the entire eyelid loses its natural appearance, becomes swollen, and sometimes inflamed. I have known cases that have been supposed to be ordinary purulent ophthalmia due to the intrusion of substances. With the slightest suspicion, therefore, of anything having entered the eye, in conjunction with any of these symptoms, I make a thorough examination. I have found it necessary to use chloroform to do this, from the irritability and tenderness that existed.

The patient's sensations are not an infallible guide to the presence of bodies within the eyelids; with a full persuasion that something yet lingers in the eye, he may be mistaken. Again, he may be entirely deceived, not any substance having entered the eye, the whole source of discomfort arising from a few enlarged conjunctival vessels about the outer angle; and it is well known that one of the symptoms of inflammation of the conjunctiva is the sensation of sand, or grit, as it is usually expressed, in the eye. On the other hand, it is not unusual that the error is on the side of the surgeon, who, imagining the substance to have been removed, directs his treatment against the supposed consecutive inflammation, while the true cause, the irritating body, is still extant. A gentleman perceiving that something had entered his eye, and having in vain tried to remove it, applied to his usual medical attendant. Nothing was found, but his suffering continued. On the following day inflammation and pain rendered him unable to attend his duties. He was cupped, confined to a dark room, and salivated. Six weeks of misery were passed in implicit obedience to the rules of his adviser, who now became not only very anxious, but actually alarmed, and requested a consultation with some one more conversant with eye diseases. This was granted, the upper lid was everted, and a portion of cigar ash removed from about the centre of the cartilage, the usual seat of small particles under the eyelid. Relief was instantaneous, the symptoms declined rapidly, and the cloudy cornea recovered its transparency.

The minuteness of bodies may cause them to be overlooked, when on the cornea, especially when over the pupil, although this is generally much contracted from the irritation, and often they cannot be discerned, except in a particular light, by the loss of polish of that portion of the cornea upon which they rest. When they merely adhere they are easily removed, the chief difficulty being in fixing the eye, which should be done as if an operation for cataract were about to be performed. This is. among the nicest manœuvres of ophthalmic surgery, and the difficulty is increased by the involuntary and strong action of the orbicularis muscle, occasioned by the irritability of the eye. When, from want of practice, or any other cause, the fingers are not efficient, the spring-wire retractor may be available. In most instances there is more than mere adhesion. When fairly embedded in the anterior elastic lamina, or deeper, some perseverance is required to extricate them ; a cataract-needle is generally employed for the dislodgment. It would be better to use some instrument, with a broader point. A small scoop, such as I have figured, is superior to everything else that I have tried. The body is sooner withdrawn with it, and, remaining on the end of the instrument, is readily removed, and very much less injury is inflicted on the eye than in the usual and repeated attempts with needles, cataract-knives, or other angularly-pointed blades. I may add that I use it for all cases, when the body is on the surface, and when it is impacted. Manipulation is as safe with this as anything else. A speck may be taken off more lightly, and certainly more readily than with a blunt instrument; but the gouge may not be sufficient. I have found it necessary to use a minute pair of forceps to extract a wood splinter. Even more than this, I have incised the cornea a little before I could get out a bit of brass, from a lathe, that had entered the cornea obliquely. Affections of the cornea should always be regarded with deep interest, as the sense of sight is more frequently impaired by the spoiling of this part of the eye than of any other.

It is advised by some surgeons, that when an attempt to remove a body thus impacted is not readily successful the endeavour should be relinquished. This is a very dangerous doctrine, and if literally acted on, would cause the sacrifice of many eyes. So long as it has not passed beyond the cornea, we should not desist, except under very peculiar circumstances. The only exception is to be found in rude attempts by mechanics, but this hardly comes under our legitimate observation. In the natural processes of separation by ulceration, or by sloughing, there is more or less risk to the integrity of the eye from opacity, or partial staphyloma; and more certainly there is danger of entire destruction of the organ from suppuration of the cornea, and it may be, of the eyeball. Even the remarkably rare occurrence of a body being encysted is not without its perils, for I have known the accompanying action prove fatal to the integrity of the retina, and destroy sight. I have seen ulceration of the cornea, and prolapse of the iris, occasioned by the presence of a particle of iron that had entered a week before, but which was so diminutive that a surgeon did not detect it. A patient had general inflammation of the eyeball from a minute bit of iron that had been lodged in the cornea for three weeks; it was readily removed, but the other eye sympathised in the inflammation. I could quote many parallel cases of danger to the eye, even when the foreign body had been superficially placed.

I must say that I have never regretted the persevering attempt to remove a body from the cornea; and I make the statement after ample opportunities of observation; for, from the immense establishment of Messrs. Cubitt, in Gray's-inn-road, with its numerous workshops and manufactories, scarcely a week passes without workmen applying to me at the Ophthalmic Hospital on account of such accidents; while the neighbouring parish of Clerkenwell, swarming with those who exercise trades whereby they are peculiarly exposed to similar injuries of the eye, affords a wide field of observation ; to say nothing of other opportunities. I am often obliged to dig into the cornea ; and I find the repair is usually complete ; and no opacity follows when the conjunctiva and the anterior elastic lamina only have been involved, and none that is practically recognisable when the gouge is carried deeper.

The following case, occurring in the practice of my friend Mr. Browne, of Belfast, shows how much may be required in these accidents, and how great may be the repair. The entire surface of the cornea, and the greater portion of the conjunctiva scleroticæ, were literally paved by fine particles of iron. A young man in an iron foundry was drilling a hole in the cylinder-case of a steam-engine ; he stooped down to observe his progress, and holding a lighted candle, there was an explosion of some gas that had collected between the cylinder and case. The eye was scorched, and the particles from the drilling thrown on its surface. The cornea was scraped of its epithelium, and the particles of iron removed to an extent that saved the eye, and rendered it useful. Deformity, however, remained, from the stains on the cornea and the presence of some of the iron in the conjunctiva, from which but a small quantity of the filings was extracted. Some of the metal was even under the conjunctiva.

The only exception, I imagine, to interfering, except to gratify a patient with any extraneous substance in the cornea, is when we find it deeply imbedded, and many days or months have elapsed without any ill effects arising—the surrounding portion of the cornea not being hazy ; and pain, vascularity, and lacrymation absent ; or when there has been a complete cessation of all acute symptoms. Several times I have been consulted about such cases. In each it was a bit of a percussion copper cap that had entered. The copper did not produce any irritation; it was not projecting beyond the surface. I decided not to interfere, because to extricate it would in all probability have been a difficult job, and to excise the cornea would have been to reduce the eye, and the operation might have been attended with complete collapse. Besides, there was time enough to operate, if irritation ensued. This is familiarly called leaving well alone—a maxim of especial value as applied to surgery.

In February, 1855, Mr. Parrott, of Clapham Common, brought his niece to me, a girl æt. 5. Four months previously she struck a copper cap between two pieces of iron, and a portion of the copper entered her right eye. The cornea was divided nearly perpendicularly; the iris had prolapsed, and the pupil was lost. Considerable irritation and inflammation followed the injury, but now the eye had recovered from the acute symptoms, and was, as is usually the case after these accidents, a little shrunken and flaccid. About the centre of the cicatrix was a minute piece of the copper, and a question was raised about its removal. The girl's mother was opposed to this, and I did not press interference, as it was not producing any irritation.

On the 30th of September, 1856, I saw a carpenter who had a bit of iron in his cornea, of two years' standing. It had never produced irritation. But these are examples of units among many thousands. I suppose in all these the process of encysting, of which I shall now speak, takes place.

Mr. Wardrop, in his "Pathology of the Human Eye," correctly observes—that it sometimes happens, after a body is imbedded in the cornea, a layer of new substance is produced over it, so that it does not excite inflammation, but remains through life in a kind of sac. He quotes a curious case in which the hard elytra of a beetle traversed in two years from the upper part of the eyeball to the centre of the cornea, immediately opposite the pupil, finally lodging there. In the case of a patient at the Central London Ophthalmic Hospital, a bit of wire was impacted at the lower part of the cornea; there was a dark-brown deposit, in the centre of which appeared a darker spot. The injury had been received sixteen years before, but as it did not occasion the least inconvenience I did not interfere.   But such phenomena, I repeat, are rare.

But the form of a body and the peculiarity of its impaction may, as Dr. Mackenzie observes, prevent its either escaping or becoming encysted; and a case of Mr. Wardrop's, reported in the " Lancet," is adduced as an example. A bit of gold wire had entered the cornea, and a small part protruded, while the larger portion was impacted within, where it had remained fourteen weeks before it was removed with a pair of forceps; but in the mean time the eye was nearly lost, and the pupil was adherent to the cornea when the patient applied to Mr. Wardrop. The portion of wire was fully three lines in length; one extremity had entered the anterior chamber, and the aqueous humour escaped at the extraction.

After a metallic fragment, especially of iron, has been removed, some rust, or mark, or stain, may remain. This is of no consequence, and should not be picked at, nor be attacked with chemical reagents; for it is soon cast off. Very little practice enables a surgeon to ascertain when the particle has been removed.

Carbonized and other substances act similarly; and without a knowledge of this, unnecessary injury may be inflicted. I have known vegetable matter produce stain.

In the " Medical Times and Gazette" of April 24th, 1852, Dr. H. Jeanneret very ingeniously proposes to dissolve particles of iron in the cornea by the chemical action of a solution of sulphate of copper, of the strength of from one to three grains to the ounce of water. This method should not give place to that of mechanical removal, but it may be of great value when a surgeon is not at hand, and relief cannot otherwise be obtained. An eyeglass filled with the solution, and held to the eye, is the proper mode of using this agent.

The employment of magnets has repeatedly been suggested as an easy and effectual means of extracting particles of iron and steel; and various shapes have been given to them—some pointed, some crescented, and so on; but they are mere playthings, and not of any practical value.   .

When abrasion of the cornea is a consequence of removing or extracting any substance, a drop of oil, as before spoken of, seems, by common consent, to be the most soothing application.

After-treatment is seldom required; the symptoms disappear as readily as they were manifested. When inflammation has been severe, and there is pain, with heat and intolerance of light, a fold of thin rag, large enough to cover the eyelids, dipped in cold water, applied, and renewed every few minutes, will soon give relief. The addition of some narcotic to the water may be useful. This, with rest to the eye, quiet of body, moderate abstinence, and perhaps slight purgation, amply suffice for every case.

In all instances, the eye should not be rubbed and irritated. The sensation of something remaining often exists long after the extraction.

I suspect that the majority of metallic particles that get imbedded in the cornea are forced in by the common habit of rubbing the eye when anything enters.

No advantage would accrue from my enumerating the various substances in the mineral, vegetable, and animal kingdom, that may enter the eye.

In connexion with the subject, the following case may be quoted. A delicate female, aged 31, had what she termed " inflammation in her eye," just five weeks before she applied to me. An examination showed a central opacity of the cornea large enough to cover the pupil, and below it a large superficial ulcer, uniformly of a dark-brown colour. The previous treatment having consisted entirely of blistering and purging, and no lotion having been employed, there was necessarily no metallic deposit or stain on the ulcer. I was at once struck with the peculiarity; and expecting that there might be prolapse of the iris, consequent on a penetrating ulcer of the cornea (called by the shocking name, " myocephalon"), I looked for such a cause. This, evidently, did not exist; and so great a resemblance did it bear to the presence of a foreign body, that I thought it requisite to attempt the removal, but only under the influence of chloroform, as great delicacy was required, as well as steadiness on the part of the patient, lest the cornea should be broken through. The attempt was fruitless, as not a particle could be detached. The colour was not due to any extraneous substance.

A tonic was prescribed, and an opiate lotion, as pain was a leading feature, and there was decided improvement in all the subjective symptoms ; but the ulceration and the colour remained the same. After a few visits, the patient ceased her attendance.

The conjunctiva may be penetrated, and a particle of matter remain between it and the sclerotica. Encysting is very likely to follow. I have seen several examples, I should say many, although I have never operated. The patients have either applied to me on account of something else, or I have met with them accidentally and spoken to them about the matter. Mr. Wardrop tells us that he has found a bit of whinstone inclosed in a sac of cellular membrane, lying close to the sclerotic coat, which had remained for ten years prior to the person's death, without occasioning the least uneasiness or even suspicion of its presence. Iron has remained encysted for years.

The sclerotica itself is often penetrated and retains bodies without much inconvenience. I have several times removed them when troublesome, by snipping through the conjunctiva, raising it from its attachment and then accomplishing the desired end. Generally it has been metal that has entered, and forceps have been required for the extraction. A young man received a portion of a percussion cap in the sclerotica, just outside the cornea, and after a week of inconvenience he returned to his work. The druggist to whom he applied detected nothing, and prescribed a wash. Nine months after, he came to me at the Ophthalmic Hospital, complaining of an occasional pricking in the eyelid. In the centre of a granulation at the site of the old injury, I saw an angle of the piece of copper, and extracted it. He had experienced no inconvenience till within a few days previous. The broken cap seemed to be working its way out.

I see a great many accidents from the percussion-cap—never

among sportsmen, but from improper use of the thing, from playing with it. I have seen five eyes destroyed in one year, and not in a single instance were the caps used in shooting; but two persons received their injury by exploding them between pieces of iron, and three from snapping them for nuts at a fair. The caps of the nut-sellers' toy are highly dangerous, being peculiarly constructed; the copper is not cleft, as in ordinary caps, but entire, to concentrate the force of the ignition. Thus they split with violence and fly about, not merely to the injury of those who use them, but to others.

LARVÆ OF INSECTS UNDER THE EYELIDS.

The larvæ of insects are sometimes deposited beneath the eyelids. In the fifteenth volume of the "Annales d'Oculistique," p. 133, it is told by M. Armand Bouilhet, that a young woman, while cutting rye, felt something impinge on the eye, and immediately began to suffer pain. M. Bouilhet thought he had to deal with some foreign body. After opening the lids he perceived a whitish point, put it on a pin to show it to the patient, and to his astonishment saw that it moved : he examined it attentively, and discovered it to be a little worm. Remembering that some flies deposit their larvæ in different parts of animals, he thought this little insect might not be the only one. He poured three drops of olive oil upon the globe of the eye, and drew out, successively, ten worms.

A child, of ten to eleven years of age, who since the preceding evening had experienced great uneasiness in the eye, was brought to M. Bouilhet. The symptoms had come on immediately after a fly had flown into the eye, though it scarcely remained a moment. The patient was sure that an insect had come in contact with the eye. M. Bouilhet examined it attentively, and discovered little worms in the recess of the upper lid. The same means were employed as in the first instance, and six worms were drawn out. As the case was spoken of as something extraordinary, a physician went to see the child, and detected other worms; he immediately sent the child back to M. Bouilhet, who took away two more.

A unique case is related by Cloquet in his "Pathologie Chirurgicale." A man, fifty years of age, who was drunk, fell asleep in the fields; flies (*musca carnaria*) deposited their ova at the orifice of the nostrils and ears, between the eyelids, and on the prepuce. The larvæ made their way into the body in these several situations; the eyes were completely destroyed, for on removing the larvæ, the lenses escaped through the perforations they had effected in the cornea. Under the cranial integuments they formed large deposits, from which they could be pressed in thousands through ulcerated openings. The miserable mortal survived for about a month in a state of imbecility; the bones of the skull were partly necrosed, and the corresponding parts of the dura mater and arachnoid membrane were in a state of inflammation.

FOREIGN BODIES WITHIN THE EYEBALL.

Accidents of this nature are rare. Surgeons of the largest experience have had but few examples in their practice.

In order that I may not unnecessarily increase these pages, and for other obvious reasons, I shall avoid quoting cases as mere curiosities, and adduce those only that serve especially and directly for illustration. At the outset, I reiterate the principle I propounded in the foregoing part of this chapter respecting substances on the surface of the eye. It is our duty, as a rule, to try to remove whatever is driven into the eye. Whenever this is practicable, an endeavour should be made to extract everything, except when it has passed out of sight, and cannot be readily felt with a probe, or ascertained to be superficial, or at least likely to be removed, in which cases the eye must, for a time, be left to take its chance; as likewise when it is so small that it is scarcely probable that it can be seized; or when it is of a exture that is likely to be absorbed; or is a soft substance which, a few h insoluble, could not be removed, as gunpowder, or its

way G

I as

d, and

back to

FOREIGN BODIES IN THE ANTERIOR CHAMBER OF THE EYE.

We have now sufficient evidence, through Mr. Lawrence and others, and I have personal knowledge of an instance, that a portion of steel, such as the point of a cataract-knife, or of a cataract-needle, provided that it be but a mere fragment, will become oxidized and absorbed in the anterior chamber, leaving the eye uninjured. So long then as an oxidizable bit of metal sufficiently small does not produce symptoms, wait and see the issue. But this does not hold good with copper or brass. These resist the saline action of the aqueous fluid, and should be taken away, and the sooner the better.

There are several examples published, to show the tolerance the eye may exhibit with bodies in this place, for days, weeks, and even years,—in one peculiar instance for sixteen years; but as a rule the end is disastrous. Except the very unlikely process of encysting should ensue, of which due notice will be taken, the eye will perish. It is suppuration that usually destroys, but generally sub-acute inflammatory action; and sometimes the function of sight is lost, with scarcely recognisable objective symptoms.

The length of time that may have elapsed since a foreign body entered the eye should be no reason against endeavouring to extract it, if its presence be injurious. In the "Dublin Medical Press" for December, 1846, Dr. Jacob tells of a bit of stone, the fourth of an inch long, and a sixth in diameter, and very sharp, that had remained loose in the anterior chamber for nearly four years, before much irritation was set up. He operated, with the hope of saving the eye from complete destruction.

Here is another example. In Ammon's "Zeitschrift," vol. iii., p. 103, we are told that a splinter of a small glass ball, which had been filled with spirits of wine, and as a joke put into the fire, flew into the left eye of a female, and became fixed in the middle of the cornea. Next day a surgeon was called, who, in attempting to extract the splinter, unfortunately drove it into the anterior chamber. For a whole year the woman suffered the severest pain. The cornea continued transparent for about six months, and her husband asserted that during that time the glass splinter was visible, free, floating, and moveable in the anterior chamber, but that, subsequently, the eye became more and more opaque, and acquired a pannus-like condition. The patient went to Vienna, where she applied to many surgeons, none of whom, however, believed in the existence of any foreign substance, as it was no longer visible. By degress the cornea became clear, and vision returned; but the severe pain, extending from the eye towards the head, remained unmigitated. At the end of five years of suffering, she again repaired to Vienna, and saw Dr. Carl Jäger, who made an incision in the cornea with a common cataract-knife, and with various forceps, probes, and other instruments, endeavoured, but in vain, to extract the body, which in consequence of bleeding from the iris was now hidden. The eye was soon in the same condition as before the operation, although less painful. In a few months, however, her sufferings returned, and again she applied to Dr. Carl Jäger, who now succeeded in detecting the piece of glass, which was of a triangular shape, measuring in its greatest diameter about five lines, covered with a light-brown coloured exudation, and extracted it with a pair of forceps. No injurious consequences followed, and vision was scarcely impaired.

Experience, and much inquiry, have convinced me that after symptoms of irritation have set in, it is a fallacy fraught with danger to wait till they subside for an opportunity to operate. The subsidence, for the most part, never arrives till the eye is destroyed, and the most threatening symptoms will rapidly subside when the irritant has been removed. Except, then, when in accordance with sound practice, we attempt first to subdue any very acute inflammatory action, there should be no delay.

But it is no easy matter to execute the operation with the least possible injury, and effectively. Attempt upon attempt is often made in vain, and a well-tutored hand only can be expected to be successful. It is an undertaking, above all others, that needs self-possession, knowledge of operations on the eyeball, and cleverness in manipulation. Chloroform is indispensable. The details must be regulated by the individual peculiarities of the case. The retraction of the eyelids, the steadying of the eyeball, and the opening of the cornea, must all be attended to as in extracting a cataract. In addition, the eyeball may be kept motionless by forceps or hooks. The cornea should be freely incised. The position, and the mode of attachment of the foreign body, are to be the data in selecting the spot for the incision. The nearer to the margin of the cornea the opening is made, the less will be the danger of protrusion of the iris ; and whether forceps, hook, or curette be used, its extremity should be blunted, to avoid injuring the textures it may come in contact with, especially the capsule of the lens ; for, if that be torn or scratched, opacity will ensue. The spoon of the curette will be found very serviceable. It cannot always be determined beforehand what shall be required. I have commenced an operation with a determination to adopt a particular course, and circumstances have arisen that required a different method. Emergencies will arise, and should be expected and provided for.

The process of encysting is always rare, and the fortunate occurrence bears but an astonishingly small proportion to the usual result. Tyrrell speaks of a small particle of granite, and, in two instances, of minute portions of copper caps, thus fortunately encased. Except for very cogent reasons, I should be disposed to leave an encysted body alone. I should not interfere so long as vision was not interrupted, or likely to be damaged by this conservative effort. But a substance so tied down, is not altogether, and for ever, out of reach of harm. Effusion of lymph, or a capsule around it, does not absolutely secure immunity from future disturbance. The cyst may be spontaneously opened, or be broken by violence, or become injurious in itself. We learn, in Mr. Middlemore's "Treatise on the Diseases of the Eye," that a man came to him with a bit of metal at the bottom of the anterior chamber. There was acute inflammation of the eyeball; this was reduced. Encysting took place in a few weeks. Two years afterwards the eye was struck, the cyst burst, and the particle set loose in the chamber. Suppuration of the eyeball threatened, but was checked by the timely extraction of the body.

A foreign body may be impacted in the iris, and be apparent, and yet it might be prudent not to interfere. Except it project, and can readily be seized, the difficulty of extraction is very great, and the operation is likely to be injurious; therefore, in general, and in the absence of symptoms, and especially when it is very minute, I should be inclined to wait, as by so doing there is afforded an opportunity for encysting, which is so likely to happen in this position. I suspect that oftentimes, when an operation is imperative, the better plan would be to excise the bit of the iris, rather than what has so often proved a most tedious and fruitless process—that of picking out the fragment, particularly when more or less covered by exudation.

When the position of the penetrating body gives tolerable assurance of its comparatively easy removal, there should be no time lost. In the " Ophthalmic Hospital Reports," is this short notice of an ineffectual attempt even under apparently favourable circumstances. A body which had pierced the iris and the cornea at their lower part, could be seen lodged in the iris, and pro-jecting into the anterior chamber. A small corneal incision was made, and the canula-forceps introduced; but in the attempt at extraction, it disappeared behind the iris, and was left.

I copy the following successful cases from the first volume of the same journal. In the first, a small piece of steel was in the upper part of the iris. It had entered eighteen months pre-viously, induced inflammation, which had lasted for a month, but did not impair vision. A fortnight before this patient came to the hospital, he had had dimness, pain, and other inflammatory symptoms. When he applied, the cornea was transparent, and the pupil active, excepting near to a small black point in the substance of the iris, midway between the pupillary and corneal edges. Mr. Dixon made an opening at the margin of the cornea nearest the black point, and seizing it with the iris-forceps, extracted a black triangular hard body, surrounded by organized lymph. After three weeks, the inflammatory symp-toms had disappeared, and the patient had recovered good vision. In the second case, the foreign body had entered the eye the day before, probably through the sclerotica: the pupil was contracted, and a small whitish nodule of lymph was visible near the inner pupillary edge. The irritation and conjunctival redness were considerable. In this case, a small opening was made at the outer edge of the cornea; and while extracting the nodule with a pair of canula-forceps, a very small black body fell into the anterior chamber, and was removed with the scoop. Four days later the eye had returned to its normal state.

Even on the iris, an encysted body may become loosened and produce all possible ill effects. In the "Dublin Quarterly Journal," 1848, page 210, is recorded an instance of a very minute scale of copper cap in the iris becoming encysted, and remaining so for eight years, during which time it produced repeated attacks of inflammation of the eyeball, and, ultimately, it exfoliated through the cornea.

The cyst itself may prove injurious. Mr. Tyrrell alludes to a case of Mr. Scott's, in which that gentleman deemed it imperative to operate, because of the growth of an enclosing cyst. A bit of iron entered the iris of a blacksmith's apprentice, and after several weeks of active disease, good vision was recovered, notwithstanding a disfigured pupil. Some months after, a small cyst formed in connexion with the injured part, and grew—with a white and tendinous-like structure—to the size of a pea, when it was thought fit to operate. The result is supposed to have been unfavourable.

When the posterior chamber of the eye has been entered, the same rule must, if possible, be followed; and the propriety of it is well exemplified by two successful cases. The first is recorded by Mr. Critchett, in the "Lancet" for April 1, 1854.

An engineer was struck with considerable violence on the left eye by a piece of metal from a lathe. He suffered very much from pain in the eyeball and dimness of vision, and on the following day applied to Mr. Critchett, who found an irregular corneal wound, which was so far closed as to retain the aqueous humour. At the pupillary margin above, there was a dark looking mark, which appeared like a foreign body. The lens was becoming milky. Judging, both from the history and the appearances, that a foreign body had entered the eye, Mr. Critchett proceeded to attempt its removal. He first introduced a small probe through the wound in the cornea, towards the dark spot on the pupillary margin, and ascertained that this appearance depended upon a slit in the pupil, caused by penetration. As traumatic cataract was forming, Mr. Critchett proceeded to remove it, and to seek for what had entered. The opening in the cornea was slightly enlarged, and the scoop of a curette introduced, with which the greater part of the lens was gradually spooned away. When the lens was thus nearly removed, a dark, oblong piece of metal suddenly came into view, lying behind and across the pupil, and resting upon the hyaloid membrane, which was evidently not wounded. A pair of delicate forceps were now introduced, for the purpose of seizing and drawing it out; but although there was no difficulty in laying hold with the blades, they slipped off whenever the least traction was made, owing to the smooth polished surface of the metal, and to its prismatic form. It was subsequently lifted out with the scoop of a curette, but, in doing so, the hyaloid membrane was wounded, and a small amount of vitreous humour escaped. The eyelids were closed, and the man was put to bed. Some slight swelling ensued, together with pain, but these symptoms gradually passed away. The state of the eye, ten weeks after, was as follows:—a faint mark of the wound in the cornea; pupil small and filled with a thin layer of lymph, and above there was slight adhesion of the iris to the cornea; a good anterior chamber; some perception of objects; the eye-ball firm and free from pain, and inflammation ever since the first week after the accident.

The second I take from the "Ophthalmic Hospital Reports" for January, 1859. A healthy young mill-stone maker applied at the Royal London Ophthalmic Hospital, February 15th, 1858, his left eye having been struck with a splinter while he was at work, on the preceding evening. The conjunctiva was red and slightly chemosed; the iris was bright and active. At the outer border of the pupil was a small but conspicuous greyish object, which projected very slightly into its area, and extended outwards, behind the iris, for about one-sixteenth of an inch. A faint linear scar about the centre of the cornea was only detected by close examination. The sight was but slightly affected. He was quite free from pain, except when out of doors.

On the supposition that the object was a splinter of stone, Mr. Bowman determined to remove it. An attempt was made to seize it with the canula-forceps, introduced through a small incision at the inner edge of the cornea; a small thread of lymph came away in the grasp of the instrument, and exposed to view a minute scale of metal, which it had enveloped. The scale was easily removed with the scoop of a curette. It was a portion of the chisel with which the man was working.

He presented himself again on the 23rd; the eye was not inflamed, the pupil was active and circular, the lens was clear, and his sight uninjured.

I have not seen anything impacted in the crystalline lens, and I find but few such accidents recorded. I suspect that opacity is the inevitable consequence. I have just read of an apparent exception, in a recent French surgical book; but as some of the statements make me doubt the correctness of the report, I shall not quote it. The correct practice, according to my idea, is to remove the foreign body—an act that involves the loss of the lens. After the forty-fifth or fiftieth year, I should extract the two together, if I possibly could. When the lens is quite opaque, it leaves its capsule more readily than when transparent or semi-opaque. In youth and in childhood, it is almost a necessary consequence that the lens be much broken up, and portions more or less displaced, to effect the object; and, therefore, the practice should be at the time to extract as much of the lenticular matter as possible. I beg to refer my reader to the operation for soft cataract for an exposition of my views on this point.

While a young farmer was at work with some iron tools, a chip of iron struck his right eye, which became a little inflamed, but got well in a week. On May the 7th, the sight got misty, and rapidly became worse. Mr. Bowman detected a minute cicatrix near the outer edge of the cornea, and observed a small black spot on the outer part of the iris. The nature of this spot was doubtful; it might be a minute ecchymosis, or a small dot of uvea, or a hole in the iris. The ophthalmoscope proved the last supposition to be the correct one. The pupil was dilated with atropine, and the lens was seen to be semi-opaque in all its superficial parts; and near its posterior surface, below the nucleus, a small fragment of iron was very plainly visible. It could also now be discerned with the naked eye, by reflected light. Mr. Bowman recommended its immediate removal; it is said the patient was placed under the influence of chloroform, and a needle was passed through the cornea backwards into the lens, the point being directed obliquely behind the bit of iron, which was then brought forward to the front of the lens, whence its removal was easily accomplished with a curette, introduced through a small incision in the border of the cornea, as in Gibson's operation. The soft lenticular matter was removed through the same opening, and a clear, black, circular pupil obtained. No inflammation followed the operation, and the patient went home in a few days with good sight.

It may be well to quote from Dr. Jacob's paper in the "Dublin Quarterly Journal" for December 9th, 1846, to show what has been observed when a piece of metal is allowed to remain in the lens. A bit of a gun-cap was projected into the lens of a boy. It did not lose its brilliancy, nor did it cause any sensible effect for two or three years beyond producing cataract, which was absorbed, and the copper lay entangled in the opaque crystalline capsule. A year after the boy came to Dr. Jacob, the copper had disappeared, the pupil was dilated, the chambers filled with blood, and the organ in fact spoiled. The cap was nowhere visible, and had probably fallen to the bottom of the eye. The doctor thought it advisable to do nothing.

Even the vitreous humour can be explored and a piece of metal extracted with safety, and to the saving of the eye.

A young cooper came under the care of Mr. Dixon, December 2nd, 1858, half-an-hour after receiving an injury of the left eye from a chip of metal. A small vertical wound, a little above the margin of the left upper eyelid, marked the spot where the iron had entered the skin. A corresponding wound of the palpebral conjunctiva was observed. In the sclerotic, nearly on a level with the upper border of the cornea, and about a line from its inner edge, was a small gaping wound, a line long, surrounded by sub-conjunctival ecchymosis, through which a vesicle of vitreous humour protruded. The pupil was active, and the patient could read large type, but saw all objects as through a slight mist.

Ophthalmoscopic examination discovered a clot of blood at the upper and inner part of the pupil, behind the lens, hanging down from the wound, and slightly waving to and fro. As the rest of the humour was clear, and the cornea and the lens transparent, a good view of the retina was obtained. Just below the optic nerve, a small round body was noticed, looking almost like a minute air-bubble, and it appeared as if it were a portion of clear lymph effused round a foreign body, which was assumed to have entered the eye ; but as there was no vascularity surrounding it, this hypothesis was doubtful. A light pad of cotton wool and a bandage were applied over the closed eye ; rest and temperance enjoined, and a sedative ordered each night.

December the 6th.—The little wound in the sclerotic was closing ; there was no pain, and not much redness of the conjunctiva. Sight was less dim than on the patient's first visit, and good-sized type was pretty easily read. At the end of ten days, the henbane was left off, and four grains of iodide of potash ordered twice a day, in decoction of bark. Sight continued to improve, and by the 30th all redness of the conjunctiva had disappeared ; the little wound in the sclerotic presented a hardly traceable grey line ; there was no intolerance of light.

Again examining with the ophthalmoscope, the little globular body could not be detected. At a sudden turn of the eyeball there started from behind the inner portion of the iris an oblong, black body, which was instantly recognised as a chip of metal. It was entangled in a few thread-like remains of clot, which kept it suspended in the vitreous humour, and allowed it to move freely backwards and forwards. After due deliberation, Mr. Dixon determined to penetrate the vitreous humour from below, and endeavour to extract the body. This he preferred to following the route it had taken in entering, lest he should break through the suspending threads, when it would fall down out of reach. As it sank backwards and disappeared whenever the recumbent position was assumed, chloroform was not used. He operated in this manner:—Standing behind the patient, who was seated in a chair close by the window, the eyelids being separated with a spring retractor, he fixed the globe of the eye by nipping up a fold of conjunctiva just above the cornea. A Jäger's lance-knife was then thrust in a little distance from the margin of the cornea, and the point directed backwards, to avoid wounding the lens. The knife was now withdrawn, and Assalini's iris-forceps introduced, with which, after one or two unsuccessful attempts, the body was grasped and extracted. It proved to be a part of the edge of a chisel, about 1-10th of an inch long, and weighed a quarter of a grain. The eyelids were immediately closed with plaster, and cold rags applied.

January 6th.—The pupil was circular and clear. The patient could read the large type on his bed-ticket. The edges of the wound had drawn together. There was a small quantity of blood extravasated beneath the conjunctiva, and but very little increased vascularity of this membrane. A week later, and the pupil was round and contractile; there was no intolerance of light, and the patient could read a pica type. A few threads of clot, quite unattached, were floating in the vitreous humour. The lens was perfectly clear, and the only appearance which could be called morbid was a slight reddening of the retina and the optic nerve, the effect probably of a slight traumatic inflammation from the operation.

March 3rd.—The lens was perfectly transparent; the retina appeared quite healthy, and the only abnormal appearance was a single opaque filament floating in the vitreous humour. The patient's sight was steadily improving.

In some concluding remarks the operator says, that the instruments he employed were not the best he could imagine for the purpose, but that they were the best at hand, and the delay of a day might have caused the body to fall on the retina. Also, that in such cases there is a certain lucky chance, without which the most skilful manipulations may fail of success. (" Ophthalmic Hospital Reports," vol. i.)

Such a fortunate result can fall to the lot of but few operators, nor is a parallel case likely to occur. Still, in allied accidents, the circumstances should be studied with a view to similar treatment.

The violence that usually accompanies the entrance of anything into the vitreous humour, so damages the choroid and the retina, and is productive of so much bleeding, that the eye scarcely escapes immediate destruction. It is here, more than in any other part, that extraneous substances pass out of sight, and, getting beyond our reach, must be left alone. We must then wait for symptoms, and not act in anticipation, as nothing can be done but freely incising the eyeball, and evacuating the vitreous humour, or resorting to " extirpation;" but so desperate a proceeding should be left to the last extremity.

All the principles that I have endeavoured to establish in the foregoing subdivisions of this chapter, apply to gun-shot wounds of the eye. There are, however, just a few special points that I wish to notice.

The ophthalmoscope dispels all the mystery that surrounded the connexion between apparently slight blows from grains of shot, and impairment or loss of sight. All this I have fully explained, and need say no more except that such blows are far more violent than credit is given for.

When a shot has been driven into the eye, and is hidden, whether it have entered through the cornea or otherwise, it is impossible to tell, in the first instance, if it be still in the eyeball, or has lodged somewhere in the orbit. In all such cases, I say, do not interfere, except to relieve some symptom. The formation of cataract, the closure of the pupil, with discolouration of the iris, and a serous state of the aqueous humour, with or without atrophy of the globe of the eye, are no evidences that a grain of shot is within or about the ocular tissues. Nay, even severe ocular pain does not confirm it; for there are some authenticated cases in which the eyeball has been extirpated for this, and no shot has been discovered. But, notwithstanding the uncertainty that must prevail, and with knowledge of the fact that a shot lodged anywhere about the orbit is capable of producing such suffering, we should by no means be deterred from removing the eye, if there be even suspicion of shot being there located, and producing irritation. More than this, when no shot has been found, extirpation has removed the pain.

A remarkable case of the impaction of a grain of duck-shot in the optic nerve, where it lodged for six years and six months, is recorded in detail in the "London Medical Gazette," for 1834, vol. xiii. The shot entered the eye at the inner side of its surface, near the cornea. Occasional and intense pain, for four years and a-half, and the serious disturbance of the functions of the other eye, induced the patient, contrary to medical advice, to have the body sought for. The lens, which is said to have been partly bony, partly calcareous, was removed with the hope of affording relief, but without benefit; pain continued, and as that most distressing complication, sympathetic ophthalmitis— which is ever to be dreaded in such cases—having evidently set in, an attempt to find the shot was made, but unsuccessfully. The sufferer now determined to have the eye extirpated, and the shot was found impacted, as the report says, in that part of the optic nerve which expands and forms the retina. The right eye was daily regaining health when the last communication was sent to Dr. Butter, the operator.

A farmer with one eye only available, was unfortunate enough to be shot by a boy, a few yards in front of him. The greater part of the charge went through his hat, but several shots lodged in his scalp, his forehead, and in the eyebrow, and he was blinded. The anterior chamber seemed occupied by blood. The eyeball was very hard and tender to touch. There was no evidence of shot having entered it, yet its state could not otherwise be accounted for. Vision was quite destroyed. I was consulted, by the recommendation of Mr. Marriott, of Kibworth, for the intense pain in the brow, frequently associated with pain in the orbit, and in the eye. Other surgeons had been consulted, and the conclusions arrived at were different to my own, which was to leave the eye alone, and to remove the shot. I extracted all that I could get at—that is, all that I could feel. Some were embedded in the bone. My patient being a very large and a remarkably fat man, they were the more concealed. Every wound healed by the first intention. Considerable relief followed; but pain, at longer intervals, still tormented him, and some months later, when the position of a few more shots could be traced, I removed them with advantage. Once again he came to me, as two that yet annoyed him could be felt, and they were the last, for four or five years have passed away without pain in the scalp, or in the eye.

It is a great satisfaction to me that I avoided extirpating the eye, which would have been useless, and must have further spoiled a fine and benevolent countenance; for notwithstanding the front of the eye is not quite natural, the pupil being closed and the iris discoloured, there is no marked disfigurement.

I strongly advise the immediate removal of shot that may have entered the appendages of the eye; and whenever any grains become perceptible, as they often will, after months and years, they should be extracted. I took out a grain from the orbit of an old gentleman, who had been shot several years ago. Slight pain attracted his attention to the long-forgotten circumstance, and he traced the shot just posterior to the head of the lacrymal duct, whence I removed it with perfect success. We have abundant evidence that irritation may be set up after portions of lead have remained quietly in various parts of the body for long periods.

CALCAREOUS, OSSEOUS, AND TRUE BONY DEPOSITS, IN THE OCULAR TISSUES, AND BETWEEN THEM.

Ossification occurring in the centre of a dense leucoma.—A girl, æt. fourteen, was brought to Mr. Bowman, with acute inflammation of a disorganized and rather shrunken eye, in which there was no perception of light. There was much pain and irritation with every movement of the eyelids. A bony spiculum was partly embedded in the opaque cornea, and partly projecting. It was readily removed with a pair of forceps, and complete relief followed.

We learn, from the rich stores of Mr. Wardrop's "Morbid Anatomy of the Eye," that he found it necessary to remove a bit of bone, which he considered to have been a partial ossification of the posterior lamina of the cornea, from the anterior chamber. He has several times also observed thin laminæ of bone discharged from the anterior chamber through ulcers in the cornea. He records, also, having seen deposit—a long shell, as he terms it—on the iris. He supposed that this was ossification of the capsule of the aqueous humour, it being then thought that there was a capsule, or sac, that lined the chambers of the eye ; an opinion that was generally entertained up to a very recent period, and still taught by some.

In the " Dublin Quarterly Journal of Medical Science," vol. xxix., for February, 1853, the reviewer of the last edition of this work speaks of particles of calcareous deposit that had been on the capsule of the lens, becoming detached, falling into the anterior chamber, resting in the angle between the iris and the cornea, and causing intolerable and incessant pain. These, together with other like particles in the posterior chamber, were removed ; the patient being chloroformed.

True bone in the human eye.—I take the particulars of this case from the sixth volume of the " Transactions of the Pathological Society of London." The specimen, exhibited by Mr. R. Taylor, was removed by Dr. Kirk, from the dead body of a man, æt. 53, of strumous and syphilitic habit. The eyesight had been lost thirty years previously, in consequence of an injury, and the eye was atrophied and irregular in form. The cornea was opaque, and marked with cicatrices. The texture of the sclerotica was unaltered. The choroid adhered to a thin shell of osseous matter, occupying the position of the hyaloid membrane. Up the interior of this shell, ran a tube continous posteriorly with the central artery of the retina, and opening in front against the capsule of the lens. Between this central pillar and the outer wall were numerous spicula of bone. The tube, and the spaces between the spicula, were filled with masses of cholesterine. The spicula contained numerous well-formed lacunæ, with their branching canaliculi.

The capsule of the lens was thickened, both anteriorly and posteriorly, but was free from calcareous deposit. The greater part of the lens was intensely hard; but at several points round its margin there remained portions of soft tissue.

The external tissue was composed of fibres arranged parallel to each other. Between the fibres were numerous rounded mineral bodies, of a distinctly crystalline nature; and interspersed among them were a number of well-formed rhombic crystals. Chemically, these mineral masses consisted of phosphate and carbonate of lime. The dense central portion of the lens presented lacunæ, with numerous canaliculi, in some instances arranged concentrically around circular spaces, believed by Dr. Kirk to be Haversian canals.

A second specimen shown at the same time was procured from the eye of a man, æt. 50, who died in Edinburgh Infirmary from disease of the liver and kidneys. The eye had been lost in youth in consequence of an injury, and was completely atrophied; the other eye had been subsequently destroyed by repeated attacks of sympathetic inflammation.

Owing to the interference of the friends, only a small portion of the atrophied eye could be secured. This consisted of sclerotica and choroid; from the latter a small scale of osseous deposit was taken, which exhibited true bony organization, and contained numerous well-developed lacunæ and canaliculi.

An example of an extensive ossification in the posterior part of the eye, was exhibited at the same Society by Mr. Obré, and is recorded in the ninth volume of the "Transactions."

For many years it has been known that such ossifications arise from inflammation of the choroid coat, being merely conversion of lymph that is thrown out on the inner side.

In Virchow's "Archiv." for 1853, p. 580, Dr. Von Wittich has published the dissection of the disorganized and shrunken eye of a man aged 60, in which the posterior part of the vitreous body appeared converted into true bone. The choroid was thrown into shrivelled folds, the capsule of the lens opaque, and the lens itself the subject of earthy deposition. Traces of the retina were found lying behind and surrounding the bony mass which occupied the posterior part of the vitreous humour. This substance was true bone, as evidenced by its numerous corpuscles.

The following specimens are to be seen in the pathological collection of the Museum of the Royal College of Surgeons —:

From a man who was blinded by lightning forty years before death.—The choroid membrane contains several small thin plates of bone at its posterior part ; the lens is absorbed, and its capsule ossified.

The eye of a blind man, in which large plates of earthy matter or bone are formed in parts of the retina and on its inner surface. There is a second specimen similar to this.

Parts of an eye dried ; the lens, converted into a mass of white compact earthy substance, nearly retains its natural size and form ; some irregular portions of earthy substance extend also from it into the vitreous humour.

In the Museum of St. Bartholomew's Hospital, there are sections of the eye of an adult, showing that the retina has disappeared, and its place become occupied by a thick layer of dense osseous substance.

The sclerotica has been found partially ossified. Mr. Middlemore alludes to the *post-mortem* examination of an idiot boy, at St. Bartholomew's, where ossification of the greater part of the globe of each eye existed.

CHAPTER VI.

A VERY grave result of wounds and injuries to the eye is sympathetic implication, which has of late received much attention.

The subject was first practically recognised by Mr. Barton of Manchester, whose practice was brought before the profession by Mr. Crompton, in the "London Medical Gazette," vol. xxi., page 175. The sympathy was produced by injury from extraneous bodies in the eye. In seven cases, a portion of copper had settled in the anterior chamber. Inflammation and disorganization of the eyeball was soon followed by failure of the functions of the other eye, together with structural changes. Mr. Barton excised the cornea, and applied a poultice, in the hope that the copper-cap would escape: this did happen, and produced great relief; but it had a greater and more valuable effect,—it saved the destruction of the other eye in every instance, although some of them seemed past all hope.

The evidence of this sympathetic action should be well understood, or disease may be attributed to sympathy, which is nothing but the same local manifestation of constitutional taint that appeared in the other eye, and secondary only in order of time. I have known many mistakes to be made in this way, to the great disadvantage of the patients. In traumatic cases the diagnosis is mostly simple. The injured eye manifests symptoms of irritation or disturbance, and there is some sign of acute or of chronic inflammation. This development of morbid

action may be slight or very apparent, but is always to be discovered; soreness under touch is always present.

The implication certainly usually shows itself early, within a
few weeks; but it may appear at any time, so long as the
irritation produced by traumatic disease lingers. Mr. Wall
of Paddington called me to a patient whose eye was fast
failing, without any very apparent cause, the symptoms being
impaired vision and spectra. The other eye had been wounded,
two years previously, with a packing-needle, the cornea torn
across, and sight destroyed. Paroxysms of pain, and tenderness
under touch, convinced me that it was producing sympathetic
disease. I was correct, and my treatment saved its fellow; it
completely restored its functions.

There may be varieties in the subjective and objective symptoms of the sympathetic attack. There may be no pain, or it
may exist with great severity. Intolerance to light is the first
common result. Some form or other of impaired sight is the
next bad omen. Loss of focal adjustment, incapability of
sustaining vision on minute objects, loss of definition, generally
called feeble sight, abundance of muscæ, spectra, flashes, stars,
corruscations, inflammatory action, loss of pupillary movements,
change of iris-colour, softening of the eyeball and shrinking,
are the later manifestations. It would seem, then, that the
morbid action travels from the retina forwards; and ultimately
the whole of the ocular tissues become involved, atrophy being
the termination.

A small lacerated wound of the eye, especially of the anterior
part, and which, to all appearance, has involved only the
cornea, the iris, and the crystalline lens, may, equally with very
great lesion, induce sympathetic disturbance. It is difficult to
understand how the smallest quantity of pus, a drop or two just
behind the cornea, or a slight change of texture of some of the
tissues of the eye, can exert so baneful an effect.

Blows without wounds or breach of surface, burns, and chemical injuries, are capable of producing the kind of action
that may excite sympathetic ophthalmitis; and this shows
that no importance is to be attributed either to the peculiarity

of any kind of wound, or to the tissue which is implicated; and all we can say is, that a variety of existing causes produce morbid changes, to which the sympathetic disease is due. I illustrate this by a case published in a paper in the "Medical Times" for October 28th, 1854, by my colleague Mr. R. Taylor, who contributed another communication on the same subject, on the 4th of November. A contribution of my own will be found under the date of February 18th, of the same year.

A man received a blow on the right eye from a piece of iron, but there was no wound of any kind. The sight was not injured at the moment, but began to fail soon, and was extinct in a year. About six years after the accident, the eye became inflamed and excessively painful. The pain continued for ten months, totally incapacitating him from work; and so severe, that for a great part of the time he scarcely had an hour of uninterrupted sleep. The other eye was excessively intolerant of light. He could not read large print, nor could he look at any object for more than a second or two. He was operated on, with complete relief from pain; and the left eye was perfectly restored in about two months. Mr. Taylor saw him five years after the operation, and the sight continued perfect. The remains of the right formed an excellent stump for an artificial eye, but he did not care to have one.

Inflammatory affections producing disorganization of the eye may develope sympathetic disease. I have seen more examples of this induced from staphyloma of the sclerotica and the cornea —that is, general enlargement, the result of purulent ophthalmia in infancy—than from any other cause. I subjoin a case.

A patient at the Ophthalmic Hospital, aged 20, had purulent ophthalmia in infancy, and lost one eye. Staphyloma formed, and the growth had been gradually increasing from childhood. About puberty, it was painful, and for the first time the sight of the other eye became a little dim. Soon after this, a blow on the staphyloma produced a sharp attack of inflammation, attended with much pain. The dimness of the other eye increased, and redness appeared. From this period there had been a gradual deterioration of vision, with occasional paroxysms of pain and

inflammation. When I saw him, there was a very large staphyloma of the sclerotica, and no trace of the cornea, but in
place of it a small cicatrix, around which the staphyloma
was very vascular, the vessels being disposed in remarkably
regular radii. The eyelids could not close over the tumour.
There was a purulent discharge. The condition of the failing
eye was this : the cornea was rather reduced ; the sclerotica
was discoloured, and full of varicose vessels ; the iris dull and
shrunken ; and the pupil adherent in several places. There
was intolerance of light, and vision was very imperfect, although
he could read.

There are not recorded many careful examinations of diseased
eyes that have set up sympathetic ophthalmitis. I therefore
introduce the following, which came under my notice in the
hospital practice of my colleague Mr. R. Taylor. The details
are in the " Transactions of the Pathological Society of London,"
vol. vi., page 302.

The patient was a woman, seventy years of age, whose eye was
extirpated, in consequence of destruction by intense inflammation. The anterior chamber was completely filled with a solid
cake of lymph. The lens was hazy, and its fibres presented the
usual appearance seen in cataract at a not very advanced stage. ·
Immediately under the capsule, both anteriorly and posteriorly,
and imbedded in the superficial lens-substance, was a layer of
peculiar bodies, varying much in configuration. The predominant form was spheroidal, but many were of the most eccentric
shapes. Under the polariser, several of the larger presented a
distinct cross ; in the smaller, the cross was faintly marked, or
absent. Tested with tincture of iodine, they assumed a deep
blue colour, gradually increasing in intensity till they became
opaque. In making the examination, every precaution was
taken to prevent fallacy.

Cretaceous degeneration of the crystalline lens, and of its
capsule, is no uncommon source of the sympathy ; and in the
numbers of the " Medical Times," above quoted, are many
examples from my practice. Osseous degeneration of these
parts always produces the same effects. With such complete

disorganization of one portion of the eye, the rest of the interior is always spoiled, and vision lost. The altered lens and its covering are generally adherent to the iris. I have traced disturbance to have commenced from its becoming loose. Similar changes of other tissues of the eye may, I suspect, set up irritation.

No general treatment, no local application, no dietary system, is of avail in checking unequivocal sympathetic ophthalmitis. Nothing of the kind can be depended on; and, while I thus speak from my own observation, I endorse the statement of all trustworthy observers. The affection can be stopped, or subdued, only by surgical treatment. A portion of the eyeball must be removed, whereby the products which have set up the irritation, or the cretaceous or ossified tissue, which has acted as a foreign body, may be got rid of; or "extirpation" resorted to. When done early, this practice works wonders. If adopted before the sympathetic action has induced palpable structural changes, it will be all effectual. At later stages, it may arrest progress, and stay the destruction. Even when the pupil has become adherent to the capsule of the lens, and the iris dull, I have seen a check. I have taken notes of so many of these cases, that I have ceased to record them.

I proved many years ago (and I think that I revived Mr. Barton's practice, which, so far as I can learn, had never been generally carried out in London by any one), that removing a portion of the eyeball will generally suffice, as it is frequently in the anterior part of the eye that the centre of the morbid action is seated. The intensity of it is more common near the point of injury, and this is mostly in the front of the organ. I have very frequently found the vitreous humour healthy; this portion of the eye, therefore, not being spoiled. With the reduction of the eyeball only, the deformity is very much less, and the case is better fitted for an artificial eye; and, in the early years of life, the destined growth of the orbit is less interfered with.

When the entire eyeball is disorganized, posteriorly as well as anteriorly, especially when there is general enlargement, extirpation is the course to be adopted.

For the manner of performing the lesser operation, that of "abscission," or reducing the eyeball, I beg to refer my reader to the chapter on "Staphyloma." It is only necessary to say besides, that when there is no staphyloma, the cornea is to be excised.

"Extirpation" of the eyeball within the ocular sheath, which is given in a distinct chapter, is what would be called a more brilliant proceeding than "abscission;" and there can be no doubt that, although the operation, so far as the practical surgery is concerned, is more prolonged and severe, the recovery may be more rapid, and the general effect perhaps less. Yet I am quite sure that, if the patient's ultimate welfare be considered, its adoption should be the rare exception. Even a button of collapsed tissues is far better than none, and a slightly reduced eyeball is vastly superior to an empty orbit; and I think it better that these should be secured, if it be even at the expense of longer time.

But will "abscission" confer advantages equally lasting with "extirpation?" is a question likely to arise in the mind of the practical man. Answering from my own experience, I say, Yes. In no case in which I have selected it as the proper operation have I been disappointed. Were I to write pages, I could not express more.

The discussion on "Sympathetic ophthalmitis" might be spread out to a great length, and extensive details given; but I think that I have said enough to guide the student, and to develope inquiry. There are yet many points about which I am seeking information; among them, I am searching after the conditions that the ophthalmoscope may reveal to us in the early stages of the disease.

CHAPTER VII.

By the term "caries," I understand interstitial absorption or softening of bone, followed by ulceration and suppuration. This may occur in any portion of the orbit, but every part is not equally liable to suffer; the circumference, especially the outer inferior angle, is most commonly involved, and distortion of the palpebræ, injury to the conjunctiva from chronic inflammation, and, in aggravated cases, damage even to the eyeball from exposure, are almost certain consequences. Besides these results, extension of the disease to the interior of the skull, by which the brain or its membranes may become involved, should be enumerated.

I shall not detail the several stages by which caries is developed; it is sufficient for this work to record the fact that it may be induced by inflammation of the contiguous soft tissues, including the periosteum, or that it may commence in the bone itself. Of the predisposing causes, struma is the most frequent; indeed, if syphilis and the abuse of mercury be put aside, there are comparatively few cases that cannot be traced to its influence. A blow is a common exciting cause.

The following is one of the instances that I have seen of caries, commencing fairly within the orbit; it is the only fatal one with which I have been concerned. A remarkably robust and powerful carter, forty-two years old, applied to me in May, 1844, with impaired vision and slight protrusion of the left eyeball, without lateral displacement. The integuments of the external canthus and of the cheek were swollen and indurated,

without either redness or pain. The other portions of the eyelids were healthy. The protrusion of the ball and the mistiness
of sight commenced three years prior to his applying to me, but
the swelling was of recent occurrence. He assured me that
from time to time as many as eight hundred leeches had been
applied, partly by the direction of a surgeon, and partly by his
own desire. I lost sight of him till January, 1845, when
paroxysms of pain induced him to return ; the eyeball was now
more prominent, its movements were restricted, vision decidedly
worse, the tumefaction greater, and the parts inflamed. He was
emaciated and very weak. Even now I could not be certain
that suppuration existed, but I made a puncture over the outer
and lower edge of the orbit, apparently the most favourable
spot, and deepened the cut through the brawny tissue to the
bone before the pus flowed, about a dessert-spoonful escaping.
Much temporary relief ensued; he became very debilitated,
went into King's College Hospital, and after much nervous
excitement, delirium, and fits of an epileptic character, coma
supervened, and he died on the 27th of February. I attended
the post-mortem examination, which was performed in the presence of Dr. Todd and Mr. Fergusson. No trace of disease
could be found within the cranium, and the interior of the
orbital parietes did not show any signs of inflammation. There
was an abscess at the outer and lower angle, which passed outwards, and involved the malar bone in its orbital and its outer
aspect, these surfaces being carious ; and a small sinus, not
involving the bone, had burrowed through the spheno-maxillary
fissure into the zygomatic fossa. The chest was not examined.
The abdominal organs seemed healthy. The duration of the
disease was very remarkable.

Henry Bird, aged eleven, was admitted into King's College
Hospital, suffering from severe cerebral symptoms, which supervened on caries of the orbit. Three years previously an abscess
formed over the left malar bone, and from time to time there
were exfoliations of bone, till the lower and outer borders of the
orbit were completely destroyed, and a deep suppurating fissure
formed. The lower jaw was rigidly closed, the lower eyelid

everted, and the cheek much swollen. He died of symptoms of pneumonia, of inflammation and compression of the brain. The following state was revealed by a *post-mortem* examination. A large portion of the left malar bone was destroyed by exfoliation ; the orbital and cerebral surfaces of the greater wing of the sphenoid bone were.carious, and the periosteum of the orbit and the dura mater, which was soft and pulpy, were separated by pus. In that part of the middle lobe of the left hemisphere opposed to the diseased bone was a circumscribed abscess, about the size of a large nut, which had opened into the sac of the arachnoid. In the left lateral sinus was about a drachm of pus. These appearances seem to indicate that the disease of the brain commenced as periostitis of the malar and sphenoid bones, and that, in affecting the upper surface of the latter, there had been, from contiguity of parts, inflammation set up in the substance of the cerebral hemisphere, producing abscess, which, by opening into the arachnoid, produced fatal arachnitis. Fuller particulars are recorded in the " Medical Times and Gazette" for October 8, 1853.

I am indebted to my friend Mr. W. O. Chalk, late Surgeon to the Margate Sea Bathing Infirmary, who has had extensive experience in diseases of the bone, for the sketch (fig. 16), from a patient under his charge with caries of the edge of the orbit. I exhibit it to show to what degree the lid may be influenced

FIG. 16.

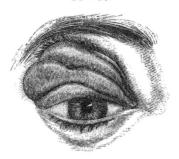

when the caries proceeds unchecked for years, as it did in this young man. It is the most marked example I have seen of ectropium of the upper eyelid from this cause.

In patients affected with caries it is useless to attempt local measures, without attending carefully to the general health, which is always seriously impaired.

Modern surgery teaches us that the process of cure may be much facilitated by removing the carious portion, which is incapable of repair, and is rarely cast off except by a very tedious process. The necessity of cutting beyond the diseased part into the new bone, which is thrown out by nature for the purpose of repairing the lesion, is well known; yet surgeons seem loth to carry out the practice in caries of the orbit, and disease, that may be cut short in a few months or weeks, is allowed to continue for years. The gouge is the instrument that must be used, and, as it is almost needless to observe, with the greatest care about those parts of the skull that are contiguous to the brain. But this should not be undertaken till there is actual necessity for it—till local and general measures have been fairly tried, and have failed,—and till sinuses, if they exist, have been efficiently opened. If this be carried out, the injurious practice of operating when the soft parts are in a state of acute inflammation is obviated, and there is secured the best period for this, the last attempt—viz., when the natural powers have made an effort at repair in the surrounding bone.

Necrosis frequently accompanies caries, and may be a natural step towards cure, the point of separation being at a spot where there is capability of healing. Here, as in other parts of the bony frame, the sequestrum may be so locked in that mechanical relief is demanded.

A patient of mine at St. Mary's Hospital, a lad eleven years of age, of a scrofulous diathesis, had caries of the upper edge of the orbit, and the surrounding soft parts being in that quiescent state that warranted interference with the bone, I scraped away the carious portion from the outer side; and while applying the gouge for a similar purpose to the inner, I discovered a necrosed piece as big as a pea, which was easily released from the enclosing cavity by a few touches with the gouge.

I subjoin a sketch, taken after cicatrization, to show how little deformity remains.

FIG. 17.

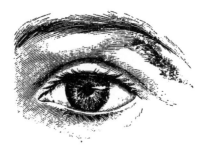

Had there been neglect in this case, a distressing ectropium must have been inevitable.

Mr. Chalk showed me a girl, who was his patient, with ectropium of the lower lid from caries, in which there had been a compensation to some extent for the lost bone. A sharp tooth-like process had been thrown out from the edge of the orbit, which wonderfully ameliorated the original depression of the tarsal edge. Since then I have seen the same thing, in less degree, in two of my hospital patients. I will mention one. A boy had chronic periostitis of the upper part of the orbit. I punctured an abscess, which discharged for three months. A deposit of bone was perceived at the orbital margin, just external to the supra-orbital foramen.

The following case of caries of the orbit was attended with the most remarkable depression of the eyelid I have ever witnessed from such a cause. L. P., aged fourteen years, at the age of three years had necrosis of the right thumb, and afterwards, in succession, of the left foot, right lower jaw, right malar bone, and, to a small extent, of the outer edge of the left orbit, from each of which places small pieces of bone came away at intervals. In consequence of the ulceration and subsequent cicatrization attendant on the disease of the cheek, the right lower eyelid was completely destroyed, with the exception of its ciliary margin, which was drawn down and firmly fixed at the bottom of a deep depression half an inch below the margin of the orbit. The eye had been in this state for six years, when she applied to my colleague Mr. Taylor at the Central London Ophthalmic Hospital. I subjoin a sketch of the deformity.

FIG. 18.

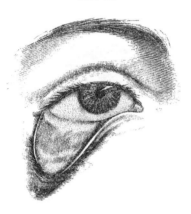

Transplantation of skin was done with success, and the eyelid restored. The eye, as represented after the operation, is given in the next chapter, under the subject of Ectropium.

Much may be done in the way of checking the extension, or even preventing the occurrence of caries, when the disease commences in the soft parts, by the timely evacuation of abscesses by free incisions, and by after-care in preventing sinuses.

Dilute nitric and phosphoric acids may be employed with advantage in those cases in which the gouge cannot be used. Mr. Bransby Cooper, who in the latter years of his life paid much attention to this subject, strongly recommended phosphoric acid diluted with an equal weight of water, as being useful in facilitating the removal of sequestra, converting the phosphate of lime into a bi-phosphate, which is more soluble and more readily acted on by the pus. This lotion is too strong to be used freely about the neighbourhood of the eye, for its accidental contact with the conjunctiva would be very painful, if not otherwise injurious; but it may be applied accurately and in small quantities with a brush, or by means of a bit of lint. Less care is needed if a much weaker solution, say one part to seven of water, is employed instead, but of course the efficacy would be much less.

That excellent surgeon showed how chemistry and the microscope assist us to diagnose disease of bone. According to him, an appreciable quantity of phosphate of lime in an ounce of pus, taken from a lumbar or psoas abscess, is an indication of a carious condition of the vertebræ. As but a small quantity of purulent fluid can be collected from an orbital abscess, I asked Mr. Cooper for an appropriate test, and he kindly told me that, if necrotic pus be placed under the microscope, an amorphous deposit will be seen, which will disappear on the addition of dilute acetic acid ; or if the pus be burnt away in a platinum spoon, the phosphate of lime will be left in the form of a greyish powder, which may be dissolved in muriatic acid without effervescence, and then precipitated by an excess of ammonia.

Mere exposure of bone from an abscess must not be mistaken for caries. Acrid, thin, and fœtid purulent discharges with unhealthy granulations, are pretty sure signs of the bone being diseased, and the probe will generally confirm these indications. The child of a noble family had several abscesses about the body, together with one at the lower and outer edge of the orbit, which was opened by a very small puncture; but little relief followed : and as the eyelids remained swollen, the eye inflamed, and bare bone was felt by the probe, it was supposed that caries existed. I made a free incision through the swollen and boggy tissues, giving a proper exit to the pus, and for a few days maintained an opening by introducing a strip of lint. The improvement was most marked, and in less than three weeks the child left town with the abscess nearly cicatrized. I have many parallel cases in my note-book. It would be useless to adduce any more.

I have received some hints from Mr. Field, the late Surgeon to the Margate Royal Sea Bathing Infirmary, respecting the lessening of the scar consequent on suppuration about the orbit. Mr. Field's vast opportunities of practical experience in this matter, and his accurate observation, entitle his recommendation to the highest respect. On the importance of the early evacuation of pus he is emphatic : and he tells me, what my own experience confirms, that strumous abscesses in the immediate neighbourhood of the orbit, when left to themselves, are always followed by a greater or less degree of ectropium. An important part of his treatment, when the bone is unaffected, is to use the caustic potash, and destroy the entire wall of the abscess, the results of which are the removal of the ill-conditioned textures, and the stimulation of the surrounding parts, whereby abundant healthy granulations are thrown out, and thus more rapid healing, and less deformity. He has even used the potash to open small abscesses, and the rapidity of cure has, he thinks, shown the value of the plan. The following is one of many similar cases treated by him :—

J. S., the subject of scrofulous disease in several parts of the body, had a painful swelling, apparently of the periosteum, extending around the outer half of the right orbit. A concentrated solution of iodine was daily applied for nearly four months, and this, together with general treatment, had the effect of somewhat reducing the swelling, but an abscess pointed at the lower part, and this was opened with potassa fusa ; a slough rather less than a sixpence separated in about a week, granulations sprang up in great abundance, and the ulcer quickly cicatrized, and did not produce ectropium.

I must make a remark about the use of the potash. Its action always extends beyond the spot touched, and more sloughing is often produced than is expected, or wished for. I never use it about the face, or neck ; for with all my care, and with the precaution of brushing over the surface acted on, with a very weak acid lotion, there is occasionally a still greater effect produced than is desirable. A much safer application is the " potassa cum calce; " merely a mechanical mixture of potash and lime, less deliquescent and more manageable than potassa fusa.

CHAPTER VIII.

AFFECTIONS OF THE EYELIDS.

ABSCESS—ERYSIPELATOUS INFLAMMATION—CARBUNCLE—HYPERTROPHY OF THE
INTEGUMENTS — SYMBLEPHARON — ANCHYLOBLEPHARON — EPICANTHUS —
PTOSIS—TRICHIASIS—ENTROPIUM—ECTROPIUM—OBSTRUCTION OF THE MEI-
BOMIAN DUCTS—CONJUNCTIVAL CALCULI.

ABSCESS, ERYSIPELATOUS INFLAMMATION, CARBUNCLE.

THE eyelids are liable to abscess, and unless the pus be early evacuated, considerable injury might ensue. Common phlegmonous abscess is not likely to be overlooked; but, from the peculiar looseness of the palpebral skin, chronic suppuration may simulate mere swelling of the integuments, and be mistaken for œdema. Through neglect, I have seen some severe cases of ectropium of the upper palpebra. Even with obscure symptoms of suppuration, a puncture should be made; for, in this situation, it is frequently by exploration only, that the fluid can be detected.

Suppuration in one of the meibomian glands is not uncommon. The discharge escapes at the mouth of the duct, in the substance of the tarsal cartilage.

In erysipelatous inflammation of the face, the palpebræ are apt to suffer from sloughing of the cellular tissue, and vigilance is required not to allow the suppurative stage to arrive, without the necessary incisions being made. The surgeon must not be deterred· from cutting freely by a dread of wounding the eyeball, although we have record of such accidents, and we read of a physician who had both of his eyeballs evacuated by a colleague. The position of the canaliculi should be ascertained, and care be taken to avoid them. The course of the lachrymal ducts, and the strip of gland that accompanies them, should also be remembered, lest they be cut, and a lachrymal fistula ensue.

All incisions in this position should be made transversely, or parallel to the natural folds of the skin, in order to lessen deformity. I frequently meet with a small abscess at the under and outer part of the upper eyelid, near the margin. It is preceded by more or less acute inflammation. If the tarsus be raised, the intensity of the action will be seen in the vicinity of the lachrymal ducts, in or about which I suspect the irritation is set up. A timely puncture will spare much suffering.

I have seen a few instances of carbuncle of the eyelids. I believe in the importance of early incision. With no small means of observation at St. Mary's and in private, and after seeing the practice of other surgeons, I am convinced, that by so doing, the best local measures are adopted for arresting the disease, and for lessening changes in the contiguous tissues.

HYPERTROPHY OF THE INTEGUMENTS OF THE EYELIDS.

All surgeons much engaged in ophthalmic practice, must have met with chronic œdema of the integuments of the upper eyelid. In an aggravated form it is rare. Once only have I found it necessary to operate.

A girl, eighteen years old, applied to me with both eyelids symmetrically affected. There was hypertrophy of the integuments from the eyebrow to the tarsal margin, and they were so depending over the lid-edge as to obscure the pupil.

The surface was traversed by tortuous veins. The affection was not congenital, but had existed four years, and was on the increase. The rest of the facial skin, although not in a diseased state, seemed coarser than natural. No exciting cause could be assigned. I operated, and removed enough to overcome the effect spoken of. There was much bleeding, but this did not prevent primary union. The personal appearance was besides much improved.   A dissection showed mere hypertrophy of the parts.

I shall relate a case of this kind, but in a more aggravated form, in the subdivision on " Ptosis."

SYMBLEPHARON, OR COMPLETE OR PARTIAL ADHESION OF THE EYELIDS TO THE EYEBALL.

When the conjunctiva is burned or scalded, or severely acted upon by escharotics, or receives a lesion that is followed directly by loss of substance, or subsequently by sloughing, or ulceration, contraction ensues ; and, according ·to the extent of the implication, the eyelid is more or less united to the globe of the eye, which is accordingly restricted in its movements, or rendered motionless.

Any operations that involve the removal of much of the conjunctiva, particularly above or below the horizontal axis of the eye, may produce this effect ; although it must be remarked, that the contraction which follows from this cause is very different in character and in extent.

Severe purulent ophthalmia may be a cause of one form of the affection.   A patient of mine, at St. Mary's Hospital, a man æt. thirty, had the entire surfaces of both eyelids intimately adherent to the eyeball, the conjunctiva oculi being dry.   I know that the treatment of inflammation of the conjunctiva by escharotics plays no unimportant part in producing these adhesions.   The nitrate of silver is often used in substance, and in very strong ointments, in a most lavish manner ; a practice which sometimes produces sloughing.   M. Desmarres, who is fully alive to this abuse of caustic, says, he has been informed by Dr. Furnari that, " during his stay in Africa, he had seen and operated on so large a number of symblepharons from that cause, that he was quite tired of them."

In connexion with this subject, I may allude to that remarkable condition of the conjunctiva, known as xeroma, or xerophthalmia, or cuticular conjunctiva ; and which has been fully treated of by my colleague Mr. R. Taylor, in a paper in the

"Edinburgh Medical and Surgical Journal," No. 198 (No. 1, New Series). In the large majority of cases which he has collected from journals, and in all which he has seen, powerful irritant and caustic applications had been at one time or another employed. Mr. Taylor attributes the disease to chronic inflammation of the sub-conjunctival cellular tissue, with exudation of lymph, which, subsequently contracting, similarly to the cicatricial tissue, gradually abolishes the palpebral sinuses, and glues the eyelids to the eyeball. He has found that the application of glycerine to the dry cornea, will, in many instances, so far restore its transparency as to afford useful vision.

Congenital symblepharon has been met with; and Mr. Wardrop has recorded a case in which it seemed owing to a cuticular condition of the conjunctiva. ("Dublin Journal of Medical Science," vol. xxviii.)

By the kindness of Mr. Fergusson, I saw a child four months old, in whom there was almost entire deficiency of the lower eyelid, and the defective portion was tied to the eyeball by cuticular-like conjunctiva, that reached just half-way up the cornea. There existed also a double harelip.

With few exceptions, all the examples of symblepharon that have come under my notice have been occasioned by the action of quicklime, or mortar. From such a cause, the accretion always takes place slowly, is extensive in proportion to the original injury, may occur even when not expected, and is not necessarily attended with the process of sloughing of the texture of the conjunctiva, and is most detrimental at the lower part of the eye. Several times I have watched the effects of quicklime from the commencement; and like every one else, I believe, who has attempted it, I have totally failed in stopping the accustomed after-effects. In each case the injury was partial, and confined to the lower part of the eyeball. The entire conjunctiva became intensely red, except where the lime had rested—that was white or whitish, from the chemical action that had taken place; this spot soon swelled, its epithelium separated in shreds, and contraction commenced. In the following very aggravated example, resulting from a burn, the lower eyelid was not only universally and closely adherent to the motionless eyeball, but was also drawn much over the cornea, which had been injured

FIG. 19.

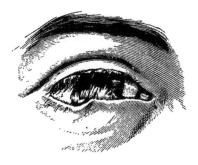

in the greater part.   The tarsal edge above, although scarred, was free.

The upper eyelid might be adherent to a considerable extent without any inconvenience.

The treatment of every variety of adhesion is difficult, and rarely successful; improvement even must depend on the extent and nature of the attachment.   When the cornea has become opaque, the question of operating should not be entertained, except, according to Dr. Mackenzie, circumstances induce us, not with any hope of restoring sight, but merely to relieve pain and a feeling of dragging, which restrains in some measure the motions even of the sound eye.

My own practice has not furnished me with an example of the " bridle form " of adhesion spoken of by some writers—that in which there is an isthmus of connexion.   The prognosis is said to be favourable.

Interference is usually very unsatisfactory when the adhesion is extensive, and perhaps also when comparatively limited, if the conjunctiva, with more or less of the sub-cellular tissue, have perished, and bands of lowly organized material form the connexion.   It is only when the tether is chiefly of conjunctiva that any success can be expected.   Experience has fully convinced me of the truth of this assertion.   In the extensively

K

implicated examples, I suspect that the cellular sheath of the eyeball, the "ocular tunic," suffers.

Failure or the return of the agglutination is not, according to my observation, due to the adhesion of the opposed surfaces, which I believe to be a very exceptional occurrence. I have said in the chapter on "Injuries," in connexion with this subject, and to which I beg to refer my reader for other remarks, that during the healing process, adhesion should rather be encouraged as likely to afford a better state for after-treatment. The divided parts come together by means of the contraction of the granulations through which they are healed, just as happens in other parts of the body in cicatrization from burns. Several times, and in spite of very great care, and under what appeared to be most favourable circumstances, I have removed the cicatrices, and carefully dissected off the bands; but the contractions have returned to the same, or even greater extent. I have adopted a plan which alone has given me a lasting favourable issue. In the first case I did, the band which tied the centre of the eyelid to the globe of the eye encroached a little on the cornea,—was narrow, soft, and loose; I merely divided it twice, and each time it returned to its former state. I then removed a small central portion of what appeared to be cicatrix, and brought the edges of the divided conjunctiva, on the eyelid and on the eyeball, severally together by sutures, and the result was very gratifying. The last time I saw the patient, several months after the operation, there was but a slight contraction at the lower part of the interior of the eyelid,—a spot where there would, I suppose, be a certain amount of puckering, in all cases of equal amount of injury, under any plan of treatment. The globe of the eye was no longer unnaturally covered by the eyelid, and the feelings of restraint to its movements were lost.

In the second I was still more fortunate, on account of a more favourable condition; for perfect success ensued. The patient, who was twenty-six years old, had, when a lad, accidentally received some quicklime in his eye; and the usual process of adhesion followed cicatrization of the conjunctival

slough. The annexed sketch accurately expresses the state
before the operation. The connecting medium, which seemed

FIG. 20.

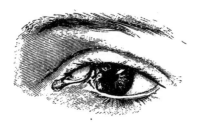

to consist entirely of conjunctiva, was long and nearly isolated.
Putting the eyelid on the stretch, I divided the band vertically
through its entire thickness, carried the incision into the tissue
below, and brought the edges of each side severally together by
three sutures. In four days the stitches were removed. In
others I have had more or less success according to the state
of the case. I know that my practice has been successfully followed by one of my colleagues.

There is a notice in the "Gazette Médicale" of 1846, of an
operation by M. Blandin that should be mentioned. A man
was burned by a drop of melted metal, and extensive ulceration
of the conjunctiva of the eyeball and lower eyelid followed.
The wound was neglected, the cartilage of the lid was destroyed,
and adhesions united the contiguous parts. The lower half of
the cornea was covered by a semi-elliptical, bluish white cicatrix,
while the upper remained clear. The eye had lost its mobility,
in a great measure, and a feeling of constraint was very
fatiguing. M. Blandin dissected the cicatrix from above downwards, turned the dense bluish white structure inwards, in the
form of a hem, so as to form a substitute for the palpebral
mucous membrane, and retained it in position by the glover's
suture. The two extremities of the thread were carried horizontally to the right and left, and fixed with a certain amount
of tension to the corresponding temples, so as to keep the

border of the eyelid free of the cornea. The sutures were removed on the fourth day. The patient was dismissed from the hospital about three weeks after the operation. The eye had quite recovered its mobility, and could be directed at will towards any object; the part of the cornea which was formerly overspread by the cicatrix, was now covered only by a delicate film of cellular tissue, which did not granulate, but daily decreased in thickness and opacity. The new eyelid had a rounded border; it was rather short, but could be approached, without difficulty, to its fellow, and effectually defended the eye from the light.

The detailed description of the eye at the time of the patient's dismissal from the hospital cannot be questioned. Yet it would be incorrect to conclude that the operation had answered. Sufficient time had not elapsed to judge of its effects; the early favourable results might have been counteracted by subsequent contraction, as too often happens in parallel instances. The report is, therefore, so far imperfect. My long intimacy with hospital practice has convinced me that the value of this description of practical surgery cannot be fairly judged of in so short a time.

I am happy in being able to adduce the particulars of a decidedly successful case, that was done on the same principle by one of my colleagues at our Ophthalmic Hospital. I assisted at it. The band of adhesion was evidently chiefly of conjunctiva. The patient, a lad of fifteen, had both eyes severely injured by lime. The condition of the right eye was this:—The eyeball was united to nearly the entire length of the lower eyelid, by a broad band, which overspread the cornea, so as almost to conceal the pupil; the little chink which was left being obscured by a faint bluish opacity. Its movements were limited, and accompanied by a disagreeable sensation of dragging and stiffness. The result of the operation was very satisfactory, and as the patient was seen by Mr. Taylor four years afterwards, the fact of its permanence is established. The palpebral sinus was restored, and the ocular movement, in every direction, decidedly free. The pupil was clear except at the upper part, where there existed the opacity alluded to, and vision was excellent.

The four following methods have been collected by M. Desmarres, and are given in his "Traité des Maladies des Yeux."

The first is that of M. Amussat. After having freely divided all existing bridles, the point of a pin, or of a cutting instrument, is daily carried to the very extremity of the division, and the pyogenic, or false membrane, torn; and this is continued until the surfaces are cicatrized, and can no longer adhere to each other.

M. Desmarres adds, that for seven years he had seen M. Lisfranc daily practise this manœuvre with his nail on the prepuce of individuals operated on for phymosis, and that he is fully satisfied of the efficacy of this method in certain cases; but he remarks, however, that the tearing of the wound sometimes produces erysipelas; that it demands continued perseverance and attention on the part of the operator for several weeks; and that the patient is often tired out before cicatrization takes place.

The second is the ligature process of M. Petrequin. A double thread is passed at one spot through the adhesions; the one is tied close to the sclerotica with great firmness, the other towards the eyelid with a less degree of tightness. The strangulation and sloughing occurring earlier at the constriction next the eyeball, that part heals before the other, and the cicatrization becomes too forward to admit of a new adhesion with the outer part. ("Supplément des Annales Oculistiques," vol. iii. p. 66.) I have tried this with much care, but without any good result.

The third is that of Professor Ammon. Two converging incisions, commencing at the free edge and carried through the entire thickness of the lid, are made to circumscribe, and thereby detach that portion to which the adhesions are connected; the incisions of course fall together in the form of the letter V. The lateral parts of the lid are then brought together by the hare-lip suture, and the central bit that has been shut out from them remains fixed to the eye, and lies between the globe and the lid. After the pins have been removed, and the union of the parts perfected, which at the soonest is in about fourteen days, the detached fragment is cut off. Two figures are given : the first to show the lines of the cuts ; the second, the appearance of the eye when the lips of the wound have been brought together.

Lastly, there is the very ingenious proposal of Professor Dieffenbach. It consists of folding the lid inwards, and placing the cuticle for a while against the globe. One incision is made from the internal angle of the eye by the side of the nose, and another equally vertical, from the external angle to the corresponding border of the orbit. The lid is detached from the globe of the eye, the cilia are cut off, and the quadrilateral piece is then turned inside to rest against the margin of the orbit, and secured by sutures which are carried from within outwards, and *vice versâ*, tied together, and further bound by small adhesive straps. When the wound on the globe is sufficiently cicatrized, the temporary and artificial entropium is removed, the lid is released, and whatever adhesion it may have formed on itself is destroyed ; it is carried back to its original position, and there retained by the twisted suture. The eyeball being then covered with the peculiar tissue from granulation, cannot renew its connexion with the recent surface of the lid, which, in its turn, acquires a solid cicatrix. This applies to the lower lid ; the upper is to be treated on the same principle.

It is evident that the attention of authors is principally directed to prevent their incisions from uniting; for they appear to consider the reunion of the divided tissue the common source of failure. This opinion I have questioned. Many mechanical contrivances have been used to check the supposed occurrence ; plates of metal and other substances have been interposed. Numerous surgeons have recorded their attempts and their failures. It is to be regretted that treatment is so often fruitless in the recent injury, and after operations, in preventing the occurrence of contraction. Mr. Tyrrell, after telling how the granulating surfaces should be exposed, three or four times a day, and any junction of granulations destroyed by a probe, the practice being continued till a new mucous or secreting membrane is formed—a state of surface which I suspect would never arrive—says, one evil that follows these injuries, which the utmost care and attention of the surgeon cannot prevent, is the contraction of the new formation as it becomes organized, so as to produce a frænum, or band, between the surfaces of the globe and the eyelid.

Professor Miller's summary of the process of repair after burns, applies to these cases :—That they heal slowly and much more by the contraction of the old surfaces, than by the formation of new ; that the new matter is imperfectly organized and liable to absorption ; and, consequently, contraction continues for some time after the completion of the cicatrix.

ANCHYLOBLEPHARON, OR ADHESION OF THE EDGES OF THE EYELIDS.

This rare affection is seen both as a congenital defect and as the result of disease and injury of the eyelids.

Of the first, an interesting example is given by M. Rognetta, in his "Cours d'Ophthalmologie," 1839, in which the eyelids were united by means of the palpebral conjunctiva, so as to form a sort of moveable veil over the cornea of about three lines in breadth, the tears flowing through a little aperture at the external angle. Mr. Travers alludes briefly to a remarkable case, a full-grown boy, whose eye was found perfect after the division, though he had been thus blind from infancy. From his remarks it seems, in this instance, to have been similar to the co-adhesion of the nymphæ or labia pudendæ in infants. Mr. Middlemore, who refers to the experience of many authors in the congenital deformity, has himself seen three cases. The defect occurred in both eyes. The eyelashes were not formed, and in the situation of the edges of the eyelid there was a narrow sulcus lined by a delicate vascular portion of skin, which admitted of extension, but not absolute separation. In one case the eyeball appeared imperfectly developed, and seemed adherent to the eyelids.

In the "Lancet" for 1840, vol. ii., the late Dr. Hocken, in his admirable Ophthalmic papers, alludes to a child who was brought to the Exeter Eye Infirmary, with a small filamentary portion of the integuments causing adhesion of the left eyelid. The band occupied the site of the junction of the outer with the middle third of the eyelid, was of the size of a common sewing thread, round, and consisted of integument. In all other respects the eye was healthy.

It would be out of place here to consider the physiological bearings of this arrest of development. To those interested in the matter, I would recommend Mr. Wilde's writings in vol. xxvii. of the "Dublin Journal of Medical Science." The treatment so plainly indicated—that of careful separation—is here easy and successful.

As an acquired state, it may be produced by any of the causes which occasion adhesion of the eyelids to the eyeball; and besides, by ulceration of the tarsal margins.

A youth, exhibiting a tolerably well-marked instance, applied to Mr. Taylor, who took the following sketch. He had long suffered from strumous ophthalmia, combined with severe ophthalmia tarsi.

FIG. 21.

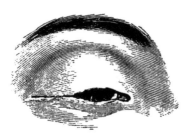

Those parts of the eyelid not in contact were quite raw; and the union that existed must have been very recent, from the ease with which the separation was effected by a common dressing probe. The ointment of the red oxide of mercury was used, and the surfaces cicatrized singly, and successfully.

It is generally stated, that, in what is called complete adhesion, there is always an aperture, however small, through which the lacrymal secretions pass. This is not, however, the case; for a man was sent to me with entire adhesion of the left eyelids, and in which not the least aperture existed. The accidental explosion of gunpowder had destroyed the globe of the eye, and in a few weeks the eyelids had united. There was not any inconvenience produced by the lacrymal secretion not having an outlet for escape; and I suspect that in its absence, there is always imperfection or destruction of other parts of the lacrymal apparatus, and especially of the conjunctiva.

The mere separation of the eyelids is simple enough, even when a director and a scalpel are required; and where there is not a passage for the entrance of the director, one must be made at the internal angle of the eye. But there is great difficulty in the prevention of fresh adhesion; and it is towards the corners of the eyelids that re-connexion usually occurs. The preventive means ordinarily prescribed are stimulating oint-ments, escharotics, and desiccative powders. Some surgeons have thought it advisable that sleep should be prohibited for twenty or more hours; or if the patient be allowed to go to bed, that he be awoke at intervals, and the dressing, whatever it may be, reapplied.

The application of goldbeater's skin, or touching the surfaces with collodion, after they have been well dried, is, I think, superior to any other method. The depression of the lower eyelid by strips of plaster, and the elevation of the upper, is a valuable adjunct; care being taken to protect the eye from dust, and where the upper eyelid is fastened up, it may be requisite to moisten the cornea with oil. I have very much mitigated several cases of most intimate union of the outer portions of the tarsi, produced by adhesion and contraction of the ulcerated surfaces from disease. In one instance, a very decided deformity was so reduced as no longer to be remark-able. I shall' allude again to the subject in connexion with "entropium."

If a suitable opportunity offer, I should try the plan that has been, as I understand, successfully adopted in webbed fingers,—that of establishing an aperture at the most remote part of the adhesion, and then dividing the remainder. The *rationale* is obvious.

Stœber has very ingeniously proposed, that after the disunion of the eyelids, a portion of conjunctiva should be raised, drawn forward to the lip of the wound, and fastened by sutures.

Dr. Mackenzie makes a distinction between close and intimate adhesion by the inosculation of ulcerated surfaces, and a bond of connexion by the intervention of coagulable lymph; and he directs, in operating on the latter, that the first incision should be made close to the edge of the under eyelid, leaving the whole of the pseudo-membrane attached to the upper, from which it is to be dissected with a pair of scissors.

We can hardly expect any benefit if we operate in this affection when the eyelids adhere to the eyeball,—a complication easily ascertained by the movements of the organ, or by any aperture that may exist; neither should we interfere when the cornea is opaque, a point less easily determined unless it can be seen: however, the capability of discerning light must be made the test, imperfect as it may be. Where one eye is sound it should be closed, and a comparison of the light-detecting power of the two may decide the question.

EPICANTHUS, OR ENCROACHMENT OF THE SKIN ON THE CORNER OF THE EYE.

In this defect, the inner canthus is covered by a crescentic fold of skin passing from the nose and covering the caruncle. Although a slight degree of this deformity is not very uncommon, an aggravated state is rare among Europeans. There are, however, varieties of our race in whom a kind of epicanthus is very frequent; and, in an article on the malformations and congenital diseases of the organs of sight, in vol. xxvii. of the "Dublin Journal," Mr. Wilde gives it as his opinion, from what he has seen of the Mongolian race, and from the examination of a great number of their crania, that this disposition of parts which we regard as a congenital malformation in the European and the Caucasian races, is allied to the natural condition of the Chinese and the Calmuc.

The abnormal fold may interfere with vision, or cause trichiasis in the upper eyelid. A marked example of the latter I have seen in an infant.

The accompanying representation of the affection is from a child nine months old, in whom the deformity was readily relieved. The fold may be reduced or pulled aside, by forcibly pinching up the intervening integuments of the nose; and hence is founded the operation of taking away a portion of skin to produce permanently such an effect. The required size of the

FIG. 22.

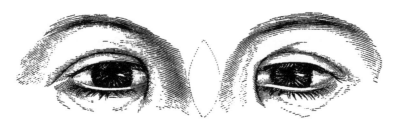

piece to be removed is tolerably ascertainable by the amount that must be pinched up to clear the eyelids. The lines on the nose in the above sketch mark the direction of the incisions, and the size of the piece of skin that I removed. Another case on which I operated, is reported in the "Medical Times" for August 27, 1853.

Latterly I have made the angle of the ellipse less obtuse, by lengthening the incisions, because there is more certainty of primary union.

After the piece is taken out—and this requires accuracy in making the incisions, which should be through the entire skin, and somewhat bevelled inwards,—the edges of the wound must be raised—that is, dissected up all round,—to allow of their easy approximation; or else, from the natural tightness of the skin in this part, there will be a strain which may endanger union by the first intention, which is so essential to success. The hare-lip suture must be used, and the pins should be entered the eighth of an inch from the edge, carried entirely through the skin, and brought out at a corresponding distance on the opposite side. Two will generally suffice. One or two sutures may be required. Instead of the ordinary coarse, clumsy, and expensive silver pin, I use sharp ones of soft steel, that are easily cut with the pliers. Common toilet pins would answer as well, and might be used, were it not for the popular objection to them on the score of their festering properties—not groundless, perhaps, when the plating is lost. At least five days should elapse before the pins are withdrawn, or else separation is risked ; but they should not remain longer, or suppuration might ensue around them, and marked scars would follow.

The defect may exist in one eye ; and should an operation be required, the above proceeding must be a little modified. One incision must be straight, the other in the form of a curve towards the affected side.

It is a commonly received, but very erroneous opinion, that a child may grow out of the deformity.

Epicanthus may be acquired,—that is, may result from the cicatrix of a wound displacing the eyelids, and pulling the skin over the corner of the eye; in which case the nature of the operation required will of course depend on a variety of circumstances.

I have seen a deficient palpebral fissure mistaken for epicanthus, and operated on for such. Eversion of the inner part of each eyelid ensued.

PTOSIS, OR FALLING OF THE UPPER EYELID.

In unison with the general arrangement of this work, those cases only of ptosis are considered in which surgical treatment is requisite—that is, when all existing causes, cerebral or otherwise, have passed away ; when the affection is congenital, with deficiency of development, or with paralysis; or when it results from direct injury to the levator palpebræ; or from feebleness of power, as in the aged.

While there is the probability of a cure by general treatment, operative measures should be kept in abeyance ; and should there be double vision or confusion of sight when the eyelid is raised, an operation is inadmissible.

Sometimes, although the eyeball is turned outwards, abducted, in consequence of paralysis of the muscles supplied by the third pair of nerves, there is no double vision. It must then be left to the patient to decide which of the two deformities he prefers—the ptosis or the outward squint. I have known the latter to be thought the least of, and the ptosis submitted to operation.

An early effect of ptosis is elevation of the eyebrow, which is produced by the frequent efforts to raise the fallen eyelid. This muscular movement is by the occipito-frontalis, and by it we are enabled to remedy the defect. The eyelid is shortened, and brought under the influence of its action.

The remedial measure is simple in execution : it consists in taking away an elliptical portion of the palpebral skin, the extent of which should be determined according to the case. Where there is partial loss of power, the removal of a small portion of skin, to tuck the eyelid up slightly, is sufficient; where the levator palpebræ is motionless, or nearly so, it must be more shortened than in the other instance, by the loss of a much larger bit. To ensure success, there should be integrity of the orbicularis palpebrarum ; for it is called on to exercise exaggerated power to compensate for the shortening of the eyelid, the closure of the eye being now principally effected by the lower eyelid rising above the ordinary level, to meet the upper. Without this, the eye would be more or less permanently open, and the eyeball exposed.

Besides the difference of circumstances in the kinds of cases to guide us in the amount of skin to be removed, and the varying degrees of the depression or falling of the eyelid, the condition of the skin itself must be taken into account—whether it is healthy, or unnaturally thickened, or loose and baggy. Of kindred importance, also, is the state of the eyebrow, whether lax or tense, and the usual action of the occipito-frontalis of the individual; for in some persons it seems motionless, when it would be useless to operate ; while in others its contractions are remarkable.

To do the operation well, an assistant is necessary. He should make the integuments tense, by raising the eyebrow and pulling down the eyelid. The piece of skin should be taken high up, the upper incision being as near to the edge of the orbit as circumstances will permit, or else the edge, rather than the body of the eyelid, will be influenced. The dissection should be made with a scalpel, the skin only raised, the orbicularis left entire; for in proportion to the destruction of the latter must the power of closing the eyelids be reduced. Sutures must be applied.

It is generally recommended, in order to be exact, that the integument should be first pinched up, and, as it were, measured with a pair of forceps, constructed for the purpose ; but for any information that may be so gained, the use of the finger and thumb will suffice.

Sometimes the skin is raised with an instrument, and cut off with a scalpel or scissors. Independently of the inaccuracy of this proceeding, a disfiguring scar is the inevitable result. This is a great contrast to my method, by which there is scarcely ever a trace of the operation.

Should there be any doubt about the extent of skin to be removed, it should be fixed at the supposed minimum, for a fault on the other side would be serious. In the earlier operations of surgeons, generally too little is removed ; and it is only after considerable practice that a proper estimate of the amount can be made.

When it is necessary to dissect away an unusually large piece of the integument, the outer portions of the incisions must not pass beyond the external angle of the eyelids, or it will be drawn unduly upwards.

I shall give two examples of congenital defect ; one of want of power in the levator palpebræ ; one of hypertrophy of the skin and subjacent cellular tissue ; and I shall add one of a state allied to ptosis from falling of the eyebrow.

W. B., Esq., aged twenty-two, was born with ptosis. In all probability the levator palpebræ was not developed. When the eyes were opened to their utmost, and directed to an object on their level, the cornea of the left was not half uncovered, but about two-thirds concealed, as shown in this sketch.

FIG. 23.

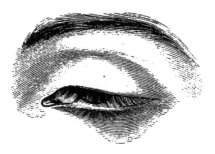

The disabled eye could be closed with ease ; and when the two were shut, they differed in no respect from each other. The eyebrows were in a line, and the skin of each eyelid wrinkled alike. .

The eyeballs were parallel, the recti muscles perfect in action, and vision was unimpaired. When he was depressed in spirits or fatigued, the eyelid always drooped more. I operated. The skin which was removed was of this size and shape.

FIG. 24.

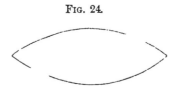

Four sutures were applied. As circumstances obliged my patient to return home next day, I withdrew them just before his departure, so that they were in only twenty-seven hours. Three weeks after, he wrote to me, saying, that there was great improvement in the usefulness and appearance of the eye; that although the eyelid was not quite as high as the other, the abstraction of any more skin would have prevented the eye from closing.

A young woman, aged twenty-two, applied to the Ophthalmic Hospital, with congenital ptosis of the left eyelid. The un- wrinkled and elongated eyelid peculiar to complete dropping was well displayed. With great effort, she could expose a small part of the eyeball. Vision was slightly impaired— being misty. The recti muscles were sound. I dissected off a large semi-lunar piece of skin. On the third day the sutures were removed. I did not see my patient for a year, and the success of the operation was very great; there was but a faint mark of the wound; the eyelid could be raised to the same height as its fellow, and when closed, only differed from it by not descending so low—the lower eyelid rising a little to meet it, and in the edge being straight and not curved.

Some deficiency in the development of the eyelid has been long noticed in congenital cases. Dr. Mackenzie says, that in some he had met with, the eyelid was the reverse of being swollen—it rather appeared atrophied, as if the levator muscle had either been originally deficient, or had wasted from disease. M. Caffe also has noticed the fact; his observations are to be found in the "Dictionnaire des Études Médicales."

A woman, aged sixty-four, infirm, and with ptosis of both eyes, applied at the Ophthalmic Hospital. There was feebleness of the levators, rather than paralysis; for with a strong effort, which she could not long maintain, both eyes could be sufficiently opened for her to see. To enable her to move about or see any- thing in which she might be engaged, it was necessary to keep one of the eyelids raised with the finger. I operated on both sides, and the poor old woman was relieved from her distressing condition. This is the only opportunity I have had of perform- ing the double operation.

This case of ptosis from hypertrophy of the skin and cellular tissue of the orbital region, I give in the patient's words :—

"The lid of my left eye drooped when I was two years old, and as years passed by, it continued to droop and to enlarge; but I felt little inconvenience until I was twelve, when the swelling had so much increased that it became a source of annoyance from the constant inquiries of persons. Then, although I could yet see downwards, I wore a shade, till twenty. I was now operated on. The hæmorrhage was considerable, and produced feebleness, that lasted for many weeks. I was afterwards introduced to Mr. Smee."

In consultation with Mr. Smee, my colleague at the Central

FIG. 25.

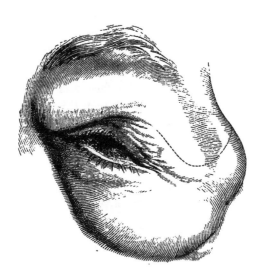

London Ophthalmic Hospital, we determined to attempt to reduce the mass, lessen the deformity, and render the eye useful. At this time the whole of the palpebral skin, the outer part of that of the brow and a portion of the temple, was swollen into a mass that hung over the eye, and nearly concealed it, —the weight closing the eyelid, and preventing its being elevated by natural efforts. All that was pendulous was circumscribed by transverse elliptical incisions by Mr. Smee, and removed. Very active bleeding ensued, and several ligatures were required.

The appearance of the excised portion was like the thickening and enlargement of the scrotum which takes place in hot climates. The actual change was hypertrophy of the skin and subjacent cellular tissue. The result was not unsatisfactory; for the deformity was greatly lessened, and the eyelid could be sufficiently raised to render the eye available. Figure 25 shows the after state of the case; the dotted line marks the course of the incisions.

During my house-surgeoncy at St. Bartholomew's Hospital, there was in attendance as an out-patient, a man of thirty, whose left eye was nearly closed from falling of the eyebrow. The skin was not unhealthy, nor could I observe any other change than paralysis of the occipito-frontalis muscle. He told me that he was born in that state. The levator palpebræ was sound, for when the eyebrow was held up the eyelid could be raised. The other side of the face was unaffected. Mr. Delamotte, Librarian to the Hospital, took this sketch of it.

FIG. 26.

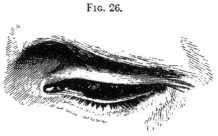

The patient was at the time sitting and looking directly at the draughtsman, who was on the same level.

I doubt not but that this man could have been relieved by removing some of the integuments of the forehead.

Some foreign surgeons regard mere looseness or relaxation of the skin as a cause of ptosis; but it is not easy to see how that can have any influence, unless increased weight be added to relaxation. Undue ponderance in any of the tissues of the eyelid will affect its movements.

When the eyeball is a little less in size than its fellow, from congenital defect, or from atrophy consequent on disease, the eyelid droops, and the state of ptosis is simulated. An operation will materially improve the personal appearance by raising the eyelid and exposing more of the globe of the eye. A young woman, a patient at the Central London Ophthalmic Hospital, availed herself of this. The eyeball was congenitally small, and the narrow aperture of the eyelids gave the usual disagreeable appearance. Mr. Taylor, whose patient she was, removed a portion of skin with very marked benefit.

In a few cases of ptosis, I have found it necessary to add a supplemental operation to that above described; for, although I had removed sufficient skin to affect the greater part of the eyelid, the inner angle yet drooped. The removal of more integument in an oblique direction over the drooping spot, has been effectual.

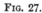

FIG. 27.

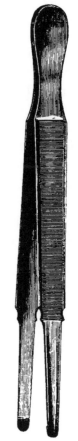

CILIA FORCEPS.

These have, on their points, a broad fine cross-cut, or file-like surface, for taking secure hold. The edges are so much rounded that they cannot cut. The points also are rounded; and, further, the blades are strong enough to admit of proper pressure being exerted at their extremities.

TRICHIASIS.

Trichiasis signifies that misdirection of the cilia or eyelashes whereby their natural position is changed, and they are turned towards the globe of the eye, and touch or rest on it more or less; thus, practically, the term is not applicable until the maldirection has arrived at a state that occasions some inconvenience or injury. It is frequently associated with " entropium," but here I shall speak of it as existing alone.

Trichiasis, although among the most common affections of the eye that call for surgical relief, demands as serious attention as any in the Ophthalmic catalogue ; for, notwithstanding it does not rapidly destroy the eye, yet, if allowed to proceed unchecked, or if merely partially relieved, it becomes, from the constant irritation and subsequent changes which it causes, one of the most destructive diseases.

The number of persons, especially among the poor, who from this cause are doomed to blindness, or impairment of sight, is by no means small.   Unfortunately, the results are not sufficiently dreaded, perhaps not known, and palliative rather than radical measures are too much recommended and adopted.

The disease is peculiarly common among the lowest orders of Irish in their own country, and may be justly ascribed to the influence of the acrid smoke of their miserable hovels, their neglect of ablution, the filth amidst which they exist, and the exposure to which the many wretched pursuits attendant on poverty subjects them.

Trichiasis varies in degree from a slight deflection of some of the cilia, just sufficient to touch the eyeball, to the inveterate implication of all except the smaller ones at the corners, which are usually exempt.

The next figure was taken from a good specimen of the affection.   A few of the cilia just touch the cornea, and a

FIG. 23.

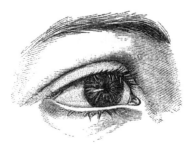

small bunch rests on the sclerotica.   The edge of the eyelid is natural, and not in the least turned in; there is, then, trichiasis, and that only.

The manner in which the more internal of the cilia deviate either in a limited number in one or more places, or along the greater length of the eyelid, has induced some surgeons to suppose that in this distichiasis, as it is called, there is actually a new production of an inner set of hairs, a supplemental development from a more internal part of the eyelid. It has been a question much discussed, whether this is, or is not the case—whether new cilia have sprung forth, or old ones have turned in. I have not myself been able to gather any facts that support the secondary creative theory; all the evidence that I can collect is adverse to it. The supposed new row is a mere deception, arising partly from the irregular, though natural, manner in which the cilia are placed, owing to the different planes in which their follicles lie; a fact which seems to be frequently overlooked, although noticed by the earlier anatomists; and partly from the more apparent isolated position of those which are turned in from their fellows that are set more externally. This distichiasis may be artificially produced, and the permanent misdirection accurately imitated in a perfectly healthy eyelid, by separating the inner row of the cilia, and bending them towards the eyeball. Again, the usual number of cilia in a healthy eyelid is not exceeded in these cases; this can be demonstrated when one eye only is affected. But the crowning argument against the growth of supplemental hairs is, that there is no such thing as a secondary formation of hair in any part of the surface of the body, the hair-follicles being all of primary development. It is well known that hair is occasionally found in the ovaries, and other situations where it is not a natural product; still this is no argument for its abnormal position on the eyelids. Its growth on parts that have been repeatedly blistered, has suggested the idea that it might likewise be generated in the eyelids as a result of chronic inflammation. Experience does not support this theory, which is advanced in ignorance of the fact that the surface of the human body at the time of birth equals, if not surpasses, in the number of hair-follicles, that of any other animal; and when, from accidental causes in after life, hair springs forth, it is owing merely to hyper-nutrition of original germs.

The utmost that can be urged is, that in the eyelid an animating influence might be exerted on dormant bulbs; but the arrangement of the parts renders most doubtful the existence of such an occult capability.

Some surgeons, who are not disposed to believe in the creation of new hairs, assert that the displaced cilia are growths from old follicles, which pierce the eyelid in the wrong place. But this is both anatomically and pathologically incorrect; for the internal cilia are close against the cartilage, and issue by the side of the edge, as near to it as it is possible.

Excluding chemical and traumatic injuries to the eyelids, most of the causes, direct and remote, that produce trichiasis, are palpable. The inversion may be a permanent state of distortion of the cilia by some mechanical means, without any diseased condition, of which the matting together of them in chronic purulent discharges from the conjunctiva, and the attendant misdirection, is an example. Or it may be an idiopathic affection, due to certain pathological changes in the edges of the eyelid itself, nearly all of which arise from strumous inflammation; not always, it is true, very apparent, but, when the trichiasis is extensive, generally well marked. I may mention that sometimes the eyelashes are twisted in many directions. The next illustration was from an unusually severe case.

FIG. 29.

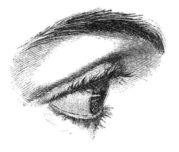

The upper eyelid, the only one affected, had been involved in chronic inflammation for three years, and was much thickened at the edge. The cilia were healthy, none of them were lost, or imperfectly formed, but they were scattered. There were two well-marked rows, the upper of which, from its unnaturally high position, had as much the appearance of a new row as the under, from its inner position, had of a supernumerary growth. Not the least interesting fact is, that a year after the sketch was taken, when the inflammatory symptoms had declined, and the edge of the eyelid was nearly reduced to a natural state, the cilia had in a great measure regained their lost relations, and the duplex arrangement was no longer recognisable, a mere bushiness remaining.

With disarrangement of the cilia there may be imperfect development, or abortive reproduction, arising from disease of the hair-follicles, or from frequent plucking. The last is a common cause.

When a malady is so apparent, it might, perhaps, seem superfluous to speak of its effect on the eyeball as a means of diagnosis, on the supposition that whenever these effects have attracted notice the cause also would be self-evident. But such is not generally the case; were it otherwise, there would be an end of that misdirected, and injurious local and general treatment so frequently adopted, in the desire to dissipate inflammatory affections of the eye, in reality owing to the presence of trichiasis, but ascribed to various causes. The cilia that fret the eye, may be so minute as to escape the observation of those unaccustomed to search for them. Even with a knowledge of their presence, their exact position may not readily be detected, and minuteness does not diminish their powers of mischief. Therefore, with the sensation of something in the eye, attended by continued inflammation of the conjunctiva, or of the cornea, or superficial ulceration of the cornea with or without opacity, and with any of these states, intolerance of light, the existence of trichiasis may be suspected. It is no uncommon circumstance for the individual who suffers from its effects to be ignorant of its presence. The following case, one of the many that I have met with, exemplifies how the true cause of opacity of the cornea may be overlooked ; and also shows what slight mechanical causes will produce the loss of lustre of that part.

A man, aged thirty-one, presented himself at the Ophthalmic Hospital, to be treated for an affection of the right eye. My attention was attracted to the condition of the cornea of the left, which was densely opaque in the upper half, and hazy in the remainder ; and the cause of which I quickly discovered in two inverted cilia of the upper eyelid, about the eighth of an inch apart, that rested on the cornea. There was scarcely any power of vision remaining. To use the man's words, the sight had been failing for several years, treatment was ineffectual, and as it was becoming more and more dim, he regarded the eye as lost. He was totally unconscious that cilia were inverted, and was sure that none had ever been plucked out in treatment—a proof that the true nature of the case had been overlooked.

A young woman had an inverted cilium in each upper eyelid that touched the cornea and produced ulceration, which ended in penetration and prolapse of the iris. After this, as the cicatrix on each eye was insensible, there was no more irritation. The appearance of the two eyes was remarkably symmetrical. The poor creature was nearly blind. She told me that all the treatment she received had been directed to the inflamed state of the eyeballs.

In Mr. Liston's museum there was a preparation exhibiting four or five delicate eyelashes, which, as in the case above, not only cost the patient her sight, but were the cause of ruin to her constitution, through the use of fruitless antiphlogistics to subdue the inflammation that they produced.

The treatment of trichiasis is palliative and temporary, or radical and permanent. Of the palliative, that alone is worthy of notice which is so naturally resorted to—the pulling out of the cilia by forceps. Of a means so generally adopted, and apparently so universally applicable, it is well to ascertain in what species of implication it is advisable to be practised, and, besides this, how long in any instance it may be persevered in. The condition of the cilia that irritate, and the state of the eyelid on which they are seated, should be taken into consideration. When the irritation is occasioned by a few well-formed, but inverted ones proceeding from a healthy eyelid, there cannot be a doubt about the propriety of using the cilia-forceps, because there may not be a return of the inversion ; and even if the hairs so treated show on their reproduction a tendency to become distorted to a like degree, their injurious effect can be anticipated, and the process of extraction repeated. It thus becomes a mere matter of consideration to the patient whether he shall submit to the periodic repetition of the process, or to a rather more severe or effectual plan, resulting in a cure. But when the extraction is followed by an increase in the number of inverted cilia, or by abortive ones, the application of the cilia-forceps has reached its limit, and, as a rule, should be discontinued. There cannot be a doubt that the continued removal of the cilia by force is very frequently hurtful to their follicles, renders the direction of them more perverse, causes abortive productions, tends to involve the contiguous follicles, to increase the trichiasis, and should not be persevered in except at the particular request of the patient. So also, where the eyelid is unhealthy, and the offending cilia, although few in number, are abortive, and grow directly inwards, extraction is contra-indicated : some effectual treatment only is admissible; for in the majority of such cases, with all the vigilance of both patient and surgeon, and weekly extraction practised, there will be an impossibility of keeping the globe of the eye exempt from their contact. The majority of such fine cilia are not in reality plucked out, but are broken off, and with any accession of growth, again exert their injurious effect, long before the eye recovers from the last irritation. Notwithstanding the gradual deterioration of the state of the eye under this palliative treatment, patients will still desire a continuance of it ; and the careful use of the forceps will greatly delay the arrival of its worst effects, while their careless application will hasten it. The proper way of using this instrument is to press on the upper or the under part of the tarsus, according to the eyelid affected, evert its edge, apply the points close to the cilium as it emerges, and pull it out in the direction of its growth.

The radical cure consists in the adoption of some operative measure by which the maldirection of the cilia is influenced, or by which they are removed or amputated, or destroyed.

The excision of a portion of the palpebral skin, in depth and extent proportionate to the required effect, to give a slight outward position to the edge of the tarsus, is a very valuable resource, applicable frequently to the upper eyelid, and nearly always practicable in the lower. It is suited to those cases in which the cilia retain their proper size, are merely slightly misdirected, and just touch the globe of the eye, and exceptionally to abortive cilia that do not grow as much towards the eyeball as usual; and, it may be, its greatest extent of application is to be found when the central cilia are affected. Its adaptation to any given case is readily decided by rendering the skin of the eyelid tense, and observing the effect. It is difficult to point out what degree of inversion may be so treated—that must be left to the judgment of the surgeon; yet this may be said, that whenever the eyeball can be just cleared by the greatest admissible amount of eversion, the principle is yet available, for in all probability there will be improvement when the irritation of the eye, and consequent swelling of the eyelid, have ceased.

I operate in this way in the worst cases; that is, when I wish to act on the entire length of the tarsus. An assistant stands behind the patient, makes the eyelid tense by drawing its external angle outwards and raising the eyebrow. With a scalpel, I cut through the skin in the direction of the lines on the eyelid in the following diagram, making the under incision the first, and, with the aid of the forceps, dissect off the flap, commencing at the inner angle, and endeavour not to interfere with the subjacent muscle. The sponge, if required, should be used by a third person when he can be commanded. I apply three or four sutures. As regards a local application, water-dressing, or greased lint, may be used. I employ nothing unless the eyelid be unhealthy, when one or the other is chosen; the latter when it is likely that trouble will not be taken to renew the wet lint sufficiently often, and to apply it neatly and properly.

The upper incision is not so readily accomplished as the under; and I recommend those who are not in the constant habit of operating, after the first incision has been made, to lay hold of the centre of the upper portion of the skin with the forceps, and draw it downwards, and thus secure it for the second cut. In operating on the right eye, as a matter of convenience the dissection should be made from the inner to the outer corner of the flap. The operation on the under lid in nowise differs in principle from that on the upper. The variation in the detail of the position of the assistant, and the advantage of making

FIG. 30.

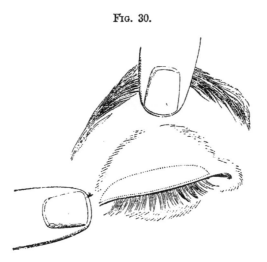

the under incision first, include the dissimilar points. Should circumstances render it necessary that the operation be performed in a recumbent position, it may be found more convenient to stand behind than at the side of the patient. All that the alteration of position requires, is to reverse the order of incisions, making the upper in each eyelid the first.

The partial operation is to be done in like manner, but it cannot be generally depended on, except a strip of skin not less long than half the width of the eyelid be removed.

After several years' experience in this operation, I am unaware of a single drawback. It does not interfere with the proper escape of the lacrymal secretions. The positions of the puncta are not altered.

A young woman, who was obliged to leave her situation from the effects of trichiasis, was sent to me. The central cilia of the upper eyelid, and the outer ones of the lower, were inverted, and rested on the cornea. The cilia-forceps had been repeatedly used. I operated on each eye. The sketch below shows the state of the eyelids seven months after the operation, and it exemplifies the peculiar adaptation of the principle to the lower eyelid, where the cilia that were completely reversed were made to clear the eyeball.

FIG. 31.

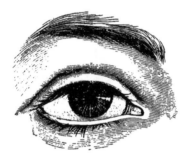

J. O., aged eleven years, came to the Central London Ophthalmic Hospital. His mother's account was, that soon after an attack of measles in infancy his eyes became weak, and never regained strength: for the last seven or eight years he had suffered from intolerance of light and lacrymation, while the inability to use his eyes had prevented his learning to read, or attending to any kind of employment. In the left eye two bunches of cilia,—one from the outer part of the eyelid, where in this instance the cilia were large and long, and the other from the centre,—rested on the globe of the eye. The cornea was opaque, the greater part densely so, with adhesion of the iris to it, in consequence of former ulceration. The pupil was nearly closed; the conjunctiva was highly inflamed, and vision almost extinct.

In the right eye a single bunch of cilia from the central part of the eyelid turned in; the whole surface of the cornea was ulcerated, but without being opaque; the conjunctiva was nearly like that of the other eye, and vision was very imperfect. In both there was thickening of the tarsi. The removal of skin on each side was sufficient to separate the cilia from the eyeballs. The first time I saw this lad after the operation, which was on the third day, he expressed great relief. He came only twice afterwards to the hospital. What might have been the nature of the early affection, or how long the trichiasis had existed, or in what order the several changes in the eye occurred, it is impossible to say.

It must be apparent that only with a knife can the skin be incised with that accuracy and closeness along the edge of the tarsus which are necessary; but even if the scissors could be equally efficacious, the conspicuous scar that is inseparable from their use, is more than enough to proscribe them.

Another measure is the excision of the cilia; it is an effectual remedy in all stages of their inversion, but the operation produces deformity, and disfiguration about the face is secondary in importance only to disease; besides, the injury that is inflicted on the meibomian glands, by some supposed to be of little importance, should induce us to reserve excision as a last or only resource—for such cases only in which the above operation is inapplicable. It is a very common impression that with care the glands may be avoided; but I cannot understand how a dissection in the living subject that shall remove the cilia in an effectual manner, can fail also to bring away a portion of the cartilage, and, therefore, to a greater or lesser extent, injure and destroy the meibomian glands. The objection applies chiefly to complete amputation. Partial excision is much less severe, and may often be advantageously resorted to when it is expedient to get rid of a cluster of eyelashes.

The following display of the cilia, by the removal of the integuments and muscle, may be a useful reminder of their position on the cartilages. The eyelids are supposed to be laid flat, and the lower cilia are turned up to afford the best view. The irregular manner in which they are planted in the dense fibro-cellular tissue, admits the entire extent of only the most superficial to be

exposed.   The specimen was taken from an adult female, and
the natural size has been preserved.

FIG. 32.

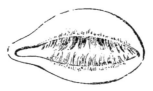

This second diagram shows the edge of the lids in profile, and
exhibits the relations of the several parts.

FIG. 33.

For the partial excision, the eyelid should be secured, as in
the foregoing diagram for the removal of the skin; an incision
made on either side of the bunch to be taken away, long
enough to reach beyond their follicles and through the skin and
orbicularis muscle, and a third transversely, at the very edge of
the eyelid, falling in with the two vertical ones, as in fig. 34;
the little flap raised and entrusted to the care of an assistant,

FIG. 34.

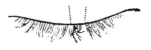

who keeps it turned up with an instrument or his finger, the
bleeding checked, the mass of follicles, with the investing tissue,
carefully hooked with the tenaculum forceps and dissected out
with the small scalpel.   The flap is then to be restored and
retained by three sutures, one on each edge.   Sometimes a strip
of court plaster will suffice.   Unless the skin be raised to a greater
extent than will merely uncover the cilia, there would be a

deficiency of space for operating efficiently, and the base of the flap, which I generally make broader than the apex, would not be sufficiently wide to insure its vitality. The destruction of healthy cilia is inevitable; no one who has dissected the edge of the eyelid, and made himself conversant with the parts, will sanction any method of operating by which it is proposed to remove a given number of irregular lashes, without injuring contiguous ones. Dr. Mackenzie performs this operation

FIG. 35.

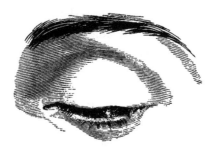

by the transverse incision only. The above illustration of partial removal from the upper eyelid, was taken four months after the operation.

The patient, a female forty years of age, had been long tormented by ten or twelve cilia that rested on the globe of the eye; they were very minute and white, and grew directly inwards. She had given a long trial to the cilia-forceps.

The partial operation may be done in two places on the same eyelid.

To remove a portion of the entire thickness of the eyelid with the cilia, is an operation of old date. It occasions much deformity. Mr. Tyrrell, who had much experience, after advising the measure, where several cilia are inverted together, says, "Such a plan is not, however, advisable when there are many cilia remaining, as the contraction of the new cicatrix is very likely to produce inversion of some of the neighbouring hairs. The patient must therefore be contented with having them extracted with forceps whenever their growth occasions the slightest irritation."

The entire excision is called for where there is inversion of the hairs in several places. The indications are to remove the cilia with as little damage as possible to the tarsal cartilage, and to leave the punctum lacrymale untouched.

When the tarsal margin is sufficiently healthy to admit of the plan, I always endeavour to save the skin by reflecting it. The eyelid is fixed as above; three incisions are made, one at each corner, and one along the margin; the skin and muscle are then raised and held back, the cilia dissected off, and a few sutures applied. It requires great caution not to allow some of them to escape; and unless the tenaculum forceps be used, and the sponge be nicely employed by the assistant, so that the operator may clearly see the several steps of his course, a few are likely to be left behind. More care is required than might be supposed.

The following diagram shows the lines the knife should take.

FIG. 36.

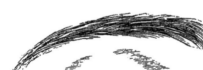

When the parts will not allow of this, there must be more of an amputation; the skin being necessarily removed with the eyelashes. An incision is made through the skin and the muscle, at about the eighth of an inch above the tarsal margin, from the outer angle, nearly to the punctum, or from within to without, according to the eye to be treated, as in the next diagram; the end seized with the forceps, made tense, and skin, muscle, and cilia all dissected off in a mass in a vertical direction. Some of the cartilage is necessarily removed. The dotted line in the engraving shows the direction to be taken. This is far preferable to cutting through the entire thickness of the eyelid.

FIG. 37.

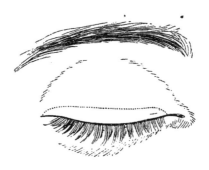

The execution is necessarily slow, from the frequent demand for the sponge. Should any of the cilia-bulbs escape detachment—a point ascertained by scrutinising the denuded surface, or the part excised—they must be removed. It is seldom that a few fine hairs at the inner corner are not left; indeed such must happen when they grow over and a little beyond the punctum; but it matters little, as they are very rarely inverted, and may be eradicated if they cause any inconvenience. The edge of the cartilage and that of the skin, may be brought together with accuracy by a few sutures.

Here is an example of double excision. The lower eyelid

FIG. 38.

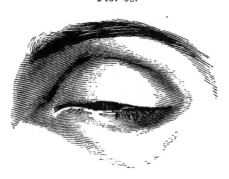

was operated on by a surgeon, long since deceased: the intention was not quite fulfilled, for the greater number of the cilia

M

escaped the knife, the central ones only having been removed;
and when there was a fresh growth of those that had been
merely cut across, trichiasis was re-established. I excised a
piece of skin, everted the tarsal margin, and rectified the evil.
I also performed entire excision on the upper eyelid. It was
considered by the artist that a sketch, with the eyelids approximated, would give the best representation.

In these several operations, some surgeons place a spatula of
wood or bone under the eyelid ; and if an operator finds any
such appliance of use, he should employ it.

Other methods of treatment have, during centuries, accumulated into a long catalogue. They consist for the most part in
different kinds of cauterization of the eyelid, or of the cilia-
bulbs, with the actual cautery, or escharotics; but the greater
part of them are obsolete, and need not be further mentioned.
Others are, in my judgment, far inferior to the surgical measures I have advanced. Mr. Wilde's ingenious .plan I have
not tried. In a paper on Entropium and Trichiasis in the
" Dublin Journal of Medical Science" for 1844, that excellent
surgeon writes: " A single lash, or one or two lashes, will
sometimes turn in upon the eye and produce the greatest annoyance: the patient gets tired of plucking them out, and applies
for surgical relief. In such cases, placing the horn-spatula
within the lid, I make an incision with a small knife down to
the root of the inverted lash, and, having waited till the hæmorrhage has ceased, I apply a point of nitrate of silver by means
of a small port-caustic, down to the bottom of the wound, and
then remove the lash ; it seldom fails, but frequently it destroys
two or three of the neighbouring cilia. Partial distichiasis
also, or more extended trichiasis, may likewise be successfully
treated by the same means."

Perhaps I ought to mention that of Dr. J. Hunter's, somewhat allied to Mr. Wilde's, and published in the " Edinburgh
Monthly Journal " for April, 1841. " A puncture is made over
the bulbs of the cilia that offend, and tartar emetic is introduced
on a probe which is charged with this substance, by first coating

it with a thin layer of sealing-wax, and dipping it when hot into the powder. The cilia are then plucked out. Sub-acute inflammation is induced, and the cilia-follicles perish."

I have seen the tartar emetic introduced on a lancet-point, after a previous incision through the edge of the eyelid. I cannot speak favourably of it.

I do not propose to improve a patient's appearance by supplying cilia for those that have been removed, either by the surgeon's hand or by disease; but I quote a passage on the subject, which occurs in a review of Dieffenbach's "Operative Surgery," in vol. xxi. of the "British and Foreign Medical Review," under the heading, "Transplantation of the Eyelashes."

"It has been established by experiment, that strong hairs freshly plucked take root when they are inserted into small oblique punctures, and protected by slips of plaster. The hair must be strong and young, not just about to fall away. Greyness of the hair is of no consequence, as it is the age of the hair, not the individual, that is to be considered. Dzondi was the first to apply these physiological facts in practical surgery, planting a row of cilia upon an artificial eyelid. Dieffenbach does not appear to have followed his example, but he says, to increase the satisfaction of the patient in a case of successful blepharoplasty, the necessary quantity of cilia might be plucked from the other eye by forceps, and inserted in small oblique punctures half a line in depth, made along the lower border of the eyelid, the parts being then covered with fine straps of plaster."

Trichiasis is often associated with slight entropium. This is treated of under the subdivision, "Entropium with trichiasis."

ENTROPIUM.

Idiopathic entropium, or turning in of the edge of the eyelid, is met with in two states: in an acute or spasmodic form, for the most part occurring in old people, and almost always confined to the lower eyelid, the tarsal margin being healthy, and the eyelid capable of being readily righted, or returned to its place ; and in a chronic form, which may affect both eyelids, is for the most part associated with more or less inflammation of the tarsal edge—whereby the cilia are mal-directed or influenced, the pliancy of the parts lost—and is generally seen in the upper eyelid.

Of the many opinions respecting the presumed origins of this derangement, some are obsolete, and need not be recounted : but others, such as relaxation of the skin of the eyelid; thickening of the palpebral conjunctiva ; shrinking of the tarsal cartilages; occasional faulty action of the orbicularis palpebrarum muscle combined with one or other of those states; are yet entertained, and ingeniously advocated by their several propounders. I ascribe the disease to faulty muscular action alone.

To say that looseness of the skin allows inversion of the tarsus, would be to affirm that, in a healthy eye, the skin is antagonistic to some power acting on the eyelids; a statement unphysiological and erroneous. The skin is never tense, but always loose, as a natural provision for unrestrained movements ; and this is especially exemplified in the upper eyelid, where the motions are freer than those of the under. Moreover, the skin here is singularly thin, and apparently devoid of elasticity ; or, at most, possesses it in a minimum degree ; and were it required to show more than this, I might point to the baggy and even sometimes pendulous state of it in advancing life, coexistent with the perfect integrity of the ocular appendages.

The supposed influence of the palpebral conjunctiva in producing inversion, has been taught for more than two hundred years ; but it appears to me, that the morbid changes it may acquire are merely the effect of the general irritation of the eye, due to the inversion ; for, in incipient entropium, I have not been able to satisfy myself of any condition that may not be seen in a healthy eye. After a time, which varies according to circumstance, when the entire conjunctiva is involved in that general inflammation which is sure to ensue in the progress of the affection, it exhibits various appearances, which, as far I can make out, differ in no respect from those the result of inflammation from other causes, and from which the eyelid does not become curved.

That the unnatural state of the eyelid might depend on some primary change in the shape of the tarsal cartilage, seems probable, and this is the theory most generally received as true. To examine into its correctness, cases should be chosen for the investigation in which the tarsal cartilages have not suffered from disease, and there will be no difficulty in finding such.

It will simplify the inquiry even more to look principally to an inverted lower eyelid, because it offers a greater facility for observation, as the natural direction of its border is outwards, and away from the globe of the eye; and any change in its direction can be better appreciated than in the upper, where the margin inclines somewhat inwards. Besides, there is a very marked difference in the size of the two cartilages, and this may throw additional light on the inquiry, the upper being considerably broader than the under, as the outline of them below shows.

FIG. 39.

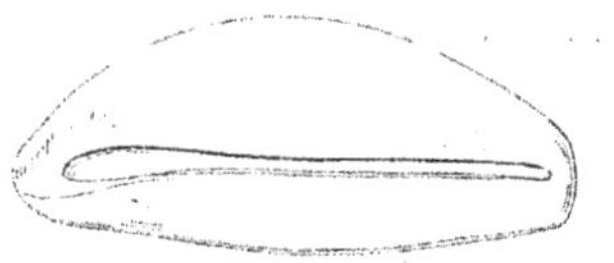

In the most marked or aggravated stage of entropium in the under eyelid, the narrow cartilage does not rest against the eyeball, as though it bound it, because it is contracted; but it is so completely turned on itself, and rolled upon the eyelid, that its position is completely reversed, and the cilia are hidden. It is dislocated in a manner which I attempt to explain by the next diagram.

It is evident, from the narrowness of the cartilage, that no curve of it, nor any kind of contraction, could produce these changes. But, more than this, I have never been able to satisfy myself that the cartilage is ever altered or modified; and if not, it cannot have any degree of influence in producing the inversion.

FIG. 40.

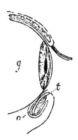

g, The eyeball.   *c*, The cilium.   *t*, The tarsal cartilage.

In entropium of the upper eyelid, the inverted cartilage rests against the eyeball, and the convexities of the cilia are then on the cornea, while their extremities are directed outwards—a position that their ends assume from the handkerchief being used in that direction during the frequent calls for its application. In some aggravated cases they lie spread out on the globe of the eye. Now, this difference in the direction of the edges of the eyelids ought not, I think, to be attributed to dissimilar causes, but to that acting on the dissimilar physical constructions of the eyelids themselves. Thus the upper cartilage is merely curved, because its breadth does not allow it to be rolled up, like the lower.

The influence of muscular power has heretofore been regarded merely as a partial and secondary cause, blended with one of the supposed primary causes that I have examined. The general opinion is, that its detrimental action is induced by tegumentary disarrangements, by relaxation, or by swelling of the skin over the eyelid, by which its influence in supporting the muscular fibres of that part is lost, while the remainder of the muscle on which the skin yet acts continues its function, and rolls the edges of the cartilage inwards. That the action of the orbicularis depends on the binding of the skin is an assertion thoroughly untenable.

The similarity of curvature in every case of entropium, the

implication of the whole eyelid, and the symmetry of the deformity, induced me to attribute all forms of the affection to one and the same cause—that of muscular action ; but doubting the power of that part of the muscle situated on the edge of the lid, which is described as the thinnest portion of the orbicularis, to exercise such an action,—and from that part alone could such effect be produced,—I made dissections, to satisfy myself of its real nature. I found that over the edges of the eyelids, for about the sixth of an inch, the muscle is thicker, perhaps twice as thick as over the remainder of them ; the fibres also were redder, larger, and more compact. In the lower eyelid the marginal portion is even greater, and the fibres lie irregularly in bundles.

This fact seems to have been generally overlooked by modern anatomists, as a reference to their works will testify.

The late Mr. Dalrymple, in his " Anatomy of the Human Eye," says :—

" The few pale and horizontal fibres which immediately cover the tarsal cartilages, and which are continued to the edge of the palpebral fissure itself, have received the name of musculus ciliaris."

About the time that I was investigating this muscular origin of entropium, one of my colleagues at the Central London Ophthalmic Hospital, showed me that he could, by the influence of the will, invert the edges of both his lower eyelids, produce the most complete entropium, and conceal his long and numerous cilia. Of course this greatly strengthened my opinion, and I did not hesitate to regard my idea of the cause of entropium as correct. After that I made some dissections to ascertain the relation of the tensor tarsi muscle to the orbicularis, and was not a little surprised to find that it has an extensive connexion with that muscle, and may justly be considered a part of it, that part which has a bony attachment. The correct anatomy, and the relations of this the supplemental portion, have hitherto, it appears to me, not been correctly understood.

Were I to speak of it as a distinct muscle, and to give the description from a well-developed example, I should say it arises as a thin plane of well-marked muscular fibres, of about the fourth of an inch in breadth, from the vertical ridge on the lacrymal bone, passes forwards and outwards towards the lacrymal sac, and bifurcates in a remarkably distinct manner, the branches proceeding towards the eyelids, and on their edges become blended with the orbicularis muscle; they can be traced to the middle of the eyelid. In their passage they distribute fibres to the posterior surfaces of the puncta, and some few would seem to surround them. The best manner of dissecting the muscle is to remove the skin from the orbicularis, then to detach the upper and outer walls of the orbit, divide the optic nerve and the muscles around, and draw the back of the eye outwards and forwards.

There is great variety in the development of this muscle, and also in the portion of the orbicularis that lies on the edges of the tarsal cartilages. Occasionally, it is scarcely possible with the naked eye to recognise the muscularity of the fibres.

It is not surprising that, as the anatomy of the tensor tarsi had not been ascertained, its physiology was only partly understood, and no pathological state conceived. As far as I can ascertain, with the exception of Dr. Physic, who took the most extended view of its action, and justly supposed that it must exert some influence on the movements of the eyelids, writers have confined its use to the apparatus for conveying away the tears. In the last edition of Dr. Quain's "Anatomy," by Dr. Sharpey, it is called " musculus sacci lacrymalis."

Although I am now satisfied as to the true cause of entropium, it is as difficult, nay, impossible, to decide what are the circumstances that bring about such unequal and prejudicial action of the orbicularis, as to account for squinting, or other deformities, the result of perverted muscular action. These occur without the perceptible influence of any cause; and the most that can be said of them is, that sometimes they follow other pathological phenomena of common occurrence. They are then regarded as excitants, and, in the case of entropium, conjunctival inflammation would, sometimes in the chronic form, seem to stand in that relation.

I have founded the treatment on what appears to me to be the pathological interpretation of the affection, and of which the indications are, to overcome the means of the inversion by dissecting away the marginal thick portion of the orbicularis, supposing that part of the muscle to be almost, or exclusively at fault; also to remove as much of the skin of the eyelid as may be necessary to produce such tension as shall overcome the deformity which other tissues of the eyelid may have acquired, from the irregular position into which they have been thrown by the muscle, and which, in many instances, become more or less influenced by any existing inflammatory state. In a few instances of acute entropium of the lower eyelid, of short duration, I have dissected out the muscular tissue only, and with success. The practice has been adopted by Mr. R. Taylor. I doubt not that it would suffice in most of these cases if done very early, but usually patients do not apply till the changes alluded to in the other parts of the eyelid have occurred, and then the skin must be removed as well.

I have been practising the operation now for many years, and have applied it to hundreds of cases, and with the most unreserved satisfaction. In acute entropium it is all-sufficient; in chronic entropium, generally nothing more is needed. When, however, the tarsal edge is very much thickened and hardened, or when there coexists severe trichiasis, it is insufficient alone: the cilia must also be excised, or perhaps even the edge of the tarsus cut off.

In an ordinary uncomplicated case I operate in this way. Let me suppose that the upper eyelid of the right eye is to be rectified. An assistant stands behind the patient, and having made the eyelid tense, by drawing it outwards and raising the brow, as is shown in the operation for trichiasis, the surgeon makes two incisions through the skin and the muscular fibres, in the course indicated by the lines in the following diagram. This will include what I shall call the ciliary portion of the muscle.

The flap thus outlined is drawn forwards, and slowly dissected by vertical strokes of the knife, from the one side to the other, and not taken away by horizontal cuts, or else the muscular portion will not be effectually removed. The wound

FIG. 41.

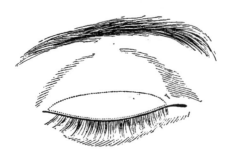

should be very carefully sponged during the operation. Any arterial jet must be checked by sufficient pressure with the finger. I have never found a ligature to be necessary. The exposed surface must be inspected; and if any muscular fibres have escaped, the forceps and knife must be re-applied. The assistant should continue the proper retraction of the skin till the knife has been laid aside, as essential to steady and effectual dissection. Three or four sutures should be used; and if a patient desire some local treatment, water-dressing may be employed. Union is always effected by first intention.

Various moral and physical states of individuals require different constitutional treatment. Those who are nervous and highly excitable had better be kept quiet for a day or two, with the eyelid in as perfect a state of rest as possible. One class of patients will resume their usual avocations directly after the operation, while another will require a cessation from all activity.

The surgeon and his assistant must take their positions according to the eye to be operated on. Sometimes, and especially if the patient be lying, the operator may find it better to stand behind; and the left eye may thus be more readily reached.

The cilia might appear to be in danger of being dissected off, but in reality they are not. A part only of the dissection is over them; and the muscle is readily raised, in consequence of its looseness, from the dense fibro-cellular tissue in which they lie.

Inversion of the upper eyelid produces severer symptoms than that of the under; because of the constant contact of the cilia with the globe of the eye in all the stages of the affection, and in certain cases from increased irritation due to thickening and induration of the tarsal edge. A feeling of something in the eye, followed by ulceration and opacity of the cornea, and either partial destruction of the eye for visual purposes, or loss of vision from opacity of the cornea, or of changes in its entire parts, resulting from general inflammation, followed by atrophy, are its consequences. A common termination is, after months, or it may be years, of suffering, for the conjunctiva to become thickened and insensible,—a kind of natural cure, or at least a conservative effect. But the course depends on the degree of the entropium, the condition of the cilia, the state of the edge of the eyelid, and the constitution on which the local irritation acts.

F. B., a pale, thin, and lax-fibred girl, aged twenty, with abundant lacrymation, and intolerance of light, suffered from entropium of both upper eyelids; the right was the more turned in of the two, and the cilia of each, except a few fine ones at the corners, rested on the globes of the eyes. The conjunctivæ were very highly inflamed. The edges of the eyelids were not in the least thickened, nor was trichiasis present; so that when their edges were turned out, the lashes were nearly in their natural position, being necessarily a little disarranged. The upper parts of both corneæ were hazy, the left being the less affected. Although of long standing, the effects were not very severe, but the mildness of the symptoms was evidently attributable to the paucity of the cilia, their delicacy and their shortness, for few of them were of ordinary length; and to this also must be ascribed her immunity from pain.

The illustration is an accurate representation of the right eye in profile, taken the day before I operated.

I removed rather more skin along with the muscle from this eye than from the left, which was treated at the same time. On

the third day the sutures were removed, and the patient left
the hospital for home.

FIG. 42.

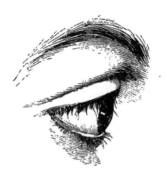

Three months after, she called to show herself. Faint scars
merely indicated the operations. The lacrymation and intolerance of light, and the conjunctival inflammation, had passed
away. The right cornea had much improved in transparency,
and the left was nearly natural, there being only a little loss of
lustre. I now discovered that she was near-sighted. The

FIG. 43.

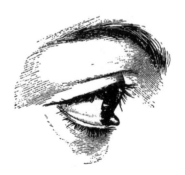

annexed sketch, taken at the latter period, shows the eyelid
righted, and the cilia raised.

E. H., a female, aged thirty, a patient at the Central London
Ophthalmic Hospital. The upper tarsal cartilage of the left eye
was inverted, and nearly all the cilia were resting on the globe

of the eye, causing considerable irritation; the cornea was ulcerated and hazy. The eyelid bore on its upper part near the orbit a large and peculiarly disfiguring scar, the result of the removal of a portion of the skin with scissors in an attempt to remedy the deformity. The right eyelid, which was divided in the middle, had been successfully operated on by snipping off a portion of skin, subsequent applications of nitric acid, and central division of the tarsus. I operated on the left eye after the manner I have advocated, and with success, as shown in Fig. 44.

FIG. 44.

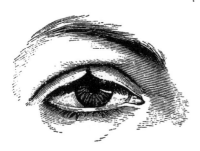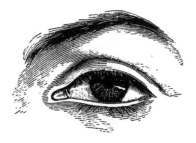

Entropium of the under eyelid is not, generally speaking, a very serious affection; the cilia are finer, shorter, and less numerous than those of the upper, and from their mode of insertion, and the lowness of the lid, they rarely come in contact with the cornea. When they do encroach on it, opacity is seldom produced, and their presence on the conjunctiva of the

FIG. 45.

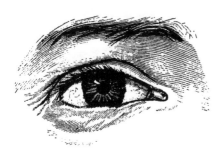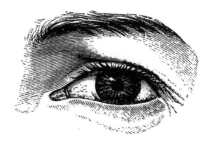

sclerotica is less irritating. In well-marked cases there may be no more inconvenience than conjunctival inflammation, with

slight lacrymation, and gumming together of the eyelids at
night. Even with complete inversion, the eyeball does not
suffer as in that of the upper eyelid; because the cilia no
longer recline upon it, and the tarsal cartilage being folded
inwards, they are put out of the way, and lie at the bottom
of the eye in the sinus of the conjunctiva. But before this
state of perfect inversion arrives, the eyeball has generally
become more or less tolerant to the contact of the cilia; because
very slight structural change in the conjunctiva, which is soon
set up, is sufficient to defend it from their irritation.

The foregoing sketch, taken from an old man, represents a case
of inversion, in which the right eyelid was completely turned
in, and the left only tilted or half inverted, with the cilia on
the globe of the eye.

M. H., aged sixty-seven. In the left eye the cilia were
thrown against the globe of the eye; some of them rested on
the cornea without sullying its transparency. The conjunctiva
was much inflamed; there was constant lacrymation, a white
frothy secretion at the edges of both the lids, and a sensation
of something in the eye. The integument just under the tarsal
cartilages bulged in a singular manner. In the right eye the
lid edge was completely inverted, there was only slight conjunctival inflammation, trifling lacrymation, and but little
uneasiness. Each affection had existed a year and a half.

The next figure was taken three months after operation.

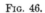

FIG. 46.

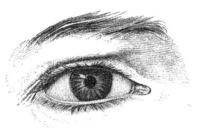
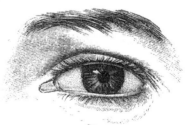

Usually, it is not requisite to dissect out more of the skin
than will admit of the easy removal of the ciliary portion of the
muscle.

It would be natural to assume that in proportion to the degree of incurvation of the tarsus must be the amount to be taken; yet that does not invariably follow. The sequence depends upon the actual condition of the tissues of the eyelid, and the means of resistance needed to overcome the inversion; and in the upper eyelid especially, the state of the cartilage is of importance, for much depends upon its flexibility, whether perfect or impaired. Where the edge of the eyelid is a little thickened and indurated, and not quite so easily acted upon; and in the entropium of the aged, where, from the retraction and reduction of the eye, perhaps also of the proper tissues of the eyelid, and the natural tendency to tegumentary folding, a larger amount must be excised, but not more than is necessary to reduce the edge of the lid to its correct position. Eversion must not be produced. The cause of the deformity being taken away, there cannot be a return of the dislocation.

It is seldom that any trace of the operation is seen after the interval of a few months, sometimes weeks, provided that the edges of the skin have been brought neatly together, and the sutures taken out on the second or third day, and not allowed to be thrown off by ulceration.

The only indication of the former existence of disease that the eyelids exhibit, is the irregular disposition and staring arrangement which the cilia acquire from having been in contact with the globe of the eye, and subjected to its movements. The greater their length, the more abundant their growth, and the longer the duration of the inversion, the more is this apparent.

I shall cursorily review some other methods of operative treatment that are practised and recommended. The operations most commonly resorted to are: the removal of a transverse portion of the skin, by pinching it up with the finger, or by the entropium forceps—an instrument invented for the purpose—and cutting it off with a pair of scissors; and the destruction of the skin by caustic, or the actual cautery, in order to produce contraction.

That some improvement occasionally follows such contraction of skin, and that more frequently in the lower than in the upper lid, I am perfectly aware; but it is apparent in incipient cases only, and then it is for the most part temporary. In all well-marked instances, the above-mentioned methods scarcely improve them in the least. It is true that excision of the skin from the lower eyelid, to a considerable extent, may always be effectual in removing an entropium from it, owing to the configuration of its cartilage, as pointed out. But then to bring about this alteration by removal of the skin alone, the eyelid must actually be depressed or everted; and thus one evil would be exchanged for another.

There is, besides, the division of the outer commissure, and the vertical incision of the cartilage at the centre, after the manner of Ware. Also the vertical cut at each angle, the horizontal incision of the conjunctiva, and the elevation of the eyelid by an instrument called the suspensorium palpebrarum—a sort of elevator, during the healing process, after Sir Philip Crampton's plan. Then the still severer method of dividing the tarsal cartilage of the upper eyelid longitudinally as well as vertically, of the under eyelid vertically only, taking away a fold of the skin besides, and fastening the eyelid to the brow, or to the cheek, by means of several fine ligatures passed through its edge, and then secured by strips of plaster, for the space of eight or ten days, as recommended and practised by the late Mr. Guthrie, followed up by frequently touching the incision with sulphate of copper to ensure healing by granulation; but all are uncertain in confirmed entropium; for, with the cicatrization, the power of the muscle is wont to be renewed, and the entropium returns. This was proved nearly fifty years ago by Mr. Saunders, who recommended, when the upper eyelid was affected, excision of the whole tarsal cartilage. Mr. Wilde, too, has pointed out the inutility of the latter. One of his cases, in the person of a young female, had been under the hands of Mr. Guthrie himself. The upper eyelid curled up, the lower fell down, and the patient suffered from all the horrors of a double ectropium. From my own personal knowledge, I could advance several instances of its utter failure,— in all, the upper eyelid had been affected. When it does succeed, and which is only, as some authors seem to admit, in incipient entropium, there is danger of the sphincter power of the orbicularis palpebrarum muscle being lost, as Mr. Wilde has shown by a remarkable instance narrated and figured. It is to be hoped that such practice is now obsolete, and will never be revived.

Another mode is the excision of the cilia ; but their removal is an evil, that should, when possible, be avoided ; and as I have before said, they cannot be excised without injury to the meihomian glands. But the ill effects of entropium are not always due to the contact of the cilia on the eyeball. In the upper eyelid, the thick and hard edge of the tarsus is in itself a source of irritation to the eyeball. I have had several such cases in adults, in whom the cilia had been lost in childhood. I have seen the same from entropium of the lower eyelid of a female, from whom the cilia had been excised five years before.

ENTROPIUM WITH TRICHIASIS.

With inversion of the upper eyelid there is not unfrequently decided trichiasis; and whether, in any particular instance, the two affections are due to the same exciting cause, or the trichiasis has been the original affection, or merely an effect of the inversion, matters nothing so far as the treatment is concerned. I am, however, inclined to regard trichiasis more frequently as an effect, because it is generally of one form, that of a separation or twisting in of the innermost cilia from their fellows, without any alteration or degeneration in the individual hairs ; and because, for the most part, the removal of the entropium is generally sufficient to take it away. It is therefore important, before operating on any case, to ascertain whether trichiasis do exist, and to learn also, if possible, whether the restoration of the eyelid to its natural position will, or will not, counteract the maldirection of the hairs. Should it not, then more skin must be taken than would

N

otherwise have been necessary, and a slight degree of eversion of the centre of the tarsal margin produced. The amount is easily determined. When it is apparent that such moderate eversion will not suffice, the treatment must depend on the degree of the trichiasis; for if it be general, the entropium and the trichiasis must be attacked by one operation, and the cilia excised at the same time, after the rules given under the head of Trichiasis.

When the trichiasis is partial, as it is for the most part, the skin and the muscle should first be dissected away, and then the irregular cilia sought for and excised. When there is a doubt about the necessity of removing them, the entropium should be alone attended to, and the result observed; because it is not always possible, before the operation has been performed, the eyelid restored, as well as recovered from any inflammation and swelling that the inversion may have induced, to ascertain with exactness to what extent the trichiasis may be benefited.

With many of the cilia broken, and some just reproduced after having been plucked out, it cannot be known what direction they may assume when grown, and such a case should be watched.

It can be very seldom that the removal of entropium from the lower eyelid does not at the same time separate any irregular cilia from contact with the globe of the eye, for a single exception only has occurred to me.

The following case will illustrate some of the foregoing points:—A. C., a female, aged forty, with entropium and partial trichiasis of both upper eyelids of three years' standing. The corneæ were clouded in their entire extent, and studded with minute ulcers. Some of her cilia had been pulled out at various times; but getting worse, and the sight being nearly lost, she came to the Ophthalmic Hospital.

I removed more skin than was merely sufficient to restore the eyelids to their natural position, and thereby everted their centres a little. In nearly all cases of partial trichiasis, the central lashes offend. In the right eye the intention was answered; but in the left, a central bundle of cilia still touched the eyeball, and four weeks afterwards I extirpated it. In six weeks she was gaining her bread as a charwoman.

I have never seen the least unpleasant result from this slight eversion of the centre of the edge of the eyelid. Excision of the cilia does not admit of being compared with it as a curative measure.

It is only by observation that an adequate idea can be formed of the rapidity and extent of the recovery of the eye, and especially the cornea, from the effects of entropium. From the moment that the cilia cease to irritate, all the distressing symptoms begin to yield; and so quickly is repair exhibited, that on the third day, the period when I remove the sutures, cases have not been directly recognised by gentlemen who have assisted me with the operation; the conjunctiva having lost its vascularity, and lacrymation being subdued.

After-treatment is wholly unnecessary; a fact which confirms the statement, that the pathological changes in the conjunctiva are merely the consequences of the entropium, and not an independent affection.

The imperfect closure of the eyelids, a state that must more or less ensue when their edges are in any degree everted, is unproductive of any inconvenience.

It may be mentioned as a matter of pathological interest, that Mr. Wilde has met with congenital entropium, which he attributes to inflammation occurring in utero.

ENTROPIUM, WITH CONSIDERABLE THICKENING OF THE TARSAL MARGIN.

When entropium of the upper eyelid is associated with considerable changes in the physical character of the tarsal edge, from long-continued inflammation, by which it has been rendered thick and very hard, in which case I suspect that disease of the fibro-cellular tissue around the cilia-follicles plays no unimportant part, the ordinary operation for an inverted eyelid is not applicable. The point can always be readily determined, by trying how far the entropium can be covered by the fingers.

Generally little or no impression can be made on it, however much the eyelid be lifted.. The tarsal edge is so hard that it feels like a bit of wire under the skin. There is not necessarily trichiasis. In some of the worst cases that I have had to treat, the eyelashes have been neither irregular nor abortive, but still they act injuriously on the eyeballs. I have seen the corneæ with all the appearance of ligamentous structure.

My practice here is to excise the cilia and the diseased tarsal margin, with scalpel and forceps, and bring the edges together with a few sutures. There need be no apprehension about passing the threads through the cartilage.

ECTROPIUM.

Ectropium, or turning out of the eyelid, is the reverse of entropium, and is more rare. In aggravated cases, and especially when both the eyelids are everted, the eyeball may suffer from exposure and want of necessary moisture. In the ordinary, ro less severe states, and where only one eyelid is everted, disfiguration, and flowing of the lacrymal secretions over the cheek, are the immediate evils. But in every degree there is a remote risk of the injurious effects of inflammation of the eyeball, from perpetual exposure of the eye, and the inability of the eyelids to wipe off or brush aside intruding particles. The exposed palpebral conjunctiva is always unnaturally and highly vascular, and so is frequently the ocular also.

The causes of ectropium may be referred to two classes—that arising from accidental circumstances, and that which springs from some morbid change within the eyelids.

The first includes abscesses about the orbit, usually at the circumference ; burns ; scalds ; chemical injuries ; ulcerations, either simple or specific, as from syphilis, lupus, sloughing after erysipelas ; wounds ; contusions ; and surgical operations. Of these, the effect of the cicatrization of abscesses is by far the most frequent ; and the most usual seat of suppuration is the lower and outer part of the edge of the orbit.

I shall, in the first instance, speak of operations on the lower eyelid.

FIG. 47.

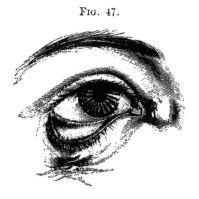

In Fig. 47 is illustrated a well-marked instance, from a child four years old. The scar on the side of the nose points out the remains of an abscess coeval with that on the cheek. Both were scrofulous, and unconnected with disease of the bone.

I select the case to illustrate the appropriate treatment of this kind of eversion. It is apparent that the great object is to procure a supply of healthy tissue to replace that which has been lost, and without which there can be no permanent improvement; so that when the eyelid is liberated and replaced, there shall be a continuity of healthy structure. The actual loss of skin from the abscess in such cases is, in fact, very slight. It is mainly the cellular tissue that is destroyed by suppuration, the contraction from the loss of which pulls aside the skin, and ties or binds it down. Merely to release the eyelid from its adhesion by any plan of dissection, and to leave the wound to be filled up, and to heal by granulation, according to the method of the ancients, would be perfectly useless; nay, the attempt might aggravate the ectropium and add to the scar.

The operation was thus performed. The cicatrix was sparingly removed, and from either extremity of the small oval wound two straight incisions were made, after the plan in the following diagram; the surrounding skin was then separated from its attachments to a considerable extent, especially on the cheek, by which it admitted of transposition, and so as to serve the place of that which had been damaged.

FIG. 48.

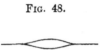

So extensively had the cellular tissue been destroyed by long suppuration, that the eyelid could not be freed and replaced till the dissection had reached nearly to the tarsal margin.

A portion of the conjunctiva was next removed from the sinus, corresponding to the everted portion of the tarsus, and the operation concluded by drawing up the eyelid as far as possible, and fixing it by means of narrow slips of plaster passed circularly from the nose to the temple. This has a double object, the removal of unhealthy tissue and the obtaining of contraction by the loss of structure, whereby the eyelid is braced up.

Cicatrization was rapid, and the improvement so far satisfactory. Some deformity remained, as the curved cartilage could not be made to accommodate itself to the eyeball ; and a few weeks later, I removed that part of the eyelid yet distorted with the tenaculum forceps and the scalpel, and applied two sutures. By any one not aware of the nature of the operation, I am sure that the former condition of the eye could never have been imagined.

FIG. 49.

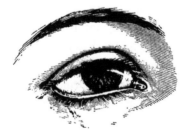

The preceding sketch shows a correct likeness of the alteration that was effected.

It may not be always necessary to shorten the tarsus, nor perhaps to excise any conjunctiva; but when either process is required, it is, I think, generally better to execute it simultaneously with the transposition of the skin. I suspect that the tarsus with its coverings is not in reality much stretched. I doubt not that it yields somewhat, but the depression must be due principally to displacement; for when it is much pulled down, and apparently lengthened, the upper eyelid is lowered.

For the removal of the piece to be effectual, it must be large enough to shorten the eyelid a little under the natural dimensions; and the following diagram gives the size of the portion that was taken in the case before us, marks its position, and shows the shape, which differs from the V form, that usually recommended. The curved sides come easily together, and make the edge level; whereas, a retiring angle is produced by

FIG. 50.

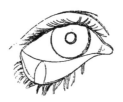

the straight incisions. I may add that the portion was taken just where the tarsus was bent and irregular, and had acquired a form not to be overcome by means that would ever bring the rest of the border to the correct line. The removal of a portion of cartilage from the outer angle, is preferable when circumstances will admit of it, and there is not a necessity for taking it at a given spot, because the scar which may follow is somewhat hidden by the natural folds of the skin.

Other methods embodying the same principle, and differing only in the direction and extent of the cuts, have been proposed and practised; but this is superior on account of the limited division of the skin, the smallness of the subsequent scar; and, from the absence of angular flaps, the greater certainty of healing by the first intention. The peculiarity, the size, and the position of the cicatrix, and the presence of more than one, will require modifications in the direction, number, and extent of the incisions.

The same details are applicable to the upper eyelid. Very great care must be taken in drawing down the borrowed skin, and the eye should not be opened until adhesion is supposed to be perfect. The cartilage also may be adherent to the bone, when of course it must be detached. The dissimilar anatomical arrangements of this lid, and the usual depth of the abscess from the surface, render it less favourable for amelioration, and the result must almost always depend on the site of the cicatrix : the more external it is, the more promising will be the issue.

A boy, twelve years old, was wounded in the upper eyelid. The cut was near the inner angle, and passed from the eyebrow to the margin of the eyelid, completely dividing the tarsal cartilage. The contraction, the eversion, and the deformity were great; but as there had been no loss of skin, but considerable puckering of it, and the distortion being evidently due to neglect of the recent injury, I recommended treatment, and promised much success. After dissecting away the cicatrix,

FIG. 51.

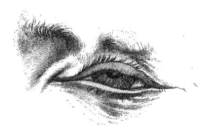

and paring the edges of the cleft portion through its entire thickness, I transposed very freely, united the parts with sutures and soft steel pins, and strapped the eyelids together. Subsequently I removed portions of the conjunctiva,—all, indeed, that had been exposed, and had undergone change in structure. The effect was beyond my expectation. The deformity was almost removed; the eyeball was no longer exposed, and the eyelid, which could now be closed and brought to meet its fellow, merely showed a small notch in the margin.

Mr. Gay requested me to meet him in consultation on a case of ectropium of the upper eyelid, caused by an accident from strong sulphuric acid. The preceding sketch shows the eye closed to the utmost that could be effected, and gives some idea of the extent of the injury.

In the ordinary state there was a stare, the eyelid was everted,

FIG. 52.

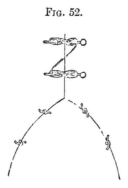

and the inside of the cartilage shown. At my recommendation Mr. Gay shaved the irregular hairs of the eyebrow, made an in_cision corresponding to the curved line, and dissected off the flap, which allowed the eyelid to descend. Then freely separating the edges of the skin on either side, he brought them together over the exposed surface, retaining them by sutures after the manner shown in Fig. 52, and dissected away a piece of conjunctiva along the edge of the tarsus. The result was more satisfactory than I had anticipated, and after four months the patient could nearly close the eye, the ectropium being removed, and the corneitis consequent on the exposure of the eyeball having disappeared.

An operator must not restrict himself to any form of flap,

although he must remember that acute angles are the more likely to slough.

Dieffenbach operates in this way. A triangular flap, including the cicatrix, being raised, the sections *a a* are extended freely on either side, to allow of the ready approximation of the two sides *b b*; these being then fixed by sutures, the two cut

FIG. 53.

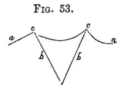

margins *a c* and *c a* are connected with the corresponding margins of the eyelid included between *c c*.

Cicatrices on the temple may produce more or less partial eversion of the corners of the eyelids; or they may not fairly evert their edges, but merely pull them away from the globe of the eye. The defect must be reduced by removing a triangular bit after the manner here shown, although a much greater

FIG. 54.

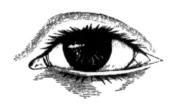

portion must be taken away, transposing the skin, and perhaps also removing a certain amount of the conjunctiva, after the method already detailed.

I have repaired cases of this kind that seemed at first to be irremediable. In an instance that occurred at St. Mary's Hospital, produced by scrofulous caries of the outer edge of the orbit, nearly half of each eyelid was almost entirely everted, and the commissure of the lids was pulled half an inch outwards. I removed the cicatrix sparingly, thoroughly transposed the integument, and applied pins and sutures. A few weeks after, I excised a considerable piece of conjunctiva from each eyelid.

The improvement was so great, that the defect was no longer noticed.

Most examples of this class, especially those of ectropium from abscess, may be treated on this plan. When, however, from much loss of skin, the eversion is excessive, transposition will seldom suffice, and skin must be borrowed by a plastic operation from a spot where its loss cannot ultimately be detrimental. But even this may be impracticable, for healthy skin may be out of reach. In a lad of eleven years of age, who was scalded in infancy, the right cheek was covered with cicatrices, and the alteration of the features actually defied immediate recognition of the exact nature of the change. The upper tarsus was dragged down below the level of the under one, and beneath it was a plane surface about an inch square, at first supposed to be an ulcer, but which was the conjunctiva; and below that and the distorted side of the mouth, a short and irregularly disposed row of cilia marked the inferior tarsus.

Plastic operations demand considerable nicety, and require for their effectual execution a well-tutored hand. Every circumstance should be promising, and the patient in good health. There are two means of operating : in the one, skin is raised from an adjacent part and twisted round to the required spot; in the other, with the maintenance of a connecting slip, the skin is slided laterally from a contiguous site. The adoption of either must be regulated by circumstances,—the situation of the part at which the skin is required, the extent of the demand, and the position from which the skin may be taken. The first is most used, because more generally applicable, and it is executed in the following manner.

FIG. 55.

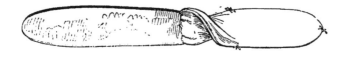

After the cicatrix has been dissected out as symmetrically as possible, with the greatest preservation of sound skin, and the eyelid liberated and carried to its place, a flap of skin, cellular and even adipose tissue of the required size, is to be raised and twisted to the place made to receive it, as is shown in the preceding diagram.

When the new bit is taken from a place in a line with the spot for which it is destined, there must be a sufficient strap or isthmus left uncut. But it is better to borrow it from a nearer point, so as to reduce the twist; because that interferes less with the circulation, and affords greater security to the preservation of vitality, while it moreover facilitates coaptation. I think that it would be still preferable to avoid the isthmus of skin by an arrangement of the following kind, the flap being taken from below or above, as occasion may require.

FIG. 56.

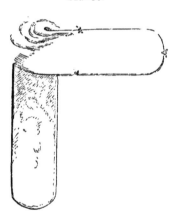

It is well not to wait till bleeding has ceased, but at once to adapt the parts and apply the sutures, as that will stop all hæmorrhage; and the risk, from the exposure and chilling of the surfaces, and the exsanguine state of the flap, is avoided. Indeed, in all operations about the eyelids, I approximate the surfaces that are to come together as quickly as possible, irrespective of bleeding; and numerous instances of uninterrupted success confirm the propriety of so doing. Perhaps the rule will hold good in all cutaneous operations. Of course union could not ensue if clots interposed; but these do not form during the dissection, neither do they afterwards, if pressure be applied.

The gap that is left should be diminished, in whatever manner may seem most expedient. The nearer the edges can be brought together, and thus maintained, so much the better ; and the quicker the surface heals the less will be the scar. When the skin has been turned completely round, or nearly so, the root may subsequently require to be divided, and made flat by a little dissection.

We must carefully guard against making the flap too small : allowance should always be given for contraction, which goes on for weeks after. A pretty just idea of what will be required, with the necessary twisting, may be attained by practising on the recently dead subject ; indeed, without such preparation, mistakes are almost certain to be made. With a little practice, however, rules of proportions will readily suggest themselves. In the case from which the first diagram was made, the place to be filled was an inch long, but the length of the flap was two inches ; less would not have been enough for the twist, and attachment sufficient to ensure vascular supply. In the second,

FIG. 57.

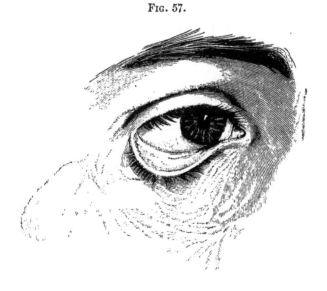

where there was neither twist nor isthmus, the proportions were different ; the flap to fill the same sized wound was an inch and three quarters. It may be well to trace out with tincture of iodine the size of the flap to be raised.

The preceding illustration of the operation shows the usual result of insufficiency of flap both in length and in breadth ; in other respects, the operation was well executed.

The patient had, in childhood, fallen into the fire; the scars about the cheek indicate the extent of injury; the outline of the flap, and the spot from which it was taken, are just visible. The transplantation was made at an hospital in London when the man was thirty years old ; and, according to his statement, half the turned down eyelid—that is, half the deformity—was removed. The tarsus had not been shortened, nor was the conjunctiva excised.

I assisted Mr. Taylor in operating in the very inveterate case of ectropium which is given in the chapter on " Caries of the Orbit," and to which I request the reader to refer. The edge of the tarsus and the conjunctiva were carefully dissected up, and the flap, which, in consequence of scars on the cheek, was taken from a spot directly opposite, placed between the tarsus and the skin. The proportions which I have given were observed, and answered well. At a later period, a part of the conjunctiva was removed. The only untoward circumstance was sloughing of a

Fig. 58.

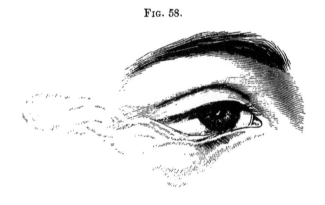

small part of the end of the flap, but that did not foil the operation, as the likeness here shows. The twist at the base adjusted itself so nicely, that an operation on it was unnecessary.

Mr. Taylor ultimately proposed to effect still further improvement, but he lost sight of the girl. Just six years later I met with this patient, and her condition was still better than when I last saw her. The removal of a bit more of the conjunctiva would have been advantageous.

The upper eyelid does not offer the same facilities for operation; although the effects of its retraction are more distressing, from the loss of covering to the eyeball; for failure through imperfect union of the flap is much more likely to ensue.

With Dieffenbach's mode of lateral sliding, I have no practical acquaintance. In vol. vii. of "The British and Foreign Medical Review," an account of it will be found, with much practical information upon plastic operations by Blandin, Zeiss, Dieffenbach, and Liston. I have borrowed the diagram from Ammon's "Zeitschrift," vol. iv., where it originally appeared. The account of the plan was first published in Casper's "Wochenschrift" for 1835; and it appears that Ammon was the first to operate on the lower eyelid. The operation is commenced by two incisions, one extending from either commissure of the tarsus; and when the lower eyelid is the subject of restoration, the incisions are so inclined towards each other as to meet at an acute angle on the cheek; or above the eyebrow, when the upper eyelid is defective. This triangular flap, of

FIG. 59.

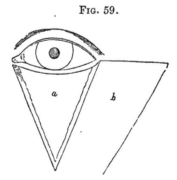

which the third side is the remnant of the former eyelid, is then dissected up and completely removed; care being taken to spare as much as possible the neighbouring nervous filaments. The space *a* thus left is that intended to be occupied by the transplanted flap, *b*.

The next step, whether for the upper or the lower eyelid, is to carry a horizontal incision from the external canthus over the zygoma, and in a straight line towards the external auditory meatus; this incision must, in any case, exceed in length the breadth of the defect in the eyelid. From the extreme outer point of this incision another is carried—when the lower eyelid is required, downwards upon the cheek; and for the upper eyelid, upwards upon the temple. In either case the incision must be nearly parallel to the outer line of the removed flap; its termination being on a level with, though slightly approximated to, the point of the same. Here, then, everything is arranged for replacing the eyelid. The new flap is gently raised, and after a careful cleansing of the prepared space, it is removed to its new position. The twisting of the broad pedicle which is thus placed inferiorly, is very slight in this operation; for that which formed the superior margin of the flap becomes the edge of the lower eyelid, the converse being the case in the upper operation. The same course as regards sutures is pursued in this as in the rhinoplastic operation. The importance of saving the ciliary margin, in the preliminary dissection, is self-evident. When that is out of the question, or when it has been originally lost, a great effort must be made to procure a conjunctival lining for the edge of the flap, and some dissection of that membrane towards the eyeball may render more of it available. The conjunctiva and the skin must be adapted by sutures.

In the "London and Edinburgh Monthly Journal" for 1843, p. 359, is an extract from the "Annales de la Chirurgie Française et Etrangère" for January 7th, 1843, of two cases of lid restoration. One was done by Dr. Baumgarten, in a child six months old, labouring under aneurism by anastomosis on the right lower eyelid; the rapid increase, encroachment on the cheek, great size, and the imminent rupture of the growth, induced its extirpation. The flap was borrowed from the temple, and slipped laterally into the required place; the upper edge was fixed to the tarsus by means of four points of suture, the inner by six, the outer remaining free. Union by the first intention followed, and on the fourth day the last suture was removed. In a week the loss of substance in the temple was repaired, and the eyelid presented a good appearance. The other was performed by Dr. Ammon. The loss of the lower eyelid was involved in the excision of a suspicious-looking tumour; the flap in this instance was also taken from the temple; primary adhesion was not effected, yet the flap survived, and in five weeks adhered, by granulations.

Not until all activity of the disease that has produced ectropium has ceased, and the eyelid has reached its maximum of eversion, should an operation be undertaken. At the same time, I must observe that it would be injudicious to delay operative measures when the proper time has arrived; because the issue would be less sure or perfect, from the longer disturbance of the tarsus.

Whenever dissections are to be made over the supra- or infra-orbital foramina, care should be taken to avoid the vessels and the nerves which they transmit.

There may be a loss of sensibility in the borrowed flap; this has occurred in all cases of plastic operations that I have seen, but it has been temporary. In a few weeks, or months, sensation has returned; and should it have been restored prior to the division of the twisted portion, this little operation will again suspend it.

A certain degree of puffiness follows the best executed of these operations; this becomes much less, and may quite disappear.

The hair-follicles may, from a cause which it is difficult to explain, be stimulated into activity, and produce hair of considerable length.

I believe that the operation of transplantation—that strictly so called; I mean the Taliacotian—has never been applied to the eyelids.

M. Jobert, in his work, "Traité de Chirurgie Plastique," proposes to supply the lost eyebrow with scalp hair—an act not likely to improve personal appearance, nor is his representation of a case prepossessing.

I have much pleasure in referring to some very excellent cases of restoration of lost parts by the late Dr. Richard Mackenzie, of the Royal Infirmary of Edinburgh, in the " Monthly Journal of Medical Science," and especially to one in the number for January, 1852, embodying restoration of the upper lip, cheek, and eyelid, the chief facts of which I subjoin. In the original there are two wood-cuts showing the former and the after state of the face.

The deformity was the result of mortification occurring during the early stage of convalescence from scarlet fever. Nearly the entire cheek and lower eyelid, the side of the nose and the half of the upper lip, were destroyed. Necrosis followed, and the nasal bones were lost, with the greater part of the superior maxillary bone.

When admitted into the hospital, the child, then seven years old, was in good health, and the parts in the neighbourhood of the extensive cicatrix in a perfectly sound condition. The absence of the lower eyelid had given rise to a vascular condition of the conjunctiva of the right eye, and the part of the cornea which was exposed was dull and slightly nebulous. In addition to the deformity of the features, the twisting and displacement of the mouth rendered her articulation very indistinct.

He attempted to restore the lost parts by bringing up a large flap, consisting of the lower lip, and of the integuments over the base of the jaw, so as to fill up the whole gap at once. The operation, however, failed, in consequence of vomiting with little cessation for thirty-six hours, the effect of chloroform. The contracted flap, nevertheless, was retained, as much as possible, in the situation of the upper lip, and his object so far attained as to bring the parts into a condition nearly similar to that of simple harelip.

About six weeks later, by the harelip operation, the edges of the cleft were brought into apposition ; perfect union was established, and the natural appearance of the upper lip was thus nearly restored.

The deformity of the face, although much diminished, was still very great, from the absence of the nose, eyelid, and greater part of the cheek. As the child herself, and her parents, were anxious that something more should be done to improve her appearance, a third operation was performed, three months after, and the gap was filled by a large flap of skin brought from over the ramus of the jaw, the base being situated over the upper part of the malar prominence, and its extremity corresponding to the angle of the jaw. This was attached by twisted and interrupted sutures to a cut surface extending from between the eyebrows along the mesial line. in the former situation of the nose, and along the upper border of the new upper lip. It retained its vitality in its entire extent, and primary union was obtained along the whole line of incision. The edges of the wound that was left were united by one or two sutures at the lower extremity of incisions. The remainder of the surface was left to granulate, and healed quickly. In addition to the improved appearance of the features, her articulation was rendered much more distinct, an advantage which was contem- plated in deciding at first as to the expediency of surgical inter ference.

The child, nothing daunted by what she had undergone, was now anxious to have her appearance still further improved by the formation of a nose. This proposal was negatived, as the operation is applicable only in adults.

The second class of cases of ectropium contains those which are the consequence or termination of disease of the eyelid itself, and occur principally in the under lid.

It is generally supposed that the eversion is owing to the contraction of the skin of the eyelid from the excoriating in- fluence of the tears. Ulcerations that penetrate the skin suffi- ciently to produce a scar, would doubtless be followed by such an effect, be the cause of that ulceration what it may ; but ulcera- tion of the exterior of the eyelid is not usually associated with ectropium. Roughness, and even excoriation of the skin, is, according to my observation, a frequent effect of eversion, and both are common in lippitudo, where eversion is absent. The direction of the tarsus somewhat indicates, also, that it is not entirely influenced by tension of the skin ; for it is not so much pulled down or away from the globe of the eye as turned outwards.

I believe it to be due to inflammation, and almost . always of a strumous kind. It exists in two forms. In the one, the conjunctiva is first inflamed, lacrymation follows, with more or less intolerance of light; afterwards the meibomian glands are involved, and the entire edge of the eyelid being implicated, the cilia drop out, or become stunted ; that state called lippitudo generally occurs, and the eversion follows. There seems to be not only actual loss of substance of the eyelid in the rounding of the edge, but the cartilage and the tarsal ligament shrink. This appears to me to receive corroboration in the circumstance that, in the lippitudo which generally precedes, it is not un-common to observe inability to close the eyelids, except with great effort. Perhaps I may venture to surmise that the inflammation which lingers about the eyelid may so far alter that portion of the orbicularis on the edge, as to impair its supporting or binding influence.

In the other, certain changes of thickness in the palpebral portion of the conjunctiva alone evert the tarsus, the edge of the eyelid, with the cilia and the glands, remaining entire. In nearly all of these cases that have come under my inspection, irritating substances had been used for conjunctival affections, and had, I believe, been the' chief cause of the eversion.

Here follows a representation of entropium of the first kind, that with considerable disease of the eyelid. It was taken from a young man of nineteen, a patient at the Ophthalmic Hospital.

Both eyes were similarly diseased. Having been the most marked case that had been at the hospital for some months, it was chosen for representation before treatment by operation, with the intention of contrasting it with the after improvement; but the patient subsequently declined my assistance. A better illustration of an aggravated case could not be desired. All the conjunctiva on the everted eyelid was thickened, and the edge of the tarsus ragged, from former ulceration. In the upper

Fig. 60.

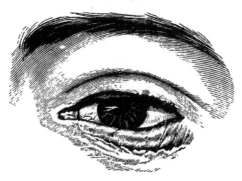

eyelid, also, there was slight eversion, and most of the cilia were lost.

Improvement might be effected in slight acute cases, by general and local treatment, by restoring the health, and the use of mild astringents ; but, in general, and always when the exposed conjunctiva is decidedly altered in structure, an operation is required.

Escharotics strong enough to produce slough have been recommended to supersede the knife, but they are inferior in effect, and objectionable also on the score of danger ; it being difficult, or even impossible, to limit their action.

I adopt in the first form ; eversion with general disease of the lid edge; excision of a portion of the conjunctiva.

The eyelid having been duly depressed, two incisions are to be made, an internal one circumscribing the inward limit, and an outward one along the tarsal margin; the isolated piece is then seized with the tenaculum forceps, and dissected away. The outer incision should be carried to the edge of the tarsus, along the entire length of the eversion, or the operation is imperfectly done.

The amount of conjunctiva to be thus removed should be regulated by circumstances which practice alone can teach. As a rule, I take away all that is permanently exposed. It must be recollected that eversion may be changed to inversion, by too lavish a dissection.   Frequent sponging is needed.   I generally apply sutures.

The following sketch was taken from a girl fifteen years old, with partial ectropium of both lower eyelids, from long existing strumous ophthalmia, which had also destroyed all the cilia.

FIG. 61.

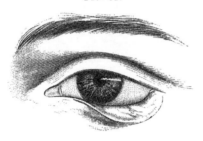

The greater part of the exposed membrane was dissected away, and with such an effect that, four months after, the eye was in that state which the second sketch accurately represents.

For so perfect a result the eyelid must have escaped ulceration, and the tarsal cartilage been but little damaged ; and then all trace of the operation is a bridle of conjunctiva,—which is a part of the ocular membrane uniting the eyelid to the globe of the eye, but does not interfere with the ocular movements.

In the second form ; that of eversion from thickening of the

FIG. 62.

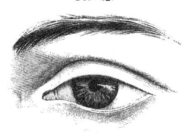

conjunctiva without tarsal disease, of which the next figure is an example ; a double operation is generally required ; the removal of the conjunctiva, and of a triangular bit of the tarsus. The contraction consequent on the first is not sufficient, except in slight cases. In an instance like the following, there is always a pucker that demands the loss of a portion of the eyelid.

FIG. 63.

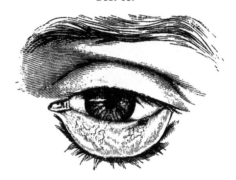

The subject of the sketch was a soldier, who had been discharged for some inflammatory affection of the eye, and who assures me that when he left the army the eyelid had not turned out, that the ectropium came on a few months after the regular application of sulphate of copper three times a week, for nine months, when he could no longer submit to it. I removed a large portion of the membrane; and six weeks later a bit of the tarsus, and united the edges by suture. So great was the improvement that the eye was not recognised by several medical men who had seen it prior to the first operation. The following sketch was taken ten days after the second.

I find it better, except under specific circumstances, not to do the double operation at once, but to wait awhile after the first; for several times, contrary to my expectation, the removal of the conjunctiva alone has sufficed.

In some of my cases I have effected still further improvement by adjusting the outer angle of the eyelids; and when the puncture is yet displaced, inverting it by removing a bit of the conjunctiva just behind, and sometimes, in addition, slitting it up. This treatment of the lacrymal conduit is fully given in the next chapter, to which I beg the reader to refer.

FIG. 64

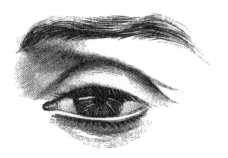

Ectropium from paralysis may be more or less benefited by the above treatment. My own experience in it is small, having operated on very few cases.

Perhaps I ought not to omit to notice that displacement of the eyelids occasionally recurring in purulent ophthalmia, and more commonly in the adult, which is, strictly speaking, eversion. They are turned inside-out by the infiltrated conjunctiva, chiefly of the eyeball; but except that scarifications are sometimes called for, it does not fall within the domain of operative surgery. I am averse to excision of any part of the chemosed conjunctiva, because I think that the contraction which must ensue might induce entropium; moreover, the practice is unnecessary, for as the severity of the disease is subdued the eyelids regain their wonted position. When the protrusion does not show evidences of decline under general treatment, or when it is very large, free incisions are beneficial.

The ectropium of the aged, which seems chiefly to depend upon the loss of sustaining power, or the support of the orbicularis muscle to the tarsus, and relaxation also of the tarsal connexions, is not generally, in this country at least, submitted to operation. The eyelid falls away from the eyeball rather than turns out. The removal of vertical portions of skin is beneficial, but a large portion must be removed. I have too, with advantage, excised a piece of the conjunctiva.

M. Desmarres supposes that in this senile defect there is some actual change in the relative position of the orbicularis, in consequence of relaxation of the skin; that there is a transposition of a part of the muscle, the greater portion of the ciliary fibres being carried to the lower, or adherent border of the tarsus by the cutaneous folds; and that the tarsus so circumstanced swings about during their contraction. He says he has proved this pathological change in a great number of cases, by actual dissection. He states also that ectropium can be produced by spasmodic action of the orbicularis; a theory that is tenable.

OBSTRUCTION OF THE MEIBOMIAN DUCTS.

Abscesses and concretions in the ducts, causing deformity or irritation, call for surgical assistance. The natural secretion may block up and close them, and be mistaken for calcareous matter. In two instances, when I thought I had taken away calculi, minute examination proved the dense masses to be of this nature.

Mr. Dalrymple removed a small tumour, larger than a pea, from beneath the tarsal cartilage of the upper eyelid of a middle-aged man. It was composed of concentric layers of hard earthy material. Its pressure had caused absorption of the cartilage and ulceration of the conjunctiva, and the friction produced pain, inflammation of the conjunctiva scleroticæ, and opacity of the upper part of the cornea. The microscope disclosed epithelium scales, closely agglutinated, thickened and hard, and containing granular earthy molecules, phosphate of lime, with a trace of the carbonate of the same earth, which could not be removed by immersion in weak muriatic acid. No amorphous earthy deposit existed around or among the scales.

It is not uncommon to find some of these ducts, and even parts of the glands, choked up with epithelium scales. For the most part no inconvenience accrues.

CONJUNCTIVAL CALCULI.

The formation of calculi on the free surface of the conjunctiva is very questionable, and many stories of the ossification of the tears are too wonderful to be repeated. All concretions found between the eyelids have probably descended from the lacrymal gland, as appears to have taken place in a well-reported case of Mr. R. H. Meade, in vol. xv. of the "London Medical Gazette." A girl of nineteen, who had been in bad health, and suffered severe headache and pain over the left eye, was bled and leeched without relief. Inflammation suddenly appeared in the left eye, with lancinating pain in the upper and outer part of the orbit, accompanied with sudden and profuse discharge of tears. Something which resembled a fragment of mortar was removed from the conjunctiva. The pain ceased, but returned in an hour after, and another bit came away. During the four following days as many as twenty-three similar pieces were discharged, after which the pain and inflammation abated. Neither abrasion nor ulceration of the conjunctiva was observed. There was tenderness in the situation of the lacrymal glands. The calculi were small, rough, very hard, and of a dirty-white colour, the largest being about a line in diameter. Through a microscope they looked like rough pieces of chalk studded with small portions of silex. They consisted principally of phosphate of lime, with a small quantity of carbonate of lime, and traces of animal matter. The author very shrewdly suspects that the calculi were formed in the lacrymal duct, and that, producing irritation, they were dispelled with the tears which they excited.

To this cause I refer a very remarkable case of the double affection, related by Walther, in Gräfe and Walther's "Journal," 1820. The rapidity of the formation of the calculi which were in the lower sinus was wonderful : in one eye, the first affected, they were removed twice, and even three times a day. But the most remarkable occurrence is their rapid cessation, under the administration of five grains of carbonate of potass four times a day, with syrup and common water, and also an infusion of viola tricolor. Some years after, the disease returned ; the upper sinus of one eye was the seat of the deposit, and potass again cured it. The term which Walther applied to these concretions, that of Dacryolites, has come into general use.

M. Desmarres has written very extensively on dacryolites and rhinolithes, in vols. vii., viii., and ix. of "Les Annales d'Oculistique."

A calculus has been removed from the caruncle.

CHAPTER IX

NÆVI.

Varieties—Pathology—Methods of Treatment.

THE term "nævus," which is now generally restricted in its application to those congenital marks or tumours characterised by peculiar vascularity, and distinguished from the mole or mother-spot, is not, as is commonly supposed, a mere exaggeration or hypertrophy of blood-vessels. Vascularity is certainly the great characteristic, and there is an inducement to arrange the disease under arterial and venous kinds, according to the supposed sort of blood with which they are filled, without reference to the nature of the vessels that contain it; but this would apply almost exclusively to those on the surface. It is better for surgical purposes to speak of them according to the positions they occupy in the body, as cutaneous, subcutaneous, and mixed.

The cutaneous is particularly well marked, and varies in extent and in level — sometimes being a stain of varying breadth, at others a conglomerate mass of vessels, forming a tumour.

The subcutaneous is generally more or less defined, but may be without definite limits, and, according to its depth from the surface, is of a light-bluish tint, or colourless. When deep, it is in all respects like a common fatty tumour, and its true nature may be so obscure as to be overlooked; our best surgeons have been deceived respecting them. It is recorded in vol. xxvi. of the "Medico-Chirurgical Transactions" that Mr. Liston proceeded, after careful examination, to extirpate from the ham what he supposed to be a fatty tumour, but which proved to be made up of erectile tissue, as he termed it. The case is well worth perusal. Mr. Fergusson gives, in his "Practical Surgery," a somewhat similar instance that occurred to himself. A supposed cyst in the cheek proved to be a subcutaneous vascular tumour. I could quote another instance that happened at one of our London hospitals, and, doubtless, many surgeons have been similarly deceived.

The mixed nævus combines the characters of both, presenting a vascular mark on the skin, with a tumour extending more or less deeply into the subjacent tissues.

In most instances of each kind, and especially in the cutaneous, when pressure is applied, the blood-vessels are more or less emptied, and when it is remitted they refill. The sensation conveyed to the finger, and the rapidity of the change, are worth little as a diagnostic of the nature of a vascular tumour.

Concerning pulsation in them, there is a difference of opinion. My own belief is, that a simple nævus, however large, does not pulsate; and for arterial thrill to be present, it must be more or less mixed with aneurism by anastomosis.

So marked an example of a congenital cutaneous nævus about the eye as that shown in the following figure, taken from a man forty years old, is seldom seen. It was at first a mere dot upon the brow, and the increase had been very slow. It was raised about three-quarters of an inch throughout its entire extent, was dark-blue, apparently filled with venous blood, dense, cold, and pulseless; did not admit of much reduction in bulk or in colour by pressure, and was subject to periodic pains.

Little was heretofore known of the structure of nævi: the difficulty of procuring proper specimens for research has, no doubt, been the bar to our knowledge; and even at this time, few dissections have been made. Mr. Birkett made a careful investigation into the structure of a subcutaneous one furnished to him by Mr. Curling. His description is in vol. xxx. of the "Medico-Chirurgical Transactions." He tells us that it is composed of areolar uniting or fibrous tissue, capillary vessels, and vessels of larger calibre, and he describes in detail their disposition. With regard to their histological relations, he concludes that there is no more reason to give them the title of vascular or blood-vessel tumours than many others which have received very different names; that they consist neither of small arteries, small veins, nor of a mixture of these vessels. They do not consist of erectile tissue, though they more closely resemble the corpus cavernosum than any other normal structure; and he classes them with the fibrous tissues, and considers that they are probably developed in a similar manner, and possess cells that are in communication with larger or smaller veins, and are nourished by arteries that may differ greatly in size.

FIG. 65.

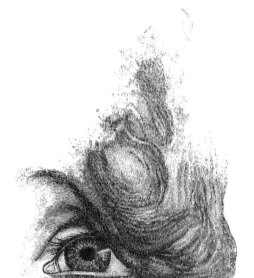

Mr. Paget is inclined to look upon nævi as erectile tumours, and meets the objection advanced in the "Lectures on Surgery," by Mr. Humphrey, of Cambridge, that they possess no power of filling themselves with blood as if by some internal force; with the remark that, since the power of true erectile tissue depends as much on the accessory structure of nerves and muscles as on the tissue itself, we may, perhaps, apply the term erectile to these tumours, remembering only that, for this, as for other structures occurring in tumours, the imitation of the natural tissue is imperfect or partial. He also states that the likeness which these tumours bear to the erectile tissue, as exemplified in the corpus cavernosum penis, is sometimes in general appearance perfect. A well-marked specimen in the Hunterian Collection is alluded to in illustration; and he adds that what he has seen, and the description which more fortunate watchers have recorded, leave him little doubt that this imitation of erectile tissue is a frequent character of such tumours. As further evidence, he remarks: " The descriptions by Mr. Wardrop and Mr. Cæsar Hawkins, and the more minute accounts of structure by Mr. Goodsir, Mr. Liston, and Rokitansky, confirm this view; and neither Mr. Birkett's, nor any other that I have met with, is discordant to it." Mr. Paget's lecture, from which this is taken, the eighth of the course, is in the " Medical Gazette " for August, 1851.

Mr. Simon, in his " Lectures on General Pathology," classes nævi under the head of vascular tumours, and describes cutaneous nævi as consisting of adventitious cavernous structure, with the interlaced columnar appearance of ordinary erectile tissue, coated with tesselated epithelium continuous with that of the adjoining vessels; the hollow intercolumnar spaces communicating, and appearing to be altered capillary channels of the part.

There is nothing positively known of the mode of their development. Rokitansky thinks that they arise as excavations in a blastema deposited in a solid form, and that the reticular structure then communicates with the original vessels of the part by penetration of their walls, and forms a diverticulum from the circulation. Mr. Simon discredits this, and considers it to be the result of true growth in the original blood-vessels of the affected part. Whether they are always congenital is still disputed; but the solution is certainly not of any surgical moment.

In the volume for 1855 of the " Bulletins de la Société Ana-tomique," there is a lucid account of a dissection of a cutaneous nævus by M. Godard, which differs essentially from those already glanced at. During life it was about the size of a cherry, and had all the characters common to superficial nævi. When removed for examination, after death, it had the appear-ance of a small disc, of a pinkish-yellow colour, made up of loose fibrous tissue, replacing the proper structures of the dermis, with which it was continuous at its periphery. It had no vascular connexion with the tissue immediately subjacent, but a large vein could be traced to it from the subcutaneous adipose tissue, dividing into smaller veinules, and in the nævus itself terminating—or rather commencing—in little venous sinuses, which together formed a small mass resembling a blackberry, both in aspect and in colour. This appearance was found to be produced by the fibrous tissue of the dermis stran-gulating these sinuses at various points, and compressing them so that the blood could not be made to pass from one pouch to another, till the little fibrous bridles were divided, when the continuity of the sinus could be traced.

Nævi may occur in any part of the body; the face is a very common seat, and they are frequently found on or near the eye-lids, and within the orbit itself. I have not met with nævi on the eyeball alone, but such examples have been recorded by Von Ammon; in one instance it was hereditary, the parents having the same defect. Mr. Wormald has met with a nævus on the iris which bled regularly at the menstrual period.

A disease so conspicuous as nævus is naturally brought under the observation of the surgeon at an early period; but, strange as it may appear, there are persons who discountenance any treatment, trusting rather to a natural cure. Of this, however, there can be no certainty, nor is a case wholly unattended with danger from accidental bleeding.

A mere stain, whether of an arterial or venous character, need excite little apprehension; and if it remain stationary, there is no call for treatment, unless it be small and a slight scar be deemed preferable. Although there is very little tendency in these simple stains to increase, there is little chance of their disappearance. I have met with them several times on the conjunctiva. With the bluish superficial nævus there is greater probability of natural cure than with the scarlet kind, and nævi show different tendencies to disappear, according to the parts in which they are situated, being more likely to decline about the neck and trunk than elsewhere; while increase is more certain when they are seated upon or in contiguity to mucous membrane. A debilitated constitution is favourable to their disappearance.

That the vitality of nævi is low is a well-known fact, and accidental injury will sometimes be followed by sloughing or ulceration. In vol. xxii. of the "London Medical Gazette," page 795, is recorded a case of extensive nævus of the upper extremity, spontaneously cured by sloughing; the destructive process commencing near the middle of the diseased portion of integument, and continuing till it arrived at the sound skin, no part of which was destroyed, as the slough ceased when that was reached; reparation then setting in and advancing with rapidity.

My own course of proceeding is unhesitatingly to adopt some treatment when a nævus of any kind, however small, shows any signs of increase; and this, knowing that the enlargement may be only temporary. If at any time surgical proceedings be delayed for the sake of watching a case, the slightest augmentation should be the signal for acting; but when time is thus allowed, there may be subcutaneous spreading without external evidence of the extension of the disease. This is especially the case with nævi about the eye and in its immediate vicinity, where, from the functional derangement they may cause, independently of ordinary evils, they require a strictness of attention scarcely demanded in any other part of the body.

Extirpation, the production of sloughing, suppuration, or adhesion of their intimate structure, are the available processes of cure; and we should endeavour to effect the removal of the disease with the least subsequent deformity, and with the slightest disturbance or destruction of the surrounding parts. It is an advantage to possess several resources of treatment from which a selection may be made, adapted to the peculiarity of the individual case.

The most simple means that can be adopted is that of pressure, but its use must be restricted to localities that will allow of counter-pressure, by an opposing surface. Many methods are employed, but no one can so generally be depended on as a metallic spring, after the manner of a truss, by which bandages, which are always objectionable, are superseded. I have adopted it with success in that form of nævus in which there is a stellate arrangement of a few vessels in the skin. I lately had a good example on the forehead of a young lady six years old, who was introduced to me by Dr. Sieveking. Mr. Abernethy was in the habit of applying cold washes along with pressure by bandage, and sometimes the growth was checked ; the nævi shrank and were no longer of consequence. Dieffenbach also employed pressure by means of a piece of tea-lead, or of a small silver coin. But pressure may irritate and eventually augment the growth, instead of effecting a cure ; moreover, it can never be thoroughly relied upon in well-marked instances, while it requires long perseverance, is troublesome in application, and irksome and annoying to the patient. Combined with Dr. Marshall Hall's plan of breaking up the interior of the tumour with a needle through one place of puncture, it may be more effectual.

Intense cold is an agent that has of late been much spoken of and recommended. Dr. James Arnott, a great enthusiast in the matter of freezing, tells me that he employed it with benefit, in a nævus the size of a sixpence, on the forehead of a child about three years old. Enlarged vessels led to it, and the very rapid growth induced the mother to bring the child to the Brighton Dispensary. It was congealed, as Dr. Arnott terms it, by the common frigorific mixture of equal parts of ice and rock salt, applied in a small network bag, for about three minutes, on three occasions, with intervals of a week. The effect was to reduce the enlargement one half, and apparently to remove all vascular excitement. The vessels which had previously led to it were no longer visible after the third application. But this cannot be received as a cure. I have given the method a full trial. With much care I have persisted with it, in individual instances of growing nævi; I have applied it as often as twenty times, on each occasion the surface being frozen, and never have I been able to arrest the increase.

A plan of cutting and searing nævi, by means of a piece of platinum wire made red-hot by a galvanic current, has been applied by Mr. Marshall. The application of heat, produced by ordinary means, has long been practised; M. Carron du Villards passes long pins through the greatest diameter of the tumour, bends them till their extremities meet, unites them by a metallic knot, and then applies the flame of a candle to the pins till they are of a white heat, moistening the tumour·during the while with oil—a practice, together with the actual cautery of M. Cloquet, not likely to be generally followed in England. Puncture with red-hot needles is, however, recommended and praetised by some English and American surgeons.

Removal by extirpation is of old ·date; it is somewhat dangerous, and not lightly to be undertaken. Allan Burns, in his "Surgical Anatomy of the Head and Neck," gives an instance of a cutaneous nævus that he removed from the eye, temple, and side of the face, in a middle-aged man. A part of the upper eyelid, and the outer part of the eyeball, including the conjunctiva and the sclerotica, were involved. Extirpation was performed, the operation being undertaken because of the growth increasing, especially in its ocular portion, and threatening to obscure the eye, and the patient's anxious desire to be relieved of it. A very tedious and intricate dissection was required, the tumour dipped in and formed attachments that could not be foretold. Success crowned his efforts, and the only resulting inconvenience was some alteration in the position of the upper eyelid, in consequence of adhesion to the eyeball and restriction of its movement.

Although extirpation may be admissible when the tumour is small and probably circumscribed, and the surrounding parts healthy, there are not many cases in which it should be preferred. Several children have died under the operation; and the possible, and very probable recurrence of severe hæmorrhage, must always be a bar to this practice. If it should seem advisable to adopt it, John Bell's maxim of not cutting into the mass, but of cutting it out, and keeping as wide away from the tumour as possible without unnecessarily destroying skin, should be observed.

Vaccination has occasionally succeeded, as has every other irritant treatment that has been tried; but I have seen it cause very rapid increase in several cases. It would seem to be most applicable where a single pustule would circumscribe the nævus. The late Dr. Gregory, of the Smallpox Hospital, who tried it most extensively, told me that, from the frequent failures he has met with, he has ceased to treat any in this manner.

Escharotics form a very powerful and efficient class of remedies, and are frequently used; potassa fusa and the strongest nitric acid being preferred. The surrounding parts should be protected by plaster, or substances that will neutralize these chemical agents. I never use the potash, on account of the liability of sloughing beyond the extent of surface touched. I have already alluded to this drug at page 124. The "Potassa c. calce" is not open to this objection; it is far more manageable, and does not deliquesce so quickly; indeed, it might be called a safe application. I have not myself employed.it in these cases.

All escharotics are exceedingly painful, and several applications are often necessary.

During the several years of my pupilage to Mr. Lawrence, he employed nitric acid in the treatment of all the cases of nævi that came to the hospital, applying it by means of a little mop of lint tied on a stick—a plan most generally adopted at St. Bartholomew's Hospital at the period of my attendance. In this way I destroyed the largest cutaneous nævus I ever saw. Mr. Hey, of Leeds, and myself, were summoned to a gentleman's seat near Northallerton, in Yorkshire, to treat a nævus on the leg of a child three months old. The nævus seemed cutaneous, was mottled with red and purple, raised about half an inch from the surface, and occupied rather more than the central third of the leg, very nearly encircling it : a thin strip of integument at the back part was sound. At birth, it was the size of a five-shilling piece, and till the child was a month old it was nearly level with the skin, and had not spread. A single application of the acid sufficed. The whole of the eschar did not separate till the expiration of three months. I did not see the child from the day I operated till two years after, in London, when not a trace of the disease remained. As the acid acts chiefly superficially, I employ it of a higher specific gravity than of the Pharmaco-pœial strength, as this lessens the necessity of re-applications.

Removal of the epidermis by a blister, and applications of a strong solution of perchloride of iron, is recommended by M. Broca, and is said by him to be remarkably efficacious in super-ficial nævi ; a single application sufficing.

Caustic, combined with subcutaneous puncture, first intro-duced by Mr. Wardrop, has been extensively employed by Sir Benjamin Brodie and other surgeons, in nævi of very large extent. Sir Benjamin punctures the tumour in several places with a narrow flat-bladed knife, breaks up the tissue, introduces a flat probe coated with nitrate of silver, and moves it about in the torn mass. He repeats this at intervals, according to the effect ; and he has thus destroyed a very large subcutaneous nævus, with a very slight amount of disfiguration. This treatment may extend over a long period, perhaps over several months.

In the year 1836 Mr. Lloyd published in the " Medical

Gazette," vol. xix., page 13, his mode of treatment by injecting irritating fluids, having, as he states, been led to its adoption for the purpose of overcoming the danger of the knife, the insufficiency of the ligature, and the disfiguration produced by escharotics. He considers the principal advantages to be, its applicability to nævi so large and so situated as to be wholly irremediable by other means, the absence of deformity and of constitutional disturbance, and the slight amount of pain occasioned.

His method was, to puncture the integument at some distance from the tumour, introduce the nozzle of a syringe, and inject the fluid. Some of the objections urged against this practice, such as the risk of extravasation of the fluid, and the liability to extensive and violent inflammation, which would be especially dangerous in the vicinity of the eye, have recently been to a considerable degree obviated by the employment of more delicate instruments, such as Pravaz's syringe, and of fluids such as solutions of perchloride of iron and of tannic acid, which are not merely irritant, but which at once coagulate the blood; and thus modified, this treatment has of late years been extensively tried. By means of Pravaz's syringe, of which the nozzle is a needle traversed by a canal, and the piston is worked by a screw, each revolution of which expels exactly one minim of fluid, the utmost precision as to the quantity and direction of the agent is ensured.

For superficial nævi, the Tinctura ferri sesquichloridi may be used; but for deeper ones, the solution of the sesquichloride prepared according to the French codex ought to be preferred, as it is less liable to set up inflammation. When this very potent remedy is thus employed for the destruction of a cutaneous nævus, the effect can be seen and estimated by the points reached becoming pale and hard. I have, however, known injection of both preparations into deep-seated nævi followed by suppuration and abscess in so many instances that I do not venture to use it about the face or the orbit.

I have often employed, with perfect success, tannic acid in subcutaneous nævi, in the proportion of one drachm of the acid to an ounce of water; not a saturated solution, as this quantity of water takes up readily two drachms. I use Anel's syringe; make an aperture at the circumference of the tumour, not larger than will admit the nozzle of the instrument, and then gently inject a few drops or more of the fluid. Sometimes I break up the structure of the nævus, and, if practicable, I think it well to empty it by gentle pressure, before injecting. No force must be used, or extravasation into healthy textures might ensue. We have it on Mr. Birkett's authority, that there is an intimate connexion subsisting between the reticular texture of the lobes of nævi and the veins, which are often large.

Perhaps the safest plan, especially for those unaccustomed to surgical operations, is always to inject with the screw piston syringe.

Commonly, a few days after the operation, a dark-coloured discharge issues from the point of puncture, but frequently the coagulated blood is gradually absorbed without this.

The circumstances that induced me to resort to tannic acid, which quickly coagulates the blood, together with my experiments, are recorded in the "Medico-Chirurgical Proceedings" for 1857-58, in the narrative of a very remarkable example of vascular tumour in the orbit. I will give here only a slight outline of the case.

The subject of the affection, a young lady, was sent to me by Mr. Square, of Plymouth, under whose care she had been. The tumour was in the left orbit. The eyeball was a little everted, much restricted in motion, and incapable of rotation inwards. The lower eyelid was prominent, of a bluish tint, traversed by large veins, and just above the edge of it appeared a part of a vascular tumour, about which there were many contorted veins, some of them as large as a crow-quill. Depressing the lid brought more of the tumour into view, and a very cursory examination now showed that the diseased mass certainly extended far into the orbit, and probably elsewhere. Vision was very much impaired. There was much pain in the part, as well as in the forehead and face, and especially at the menstrual period. She had not been able to lie flat in bed for many months, and this, as well as general distress, made her very anxious for relief. Some years before, she had consulted Sir Benjamin Brodie, Messrs. Lawrence, Tyrrell, and Dalrymple, all of whom advised delay. An attempt was subsequently made to arrest the growth by some surgical treatment, but ineffectually.

I determined to inject with tannic acid. On the 16th of October, 1856, in the presence of Mr. Square, and some other surgeons, I made a small opening into one of the most prominent veins, introduced the coarse nozzle of an Anel's syringe, and rapidly injected the syringeful of a solution of tannic acid. Hæmorrhage, which was for a few seconds copious, ceased at once, and the tumour became solid. Except for the escape of blood, the quantity of injection could not, I suppose, have passed in so readily.

Severe inflammatory action, abscess, with discharge of the solidified blood, and great constitutional fever, followed the operation. In three months the abscess had healed, the eyeball had sunk to its natural level, the tumour was destroyed, and all the distress occasioned by it had passed away. At this date the cure is still complete. The ocular movements are restricted, and there is no vision, but the eyeball looks quite natural.

My patient is well satisfied with the result.

The ligature in various forms; to cause strangulation and sloughing, is the remedy I most commonly use, and is most to be relied upon. It is applicable to every kind of nævus, although not to every case; and it may be used in combination with other modes of treatment. The most simple means of application is to introduce one or more pins of soft steel across the bottom of the tumour, and with a string of suitable strength, and sufficiently long to be securely held, to tie it very tightly, cutting off, of course, the pin-points. Some surgeons leave the part to slough off; but the cure is equally well effected, and a less scar is left, by releasing the ligature, and withdrawing the pins at an early period; that is, so soon as the surface of the part is blackened over, and the superficies evinces a loss of vitality, by which time the entire nævus is generally destroyed. As tying the skin gives great pain, and will in children produce constitutional disturbance, a channel should be cut for the ligature, unless the nævus is small. A single ligature will suffice only when the nævus is superficial and narrow; if it be broad, the centre cannot be constricted, except more than one noose or tie be used. A double ligature is applied by a needle set in a handle, which is passed through the nævus, and each half separately tied. Sometimes more ligatures are

FIG. 66.

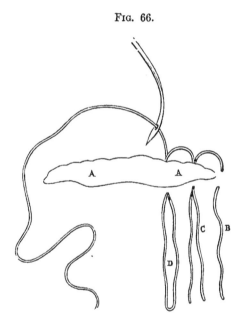

A, A, Projecting nævus to be tied.
B, Single ligature, passed beyond the limits of the growth.
C, Cut extremity of the first loop, to form a knot with B.
D, Third loop, uncut.

required, in which case the needle must be passed across at short intervals, so that the entire growth may be traversed, and every part included within the circles of the thread, as above represented.

If a nævus be superficial, there is not any difficulty in thus treating it; if deep, the ligatures must be kept down by being tied under pins previously introduced as deeply as it is necessary that strangulation should be effected. A multiplicity of ligatures may be conveniently replaced in particular instances, especially when the mass is round, by certain forms of noose. Mr. Fergusson has suggested one, which is figured in his work on "Surgery." This I have modified a little, so as to make it more symmetrical; as double ties work better when made uniformly, and by my arrangement of the threads there is less likelihood of mistake being made, by the wrong ends being taken up. The annexed diagram shows the arrangement of the noose, which is tied in the following manner:—A nævus needle, with

FIG. 67.

an eye sufficiently large to be readily threaded, armed with a double thread, is passed obliquely from left to right across and under the mass. The bow of the thread is divided, the thread disengaged, and the needle withdrawn; the needle is again threaded with the upper end of the thread on the right side, brought round on the right, entered midway between the two punctures, and carried directly across; the thread is disengaged, the needle not yet withdrawn, but first threaded with the lower end of the thread, on the left side of the first puncture, and then drawn back. If these directions have been correctly followed, the tie will have the form shown in Fig. 68.

For the subcutaneous class, tying is peculiarly adapted. The late Mr. Liston was most successful with it, reflecting the skin, usually by a cross incision, and then strangulating the nævus. After the tumour has been exposed, it should be pulled well up before being tied. The bleeding is usually not so profuse as might be expected, deep nævi being generally surrounded by a sort of fibrous capsule, which isolates them, and renders the

FIG. 68.

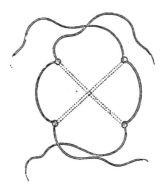

integument easy to be detached. Mr. Henry Smith operated on one as large as an orange, situated on the scapula, in which this fibrous capsule or investment was very distinct. To check any after-oozing of blood, Mr. Liston used to wrap a piece of lint tightly around the base of the tumour, and secure it by a single knot.

Another method that may be adopted when the tumour is small, and does not lie very deep, is to cut through the surface and make a channel for the ligatures to sink into. Either of these plans must be selected, according to existing circumstances: the state of the skin, the depth, the form, the extent, and the position of the nævus being the points for guidance.

But nævi may be tied without breaking the skin, except at the punctures where the ligature is introduced. This is a great advantage when the skin is healthy. The subjoined diagram, which I copy from a paper by Mr. Curling, is intended to show a mixed nævus of the lower eyelid so treated. Setons had failed in his hands, and another surgeon had applied escharotics several times.

Of the case he writes, " I took a slightly-curved needle, armed

with a strong silk ligature, and inserted it at the outer margin
of the lid, passed it close beneath the skin transversely across
near the margin of the palpebra, bringing it out at the inner
side of the swelling. I then re-inserted it at the point of exit,
carrying it in like manner close underneath the skin downward,
and bringing it out below the lowest part of the nævus. The
needle was again introduced at the point of exit, and carried
upwards beneath the skin to the point at which it was first
inserted, thus encircling subcutaneously the whole of the morbid
growth. The ligatures were then drawn tight." The nævus
was entirely obliterated.

FIG. 69.

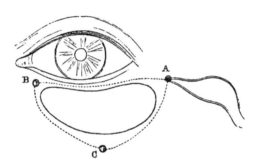

A, Point at which the ligature was introduced.
B, Point at which the ligature was brought out and again inserted.
C, Second point of exit and third of insertion.
The dotted line marks the course of the ligature subcutaneously.

Mr. Startin has lately tied nævi under the skin in a manner
which differs from the above only in the slowness of the process:
an elastic band being tied to the ligature, passed round the
nævus, and by the action of which the ligature cuts its way out
in a few days.

Like the ordinary superficial ligature, the subcutaneous one
may be multiple, or the noose I have described may be tied
subcutaneously. The first time I effected this, which is a complex process, was in a child a few months old, with a large
subcutaneous nævus between the side of the nose and the
eyelid. Several kinds of treatment had been ineffectually tried,

and the disease was rapidly progressing. I carried the ligatures close to the bone. The disease was destroyed. It will be found easier, when it is desirable to save skin, not to make this noose altogether subcutaneous, but to cut the surface for a part of the ligature to enter, when the size of the nævus would seem to require it. I suspect that certain favourable conditions should be present to render the subcutaneous tying efficient, and especially those of unusual prominence, with little depth of the part to be tied. The insertion of pins for the ligature to pass under would in a manner overcome the tendency to embrace only the super- ficies of the tumour, but it would render the subcutaneous tie very difficult.

The twisted or harelip suture is often resorted to by some surgeons. A pin is passed through the tumour, and a thread carried over it, in a figure of 8. If the object be to cut off the supply of blood, several pins are generally used, and made to circumscribe the base of the nævus. This suture should not be used merely as a means of exciting inflammation, since it is less effectual for this purpose than a method yet to be described, the seton, and is sure to be attended by a well-marked scar, should the pin be allowed to ulcerate its way out.

The last to be noticed of the means in general use is the seton, which is very useful, and is followed by less scar than any other surgical measure, except subcutaneous tying. Like many others, it is uncertain, but its failure is unattended with any disadvantage save disappointment, while it does not render the nævus at all less fit for other treatment. It is applicable to all species of nævus, and, as with all setons used to excite inflam- mation, the degree can generally be regulated. Threads of various materials and size are passed by a needle in several directions, and at different depths; and they may be charged with irritant fluids, such as a solution of lunar caustic, caustic potass, or with perchloride of iron, croton oil, or tincture of cantharides. It is usually mentioned as a precaution against hæmorrhage, that the seton should fill the wound made for it.

A remarkable instance of the usefulness of the seton on a

large scale is given by Mr. Fergusson, in his "Practical Surgery" (second edition). A tumour was situated between the trochanter major and the external condyle, of three or four inches at least in diameter, its exact limits being indefinite, with large pulsating vessels passing into it at all sides. Small ulcers formed, and bled on any unusual effort; excision was out of the question, and incision equally so, while its breadth, flatness, and supposed depth, prevented any attempt to produce sloughing by ligature. The parts were not favourable for pressure, and vaccination or caustic seemed insufficient for a tumour of such bulk. The twisted suture had been used with some effect, but still a formidable part of the disease remained. Mr. Fergusson passed several large cords as setons; these had a favourable influence, but the inflammation excited was not sufficient for the cure. By means of long slender needles, single threads were introduced in all directions, more active inflammation ensued, the tumour became smaller and firmer, the pulsation was less, and the thrill lost. The lad was watched for a year and a half, but there was no indication of disease likely to trouble him, and he went to sea.

In contrast to the severity of the last case may be mentioned that of the infant daughter of a. medical friend, born with a

FIG. 70.

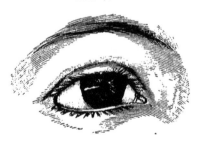

nævus at the inner angle of the eye, not larger than a pin's head, which rapidly increased, and in six weeks had acquired the size of a bean. Three twisted threads, which had been moistened in a solution of caustic potash, were passed into it with a curved needle, and retained for three days. Very slight inflammation was excited, a healthy eschar formed, and the nævus was cured. Neither contraction of surrounding skin, nor of the cartilage of the lid, followed ; the lacrymal duct was uninjured, and the scar is just perceptible, as the figure indicates.

Very slight degree of contraction of the soft parts at the internal angle of the eye would have drawn the puncta lacrymalia away from the globe, and might, if considerable, have been injurious to the lacrymal apparatus.

In this review of remedies,· little more than slight allusion has been made to the mixed nævus, the tumour involving both skin and subcutaneous tissue, and which is most difficult to be eradicated. The following condensed notes of such a case show how all treatment was baffled, and the value of this example is enhanced by the fact that the surgeons who exercised their skill had attained the highest eminence in their profession, and were in the frequent habit of treating every variety of the disease. Two distinct red spots, not larger than the point of a pin, were discovered fourteen days after birth, on the lower eyelid ; they increased, but were not treated till the child was nine weeks old. June 11th, 1849, Mr. Key applied potassa fusa without decided effect, a very small portion only having been used, through fear of the escharotic entering the eye. June 18th, the potass was again applied, and repeated on the 21st, the 26th, and the 30th of June, and on the 5th and 9th of July. It was now considered necessary to use nitrate of silver from time to time. The family left town for another residence ; and as the nævus still increased, Mr. Key was written to, and he ordered the tincture of iodine. On the 13th August, being sent for, he was greatly surprised to find how much the nævus had augmented. Before the next appointed consultation, this able surgeon was removed from his sphere of usefulness. Mr. Coulson was now consulted, and employed the ligature, endeavouring to strangulate the greater part of the growth, and succeeded in destroying a considerable portion. He afterwards used nitric acid, which unfortunately excited

a violent ophthalmia, followed by an abscess within the lid.
March 13th, Sir Benjamin Brodie and Mr. Coulson attended,
and the baronet's method of puncturing and using caustic was
four times adopted; April 6th being the period of the last
application, still the disease crept on, and by Mr. Coulson's
request, I was now consulted. I found the cheek much scarred,
and the cutaneous portion of the nævus nearly destroyed, but
the subcutaneous part was in full activity ; the space from the
external angle of the eye to the angle of the mouth, and to the
side of the nose, was occupied by it ; the bridge of the nose was
also traversed, and a narrow portion was stealing under the
other eyelid. It was no easy matter to decide on what should be
done, on account of the very great extent, the peculiarly irregular outline, and the position of the disease, and the probability of eversion of the eyelid, should sloughing ensue. There
had been a slight amount of eversion after the ligature by
Mr. Coulson, but this had passed away. I decided on passing
some fifteen or twenty threads in many directions, as a first
trial. The day was arranged for this, but afterwards postponed,
as the child had a severe and dangerous attack of measles, and
I have not since heard of it.

Tying the common carotid artery on the side corresponding
to a nævus has been practised, when the position of the disease
about the head or face, or other circumstances, forbade the
adoption of any of the foregoing means ; or when local measures alone have been unavailing—the probability of coagulation
occurring in the diseased part being the ground on which the
practice is founded. I was informed by Mr. Wardrop that, of
six instances in which he tied this artery, three were for nævi.
Two proved unsuccessful. The third was in an infant five
months old : the disease covered one half of the root of the
nose, the eyebrow, and the upper eyelid. The eyelid could not
be sufficiently raised to expose the eyeball, nor could the precise
limits of the tumour in the orbit be traced, but it seemed to
penetrate deeply. The colour was pale-blue, and numerous
tortuous veins were in the integument. It did not pulsate, was

doughy and inelastic, and capable of great diminution by pressure. Complete success ensued.

A case by Dr. Arenat, communicated to the Medico-Chirurgical Society by Mr. Wardrop, illustrated the necessity of tying the carotid, as a preparatory measure to other treatment. A man who had from birth several nævi in different parts of his body, received a blow on one of them, situated on the right temple. It increased rapidly in size, acquiring a prodigious bulk in the space of two hours after the injury. The carotid artery was ligatured. The tumour burst during the operation, and the loss of blood was calculated at not less than eight pounds. On the next day the tumour was entirely empty of blood, a considerable portion of skin was cut away, and about twelve small arteries tied. Success followed.

The severity of some cases has necessitated the tying of both carotids. Möller practised it on a child four years old with success; and in a child three years of age, Mott obtaining only imperfect results from tying one common carotid artery, subsequently tied that on the other side. It would be useless to multiply examples, for enough has been advanced to prove the legitimacy of this proceeding, which has been frequently successful. Sometimes when the disease has not been removed, it has been checked, and reduced to a harmless state; yet in some few cases, tying the carotid artery, with all practicable local measures, has failed.

DILATED AND TORTUOUS VEINS.

Certain diseased conditions of the veins may resemble nævi, and are not unlikely to be confounded with them, whether on the skin or beneath it: the parts about the eye are as likely to be the seat of such morbid changes as other regions of the body. Other non-pulsating and non-malignant vascular tumours are, no doubt, met with, which do not strictly fall under any of the denominations now considered.

A delicate young man, aged twenty, an undergraduate of Oxford, consulted Mr. Lawrence, for an oblong, pulseless, blue-

coloured vascular tumour of four years' duration, situated in
front of the abdomen over the lowest ribs of the right side; it
was firm, having been frequently cauterized; and the blood
when squeezed out by pressure did not readily enter it again.
The whole mass, including some diseased integument, was
removed; the bleeding was inconsiderable, and one small cutaneous artery only was tied. The tumour consisted of a number
of tortuous and dilated vessels, which, from the thinness of
their walls, the collapsed state of the cut extremities, the want
of pulsation during life, and the general varicose appearance,
were concluded to be veins; they contained a thin watery
yellowish-red fluid, which, under the microscope, was seen to
contain blood-discs in small quantity, altered in shape and
jagged at their edges; granules, probably the remains of
decomposed blood-discs, epithelium, and fatty matter. The
wound healed without a bad symptom, and the gentleman left
town in a fortnight. The Report by Mr. Coote is in "The
Transactions of the Abernethian Society, St. Bartholomew's
Hospital."

In connexion with this subject, I must allude to a Clinical
Lecture, by Mr. Lawrence, published in the "Medical Times"
for 1850, on Cystic Tumours, their frequent connexion with
diseased vessels, and their supposed development from congenital nævi.

In the case of a tumour, to all appearance consisting entirely
of veins, Mr. Storks—whose retirement from the profession all
who knew him must deplore—tied the common carotid artery,
with the effect of greatly diminishing the mass, but it was
necessary afterwards to attack it with the twisted suture, by
which it was entirely destroyed. A drawing illustrative of the
case is to be found in the fifth and following editions of Dr.
Druitt's "Surgeon's Vade-mecum."

ANEURISM BY ANASTOMOSIS.

The affection which has received this name is nearly allied to
that just described; and, indeed, cases are not uncommonly met

with in which the characteristics of the two are combined. In its best marked form, aneurism by anastomosis consists of a mass of dilated and tortuous arteries, freely anastomosing, and forming a tumour, in which pulsation is perceptible; giving also to the hand placed on it a thrilling sensation, while, by means of the stethoscope, a loud whizzing or buzzing bruit is heard.

John Bell, who first drew attention to the true nature of this disease, which had previously been wholly misunderstood, and frequently confounded with other affections — even those of malignant nature,—included under the term "Aneurism by Anastomosis," invented by him, other morbid growths of diverse character, as is evident both from his description of their structure and from the account he gives of cases. He describes aneurism by anastomosis as consisting of small active arteries, absorbing veins, and intervening cells; and he says that in the course of the disease various sacs are formed, which sometimes contain serum, sometimes blood. Again, he speaks of some of these tumours as cellular and stringy, with uniform firmness. One is mentioned as having burst, and discharged three pounds of serum, and no blood ; and others are described as superficial, and of large dimensions, without pulsation, or exhibiting it only at times.

There can be little doubt that the subcutaneous nævus was included in this class, and even now some practical surgeons retain Bell's name, "aneurism by or from anastomosis," for all vascular tumours, and define nævus to be a mole or mother's-spot ; but anatomy, so far as it has gone, convinces us that there are important varieties of vascular tumours, and Mr. Bell's term is now properly restricted to such tumours as are made up chiefly of arteries.

The latest and most perfect examination of such a tumour that I have been able to meet with, is by Mr. Holmes Coote, who inspected a pulsating tumour, said to have been congenital, taken from the lip of a gentleman, aged forty-four, by Mr. Lawrence, in 1847. It consisted of arteries, the natural diameter of which would have been that of a large pin, dilated for about an inch of their course into thin-walled sinuses or canals, of about the calibre of the radial artery. They communicated freely, and were lodged in the natural structure of the lip, to which they were attached by loose areolar tissue.. Upon the divided surfaces there were the cut orifices of eight arteries, some of them of considerable size. Other observers have spoken of convolutions with dilatation of the vessels.

John Bell, who was a bold surgeon in the true sense of the word, scarcely recognised the danger of removing these aneurisms by the knife; he gives some admirable and practical accounts of his operations, and recommends us to proceed so as at once to reach the source whence the tumour receives its supply, to disregard the bleeding from the first incision, and save blood ultimately by making the operation rapid. Success in effecting this must depend on the sudden alteration of the blood-vessels from that state of dilatation which constitutes the disease, to their natural calibre. When the vessels are shaded off in their varicose condition to some distance around, extirpation is attended with great danger. The circumstances calling for excision must be peculiar, and the necessity for this procedure is therefore rare.

The resources of the surgeon are, however. frequently taxed to the utmost in the treatment of this formidable affection. The most energetic local measures—pressure, strangulation, ligature of the vessels passing into the tumour—frequently fail to effect a cure; and even the bolder procedure of tying the main artery supplying the region of the body on which the growth is situated is sometimes ineffectual, especially when the tumour is about the head or face.

Examples of failure after tying local vessels are to be found in cases recorded by Messrs. Lawrence, Warren, Bell, Sir Benjamin Brodie, and others; and Dr. Massey, of America, as we are told in Mr. Cooper's "Surgical Dictionary," tied both common carotid arteries, with an interval of twelve days, for a large pulsating congenital tumour upon the head of a man, and was obliged ultimately to dissect the diseased structure away.

A remarkable case is related by Mr. Colles, in the "Dublin

Hospital Gazette " for 1858, of a young man who had almost all his life been under treatment for a large arterial tumour lying on the right parietal bone. Pressure, ligature of the posterior auricular artery, and subsequently of the carotid, had been tried without effect. Six large arteries which could be felt leading to it were obliterated by the twisted suture; and this failing, the entire growth was surrounded with a circle of fourteen pins and twisted sutures, and these were allowed to cut their way out—a process which required six weeks. This was only partially successful, and setons were tried; at first simple, then of woollen thread dipped in solution of sulphate of copper. By this means inflammation was set up, and an abscess formed; but it was still found necessary to apply caustic freely before a cure could be effected.

Several cases have been recorded as aneurism by anastomosis in the orbit; it has, however, been shown by Mr. Nunneley, of Leeds, in an able paper in vol. xlii. of the " Medico-Chirurgical Transactions," that this has not been their true nature, but that the affection is really exceedingly rare. Referring to these, and especially to those of Mr. Travers, recorded in vol. ii. of the " Transactions," and of Mr. Dalrymple, in vol. vi., which originally gave rise to the erroneous idea which has since prevailed respecting them, he says:—" In hardly one particular do these cases of disease in the orbit resemble aneurism by dilatation, or enlargement of the small blood-vessels in any other part of the body. 1st. It is very doubtful if aneurism by anastomosis is ever developed unless it has a congenital origin. 2nd. Aneurism by anastomosis does not appear suddenly; and when it is noticed, its increase is usually slow and gradual. 3rd. It is not caused by direct violence. 4th. All the blood-vessels in the neighbourhood of aneurism by anastomosis appear to participate more or less in the increased action, as active agents, and not merely as passively dilated tubes. 5th. It is almost always, if not invariably, connected with the cutaneous or subcutaneous tissues. 6th. The result, where a single large distant artery has been tied in aneurism by anastomosis, is not such as to lead to the supposition that all pulsation and tumefaction would instantly disappear on ligature of the carotid, if such a disease existed in the orbit; though a cure might follow, the effect would be more gradual." In contrast with these statements, he points out—1st. That with certain exceptions all the cases were in adults. 2nd. The want of evidence of congenital undeveloped disease of the blood-vessels. 3rd. The sudden access and frequently traumatic origin of the disease. 4th. The merely passive dilatation of the neighbouring vessels. 5th. The depth of the disease from the cutaneous surface. 6th. The sudden arrest of the pulsation, thrill, and tumefaction on ligature of the carotid.

Dr. Valentine Mott had a case in which aneurism by anastomosis of the orbit extended over the bridge of the nose, and Dr. Wood (both of America) another, in which nævus commencing near the angle of the eye involved the orbit ; but, to quote again Mr. Nunneley, " the integuments about the orbit were so involved that the affection should rather be regarded as that so frequently found in the integuments of the head and face, accidentally involving the orbit, than as aneurism of the orbit itself." In both these instances also, the carotid was tied with success.

The following case, in which, as the disease could not be attacked locally, I tied the carotid, seems to have been one of aneurism by anastomosis in the orbit, and so far as I know it is unique.

A remarkably fine girl, two months old, was brought to me at the Central London Ophthalmic Hospital, in 1851, with a slight prominence of the right eye, which had been discovered within a month after birth. There was no indication of any particular disease, and after a few visits, the infant was not again brought till she was four months old. At that time the eye was prominent, the eyelids swollen, the cheek puffy, and the conjunctiva thickly set with large bright-red vessels. Pressure on the eyeball lessened the protrusion for a few seconds, while crying rendered the eye more vascular, and caused great temporary protrusion. In a fortnight there was an increase of all the symptoms ; pulsation was felt, and the stethoscope applied over the eye detected an arterial souffle, not heard at the other orbit. Those of my colleagues at St. Mary's Hospital who examined the case, agreed with me that there was an aneurism by anastomosis. Cold lotion had been constantly applied for three weeks without effect. It was not considered prudent to apply pressure, on account of the pain which it seemed to produce. The following figure conveys a good idea of the prominence of the eye.

FIG. 71.

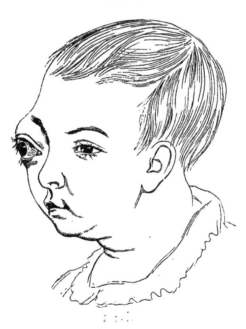

On the 5th of June, when the child was four months and three weeks old, with the assistance of Mr. Coulson, Mr. Browne, of Belfast, and Mr. R. Taylor, I proceeded to tie the common carotid artery, Dr. Snow administering chloroform. The incision was made an inch and three quarters long, over the course of the artery. The undeveloped state of the muscles of the neck, and the adhesion of their surfaces peculiar to infancy, rendered the use of the knife necessary for their separation : only a very small portion of the internal jugular vein was seen. The ligature was passed, but not tied till the effect of the chloroform had subsided. This was observed as a precautionary measure, but there was not the slightest perceptible effect on the brain when the circulation was checked. Only a few drops of blood were lost.

As soon as the child had become insensible under the influence of chloroform, the protrusion of the eyeball was greatly lessened.

June 6th.—The protrusion remains the same.

7th.—The wound seems to have healed by the first intention. The protrusion of the eyeball is sensibly diminished; the surrounding integuments have a less swollen appearance. The child was sick twice or thrice during the night.

June 10th.—The protrusion of the eyeball is gradually decreasing, and the child can now easily close the eyelids when asleep, which she could not do prior to the operation. There has not been any more sickness.

The sutures were removed on the fourth day, and, except where the ligature passed out, there was perfect union.

Pressure was now applied by means of pads, retained by an elastic bandage around the head.

The last time I saw the child was in February, 1854. I then took it to St. Mary's Hospital, to show it to my colleagues, and to the pupils. It was well grown and intelligent. She had never evinced the least symptom of cerebral disturbance or disordered intellect. Vision was perfect. The eyeball was yet a little prominent, but not so much as to constitute a deformity, and not thrown out of its axis: the movements were natural. The pupil was of the same size as that of the other eye, and the iris moved readily. A few tortuous vessels, deeply placed in the conjunctival sulci, marked the site of the disease ; but to get a view of them, the lids required to be everted. The vascular supply to the two sides of the face appeared to be alike. The scar of the incision in the neck was still seen, but was very small.

An objection to my procedure in this case was taken by some surgeons, who thought the rapidity of the establishment of the collateral circulation at that early period of life, would render

the operation useless, and that the disease would progress unin-
terruptedly. The result has fortunately disproved the apprehension, and certainly adds value to the remarks of Professor
Miller concerning the deligation of arteries in such cases, " that
the circulation is weakened in the tumour, not arrested; and
coagulation may partly occur, causing obliteration; but what is
more probable, that the dilated vessels merely recover their
normal calibre, and remain pervious. Immediately after the
main artery's deligation they are comparatively empty, and
remain so until the collateral circulation is fully established;
and, their tone never having been lost, they naturally contract,
and accommodate themselves to their reduced contents. By the
time the circulation is fully restored, they may have become
confirmed in their diminished bulk; the heart's impulse being
still modified, re-distension will not occur."

CHAPTER X.

ANEURISM of the ophthalmic artery; aneurism of that part of the carotid between its exit from the petrous portion of the temporal bone and its division, which lies in the cavernous sinus; and, it must be added, other diseased conditions, of more obscure character, about this sinus, all give rise to the same, or very similar symptoms—protrusion of the eyeball, pulsation, and bruit.

Mr. Guthrie gives an example in his work on the "Operative Surgery of the Eye," in which the eye had gradually protruded till it seemed to be out of the orbit; vision, however, being scarcely affected; a hissing noise in the head being also present. After the death of the patient, an aneurism of the ophthalmic artery was discovered, on each side, of about the size of a large nut; the ophthalmic vein was greatly enlarged, and obstructed near where it passes through the foramen lacerum orbitale anterius. A great increase in size of the four recti muscles, accompanied by an almost cartilaginous hardness, also added to the protrusion of the eye.

In a paper by Mr. Nunneley, in the "Medico-Chirurgical Transactions," referred to in the foregoing chapter, is related a case of an old woman of sixty-five, who, stooping down to tie her shoe, felt something give way in her left eye, suddenly, "as the crack of a gun." She had, at once, great pain and buzzing noise in the head; she became confused, and deaf on that side. The eyeball protruded, and felt as if it would burst.

The eyelids became swollen and congested; the eye was damaged, and sight lost: pulsation and bruit were present.

The carotid was tied, and next day the left eye was level with the other, the congestion less, and the sight improved. She died sixteen days after the operation, from the effects of repeated hæmorrhage. It was found that the ophthalmic artery, though atheromatous and dilated, presented no aneurism; but at the bend of the carotid, as it issued from the bony canal, in the temporal bone, was a slight dilatation, and around and within the dilated part a coagulum of about the size of a horse-bean. The brain over this point was softened and broken down.

In another instance, reported by Mr. Hulke, in which all the signs of orbital aneurism were present, protrusion, pulsation, and bruit, the carotid was ligatured by Mr. Bowman, with the effect of diminishing these symptoms, at first, but in about thirteen days after the operation the eye again became prominent, congested, and everted; there was, however, no return of the pulsation. Death took place on the nineteenth day, and the only disease to account for the symptoms was inflammation of the dura mater about the cavernous and other sinuses at the base of the skull, with coagula in their canals. The carotid was of natural size, the ophthalmic artery was not more dilated, nor were its branches more numerous, or larger than usual, but the ophthalmic vein was much enlarged, and had the appearance of a varix.

These cases, each of which is individually of great interest, are mutually illustrative, and together they indicate the essential conditions on which the symptoms attributed to aneurism by anastomosis in the orbit depend, and throw light on the entire series of cases in which this affection has been considered to exist. The symptoms in all three were similar; the pathological condition, as revealed by *post-mortem* examination, different in each;—in one, aneurism of the ophthalmic artery; in another, aneurism of the carotid in the cavernous sinus; in the third, phlebitis of the cavernous and other sinuses, with inflammation of the adjacent dura mater. In all, however, there is one common character—obstruction to the return of blood by the ophthalmic vein; and this must be held as sufficient, not only to cause the protrusion of the eyeball, but also the pulsatile movement which is communicated to it by the ophthalmic artery. Under these circumstances, as is pointed out by Mr. Hulke, in his interesting remarks on the case reported by him, "the pulsation of the ophthalmic artery must be attended by a general momentary increase of the whole quantity of blood in the orbit, because its exit through the ophthalmic vein is cut off, and the resisting bony walls of the orbit could permit a distension in front only." There is no doubt, however, that aneurism within the orbit would give rise to all the symptoms, independently of the venous obstruction.

As has been before stated, most of the cases reported as aneurism by anastomosis in the orbit, must be set down as orbital, or intra-cranial aneurism. That of Mr. Travers was as follows:—A female, aged thirty-four, far advanced in pregnancy, felt a sudden snap in the left side of the forehead, attended with pain, followed, at once, by swelling of the eyelids and ophthalmia, and subsequently by protrusion of the eyeball, with an evident tumour in the upper-part of the orbit, pulsation, thrill, and a constant noise in the head, resembling the blowing of a pair of bellows. The carotid was tied, with immediate good results, and ultimate cure. It is not necessary again to go over the grounds on which the diagnosis of so eminent a surgeon as Mr. Travers has been set aside, and this case quoted as an instance of orbital, or intra-cranial aneurism; they are fully stated under the head of "Aneurism by Anastomosis."

The disease under consideration has frequently a traumatic origin. A case of this kind was treated by Mr. Busk, and is recorded in vol. xxii. of the "Medico-Chirurgical Transactions." A seaman aged twenty was admitted into the Seamen's Hospital, July 13th, 1835, with severe concussion of the brain. The eyelids and integuments about the left eye were swollen, the pupil dilated and motionless, and the orbital muscles paralysed.

The eye became inflamed from constant exposure, and the cornea suffered from ulceration and the deposit of pus between its layers. Some months after the accident the eye became prominent. On the 1st of February distinct pulsation was for the first time made out, and a firm pulsating tumour was detected at the inner and upper part of the orbit. The pulsation was accompanied by a very distinct thrill, and the stethoscope conveyed a loud whizzing sound. Pressure on the carotid artery arrested the pulsation, and on February 2nd this vessel was ligatured. On the 15th the ligature came away ; on the 28th, there was scarcely any prominence of the eye, and the patient was discharged. Some years afterwards when he was seen by Mr. Busk, there was no trace of the tumour, nor could pulsation be detected.

The treatment to be adopted in instances of this kind has been sufficiently indicated by the cases related, — ligature of the common carotid. This operation for disease in the orbit was first performed in this country by Mr. Travers in the case quoted. It has since been done by Mr. Dalrymple (" Medico-Chirurgical Transactions," vol. vi.), by Mr. Busk and Mr. Scott (vol. xxii.), by Mr. Curling (vol. xxxvii.), by Dr. Van Buren, by Dr. Mott, by Jobert, and by Velpeau ("Bibliothèque du Médecin Praticien") ; also recently by Mr. Nunneley, of Leeds, to whom the profession is much indebted for scientific and accurate ideas respecting this disease ; in four cases, which are recorded in vol. xlii. of the " Medico-Chirurgical Transactions ;" and by Mr. Bowman, in the case reported by Mr. Hulke. Of these, Mr. Busk's, Mr. Scott's, Mr. Curling's, Dr. Van Buren's, Velpeau's, one of Mr. Nunneley's, and Mr. Bowman's, were traumatic. Of those not due to injury, it is worthy of remark, as Mr. Nunneley has pointed out, that in the majority of instances the patients were women, and advanced in pregnancy, and that the disease affected the left side. The operation has been successful in all the cases, except the two of which the pathological appearances are detailed above. Pulsation, however, may return after a longer or shorter interval in the same or opposite orbit ; and in No. 10

of the Ophthalmic reports, the case of a sailor is mentioned by Mr. Poland, in whom protrusion of the left eye with thrill and bruit came on four years after ligature of the right carotid by Dr. Mott, for a similar affection of the right eye coming on after an injury to the head.

It will be an interesting subject for future investigation to ascertain the signs by which intra-cranial and orbital aneurisms may be distinguished from each other, and from obstruction to the return of blood by the ophthalmic vein. It seems probable that, in the cases which most closely simulate aneurism by anastomosis—as when the pulsation seems to spread beyond the margin of the orbit, or where it reappears after ligature of the carotid—the cause will be found to be venous obstructions, either from pressure on the ophthalmic vein or from disease in the cavernous sinus; and when the affection has a traumatic origin from blows on the head, it is more likely to be the carotid artery that is injured when in close relation with the bone in the cavernous sinus, than the ophthalmic, lodged in the soft tissues of the orbit ; so that I should expect the intra-cranial origin of orbital pulsation to be by far the most frequent.

CHAPTER XI.

TUMOURS.

TUMOURS OF THE EYELID.

WITH the view to prevent bleeding during the removal of
tumours of the eyelids, M. Desmarres has invented an instrument, a kind of forceps with rings at the extremities, between
which the eyelid is placed, and the rings made to press on it by
a screw in the handle, which draws them together. It cannot
be employed without much pain and some violence to the parts.
I do not use it, but some surgeons speak of it in high terms.

STYE.

This miniature boil is too generally known to need much
description. Its uniform appearance, and its accustomed position
at the margin of the tarsus among the cilia, some of which are
sure to be displaced, probably from its origin in one of the cilia-
follicles, with soreness of the eyelid, and accompanying inflammation of the conjunctiva, render it little likely to be mistaken.
Stye is generally an indication of an unhealthy constitution,

and is common in strumous and enfeebled subjects, or in any class of individuals whose health is broken down. With the predisposition of impaired health it is very prone to appear, if there be long-continued employment of the eyes by artificial light, and especially if there co-exist derangement of the digestive organs.

The progress of a stye is usually sufficiently slow to allow of time for treatment, and oftentimes the prevention of suppuration. We must enjoin rest of the eye, frequent applications of cold lotions to the exterior of the eyelid, sedatives to the conjunctiva, and such means as will recruit the system. Plucking out the cilia that seem most affected is said to be advantageous.

It is only when the stye has nearly arrived at its climax that an opening is useful. The usually slow and tedious suppuration, generally attended with a little slough of the cellular tissue, may then be considerably shortened by an incision, and the use of a stimulating ointment.

HORNS.

I have met with a few specimens of the growth or deposit of inspissated sebaceous matter on the eyelids, that are called horns. They have all been small, time being wanting to give them the more marked characteristic horny appearance to which they owe their name, and of which the scalp furnishes the best examples.

It is uncalled for here to say more of their structure than that these dense appendages owe their existence to the drying and hardening, as fast as it escapes, of the contents of the encysted tumours, or of the sebaceous follicles that supply the soft material. To those who desire extended information on the pathology of the subject, I recommend the perusal of a very excellent paper by Mr. Erasmus Wilson, published in vol. xxvi. of the " Medico-Chirurgical Transactions," descriptive of a horn developed from the human body, with observations on the pathology of certain disorders of the sebaceous glands.

A single stroke of the knife will be sufficient to remove a

horn from the lid. The excrescence being pulled forwards, the separation should be made through the integuments, that the cyst from which it grows may be entirely taken away, or a return of the disease is risked. A scar may be prevented by the use of sutures.

WARTS.

These growths are very uncommon about the eyelids, and when on their margins are, for the most part, slender. A marked example of the entire edge of each, thickly set with large ones, occurred in an old man, a patient at the Ophthalmic Hospital.

Some have been remarkable from their size; and Heister mentions one that was large enough to restrict the motions of the upper eyelid. Dr. Jacob showed a specimen to the Dublin Surgical Society, a full report of which is in the "Dublin Medical Press," of one taken from the lower eyelid, and at first supposed to be a malignant growth, but which, after being carefully cleansed, proved to be a gigantic wart. The surface was covered with a cream-coloured structure, made up of coarse fibres which stood out fully the eighth of an inch perpendicularly from the surface, and which he considered as a cuticular or epidermoid growth. The patient, who was eighty years of age, died after its removal, from erysipelas of the face.

Except a wart have a very small base, snipping it off is not sufficient, unless the entire thickness of the skin be cut through, for it will return; some caustic must be applied in addition.

When beyond the ordinary size, I think it better to try, in the first instance, the effect of an escharotic, as less damage will accrue to the parts. One drachm of muriatic acid with three drachms of the muriated tincture of iron is said to be very effectual. Many other applications will succeed. Excision should be the last resource, on account of the injury that must be inflicted on the tarsus.

MOLLUSCUM, OR GLANDIFORM TUMOUR, SOMETIMES DESCRIBED AS
ALBUMINOUS TUMOUR.

A kind of tumour common in children, and now generally
called glandiform, being so named by Mr. Tyrrell, from its
resemblance to a salivary gland, occurs about the eyelids, and
frequently also on the face coincidently. It is rarely solitary;
there are several seen in different stages of development; some
of them may have softened in the centre and suppurated,
and having burst their envelope, protrude, and become surrounded with an incrustation which makes them look like warty
growths.

When fully formed, its appearance is characteristic, being
mottled, and the gland-like structure is at once recognisable.
In a very recent state it resembles a sebaceous tumour.

The subjoined figure, from a girl seven years old, represents
two of them in the lower eyelid, the larger of which was partly
covered with black incrustation, from beneath which a little pus

Fig. 72.

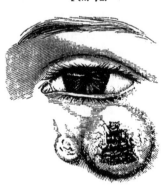

escaped. This patient had no more of them; but her sister's
face was covered, and a third member of the family, the mother,
had also a few.

The treatment consists in cutting the mass across by a free
incision, and squeezing out its contents with the thumb-nails.
If the cyst do not separate at the same time, the forceps must
be used for its extraction.

STEATOMATOUS TUMOUR.

This surface deposit of steatomatous matter, generally called milium, from its resemblance to a millet-seed, is not confined to the eyelids ; it appears also on the cheeks, and frequently in great numbers. It evidently originates in obstruction to a sebaceous follicle, which as it becomes distended gets thicker and stronger; in fact, it grows. In size it is seldom beyond that of a pin's head, except when it grows at the edge of the eyelid, about the junction of the cuticular and mucous membranes, or between the eye and the nose, when its usual limit may be far exceeded, as in this sketch, taken from a lady of seventy.

FIG. 73.

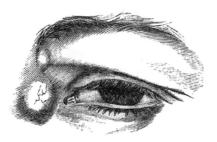

Here it was like a small bladder of lard, apparently covered only by cuticle, and retaining for a while any form into which it was pressed. Whether small or large, the treatment is to cut it across, squeeze out the contents, and apply plaster. Generally the cyst gives no trouble, and requires no special treatment. When it is thicker than usual, and evidently should be got rid of, but is yet too delicate to dissect out, nitrate of silver should be applied.

VESICULAR TUMOUR.

This is perhaps the best name for the small cyst containing fluid, and occurring about the lids, and which may perhaps, like the above, originate in a sebaceous follicle. The contents vary, being sometimes watery, sometimes glairy. I removed one

R 2

about the size of a pea, that had been growing for twenty-six years, and was filled with a glairy matter, from the surface of the upper eyelid of an elderly lady. Figure 74 shows one of a

FIG. 74.

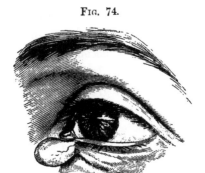

peculiar form, that had existed for five years, and was filled with serum. I have seen one at the outer corner of the eye which overlapped the edges of the eyelids, and interfered with sight. The old gentleman, who had carried it for a quarter of a century, could never make up his mind to have it removed, although he greatly wished to be relieved from the inconvenience and the deformity resulting from it.

When small, a simple puncture will effect a cure; but otherwise the cyst must be removed or cauterized, or there will be reproduction.

TARSAL, OR MEIBOMIAN TUMOUR.

I would speak of this as a hard, spherical, well-defined tumour, varying in size from a grain of small shot to that of a pea, and limited to a situation on the eyelid, in the space between the cilia bulbs, and the upper margin of the tarsal cartilage. It corresponds, therefore, to the position of the Meibomian glands, does not grow at the lid edge, and is immoveable. It is inadherent to the skin, which may or may not' be traversed by enlarged blood-vessels, being usually solitary, and for the most part occurring on the upper eyelid; yet acquiring the largest dimensions on the under one, where the skin is generally in the natural state; not unfrequently giving, on the internal surface of the eyelid, indication of its existence by a spot of preternatural redness, and at a later period, discoloration, or a darkish speck, and at a very advanced stage there may be a small fungus.

The position differs, therefore, from that of a stye in being above the edge of the tarsus, and clear of the cilia, as the figure shows.

FIG. 75.

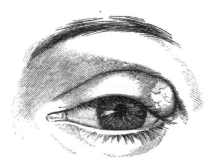

Debility of constitution favours its development; but its connexion with a vitiated state of health is not so marked as in stye, with which it may co-exist. Perhaps it is most commonly seen in middle-aged persons with acne about the face. Several

FIG. 76.

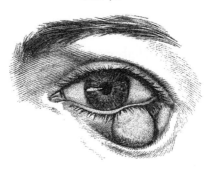

may be on the same eyelid, and both eyes may be affected alike. It is of remarkably slow growth, and many months may elapse before it attains to the size of that depicted in fig. 75.

The second illustration shows one on the lower eyelid, of unusual dimensions.

Probably, if left alone, the tumour would grow still larger, for spontaneous cure by suppuration or bursting is rare. In the Hunterian Collection of the College of Surgeons is a cyst, taken from an eyelid, three quarters of an inch in diameter, and which seems to be a tarsal tumour.

It is produced by one of the acini of the Meibomian follicles becoming enlarged and filled by sebaceous matter. The follicles are not either on the outside nor on the inside of the fibro-cartilage of the eyelid, but in its very substance.

I shall give the morbid anatomy of one that I removed from the living body, and examined with Dr. Druitt. Externally there was a dense, fibrous cyst, continuous with the fibrous tissue of the eyelid; within this, a layer of fibro-plastic matter, soft, pink, abundantly supplied with vessels from the fibrous cyst, composed of fibro-plastic cells, with a very little intercellular fibrillary matter; within this, again, a thin pellucid cyst, containing a puriform fluid, made up of pus globules, epithelium cells loaded with oil, and in the centre a perfectly round pellet of sebaceous matter.

In all probability the following is the order of development. First, the formation in a Meibomian follicle, of a pellet of hard sebaceous matter. Second, the secretion of a more copious epithelium and fluid matter around. Third, the addition of fibro-plastic matter around the obstructed gland follicle, distending the loculus of fibrous membrane into a cyst.

It is well known that Meibomian tumours may contain dissimilar substances. We meet with glairy, sebaceous, creamy, or purulent deposits, and the amount does not always bear a uniform relation to the size of the tumour, there being sometimes scarcely any fluid in a very large one, the sac being filled with a solid material. On this point, I venture to suggest that some of these characters depend on the changes effected in the fibro-plastic material that is deposited. For instance, with the onward development of the plastic material, white or yellow fibrous tissue is produced, as in the tumour commonly called polypus; hence, the more solid tumour. Or, if it degenerate and undergo retrograde metamorphosis, the cells are converted into pus or pyoid cells, and the intercellular tissue into a creamy fluid.

No effect can be produced by medical treatment, and therefore an early operation is necessary.

As the requisite measure may, for the most part, be done within the eyelid, it is advisable for it to be so effected. When, therefore, the tumour is small, does not stand out in relief, and its position is well marked within, I evert the tarsus, puncture it, and move about the point of the knife, so as to break up the adventitious cyst. I endeavour also to squeeze out any of the contents that are likely to be so evacuated. Two or three days after, I again stir about the cavity with a sharp-pointed probe.

The patient should be warned not to expect an immediate reduction; for, with the swelling that ensues, the tumour may seem as large, or larger, than before. It is only after a few days that the reduction is apparent, and generally not for a few weeks that all trace of it is lost. In some hundreds of these operations, I have seen but a few instances of a fungus springing up from the wound. In one case, it passed from the under eyelid up in front of the cornea. If very small, I touch it with an escharotic, then dry the surface, and protect the other parts by oil, or any other suitable substance. If large, I use the scissors, and perhaps apply an escharotic as well.

When, however, the tumour is large, and well developed externally, I divide it outside, cutting freely through the integument, squeeze out the secretion with my thumb-nails, and if I can pull away the cyst with the forceps, or if I think it necessary, dissect it out. There need be no fear respecting the formation of a scar, for if the incision be made horizontally, and the edges be brought together by a strip of plaster, no trace of the operation is left.

POLYPI AND WARTS.

Growths and excrescences of all kinds from the conjunctiva are decidedly rare. I have met with warts on the palpebral portion of the membrane, and these may become quite gigantic, for instances are recorded of some having overspread the globe of the eye, and protruded from within the eyelids. A small flat red vegetation sometimes appears just within the margin of the lower eyelid, and, if allowed to grow, may rise above its level. It is most frequent just before adult age, and it is often supposed to be of a cancerous nature : it is readily and effectually destroyed by a few touches with any caustic substance. Mr. Tyrrell described an affection which seems identical with this as an enlargement of the Meibomian glands.

A soft gelatinous mass, exactly like a nasal polypus, growing with a narrow base from the ocular conjunctiva, was pointed out to me by Mr. Smee ; a snip with the scissors readily separated it.

There are growths which seem like vascular prolongations of conjunctiva, with long but very delicate pedicles, so slight that, in one instance which I have seen, during an examination of the body the pedicle broke.

I once examined a small cartilaginous tumour that was developed in the substance of the conjunctiva, and lay near the caruncle. I have met with productions of the same kind in the dog.

A youth of eighteen had two peculiar tumours which appeared

FIG. 77.

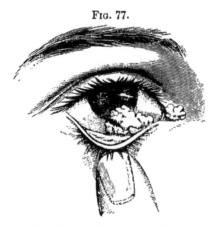

to have their seat in the conjunctiva ; the one, of a red colour, and having a mulberry, wart-like look, was on the inner surface of the upper lid, and overlapped and destroyed the punctum. The other, also red, and possessing more of a fungous appearance, overlapped and obscured a part of the cornea, but did not adhere to it; it was sufficiently wide to appear connected with the caruncle, but was found, when the tarsus was depressed, to have its base in the conjunctiva at the sinus of the eyelid, and to receive a remarkably large supply of blood-vessels from the sclerotica.

The preceding figure shows the relations of both of them.

A slight purulent discharge from the conjunctiva was all the inconvenience they produced. · It is probable that they were congenital. I removed both with the scissors, and sent the larger for microscopic examination to Dr. Sieveking, who reported it to consist "of nucleated cells, without any other constituents or stroma; the cells, varying in number, size, and shape, being oval, slightly angular, caudate, and some bifid at the extremity. Others had more irregular forms, apparently adapting themselves to the adjacent cells. There was an absence of the appearance seen in the epidermal growths, and, with few exceptions, the cells contained a distinct nucleus, with one or more dark spots, with nucleoli. Some cells that were much elongated had not any nucleus. The cells, as well as the nuclei, appeared granular, and much resembled the fibro-plastic cells figured by Lebert (Plate xiii., 'Physiologie Pathologique'), while the bifid cells had a cancerous appearance. Treated with acetic acid the cells became transparent, and the nuclei, swelling well out, became more defined and darker." The examination was with a power of four hundred diameters.

Dr. Sieveking took a sketch with his accustomed accuracy of delineation, in which he contrasted this abnormal product with the regular cells of healthy conjunctival epithelium. Nine months after the operation, there was not the least indication of the disease returning.

A man, aged sixty-four years, applied to the Central London Ophthalmic Hospital, with a circumscribed black mass about the size of an almond growing lengthwise on the interior of the

left lower eyelid, which it partially everted. The attachment
seemed slight; indeed the peculiarly well-defined base induced
the idea that the mass might be readily pulled away. The conjunctiva around and on the lower part of the eyeball, was of a
dirty brown colour. Vision was perfect. Two years prior, the
disease was discovered as a little black pimple ; and from its
commencement to his application, there had been no pain, but
merely inconvenience from the restriction to the movements of
the eyelids. He had consulted several surgeons, among whom
were Mr. Lloyd and Mr. Coulson.

I did not again see him for three years, when he reapplied at
the Ophthalmic Hospital. In the interval he had been to many
hospitals and dispensaries, where removal of the eyelid and the
eyeball had been repeatedly advised. The growth had increased
so as to cover the globe, while a piece, about the size of
a nutmeg, protruded from between the eyelids, and was with
some difficulty pulled aside to expose the cornea, which was
hazy. I wished to admit him into the house, and then carefully to examine the eye while he was under the influence of
chloroform ; and he went home with the avowed intention of
procuring some personal articles, but never returned : having
left a wrong address, I could not find him, and his fate is
unknown to me. It is probable, but not certain, that the
disease was melanosis. The duration of the affection, however,
without the surrounding parts being implicated, the absence
of pain, and the apparent isolation of the affection—for the
absorbent glands about the face were unaffected—may be taken
as some evidence against that opinion, although a strong suspicion of malignancy must still remain.

This case bears upon the writings of Dr. Jacob, of Dublin, in
the " Dublin Medical Press," in which he urges surgeons to
investigate more fully the nature of tumours of the eye and the
orbit, it being his opinion that many which are supposed to be
malignant are not so in reality, although they may not be
amenable to medical treatment, and would spread or grow to
any size unless removed by the knife or escharotics. His remarks have particular reference to what we are accustomed to

call melanotic tumours. He argues that the blackness of a disordered mass affords no clue to its true character. He had seen,
in old persons, deposits of black matter under the conjunctiva
without disease; and the fact of a growth not healing, in no
way proved the existence of a malignant disease, as he instances
in sores and warts that continue to increase under any kind of
medical treatment. In one of the two cases alluded to, a black
spongy tumour, two inches in diameter, overlapped the lids in
all directions, so as nearly to close the whole opening of the
orbit. The surface was lobulated, and appeared to have been
compressed by the bandage with which it had been covered, and
bled slightly when the adherent dressing was removed. It
appeared to be attached to the eyeball by a cylindrical stalk,
which was slightly enclosed by the eyelids. Being prepared to
remove the contents of the orbit, if necessary, Dr. Jacob drew
his knife across this, as a preliminary step of the operation,
and found that he had incised a healthy eyeball, the disease
being confined to the conjunctiva of the cornea, and of the
sclerotica. It was, in fact, a tegumentary growth from the
front of the eye. The divided eyeball healed kindly. Sufficient
time had not elapsed to enable him to pronounce as to the true
nature of the disease, whether it was to be considered malignant
or not. Its black colour, spongy texture, and slightly lobulated
appearance, did not convince him that it was a fungoid growth
of a fatal nature; although it might have produced death by
growing to a mass which could not be arrested or reduced by
remedies.

Pathology will certainly have advanced a step when a means
of accurate diagnosis shall be discovered, between melanosis of
a malignant character, and black tumours that are not malignant. I shall discuss this subject fully in the chapter on
malignant diseases of the eye, and to which I beg to refer the
reader.

The caruncle and the semilunar fold are very rarely the seat
of surgical operation. I have been applied to by a patient to
have a part of both structures removed, from enlargement following a long and severe attack of granular eyelids, and I had

some difficulty in dissuading him from it. There was a diminution of the swelling on leaving off the escharotics that had been
applied for their reduction, which were certainly causing it to
increase.

I have seen the caruncle so large, from chronic inflammation
of the conjunctiva, consequent on residence in the tropics, that
it displaced the eyelid and the punctum, and produced epiphora.
I proposed to remove it, but this was objected to.

Warty growths or polypi may issue from either of these parts.
Abscesses also form in them.

PTERYGIUM.

This affection, laboriously described by authors, derived its
name from the supposed likeness to the wing of an insect, and
has been divided into four varieties—the cellular, the vascular,
the fatty, and the fleshy; but pathology warrants no such
arrangement, while distinction for the sake of description is
useless. At different periods of its growth, different appearances
may exist : one that is thin may become thick, and one half of
the growth may be transparent and delicate, while the other is
like a piece of muscle.

The disease consists essentially of thickening of the conjunctiva and of the sub-conjunctival cellular tissue, with
increased vascularity. I have seen a little white fibrous tissue,
and even fat granules, in some of old standing. The various
aspects it presents in thickness, and in colour, depend on the
greater or lesser degree of those changes. It must retard
rather than advance the knowledge of the subject, to speak of
membranous, coriaceous, and cartilaginous pterygia, each of
which has been formally written on.

The following sketch, taken from a gentleman of colour, from
the Island of St. Kitts, exhibits a very marked specimen.

The position is the ordinary one, at the inner corner of the
eye, with the base connected with the semilunar fold and
caruncle, from which it would seem to grow. The form also is
that which is most usual.

In other instances the edges may be unequal and indefinite, and the base may be at the cornea ; even a bifurcated pterygium has been met with.

FIG. 78.

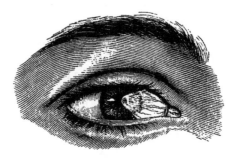

The extent or size also differs ; the greater part of the sclerotica may be covered, and the whole of the cornea veiled. Then more than one may exist in the same eye ; four have been seen several times, and Velpeau has described five.

Both eyes may be symmetrically affected.

There is a peculiarity in warm climates that renders ptery-gium common. Rognetta says that it may be met with at every step in Calabria; and the large number of operations cited by some foreign authors shows that it abounds in certain countries. Nearly all that have come under my own notice have been in natives of the tropics, Creoles, or those who have resided in hot latitudes.

Of the few exceptions, one was in a girl, a Londoner, fourteen years old, the pterygium being at the inner corner of the eye, and encroaching on the cornea. Another was in a boy twelve years old, and arose from the irritation of some slaked lime that had entered the eye. Months after the accident he was brought to me with a well-marked triangular pterygium, at the lower part of the eyeball, the rarest position for one to grow. There was not the slightest adhesion of the eyelid to the globe, nor could any of my colleagues at the Ophthalmic Hospital, or myself, determine any difference between it and an ordinary pterygium, except in the rapidity of growth. I watched it for three months, using astringents, until the increase in the corneal portion demanded operation. A third was in a stoker, about twenty years old, at one of the London gas works.

The origin of these adventitious productions is attributed to idiopathic inflammation of the eye, and to the effect produced by the entrance of irritating substances; and there can be no doubt about the general correctness of these views.

It is usually after the adult period that pterygium appears; yet it has been seen immediately after birth by Mr. Wardrop, when doubtless it must have been congenital. It is seldom, in these latitudes at least, that we have an opportunity of observing its commencement and progress. Mr. Wardrop, in his work on the Eye, gives a drawing of one that he saw from a very early period, and watched for upwards of eight years. Its first appearance was that of a small globule of fat near the junction of the cornea and the sclerotica; it then became larger, so that its base adhered to the semilunar fold, and its apex passed over the edge of the cornea.

The usual absence of any inconvenience in the earlier periods of the affection, for it arises and proceeds without any attendant symptoms, except inflammation of the conjunctiva; its slow growth, increasing but little in the course of years, and when it has overlapped the cornea, its tendency to progress still slower, have induced some surgeons to recommend non-interference. I have seen it stated that pterygium never passes over the cornea so far as to injure the sight. I have met with several examples that prove the fallacy of the assertion. In the above illustration there was an instance of it. Twice I have seen it pass quite over the pupil and render the eye useless. If the disease should become stationary from the change of climate, or from treatment, the question of operating may be left to be determined by the individual, for personal appearance alone is concerned; but when there are symptoms of augmentation, I advise the removal of it, for the operation is more severe the longer it is postponed, and the result must be less perfect.

Excision alone can be depended upon. A mere division by

cutting across the pterygium is insufficient, and may irritate it. Mr. Wardrop tells of a young gentleman who had a common triangular-shaped one from early life, which rapidly increased in growth and development under repeated scarifications. The mass was so large as to separate the tarsi, and involve the semilunar fold, and lacrymal caruncle. The greater part must be removed; yet it is advisable generally, not to touch the portion on the cornea, from the danger of injuring that strue- ture; for after the supply of blood has been cut off, that will decline.

The eyelids having been separated, the pterygium should be seized at the apex with the tenaculum forceps, and dissected off towards the base, care being taken that the edges are cut through. When operating at the inner corner of the eye, the dissection should not be continued quite to the caruncle; for in the process of repair, that body, as well as the semilunar fold, would be injured or lost. When the cornea is encroached on, the division should be at its margin.

With a view to saving the conjunctiva, Scarpa advises that when internal pterygia of the usual form have a very extensive base, they should not be severed near the broader part; and the advice is valuable, for with a great loss of that membrane, an elevated cicatrix arises, and confines the eyeball to the caruncle, preventing freedom to its outward movement. When a pterygium is adherent to the sclerotica, it must be removed at the expense of denuding this coat of the eye.

I apply sutures. I dissect up the conjunctiva slightly on each side, and put in one or two stitches at the very margin, and so bring the edges together. If the space left were too large to allow of accurate adaptation, I should still adopt the practice, as the process of healing would thereby be expedited. If the threads do not fall out in four days, in which case, in all probability, some of the subconjunctival tissue would be included, I remove them. I shall allude again to the subject of stitching the conjunctiva, in the operation for squint, and speak of its advantages.

A captain in the royal navy, who had been stationed in the

West Indies, consulted me for a pterygium that had existed
several years, and was gradually increasing; its peculiarities
are here shown. It was irregular, and the part involving the

FIG. 79.

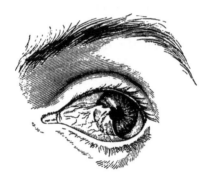

front of the eyeball was thicker than the rest. I operated,
removing a portion around the circumference of the cornea.
A dissection that would have embraced the whole of the base,
must have been followed by considerable contraction of the
conjunctiva. Even with the very limited excision, there was
for a while a sense of stiffness when the eye was turned out, but
this gradually passed off. As the corneal portion was diminishing rather slowly, I was induced to touch it with a mild
escharotic, to hasten the process, and thereby to relieve my
patient's anxiety.

Here, as in every case in which I have removed a pterygium
that had passed to the cornea, this coat remained more or less
opaque, nearly to the extent traversed by the growth. I say
nearly, for the cicatrix left from the decline of the growth is
always less than the size of the original mass. I operated on a
soldier, and four years after, the mark on the cornea was a
third less than the portion of pterygium left. Mr. Travers
gives a more favourable account of one of his operations. The
disease, in that instance, originating from beneath the whole
base of the upper eyelid, was of a triangular form, extending to
the lower margin of the cornea, of sarcomatous density, about
one line thick, and forming a fold when the eye was directed

upwards. It was, he says, completely cured by the operation of dividing and detaching it at the base;—the patient recovered her sight, and ultimately no vestige of the disease remained.

The swelling of the parts, together with the slight inflammation caused by the operation, soon subside. It is seldom, when the pterygium has been large, that the spot on which it grew recovers its normal appearance altogether. There is generally preternatural vascularity, but this becomes much less in time.

PTERYGIUM PINGUE.

This is the term applied to a little whitish-yellow tumour that is generally situated on the sclerotic coat, just internal to the cornea, and has its seat in the conjunctiva and sub-conjunctival cellular tissue. It may grow on the eyeball external to the cornea. The name, like most of the names of diseases of the eye, is badly chosen and incorrect; indeed, in this instance it is doubly wrong, for the affection has not the least resemblance to a little wing, and it does not consist of fat, but is of an albuminous nature. Like pterygium it is very common in tropical countries, yet it is not very uncommon in temperate latitudes. I meet with examples of it yearly, yet I know but of one instance in which it encroached on the cornea, and then merely the margin of it was overlapped. So inoffensive and innocuous are these growths, that it is a matter for the persons possessing them rather than the surgeon, to decide about their removal. There is involved merely the question of taking away a little blemish or deformity, and no risk of any kind attends the operation, which is simple enough. The tumour is seized with the tenaculum forceps, drawn forwards, cut off with the curved scissors, and a suture applied.

TUMOURS INVOLVING THE CORNEA AND THE SCLEROTICA.

TUMOURS OF THE SCLEROTICA.

Those tumours which are incorporated with the sclerotica, or with it and the conjunctiva, are not so readily got rid of as those involving the conjunctiva alone; nor is their removal unattended with danger. The figure shows two, that in all

FIG. 80.

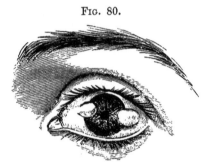

external appearances resembled the structure of the sclerotic coat.

In this instance the conjunctiva was adherent, as it has been in all the cases that I have seen. The tumours were congenital, the cornea was not encroached on till puberty; the individual being thirty when I took the sketch.

While I was attending the practice of Mr. Tyrrell, a young man came to the Royal London Ophthalmic Hospital with two of them in one eye, only one of which encroached on the cornea. This induced some remarks from my much-respected teacher on the manner of their incorporation with the sclerotica, to the effect that twice he had seen attempts at their excision; in one instance, the vitreous humour escaped, and the eye collapsed; in the other, the operator desisted when he found the true nature of the tumour. But cases are recorded of their successful extirpation.

Mr. Lawrence gives in the second edition of his ophthalmic work, two cases of tumours on the sclerotica that admitted of removal. A child ten years old had a semi-transparent firm oval swelling about the size of a pea on the sclerotica, close to the margin of the cornea, of some years' duration. Evacuation of the contents had been tried; and now, in opposition to the opinion of other gentlemen who saw the case, the cyst was punctured, and the prominent part cut away with curved scissors. It was thin but tough, the sides being firm enough to retain the figure of the tumour. The interior was smooth, and a round aperture was observed in the middle of the basis, apparently passing through the sclerotica. The wound quickly healed. The next is a case of a larger growth. A gentleman about thirty years of age, of full habit and robust frame, had a cyst on the sclerotica as large as an almond, producing irritation in the motions of the eye. An operation was performed as in the last case; but the patient was not seen again.

Scrofulous tubercles growing from the sclerotica, and elevating the conjunctiva, have been described by Dr. Mackenzie. They are whitish or yellowish, appear as if about to suppurate, but continue firm, increase slowly to perhaps the size of a hazel-nut, and burst, but do not suppurate. If left to themselves they are apt to induce disorganization and atrophy of the eyeball. If extirpation is attempted, the diseased mass is found to be soft and easily torn.

TUMOURS OF THE CORNEA.

We learn, from the publication of several cases, that the true tissue of the cornea may remain uninfluenced by growths that appear upon it, the epithelial covering alone being implicated. In an instance of this kind of surface tumour that occurred to Mr. Travers, he extirpated the anterior half of the eyeball, and the cornea and sclerotica proved to be entire; the morbid growth only lay upon and adhered to the cornea. A small portion of the sclerotic surface had acquired a lobulated appearance, and delicate white bands, the only vestige of the conjunctiva, were seen intersecting the lobules at irregular distances, in the form of septa. A case operated on by Sir A. Cooper, and mentioned in Mr. Travers's work, is nearly parallel, and other surgeons have met with similar examples.

In the fourth plate of the first volume of Mr. Wardrop's work on the eye, second edition, are two well-executed drawings of tumours involving the front of the eyeball. One is called tumour of the corneal conjunctiva; and here the growth covers one-half of the corneal surface, having, as the author describes it, no regular form, and a fine granulated texture. The other consists of a warty excrescence, occupying two-thirds of the cornea, and having an unequal surface of a peculiar dark brown colour, and of a soft texture. Other instances are recorded by authors, in some of which the tumour involved the whole cornea, and had attained the size of a hen's egg. In the Museum of the Royal College of Surgeons, is the anterior half of an eye from Sir A. Cooper's collection, with a large and broad wart-like growth covering the superficies of the cornea, and a small portion of the sclerotica around, and standing out in relief for about half an inch.

We must endeavour to remove a growth when it involves the cornea, and threatens to overspread the pupil; there should be no delay when an excrescence is steadily increasing, or has already in any way interfered with vision. As much as possible should be excised with the knife or scissors.

Escharotics should be used only when positively demanded, for they are less admissible here than in any part of the human frame. Caustic potass and the mineral acids are in general unsafe agents about the eyeball, for unless great care be exercised, they are apt to run beyond the spot to which they should be restricted. I have seen the potash applied to a little tumour of the sclerotica near the margin of the cornea, and although, as a precaution, the cornea was oiled, yet the caustic spread to it, and produced opacity. Again, strong escharotics may produce a deeper slough than is required; and however unimportant going a little beyond bounds might be in other parts of the body, precision must here be secured. The "potassa cum calce" of the London Pharmacopœia, is more manageable and safer, and should be used in preference (see page 124). But the milder caustics, such as nitrate of silver, sulphate of copper, and dilute acids, should be first tried, and

always, when practicable, with the precaution of shielding any
transparent part of the cornea with such substances in themselves harmless, as have the power of neutralizing the agent.
During this process the eyelids should be held open by an
assistant, and before they are set free, any superfluous portion of
the escharotic wiped off. It is well to grease the surfaces that
have been cauterized, lest they affect the parts with which they
naturally come into contact.

When the entire cornea is covered by the tumour, an attempt should be made to restore, as far as may be, its transparency, by cautiously excising all that can be so treated,
and leaving that which cannot be removed without injuring
it, to be further acted on by mild escharotics. It may be that
a partial operation will suffice; the thin portion left behind
may be removed by absorption.

A chimney sweeper, thirty years old, applied to me with
warty growths on each cornea. In the right eye, the pupil
was entirely obscured, and the greater part of the cornea
covered. In the left, the lower portion of the cornea only was
involved, and but half of the pupil eclipsed. I scraped off the
excrescences completely, and applied oil. There was a little
bleeding. As they were reproduced, I repeated the process three
times in two years. The effect in completely stopping the
spreading of the warts was beyond doubt. Scrotal cancer now
appeared, and the poor sufferer soon died from hæmorrhage
consequent on cancerous ulceration in the groin.

Another instance of warty opacity of the cornea relieved by
operation, is given by Mr. Bowman in his "Lectures on the
Anatomy of the Parts concerned in the Operations on the Eye."
The growth is spoken of as an old standing prominent opacity
of the right cornea, lying in a transverse position, just below
the centre, and extending across, corresponding to the interval
between the eyelids, with a rough surface like that of a soft
corn, and having the iris adherent to it. It fretted the eyelids,
and kept up inflammation; was of four years' standing, and had
followed a severe ophthalmia. Astringents were of no avail.
The opacity was sliced off to the level of the cornea. It

contained a great abundance of papillæ, covered with thick epithelium. The report concludes with saying that the part is much flatter and the sight improved.

The testimony of British and Continental surgeons establishes the fact that the cornea may regain its transparency after the removal of a growth from its surface. I have already spoken of this, in connexion with pterygium. That it possesses considerable power of repair is a fact often manifested. I have seen restoration by transparent matter, after partial loss of the entire thickness. In a girl twelve years old, an ulcer penetrated the cornea, and the aqueous humour escaped; in five months there was not a trace of any opacity. I have seen exactly the same result, but on a much larger scale, in gonorrhœal ophthalmia; and Mr. Tyrrell gives a good example occurring in the same disease, where the destruction of a considerable portion of each cornea was not followed by the formation of opaque cicatrices. In one eye, by the separation of the sloughs, the anterior chamber was opened, and a prolapse of the iris induced; nevertheless the cavities in both corneæ were gradually filled up with a perfectly transparent substance resembling very much the original texture. The case is reported at p. 261, of the first volume of his work.

Many authors have recorded cases of hair growing from tumours on the surface of the eyeball. I have in my possession a drawing that was taken of such a case by Mr. Field, of Brighton. The tumour, the size of a large pea, was largely supplied by blood-vessels, and grew partly on the cornea, and partly on the sclerotica. Mr. Wardrop has delineated a beautiful specimen; the tumour, the size of a horse-bean, appears to have been connected with the cornea only, for it is said that but a small portion of it adhered, and this seemed to grow from the cornea; the remainder rested on the white of the eye next to the temporal angle of the orbit, and contained upwards of twelve long and very strong hairs, which had appeared when the patient's beard began to grow. Hair has been met with on the caruncle, and on the conjunctiva. Hairy tumours are not very uncommon in the lower animals, and most museums possess specimens. In that of St. Bartholomew's Hospital, is the eyeball of an ox, in which there is a tumour on the outer half of the cornea and sclerotica, apparently made up of fat and condensed cellular tissue, and covered by skin, which is lost in the conjunctiva around, giving rise to long hairs, with their hair-bulbs. The other parts of the eye were healthy. I have seen similar examples in sheep.

Other tumours, which it would not be easy to classify, that are spoken of as fleshy, fatty, and albuminous, have been met with on the surface of the eyeball, and some of them have attained to a very great size. One of a fungus kind, so large as to advance like a mushroom, and cover the whole eyeball, proceeded originally, as the author, Maitre Jean, describes, from the iris through an ulcer of the cornea. Bouttatz's celebrated case of tumour beneath the conjunctiva, mentioned by Abernethy in his Surgical Observations on Tumours, was seven inches long and three and a half in circumference, and weighed two pounds and a half. It is supposed to have been the pancreatic sarcoma of Abernethy.

It is remarkable that the cornea is much less frequently the seat of tumours of any kind than the sclerotica.

Little further is required to be said of the surgical treatment of these diseases, than is comprised in the principles already laid down; that is to say, to remove by dissection, if possible, the whole of the morbid growth; but when the connexion with the cornea, or the sclerotica, is such as to render that impracticable without cutting either of them through, to consider whether it would not be well to remove a part of the growth, and trust to the reduction and disappearance of the remainder; or, afterwards to apply an escharotic. This has special reference to saving the eyeball, for its preservation ought ever to be sought after when it is possible to be effected with the patient's safety.

When the eyeball must be cut across in its anterior part, a large portion of the eye may yet be saved, if the practice recommended in the chapter on " Staphyloma," for the removal of staphyloma corneæ be followed.

When, however, a portion of sclerotica, together with the cornea, must necessarily be sacrificed, I think that, in most cases, it will be found better to extirpate the entire globe within the ocular sheath, as given in the chapter on " Extirpation of the Eyeball;" an operation of very recent date, and of little severity, compared with the old plan of clearing out the orbit.

TUMOURS OF THE ORBIT.

Abnormal growths about the orbit constituting tumours, and capable of being extirpated, should be removed early, more particularly those that encroach on, actually enter, or are entirely within the orbit. The exceptional cases are few. The circumstances therefore that are received as contra-indications should be palpable. It would be bad surgery to undertake an operation for a comparatively insignificant tumour, one perhaps that merely protrudes the eye, but does not threaten mischief, when the effect would in all probability be injury or destruction of sight. At the same time the sacrifice of the eyeball must not be regarded, if cerebral symptoms should arise from pressure on the brain through the roof of the orbit, from expansion of that cavity, or from absorption of its walls.

Much valuable time is frequently lost in attempts to disperse tumours by local applications and medicines; indeed, great faith in drugs is necessary to suppose that they can remove encysted, fatty, and osseous growths.

The size, figure, and position of the tumour to be removed must determine the direction, the form, the number, and the extent of the incisions ; and although no special rule can be laid down on this head, yet it may be stated generally, that the preliminary ones through the skin should be sufficiently extensive to facilitate the intended dissection, and that it is better to divide the eyelids at their external commissure, than vertically ; while the latter is preferable to separation at the internal commissure. Further, the eyelids should be left intact whenever a tumour can be removed by dissecting within them. It may also be observed, that all external cuts should be made with reference to the least after-disfiguration, and this may for the most part be effected by horizontal incisions, a little curved, to correspond with the wrinkles about the eye.

Healthy integument scarcely ever requires to be removed, except in pendulous tumours; and it is important to save cellular tissue in order to lessen contraction during the healing process.

The position of the levator palpebræ must be remembered, for an operation should not be commenced beneath it, for the removal of a tumour which lies above, and *vice versâ*, for ptosis will follow the division of the muscle. It is also advisable that the scalp should not be cut, on account of its great liability to erysipelas; but the superior palpebra may be so attenuated that an incision might risk its vitality; in which case it would certainly be much better that there be division of the cranial integuments.

I have observed that an extensive dissection about the upper eyelid, followed by suppuration, is apt to cause ptosis; the cause apparently being infiltration and condensation of the skin and subjacent tissue, and perhaps, too, that of the levator muscle, rather than loss of nerve force. There seem to be two ways of avoiding this; to be scrupulously careful not to involve the eyelid in any operation, more than is absolutely necessary; and to use all means to secure primary adhesion. When the wound is large, and there is a tendency to oozing of blood, the surfaces should not be brought together, until all bleeding has ceased, to insure which it may be better in some cases to wait some hours till they are glazed. No more sutures should be used than are actually required. Erysipelatous attacks should meet with prompt treatment. All this surely inculcates the necessity for removing tumours while they are small.

The scalpel which I have figured is, from its size and shape, particularly adapted for operations about the orbit; and, small as the blade is, I have found it safer when dissecting deeply, to blunt the greater part, and use the point alone, so as to pick rather than to cut.

A syringe, such as that figured in the chapter on diseases of the excretory lacrymal apparatus, may be found very useful; for a jet of water will often, by washing away the blood and clots, expose parts when a sponge cannot well reach them.

Small, bent, metal spatulas, are necessary to pull aside the eyeball, and also, at times, to protect it from injury, and to guard other parts.

A tenaculum forceps with points of the size and shape that have been figured, together with curved scissors, complete the instruments necessary for the removal of any soft tumour about the eye.

The upper and outer part of the circumference of the orbit is a frequent site of tumours, which are mostly encysted. The steatomatous variety chiefly prevails. The cyst is usually thin and often contains hair, either loose, imperfectly formed, and mixed with the fatty contents, or growing from the cyst-wall, with bulbs of nearly natural size. Lebert has detected in it the minute structures of skin. But it may be dense and even semi-cartilaginous; hence it is that the growth, from its hard-

FIG. 81.

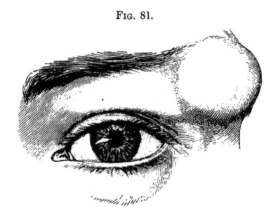

ness, might be mistaken for a fibrous tumour. The aecompanying sketch conveys a good idea of the form and position of this class; the locality, however, may vary; some of them are just within the orbital ridge; some quite under it.

It is congenital and adherent.

If an attempt be made to remove it entire, the edge of the knife must be kept rather away from the surface after the superficial dissection has been completed, which is contrary to the general rule for the extirpation of solid tumours, or in all probability the cyst will be cut into. This is very likely to happen even in the first incision also, except to a practised hand, if the integuments be not pinched up and divided from within outwards.

I never undertake now to dissect out the tumour unbroken, for it is most difficult to effect, except a very large preliminary incision be made; even then, it is frequently cut into at the base. Instead, therefore, I tighten the integuments, transfix it, and cut outwards, then squeeze out the contents, and dissect away the cyst with tenaculum forceps and scalpel. The operation is thus more certainly and expeditiously executed. More than this, primary union is almost certain, and should it not occur, the smallest possible scar only is left. I have seen very tedious suppuration after prolonged dissections in the ordinary way.

I operated on the largest specimen of this class that I have seen. It was situated partly over the eye, and partly on the temple, and of eighteen years' growth. A few years before, there had been an ineffectual attempt at its removal, the reproduction soon following the operation. I proceeded as I have advised, cutting through it from within outwards. The incision passed through the old cicatrix. Without any difficulty I then removed the cyst, which was as usual in contact with the periosteum. There was not any indentation of bone. The temporal artery ramified over it, and was of course divided. Some ligatures were applied.

I have removed but few of these tumours at the inner canthus.

The pendulous and unattached cystic growths in this situation are not congenital.

I have not met with a single bad result from the extirpation of an encysted tumour external to the orbit, although I have removed over fifty. I find that Mr. Tyrrell mentions two cases, and alludes to others, where exfoliation of bone followed. In consequence of this he felt little disposed to meddle with those that were "intimately connected with the periosteum," a condition which he thought to be usually indicated by indentation of the bone. This has been frequently quoted. I have no fear of such consequences when the operation is carefully executed as I direct, and the edges of the wound brought together in an accurate manner by sutures, and not barbarously stuffed, as is so often done, with lint or charpie. I have always found the sensation of indentation of bone around the tumour to be deceptive, and to be of the same character as that which occurs when the scalp is elevated from the skull by effused blood. Any little depression that might exist could never be detected by an external examination.

Other kinds of tumours of a solid nature about the circumference of the orbit, are, like the encysted congenital, beneath the orbicularis muscle; they may, too, be adherent. I assisted Mr. Coulson to remove a fibrous one that was firmly attached to the external angular process.

When a tumour takes its rise within the orbit, much knowledge, surgical and anatomical, is required to decide, with any approach to correctness, what are its relations. The difficulty of diagnosis has been diminished by Dr. O'Ferrall's investigation in connexion with the cellular sheath of the eyeball, the anatomy of which should be known by all those who undertake these operations.

So early as 1804 this "ocular tunic" was demonstrated by Tenon, who called it "the tunic of the eye." Since then other anatomists, among whom are Dr. O'Ferrall, Bonnet, and Dalrymple, have described it; but to Dr. O'Ferrall is due the merit of a surgical application. His memoir on the subject is in vol. xix. of the "Dublin Journal of Medical Science."

It is a distinct tunic of a white colour and fibrous consistence, continuous in front with the posterior margins of the tarsal cartilages, and, extending backwards, adheres to the optic nerve as this penetrates into the sclerotica. The sharp end of a probe, or of a director, will be sufficient to separate it from the eyeball, by breaking the fine cellular tissue which connects them. Within, it is smooth, facilitating the ocular movements; externally, loose and cellular. The muscular portions of the recti muscles lie at the outside of this tunic, which insulates and protects the eyeball in the most perfect manner possible. Half an inch posterior to its anterior margin are six well-defined openings, through which the tendons of the muscles pass to

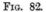

FIG. 82.

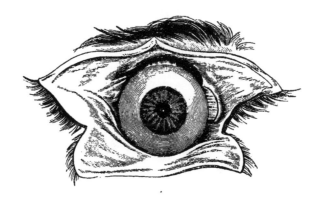

their insertions in the sclerotic coat, and over which they play as through a pulley, and get their force properly directed; securing rotation and opposing retraction, which would otherwise predominate.

The readiest way of exposing the sheath is to cut through the palpebræ vertically, to turn back the separated parts, and to divide the conjunctiva at its angles of reflection, from the internal surfaces of the eyelids to the ball of the eye. The preceding drawing is taken from a dissection I made in this manner. Two only of the recti muscles are visible; for, as the eye was in this instance very deep in the orbit, and the insertion of the other muscles could not be seen as the parts lie, to exhibit them it would have been necessary to cut away a portion

of the orbit, and then the connexion of the sheath with the
eyelids would have been destroyed.

Among other excellent observations respecting tumours, Dr.
O'Ferrall remarks that the projection of the palpebræ will not
always suggest the exact locality of a tumour that displaces the
eyeball. The eyelid may be thrown forward in such a manner
as to cause the supposition that the morbid growth is nearer to
the orbit than to the globe of the eye, and very little covered
by soft parts; and if a careful examination be not premised,
external appearances will mislead, and a tumour that is supposed to be superficial, may prove to be in actual contact with
the eyeball. Moreover, that tumours may form internally, as
well as externally, to the ocular sheath.

When an encysted tumour is not tense, its nature is unmistakeable; but when tight or hard, especially if the cyst be thick,
it may be erroneously considered a solid mass.

Figure 83 is a profile view of a fibro-cystic tumour within

FIG. 83.

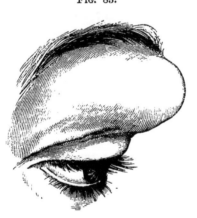

the orbit of a female forty-two years old; it was at once recognised as situated between the roof of the orbit and the muscles.
The ocular movements were not interfered with till the pressure from above thrust the eye downwards and outwards, when
they were nearly altogether arrested. It was hard and immovable, projected far beyond the brow, which was raised,

while the orbital limit passed beyond the reach of the finger. There had been an unsuccessful attempt at removal ten years before, and the patient now sought relief only because the sight was nearly extinct. She deprecated the idea that the tumour was removable, and it required no little persuasion to induce her to submit to the operation.

I divided the skin crucially, and removed the mass entire. The orbital portion was flattened, reached to the centre of the orbit, and adhered to the periosteum. The bleeding was very free, and difficult to suppress.

My patient's recovery was slow, the wound being six weeks in healing; but before that time the position of the eye was quite restored, and vision had returned. Three years after, I had the gratification of learning that the cure was, up to that period, permanent.

Of tumours in the orbit, the solid are less common than the encysted. Glandular enlargements are unknown, it would seem, from an absence of absorbent glands here. It is to be regretted that the usual description of most of them has been imperfect and indefinite; the expression sarcomatous has been too indiscriminately used. The following account of one so called, situated within the "ocular tunic," is given by Dr. O'Ferrall, in vol. xix. of the "Dublin Journal." A woman, twenty-eight years old, had the right eyeball displaced upwards and inwards, and it was slightly prominent; the lower lid was thrown forward, and covered a firm tumour which could be felt through its substance, and under the conjunctiva, when the eyelid was depressed. A free incision was carried along the inferior palpebral sinus, the tumour exposed, hooked, drawn forwards, and detached by a few slight touches of the scalpel. A process remained, which passed backwards in close contact with the eyeball; by drawing downwards and forwards the ocular sheath, it was brought more fully into view, and readily separated by the sharp end of a probe. The wound healed in a few days, and vision, which had been nearly lost, was soon regained. The tumour was lobulated, and well circumscribed by cellular tissue.

The combination of encysted tumour with solid growth, has been met with, but an example has not come under my own observation.

Solid and encysted tumours, but particularly the latter, may, from their extent, the positions in which they may grow, or into which they may be thrown by the resistance offered to them, especially if they lie behind the eyeball, be very difficult to eradicate. Complete extirpation is desirable, for without it there must be an amount of uncertainty as to the result ; yet unfortunately, it is not always practicable. However, I have known some abandoned in despair, when a little more patience and confidence on the part of the surgeon would have completed the operation. It is a common error with those who are not in the constant habit of operating, to fancy parts of the body to be more superficial than they really are, and from the same false impression they often imagine tumours to be deeper seated than they prove to be.

The following history of an operation by Mr. Barnes, of Exeter, recorded in vol. xi. of the " Medico-Chirurgical Transactions," shows how much an able surgeon can effect within the narrow limit of the orbit.

A tumour occupied a considerable portion of the orbit, and pushed the eyeball upwards so as almost to hide it behind the upper eyelid. It appeared to extend to a considerable depth, and projected so much as to constitute a very striking deformity. A superficial groove, running obliquely across the upper surface, formed a slight line of division between the more prominent and moveable part, and that more immediately under. This front portion could be moulded into different shapes by the fingers ; the posterior was more elastic. It adhered firmly to the outer angle, and part of the lower edge of the orbit; in most other points it was but loosely connected with the surrounding parts. The swelling was observed in infancy—the patient being now seventeen years old,—and was then not larger than a pea ; the principal increase was within the last four or five years. It was painless, and the eyeball was sound, but vision was lost, from the pupil being covered. The next, or hidden part of this very remarkable growth, was revealed at the operation. It extended to the bottom of the orbit, and occupied more of this cavity than the eye itself; and as it was impracticable to proceed far in the dissection, without greatly endangering the eyeball, the contents of it were partially evacuated, to obtain room, and the sac separated from its deeper attachments. Towards the posterior point on the inner side, and more than an inch from the edge of the orbit, the sac felt as if it embraced a sharp bony process, projecting outwards nearly in a perpendicular direction, and apparently attached to the periosteum : it proved to be a tooth, in form and size like one of the supernumerary teeth sometimes found in the palate. The crown, with the enamel, was within the sac ; the root, with its dental vessels, was attached to the orbit. The two cysts were distinct ; the front one had a chalky matter on some parts of it, and contained a compact lardaceous yellow substance ; the other, which in the interior was smooth, excepting a part near the tooth, contained a whey-coloured fluid, and a yellow curdy substance. The patient did well ; he could not move the eye downwards, or freely in any direction, but vision was perfect.

Even in the present day, when so much of the former difficulty of operating is removed by chloroform—a difficulty which Mr. Wardrop and others combated by bleeding patients to fainting,—and with all the advantages of superior appliances, and better knowledge of the anatomy of the ocular appendages, the relations of a tumour may render its detachment impossible, without some of the contents of the orbit being also taken away, not even excepting the globe of the eye.

In the second volume of the "Lancet" for 1827-8, Dr. Bushe records an instance, in which the right eye and a large encysted tumour were removed. The connexions with the eyeball were inseparable, and during the operation it appeared that the superior and posterior part of the orbit had been absorbed by the tumour, which pressed on the anterior lobe of the brain. Alarming cerebral symptoms had arisen, and partial paralysis of the left side of the face, and of the left upper extremity, was established. In ten days the wound had nearly healed, and the little patient was walking about without any inconvenience. Encysted tumours may even pass beyond the orbit. Thus, in the " London Medical Gazette," vol. v., Dr. Hall has given an abstract of a case that occurred to Delpech, where a tumour passed through the optic foramen into the cavity of the skull, and was imbedded in the left anterior lobe of the brain. Death ensued from the puncture of the cyst, which had formed a large projection between the eyelids. In another instance that occurred to Delpech, a cyst which followed the ocular movements, and seemed to belong to the globe of the eye, had also intimate connexions within the orbit.

Dr. Monteath, in his translation of " Weller's Manual," tells of a large hard tumour, completely encircling the optic nerve, and resting on the posterior surface of the eyeball, but not connected with it, except through the nerve and cellular tissue. Such connexions were inseparable ; and when, in the course of dissection, this difficulty appeared, the eye, with the tumour, was extirpated.

A tumour intimately connected with the orbital contents is in the Museum of St. Bartholomew's Hospital, and is much more marked and peculiar in its relations than any I have seen : it is firm, compact, and lobulated, and adheres to the back part and sides of the sclerotica ; the optic nerve, which is elongated, passes through its axis ; and the recti muscles, quite unaltered, adhere to it externally. The humours of the eye escaped through an ulcerated opening in the cornea. The retina and the choroid are collapsed, and occupy the axis of the eye between the entrance of the optic nerve and the iris ; and the space thus left between the choroid and the sclerotica contains a firm clot of blood.

A fibrous tumour, preserved by Mr. Liston, and now the property of the College of Surgeons, filled the orbit, surrounded the optic nerve and the eyeball, and extended forwards as far as the conjunctiva.

If a dense tumour do not actually surround the optic nerve, nor particularly adhere to the orbit, it may be drawn forward to an almost incredible extent, and its removal be thereby facilitated.

Even with slight hopes of success, an attempt should be made to remove a cyst that is growing or injurious. In an instance which occurred to myself, after the greater portion of the tumour had been detached, the evacuation of its contents enabled the dissection to be completed, which would otherwise have been impossible.

Whether in any instance the eyeball should be taken away with a morbid growth, must depend on the nature of the tumour, and other circumstances of the case. The probability of so dire a contingency should, as far as possible, be considered before operating. But this applies more especially to solid tumours; since the nature of the case must be peculiar which would necessitate extirpation of the eye before trying the effect of the partial removal of the cyst, or other means for its destruction.

When fluctuation indicates the presence of an encysted tumour, which declares its depth and central position in the orbit by thrusting the eye directly forwards, the practice should be to open it by as free an incision as possible, and not merely to puncture: we must wait the result, which is ever uncertain. But it will be favourable or not, according to the nature of the tumour, the state of its walls, and the character of its contents. The common termination of those that are thin-walled is the destruction of the secreting membrane by suppuration; a delicate cyst will break down rapidly, and it is said that the cyst-walls may adhere. I do not, in the first instance, attempt to produce suppuration by the introduction of lint and other substances, or the application of an escharotic; I rather trust to a natural process, lest the consecutive inflammation prove very severe; at the same time I do not hesitate, when I think it necessary to prevent premature closure, to insert in the opening, for a day or two, a few shreds of lint.

A boy, fourteen years of age, had a protruding eyeball; and

the suspicion of fluctuation induced the late Mr. Scott to make an exploratory puncture: a creamy fluid escaped, and for several weeks a purulent discharge continued, until the escape of a small cyst, which was evidently the contracted sac of the original tumour, effected a cure.

It is a very prevalent plan in Paris to inject orbital cysts with iodine, just as lumbar and other abscesses are treated; and notices of the practice have appeared within the last few years in the several English and French journals. My personal knowledge of the treatment is confined to a few cases. Mr. Gay asked me to see with him a patient in whom he had opened an encysted orbital tumour two months previously, and I recollected at once that the man had been under my own care some time before with the same complaint. His eyeball was then prominent, and thrust forwards and outwards, and, detecting a fluctuating tumour, I opened it. After a few attendances, the aperture healed, and the eye became less prominent. About a year after, the globe of the eye again came forward, and when he applied to Mr. Gay it was most remarkably protruded, turned considerably outwards, and fixed. Vision was nearly extinct. The eye had now receded but little, although the discharge, which was creamy, had lessened. The aperture was just above the upper eyelid, and near to the inner canthus. A probe could be passed to the apex of the orbit, and when bent with an elbow of half an inch, could be turned completely round, showing the extent of the cavity. I recommended the injection of sulphate of zinc, two grains to the ounce—for I greatly prefer this preparation to tincture of iodine—to be used twice daily, and in a week the discharge ceased. A month later, the eye was very much less protruded, and vision was returning.

I lately successfully treated, in private, a case like the above. The cyst passed to the apex of the orbit, and opened by a fine orifice, just under the eyebrow. There had been spontaneous evacuation of the contents several months before, and the thin purulent discharge had existed ever since. I enlarged the aperture, and directed a zinc injection of the above strength to be used daily.

Hydatids, acephalocysts, and echinococci, have been met with in the orbit, where, of course, their nature was not determined till a puncture or an incision was made ; for they produced symptoms the same as those arising from any other kind of fluid tumour. Mr. Lawrence met with an instance in a man forty-two years old ; the globe of the eye was protruded, and the discovery of a small, firm protuberance under the superciliary ridge, which seemed to be part of a deeply-situated swelling, induced him to recommend extirpation as the only chance of relief. This was refused; the disease increased, the eyeball was turned completely out of the orbit, and sight was destroyed. A puncture was made, clear watery fluid escaped, and two days after, a soft opaque white substance, which protruded in the aperture, was extracted, and proved to be a hydatid; others were discharged, and ultimately, by enlarging the aperture and injecting water into the sac, half a teacupful was removed. The cyst suppurated. The opening closed in a month, the eye returned to its natural position, and all uneasiness ceased. A little motion of the iris, and slight perception of light, returned. The particulars of the case are in the " Medico-Chirurgical Transactions," vol. xvii.

Fatty tumours, growing either in or about the orbit, acquire importance on account both of their unsightliness, and because they are very liable to compress or displace the eyeball. They appear to be most common in this locality in early life, and are probably frequently congenital. I have met with several of small size just under the ocular conjunctiva, in the space between the external and inferior recti.

If possible, they should be removed within the eyelid. When they are adherent to the conjunctiva, the attached portion of the membrane should be excised with them.

A young girl applied to Mr. Simon, of St. Thomas's Hospital, with symptoms of an orbital tumour. The eyelid was pushed out, but the eyeball, excepting having been turned a little down, was not much displaced. Mr. Simon made a free incision beneath the eyebrow, and quickly exposed a large mass of clear white fat. The edges of the wound being held widely asunder, the deep attachments were carefully divided, and the whole mass removed. It was about the size of a walnut. The wound healed kindly, and no ill effects remained.

The following case, which came under my care at St. Mary's Hospital, was of interest, not only on account of the orbital encroachments of the tumour, but from the difficulty attending its exact diagnosis. Fatty tumours, it is well known, differ much as to firmness : in some the fibro-cellular septa are very delicate, and the loculi containing pure fatty material very large ; in others, the ultimate lobules are minutely subdivided, forming granular fat, and the proportion of fibro-cellular tissue to fat, very considerable. The latter kind are often difficult to distinguish from tumours of other classes, since they possess none of the softness and pseudo-fluctuation of fat. The knowledge of the existence of this variety of firm adipose tumours, also, frequently makes the diagnosis of those of other kinds doubtful, more especially of some forms of the erectile class.

Anne B., aged twenty-five, applied on account of a tumour about the size of a walnut, overlying the upper border of the right orbit, elevating the eyebrow, depressing the eyelid, extending into the orbit, and slightly protruding the eyeball. It had firm attachments, and felt dense and solid; the skin covering it could be pinched up, excepting in a few parts, where, in the lines of cicatrices of former treatment, it was adherent. There were several large tortuous veins over it. The disease had existed from birth, but had increased very slowly. Till she was about the age of fourteen it was in the forehead, and then seemed to drop. This is not altogether an imaginary thing, for there can be no doubt that fatty tumours may shift their position. It was quite painless, and annoyed her only by the deformity. Pressure seemed a little to reduce its volume ; and when the jugulars were compressed, it appeared to swell. She also believed that, when she was excited, it generally filled out more than usual. She had been under the care of a surgeon a few months ago, who told her it was a nævus, and treated it with setons. I made a free incision over the long axis, and soon found that it consisted of an encapsuled mass of very dense fat. That part which lay over the frontal bone had contracted very firm adhesions, and required to be dissected away; but the lobule which extended into the orbit was not adherent, and came away by mere traction. Very active hæmorrhage took place, and several vessels required ligature. Recovery was rapid. I saw my patient three years afterwards, and she was well, and happy in having been operated on.

An interesting instance of symmetrical tumours of this kind, in both orbits, is given by Mr. Bowman, in the "Provincial Medical and Surgical Journal of Medicine." The swelling was nearly limited to the outer half of each eyelid, and extended from the brow to within a quarter of an inch of the tarsal border, where it ceased by a groove, over which hung the relaxed and distended integument. They were quite soft, as if from œdema of the parts subjacent to the skin, and pressure did not meet with any resistance, nor did indentation ensue. In one a seton was passed to produce consolidation of the parts, under the conviction of there being œdema only, and afterwards medicines and low diet were enjoined. Subsequently an operation was undertaken to remove a piece of the supposed infiltrated tissues; the skin, orbicularis muscle, and fascia were divided, and there fell forward a mass of fat as large as an almond, in pellets or lobes, resembling the fat in the orbit. The second eye was operated upon, and both did well.

The condition of the eyelids, respecting bulging or distension, as noticed above, is, as Dr. O'Ferrall has shown, diagnostic of disease in the cellular tissue of the orbit, external to and above the "ocular tunic." I shall refer to it more particularly in my chapter on Protrusion of the Eyeball.

A unique case of an encysted oily tumour in the orbit is copied into the Catalogue of the Museum of the Royal College of Surgeons, from a manuscript volume of cases in Medicine and Surgery by Sir E. Home. A young gentleman had a small tumour in the upper part of the orbit, at first no larger than a pea, but which increased and extended towards the nose, and pressed down the upper eyelid, keeping the eye half shut, yet unattended with pain. Reading by candlelight induced uneasiness of the eye, with throbbing. It was not firmly attached to the orbit, and evidently contained fluid, and poured forth, on puncture, pure oil perfectly clear and sweet, that burned with a very clear light, did not mix with water, and when exposed to cold became as solid as human fat.

Although rather out of place here, but in pathological connexion with the above, I may mention, that I dissected out a cyst from over the external angular process of the frontal bone, the usual position of steatomatous tumours, that contained, to all appearance, pure oil.

I am aware only of the following instance of tuberculous matter being deposited around the circumference of the orbit, and constituting a tumour. A pale and most miserable-looking

FIG. 84.

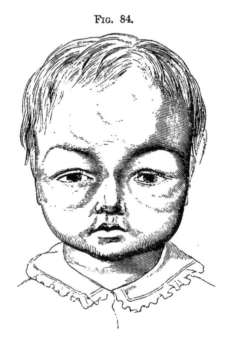

child, eight months old, was brought to the Central London Ophthalmic Hospital, on the 29th of December, 1851, with a

hard swelling of the eyelids, something resembling that attendant upon infantile purulent ophthalmia, but having a wider
circumference. The scalp, the trunk, and the limbs displayed several swellings of similar physical characters; the
lobes of the ears were enlarged, and very hard; the testicles
were four or five times their natural size, and of stony hardness;
and the foreskin was about as large as a pigeon's egg. A few
weeks later the orbital tumours increased and became livid, at
which period the foregoing sketch was taken.

I had no doubt of the tuberculous nature of the many swellings about the body, and an inspection a day after death, which
occurred on the 17th of February following, confirmed my
suspicion. There was an increase of all the deposits. The
eyes were closed so tightly by the distended palpebræ, that a
sight of the eyeballs could not be obtained; the head and face
being swollen to more than twice their natural size, there was
the most hideous deformity. The entire frame was distressingly
misshapen.

The following is an account of a minute examination of some of
the morbid product, masses of which were in every part of the
patient's body. It was of a whitish, pinky, moist, glistening
appearance, juicy, soft, and of homogeneous consistence;
closely resembling, in its external characters, encephaloid
matter. It consisted of granular corpuscles (nuclei), of
from $\frac{1}{5000}$ of an inch, with a very small number, comparatively, of nucleated corpuscles, or cells, of about $\frac{1}{1000}$ part of
an inch. There were no traces of oil, or fibrous or fibroid
tissues. Both the nuclei and cells were circular or oval. Re-
examined by daylight, a very delicate granular stroma was found
to surround the nuclei and cells; many of the small corpuscles
exhibited a complete nucleus, while in the larger cells two or
three nuclei could be counted, and these were well-defined and
darkly granulated. It was therefore infiltration of tuberculous
matter. The heart was exhibited by myself at the Pathological
Society of London, as a rare specimen of tuberculous deposit
in that organ. Except the lungs, which were healthy, every
other internal organ gave manifestation of this remarkable

example of mal-nutrition. The child was perfectly healthy till five months old, when the eyes began to be affected, and then the disease appeared in other parts of the body.

I was requested by Mr. Francis A. Bulley, of Reading, to meet him in consultation on a patient who seemed in danger of having his eyes closed by a series of small tumours around the edge of each orbit, and to consider the propriety of a surgical operation for his relief. The palpebræ of each eye, but particularly of the left, were so pushed together, and the eyeball so covered, that vision was much interfered with. The tumours were irregular in form, of a stony hardness, varying in size; the largest being about the bigness of a marble, and appeared to arise just within the edge of the orbit, and very moveable. The symmetry of the disease was very striking. The orbital affection, however, was but a small portion of similar disease in many parts of the body. Mr. Bulley has very kindly furnished me with a history of the case, which I shall give in his own words, without an apology for its length.

" Mr. M., aged 46, consulted me on the 28th of December, 1846, on account of some very hard moveable tumours occupying the lower part of the cheeks, and extending from the lobe of each ear some distance down the fore part of the neck towards the larynx. There were three or four of these on each side, the skin of the natural colour being easily moveable over them, and the swellings themselves, although closely in apposition, distinctly moveable upon each other ; they were as hard as ordinary scirrhus.

" There was a slight appearance of fulness of the upper eyelids at this time, but no perceptible deposit in their tissues. On examining the groins, which I understood were affected by the same kind of disease, I found a tumour of about the size of a hen's egg, situated just below Poupart's ligament, on each side, of the same scirrhous hardness as on the face, and perfectly moveable, with the skin over them, as well as over those of the face, completely unaffected by disease. These latter tumours had a remarkably symmetrical appearance. There were several smaller subcutaneous deposits of the same nature in different parts of the body. His skin was clammy to the feel, and had a general anæmic appearance. The swellings on the face had commenced about five years before I saw him, and had been gradually increasing up to that time. Those in the groin had been more recently developed.

"He had never suffered any particular pain in any of the swellings, only a slight aching sensation at times.

"He was weak, and his pulse feeble, and there was a certain hurry in his breathing when he talked or exerted himself. His extremities were habitually cold. Prior to the appearance of some secondary venereal symptoms, he had always enjoyed robust health, and had never displayed the slightest symptom of any scrofulous contamination of his system; he had, however, suffered on several occasions from primary syphilitic disease, to which he seemed to have been peculiarly susceptible. On the last occasion of this kind, he had had a chancre *apparently* cured by the application of the nitrate of silver, which, being followed by secondary symptoms, he considered to be the remote cause of the deposits under which he was now suffering.

"He had been engaged for many years as a commercial traveller, and during this period had lived very freely, and been much exposed to vicissitudes of weather. Shortly after the apparent cure of the last chancre by the caustic, unequivocal symptoms of constitutional contamination presented themselves in the form of extensive ulceration of the cuticle over the whole body, but more particularly affecting the hairy scalp, sore throat, and wandering pains in the limbs, for which he underwent a course of mercury, while at the same time he continued his usual occupation as a traveller, constantly exposed to bad weather, and living in the same free, careless manner as he had been used to do. The result of this carelessness was, that the secondary symptoms were not improved, and he was attacked with pulmonary inflammation. On his recovering from this, his venereal symptoms continuing, he consulted an eminent surgeon in London, who, notwithstanding his weakened state, administered mercury to such an extent that in a short time his gums became affected, and an unhealthy-looking ulcer, which ultimately acquired the size of a half-crown piece, appeared upon the inside of the left cheek; his throat became much sorer than it ever had been before; his face became puffed up and swelled in an extraordinary degree, but there was no salivation.

"Having now relinquished his occupation as a traveller, and partially recovered from the effects of the mercurial treatment, he found that, although the secondary symptoms were subdued, the swelling of the face did not entirely subside, and some small tumours began to be developed in the subcutaneous cellular tissue of the part, which had been gradually enlarging up to the time when I first saw him. I have not observed any particular alteration in these tumours since I first attended him —now nearly five years—except that about two years ago they appeared to have become somewhat smaller. He has occasionally suffered from slight periosteal pains in the ulna and tibia, which have been subdued by the use of hydriodate of potash lotions, and he has been much troubled with night perspirations, which weakened him very much. It was about four or five months ago that these perspirations somewhat suddenly ceased, when I for the first time observed that a morbid deposit, of a similar character to those in the other parts of the body, but not quite so dense in its structure, had begun to be developed in the cellular tissue of the left upper eyelid, which was shortly afterwards followed by a similar appearance in the opposite lid, occasioning a considerable projection of the skin covering the lids, and causing great difficulty in uncovering the eyes.

"Immediately after this, other swellings formed in the cellular tissue of the lower lids, which, lifting their ciliary edges upwards, have caused their approximation to the upper lids to such an extent as almost to close the eyes. These tumours, placed external to the tarsi, are of a flattened shape, and moveable, and extend some little distance beneath the superciliary ridges of the frontal bone; they are of a somewhat softer texture than those upon the face, and are entirely unattended by pain, but their contiguity to the eyeballs gives rise to occasional attacks of conjunctival irritation of their surfaces, which, extending to the ciliary margins of the lids, occasions a purulent discharge, by which they are glued together in the morning. I should mention that, simultaneously with the development of these tumours on the cessation of the profuse diaphoresis, to which the patient had previously been subject, the lowest portion of the cervical swellings also began to enlarge, and to press upon the larynx, occasioning an alteration in his voice, and some difficulty in respiration, which is now evidently impeded by the contiguity of the morbid growth."

I regret that I could not procure a sketch of this person, whose appearance, with tumours around the eyes, at the side of the face, and under the jaws, was very remarkable. As some of these on the chest had rather decreased with the improvement of the general health, and others, especially the orbital ones, were stationary, it was decided that no operation should be undertaken on these, unless there was a decided increase, whereby the eyes would be closed, but to adopt such general means as seemed necessary to improve his depressed state of vitality, for the patient was greatly depressed and very feeble. He died soon after.

Exostosis of the orbit is rare. All parts of the orbit are alike liable to it, and, as with exostosis in other situations, it varies in size and other physical properties, in the mode of attachment, having a narrow or a broad connexion with the skull, and in density; whence the division into varieties according as it is ivory-like, made up of bone and cartilage, or of bone and fibrous tissue.

When an exostosis in the orbit is hidden from the touch, there is no point of diagnosis by which it can be distinguished from any other tumour that protrudes the eyeball. It may be painless, or very painful, this being due to its position, whether pressing on a nerve or not. The slowness of growth is the only circumstance that may cause a suspicion of its nature. Neither can it always be determined whether an exostosis will admit of being removed till a portion of it has been exposed, and the nature and extent of its attachment ascertained.

In what may be called the simple form of exostosis, that

which is mere bony texture growing at the extremity by a plate of cartilage, division at the neck suffices. In that composed of a fibro-cartilaginous structure within the expanded bone, either the bone to which it is attached must be removed, or the tumour completely extirpated.

No very precise rules can be laid down for the manner of operating; but this may be said, that more may be done with the bone forceps, especially if the base of the tumour be small, than with any other instrument, and the forceps should have short and narrow blades, and long handles. It is judicious to be prepared with two pairs, one straight, the other convex or angular. In addition to these, there should be provided a variety of small saws and gouges, of different shapes and sizes; in short, all the modern instruments that are used for operations on diseased bones. The upper wall of the orbit, and the inner, require the greatest care in operating, but, as elsewhere, the surface throwing out an exostosis is generally thickened.

A carter, forty years of age, was admitted under my care at St. Mary's Hospital having an exostosis growing from the upper edge of the orbit, with a very broad base, and flattened. The greatest point of projection was two inches. The upper part was covered by the eyebrow, which was considerably thrown up; the lower dipped into the orbit, touched the globe of the eye, and thrust it downwards and outwards, protruding it about half an inch beyond its fellow, thereby nearly destroying vision. The inner boundary and the outer were less marked. The surface was tuberculated, hard as stone; the skin moveable, and traversed by a few vessels. The following figure gives an idea of its extent.

When quite a lad he had fallen down stairs, and pitched on the front of his head; two months afterwards a little swelling appeared on the orbital ridge, and gradually increasing, developed the growth. There was no doubt as to its true nature; hardness, immobility, slow growth, continuity with the bone, and absence of pain and inflammation, sufficiently marked the character.

Chloroform having been administered, I made an incision in

the line of the eyebrow, which had been previously shaved, along the entire superior edge of the tumour, a second from the inner extremity of that to the root of the nose, and a third from the outer extremity to a little below the level of the outer corner of the eyelid. I then dissected the flap downwards till

Fig. 85.

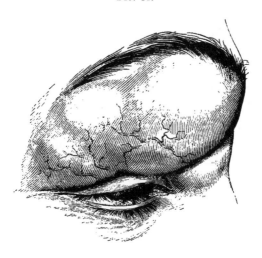

the lower part of the tumour was reached, when I passed a narrow saw between it and the eyeball, and sawed through the tumour from below upwards circularly, endeavouring to follow the natural line of the brow. The texture of the mass was like ivory, and a very long time was occupied in cutting through it. The integuments were brought together by suture; a course to be adopted only when the exostosis is superficial. Besides being allowable here, it saved the integument. Union by the first intention followed throughout the lines of incision, except at a central spot of the transverse cut, through which healthy pus was discharged for eight weeks. After a year the eye was restored to its place, the sight returned, and very little indication existed of what had been done. The eyebrow, which concealed much of the scar, descended to its proper level, and the eyelid could be raised nearly like its fellow.

Numerous instances are on record of the abandonment of

operations commenced on ivory exostoses, solely in consequence of their hardness.

I met with an instance of an exostosis on the orbital edge of the lower maxilla, but the patient ceased his attendance before anything was done for him. Other slight examples that I have seen need not be mentioned.

The orbital cavities may be greatly reduced, or almost closed, by hypertrophy of the orbital bones, in common with the hypertrophy of other facial and cranial bones. In the skull of a Peruvian exhibited in the Museum of the Royal College of Surgeons, all the bones of the face are enlarged and thickened in a remarkable manner, and the orbits are nearly closed. In the same museum is another remarkable example of two osseous tumours which completely fill both orbits, which I here illus-

FIG. 86.

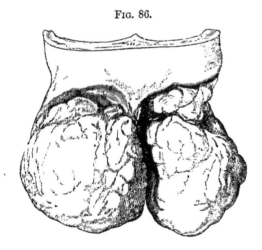

trate; the cavities of the nose, and probably the antra, extend as far as the pterygoid plates of the sphenoid bone, project more than three inches in front of the face, and jut out an inch beyond the malar bones. They are almost symmetrical, of an irregular rounded form, deeply lobed, somewhat nodulated, and their surfaces perforated apparently for blood-vessels. The individual was a man of sixty; it was supposed that the disease began eighteen years before his death, in consequence of repeated blows received on the face in prize-fighting; and during its growth he suffered much pain in the eyes, face, and head. His eyes projected from the orbits; the right, after inflammation and sloughing of the cornea, shrivelled; the left was accidentally burst by a blow while it was in a state of inflammation. During the last two years of his life he occasionally showed symptoms of insanity; and he died suddenly of apoplexy. The cranial bones were very thick and hard, and all their sutures were obliterated. The periosteal covering of the tumours was dense and hard.

A third specimen, in the same collection, and more striking from its magnitude, exemplifies how a growth from a neighbouring part may be of an equally serious nature with one originating in the orbit itself. The tumour is connected with

FIG. 87.

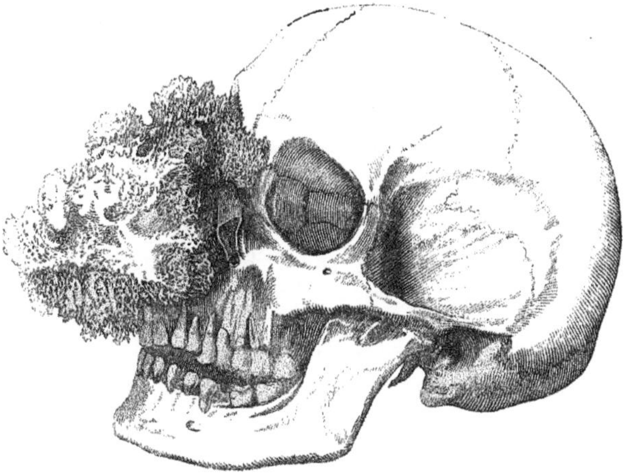

the right side of the face, and has its origin in the antrum. It was five years in progress, and had destroyed all the right orbit except its roof, and involved or destroyed the right malar, superior maxillary, and frontal bones. The part which remained after maceration consists of an oval mass of light cancellous bone about five inches in diameter, and four inches in length (fig. 87). It might have been removed even in its latest stage,

and certainly with ease and every prospect of success at an early
period. Other cases, nearly parallel, have been met with, and
need not be dwelt on, as these examples suffice for illustration.

A spontaneous separation of a large exostosis situated between
the nostril and the orbit, and weighing fourteen ounces and
three quarters, is recorded in vol. i. of the "Guy's Hospital
Reports." In the same Journal there is a case by Mr. Morgan,
of an exostosis from the superior maxilla that interfered with
the eye. Several instances are recorded of the exfoliation of
these growths after abandoned attempts at their removal; and
it has been injudiciously suggested, always to endeavour to
produce exfoliation as the means of cure, by exposing a part of
the tumour and applying an escharotic.

The general result of operations about the orbit for the
removal of tumours, is much more favourable than might be
anticipated from their peculiar locality and close proximity to
the brain. The operations do not seem to be more dangerous
than those in general about the head and upper part of the
face, which are never devoid of risk. Nevertheless, death has
followed simple puncture, partial removal, and complete extirpation of orbital tumours, both encysted and solid. The
excision of exostoses is, perhaps, attended with the most danger,
especially when growing from the orbital plate of the frontal
bone.

To guard against unsuccessful results, the utmost vigilance
must be bestowed on the preparatory and after-treatment of the
patient; and an essential part of the latter is perfect rest of the
body, and of the eye, for many days. The slightest appearance
of erysipelas should be carefully attended to, and any collections of matter early and freely evacuated.

My friend Mr. Borlase Childs removed an enormous ivory
exostosis, from the upper edge of the orbit, in his accustomed
superior style of operating. Seven years after, a growth of bone
appeared around the site, and grew within and without the
orbit. The eyeball was thrust out and destroyed. Mr. Childs
again operated. The mass was as hard as before. It quite

filled the orbit, and had pressed up the roof considerably. There were no cerebral symptoms. The woman continues well.

The recovery of the position of the eye, after the cause of protrusion has been removed, and the restoration of sight, not only when impaired, but when it seemed to have been lost, are truly astonishing, and establish important facts for the admissibility of operating; but both have their bounds, beyond which a favourable result is impossible.

So long as the structural integrity of the eyeball remains, the transparent media being unaffected, there may be hope of entire return of vision; and the less the amount of it destroyed, the greater the chance of this.

In one of the cases of orbital tumours related and figured by Dr. O'Ferrall, in the "Dublin Hospital Gazette,"—and all of his cases are very valuable,—the eyeball lay naked on the cheek an inch below the tarsal margin of the eyelid, was in constant movement, and occasioned much pain. The elongation and tension of the muscles and nerves seemed to be the chief cause of the patient's great suffering. The dislocated globe was removed, and a decided amendment of all the symptoms followed. When an eye cannot, unaided, recover its position, the use of a compress in the direction of the axis of its protrusion may be perfectly successful.

ENLARGEMENT OF THE LACRYMAL GLAND. EXTIRPATION OF THE
    GLAND IN A DISEASED AND IN A HEALTHY STATE. MORBID
    GROWTHS CONNECTED WITH THE GLAND. DILATATION OF
    THE GLAND DUCTS.

The lacrymal gland is not unfrequently affected with acute and subacute inflammation; several cases of which are reported from my practice in the "Medical Times and Gazette" for April 1, 1854. It, however, seldom falls within the domain of practical surgery, less frequently than the other ocular appendages; and the most common change requiring operation is that of enlargement with increase in density. The rarity of this condition in any degree, however, is very striking, and I have met with but comparatively few cases; in one instance both glands were enlarged; but not once have I deemed it requisite to operate.

Our most experienced surgeons confirm the slight susceptibility to disease. Mr. Tyrrell states in his work that he has met with but two cases. Other English writers give similar testimony as to its infrequency, but some continental authors have spoken of it as rather common. All the specimens that I have examined seemed to be those of mere increase of size, and sometimes with induration also: two of them are in the museum at St. Bartholomew's, and both had been extirpated during life; one is enlarged so as to form an oval mass, an inch in length, and more than an inch in breadth; it retains its lobular form and glandular appearance, and there is apparently simple hypertrophy without any decided change of structure. The patient was forty-five years old, and the disease had been in progress for several years: she recovered from the operation. The other specimen will be spoken of presently, in the details of the case quoted from the work of Mr. Lawrence, who was the operator.

A tumour in the situation of the gland, protruding the eye, and thrusting it into a position according to the form and degree of its enlargement, is the symptom that indicates the nature of the affection; yet it is evident that this is not unequivocal, for any other tumour may show the same signs, and the removal of several has been undertaken under the erroneous impression of an enlarged lacrymal gland being the disease.

There may, or may not, be subjective symptoms; pain or inconvenience of some kind is usually present; yet these may be produced by a tumour contiguous to, or developed in the gland. Preternatural lacrymation, an early attendant on a tumour in the situation of the gland, together with a lobulated surface of the tumour, seems to be the most probable diagnostic; but both may be absent, and a lobulated surface is not uncommon to adventitious growths.

When damaged vision or conspicuous deformity results from

the enlargement, and general means have failed to reduce it, removal by operation should be the remedy.

It is a necessary precaution in operating, to proceed slowly and to endeavour carefully to ascertain the limit of the mass, and to confine the dissection to it; for if an adventitious growth only be present, and it touches or is attached to the gland, the latter may be saved; otherwise, through carelessness, it might be injured or actually removed. I have seen the gland sacrificed more than once, and Mr. Tyrrell mentions having witnessed the same accident; the operator, in that instance, considering that he was dealing with a diseased gland, and being rapid in his execution, removed the healthy gland together with a steatomatous tumour. The rules already laid down in this chapter for the operations on orbital tumours in general, apply also to the extirpation of a diseased lacrymal gland, and need not be repeated.

This is the other example at St. Bartholomew's that I have alluded to. A young man was struck violently on the eyelid with an apple; pain, swelling of the eyelid, and a copious lacrymal discharge followed; the eyeball protruded, and, covered by the extended eyelids, seemed to reach half way between the orbit and the nose. A hard unyielding tumour, with a lobulated surface, was found projecting at its upper and outer part a little beyond the margin of the orbit, and whether it moved or not was questionable. Mr. Lawrence made free incisions, exposed the tumour, and removed it from the surrounding connexions, which were cellular, and it proved to be the lacrymal gland, very much enlarged, and altered to a compact homogeneous texture of a light yellow colour, with an appearance at one point, of radiated fibres. It is said that it approached in firmness to cartilage, and altogether closely resembled the firmest part of a scirrhous mammary gland. A large quantity of blood was lost, and one vessel was tied. The wound united by adhesion. The eye receded to its natural position and moved freely; its surface and that of the eyelids being moist, as usual. The operation was performed in 1826, and in 1839 Mr. Lawrence saw the patient, when a hard swelling had formed about the cicatrix under the superciliary ridge, but no inconvenience resulted. The same authority gives the particulars of another patient, who came to him with a hard tumour in the situation of the lacrymal gland, projecting under the edge of the orbit, close to the bone, and hardly moveable. The eye protruded about an inch beyond the level of the other, and was thrust downwards. The upper eyelid, which was swollen and covered the eye, still retained its power of motion. The disease commenced five years previously, with headache, slight temporary pain about the eye, and an almost continual flow of tears. The largest print could not be distinguished with the affected eye. The diseased gland was removed : it was connected by loose cellular tissue to the surrounding parts ; by a short close texture to the bone ; was equal in size to a large walnut ; slightly tuberculated on the surface ; of a light yellowish brown colour ; firm ; nearly homogeneous in texture, but not so hard as scirrhus. Free bleeding ensued, but no vessels were tied. In this case there was union by the first intention, and the patient was able to attend to his affairs in a week. In five months the position of the eye was nearly natural, and ordinary-sized print could be read. The gentleman was seen two years after, and continued well.

A case by Mr. Pemberton, in the "Dublin Journal" for 1847, possesses interest. The eye was quite concealed by a growth of ten years' standing, but not protruded. An operation was undertaken, and the removed mass, of the size of a large orange, consisted of two lobules, the smaller lying deep in the orbit, and said to be made up of dense fibrous tissue of homogeneous structure and whitish colour. The operation was easily performed, and very little blood lost. Several other instances of like operations are on record.

In Mr. Travers's work a case is mentioned in which the lacrymal gland is said to have been greatly enlarged, and in a scirrhous state : the patient from whom it was removed continued well after the interval of some years.

In one of Mr. Todd's cases in the "Dublin Hospital Reports," the gland, almost as firm as cartilage but more elastic, had lobes with deep fissures between them, and contained cartilaginous cysts filled with glairy fluid, the interspaces containing a firm fatty substance, traversed by a few membranous bands. In Dr. O'Beirne's case, in the same Reports, the surface was granular, of a pink colour, and the interior of the gland presented a cartilaginous centre, from which septa passed to the circumference.

The particulars of many other cases are published, but the majority of them are recorded in such a manner as to render them useless so far as pathology is concerned.

Several of the above cases exhibit changes that have been, and would be still called, by some surgeons, scirrhus, and therefore malignant. There cannot be a doubt that this term has been too indiscriminately applied to mere enlargement of the gland, and this is in keeping with the heretofore general latitude of expression, and looseness of description, concerning the supposed cancerous deposits in other parts of the body, arising from the imperfection of the means of defining and discriminating the new product. Those who reject the idea of malignant degenerations of the lacrymal gland, usually found their opinions on the want of the ordinary concomitants of cancerous disease, such as the ulceration, the enlarged absorbent glands, the adhesion to and implication of the surrounding parts, and the absence of return of the disease after operation; and certainly, if these be insisted upon as data for diagnosis, the mass of evidence at command is against the existence of malignancy. What was the secondary formation in the first case, quoted from Mr. Lawrence, cannot be determined; but for further inquiries on this matter, I must refer to the chapter on Malignant Affections of the Eye.

A knowledge of the state of the eye after the operation is interesting. Mr. Tyrrell states, in the first volume of his practical work, that he had thrice inspected the conjunctiva after the removal of the gland, when, of course, no secretion of tears could take place, and that in each instance it retained its usual brilliancy and moisture, proving that it secreted its own proper fluid, and that the humidity of the eye is not, as some have supposed, alone dependent on the secretion of the lacrymal gland.

Dr. Halpin, desirous, as he informs us in the " Dublin Journal of Medical Science," of ascertaining whether tears could flow from an eye deprived of its lacrymal gland, dipped the blunt end of a probe into tincture of opium, and touched the conjunctiva with it : immediately the right eye, the sound one, became suffused with tears, which flowed over the cheek ; in thirty seconds the probe was re-applied; after sixty seconds a drop of fluid fell from the left eye ; in thirty seconds more, another drop.

Weeping must certainly be taken as the most conclusive proof that a lacrymal gland yet remains; but increased conjunctival secretion must not be mistaken for tears.

Extirpation of a healthy lacrymal gland may be required when the natural channels that convey away the tears are lost. Mr. Dixon informed me that he removed it in a patient whose eyelids were united at the corners, after an accident with gunpowder, so as to leave but a small central aperture, there being no means of escape for the tears but over the cheek; and the operation, under like circumstances, has been performed by several other surgeons.

An incision in the eyelid, corresponding to the margin of the orbit opposite the centre of the orbital ridge, sufficiently external to avoid the frontal nerve, and ending a little below the superior external angle, will afford ample room for the operation. The fibres of the orbicularis and the fascia beneath it being divided, a portion of the gland comes into view. It will be remembered that the gland possesses two lobes : the one, which may be called orbital, nearly three quarters of an inch long, is in relation above to the lacrymal fossa of the frontal bone, and below to the upper and outer part of the eye, and superior and external recti, and receives its vessels and nerves behind; the other, a palpebral portion, smaller, seated on the eyelid, reaching as far as the tarsal cartilage, and having a sort of capsule. If the orbital portion be drawn forwards with the tenaculum forceps, the separation of it is as easily effected as that of the smaller division, which is in front.

The annexed diagram of the eye, with the position of the gland traced in a dotted line, may be useful.

FIG. 88.

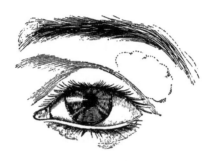

The lesser or palpebral portion may be overlooked during an operation. A surgeon being desirous of stopping the inconvenience of the entire flow of tears over the cheek from irremediable injury of the canaliculi by a burn, proceeded to remove the gland, and did not discover his insufficient anatomical knowledge until the patient's continued power of weeping proved that a part had been left behind,—that which was in the eyelid.

An accurate report of a glandular tumour in the orbit, in connexion with the lacrymal gland, of which the following is a condensation, is given by Mr. Savory, in "The Medical Times and Gazette" for February 21, 1857.

The subject was a man seventy-eight years of age. It was just two years and a half from the first symptoms—inflammation of the conjunctiva with chemosis—till the tumour protruded from the orbit as a mass of the size of an egg, and concealed the eyeball, except a small portion of the cornea, which was opaque; when death ensued. There was a strong suspicion of malignancy. The *post-mortem* examination is valuable.

The brain and all the structures in the immediate vicinity of the orbit were healthy. The eyelids and the conjunctiva (which was thickened and condensed, not otherwise altered) were easily dissected off the point of the tumour. Nearly in the centre of the mass, the shrunken and flaccid globe was imbedded. It and the optic nerve were easily separated; the latter was considerably elongated. The muscles could be traced. No portion of the lacrymal gland could be distinguished. It was of an uniform structure throughout; soft, somewhat elastic, easily torn with the needle, and the separated portions readily broke up and mingled with water. When the cut surface was scraped, a thick, white, opaque fluid appeared. It was composed entirely of gland cells and nuclei. Several portions of it were examined, and exhibited little else than clusters of gland cells, which were broken up at once by the gentlest manipulation. They were remarkably uniform in size and shape. It was very difficult to distinguish anything like a lobular arrangement, and scarcely a trace of connective tissue could be discerned. It measured three inches in length, and two inches in breadth and depth.

Cysts have been supposed to be developed in the lacrymal gland, and Schmidt describes them under the class of hydatids; but since he wrote, in 1803, little has been said on the subject, except to question the nature of the disease he describes, and the correctness of his pathological reasoning, which is too obsolete to be quoted. I suspect that his cases were merely cysts in the neighbourhood of the gland, and more or less attached to it; and it matters little whether it be the one or the other, for the treatment, that of removal, is identical. The existence of a fistula, or enlargement when crying, would be diagnostic of glandular disease.

The dilatation of the gland-ducts into a fluid tumour may occur; there are conditions that admit of it. We have a parallel example in ranula. I have seen many cases. Desmarres speaks of it, copying from Chelius, as of a size varying from a hazel-nut to a filbert. Stœber's account of it is—a circumscribed tumour, elastic, and painless, of the volume of a pigeon's egg, and becoming enlarged if a secretion of tears be

called forth. These allusions relate, of course, to mere magnitude. The complete destruction of the dilated duct can alone
be depended on for a cure, and the most certain plan is to
dissect it away, by operating within the eyelid, or else there will
be the formation of a fistulous aperture.

Mr. Coulson sent me a gentleman with some of those ducts
on both sides, much dilated. They were just apparent externally as slight tumours, but were very marked when the eyelid
was raised, and looked like ordinary cysts. They had been
discovered a few years before, and grew but very slowly. They
scarcely produced any discomfort; but as the possessor, who was
a medical man, was determined to be relieved from them, I
retracted the eyelid, transfixed each with a curved needle, and
cut it off. This was successful.

CHAPTER XII.

PROTRUSION OF THE EYEBALL.

PROTRUSION OF THE EYEBALL FROM CAUSES WITHIN THE ORBIT.

I VENTURE to group, under the general head of protrusion of
the globe of the eye, several affections of the orbit, that are for
the most part obscure, protrusion being the universal, and often
the only apparent symptom. To class them otherwise would
involve subdivisions and unnecessary repetitions, without any
practical advantage.

ANÆMIA.

The projecting eyeballs of the anæmic person, although not
actually requiring practical surgery, ought not to be passed over
here, as a knowledge of all the causes that may protrude the

eye is essential for the correct diagnosis of surgical diseases of the orbit.

I am indebted for much information on the disease to an excellent communication by Dr. James Begbie, in the "Edinburgh Monthly Journal" for February, 1849; and I draw many of the following facts from a paper by my colleague, Mr. Taylor, "On Anæmic Protrusion of the Eyeball," in the "Medical Times and Gazette" for May 24th, 1856.

The following case, one of the earliest I noted down, will suffice to give a general idea of the nature of the complaint.

When surgeon to the St. Pancras Royal General Dispensary, Dr. Ballard, one of my colleagues, transferred to me a female patient, whose eyeballs were so prominent that when in the street she was obliged to cover them to prevent the inquisitive gaze of passengers. She was twenty-two years of age, of a sandy complexion, and pale; possessing that peculiar hysterical manner of looking vaguely about, and rolling the eyes while speaking. The eyelids, which were puffy, could not be closed, except the eyeballs were previously pressed upon for a few minutes with the palm of the hand. The conjunctivæ were unnaturally vascular; the pupils rather dilated; vision was unimpaired.

The whole of the thyroid gland was enlarged; the impulse of the heart was great, and the sounds loud, being audible over the entire chest and in the large vessels, and a systolic venous murmur was perceptible. The pulse was very quick, but its habitual state could not be judged of, for whenever I saw the woman she became excited.

The important part in the history of the case is, that the ophthalmic symptoms, those of the heart, and of the thyroid body, all appeared about the same time. A tonic plan of treatment was agreed upon and prescribed, but the result is unknown to me, for a fortnight after the patient ceased to attend.

Mr. Taylor in his paper relates four cases which came under his care at the Ophthalmic Hospital, and condenses the particulars of twenty-one which he has collected from various journals. Of these twenty-five, twenty were females and four males; of one the sex is not mentioned, but from the context the patient appears to have been a male. Three deaths had occurred, in each instance in males. In two there was a *post-mortem* examination. Both of these had long suffered from extensive organic disease. In one, related by Sir Henry Marsh, there was considerable dilatation with hypertrophy, chiefly of the left side of the heart, and some amount of valvular disease, chiefly of the right. The right internal jugular vein was very much dilated. In the second, detailed by Dr. Begbie, the heart was large, soft, and flaccid: all the cavities, but especially the ventricles, were dilated; the valves were larger than usual, having accommodated themselves to the increased size of the cavities, but they were otherwise normal. The internal jugular veins were much dilated.

As a rule, however, it does not appear that organic disease of the heart is at all necessary to the production of this peculiar condition of the eyeball. The palpitation, which is invariably complained of, is due to anæmia. This, in the few instances in which the affection occurs in males, may result from extensive disease of the internal organs, from excessive and long-continued loss of blood from piles, or from any other cause productive of destruction of the red globules. In females, the starting-point of the disease is almost invariably some form of exhausting discharge in connexion with the uterine organs.

The size of the thyroid varies very much. In some the enlargement is very great, in others slight—even scarcely perceptible. In all the recorded cases, with one exception, the enlargement was due to simple hypertrophy of the normal glandular structures. In the exceptional case, given by Mr. MacDonnell ("Dublin Journal of Medical Science," vol. xxvii., p. 200), the goitre was of the cystic variety, and had attained a considerable size.

Of the actual nature of the change in the orbit causing the protrusion, we are certainly ignorant. It has been attributed to inflammatory swelling of the orbital contents, not sufficiently active to produce suppuration, or to cause effusion into the orbital cellular texture; and to loss of tonicity in the orbital muscles, so that the globes, as it were, drop forwards. The last is, perhaps, the least likely of these unlikely things. There is not any loss of voluntary power, which I think would be inevitable, were there loss of tonicity in the orbital muscles; and the freest movements of the eyes may be combined with the greatest protrusion. Again, in the most debilitating diseases, with perfect muscular prostration, the eyeballs do not protrude.

I am inclined to attribute the cause to congestion of the deep-seated veins of the orbit, which I think offers a better explanation than any other of the variable amount of the exophthalmia, and of the readiness with which the eyeballs can be replaced by gentle pressure. Mr. Taylor, adopting Dr. Marshall Hall's views, as to the spasmodic contraction of the muscles of the neck in paroxysmal and convulsive diseases, suggests that this may be the cause of the impeded return of the blood from the head; and this view is supported by the fact that, in the only two *post-mortem* examinations that have been made, the internal jugular veins were found to be much dilated, as though there had long been some cause of obstruction at the lower part of their course; and, as in neither case was there any solid growth which could have impeded the circulation, it is not unreasonable to suppose that the obstacle was due to muscular spasm. This theory seems worthy of farther investigation.

From what has been said as to the cause of this disease, it will be obvious that the treatment must be directed towards overcoming the exciting cause of the anæmia, which, in the great majority of instances, depends upon uterine disorder. In addition to the special means which may be adopted for this purpose, pure air, nutritious food, and some preparation of iron, will be invariably found useful; and those who believe in its efficacy may apply iodine locally over the thyroid gland. I have not seen complete recovery in any case, although several are recorded; but I have met with considerable amelioration; and in all that I have treated, improvement has followed the steady employment of the means I suggest.

RHEUMATIC INFLAMMATION OF THE "OCULAR TUNIC."

The knowledge which we possess on orbital affections, from
the investigations of the anatomy of the contents of the orbit
by Dr. O'Ferrall, goes far to assist in the diagnosis of the causes
that protrude the eye; but it remains for me to mention, that
the anatomy of the eyelid also is subservient to this end. Dr.
O'Ferrall shows that under the orbicularis muscle is a distinct
layer of fascia, and that this is the first element of the eyelid
that enters the orbit; that there is another layer of fascia
beneath the levator palpebræ, which also enters it, and uniting
with that above, forms a sheath for the accommodation and
support of the muscle; and he points out the attachment of the
"ocular tunic," described in the chapter on "Tumours," to the
orbital margin of the tarsal cartilages. This anatomical
arrangement he then traces on the outer surface of the eyelid in
the two portions separated by the natural fold of the skin, the
upper portion constituting about one-third of the surface of the
lid, the lower the remaining two-thirds. From these he makes
the pathological deduction, that certain forms of disease within
the orbit that are seated either in, or internal to the motor
apparatus—that is, in the substance of, or within the cavity of
the "ocular tunic"—extend their effects to the lower portion
of the eyelid with which they are continuous, and that certain
other affections situated external to the motor apparatus—which
is that part of the orbit containing the fat—will show themselves by inflammation or other changes in the upper division
of the same. A short notice of some of his cases in exempli-
fication will add value to these original anatomical and
pathological hints, and I shall give concisely the particulars
of two of protrusion of the eyeball from rheumatic inflammation of the "ocular tunic."

A man, thirty-two years old, had violent inflammation, and
considerable protrusion of the right eye; the cornea and the
iris seemed healthy, but vision was confused; the conjunctiva
was chemosed, but not vascular; the eyelids were swollen and

red, the upper one dusky with distended veins; the lower part of it so much tumefied that the cilia appeared to grow at an unusual distance from each other, and its transverse diameter was considerably increased. From the superciliary ridge to the inflamed portion of the eyelid, there was an interval about half an inch deep along the whole breadth of the lid, where there was neither redness nor swelling. There was agonizing pain in the eyeball, and while a little moderate pressure of the palm of the hand against the whole tumour gave some relief, the patient could not bear pressure by the finger of another person, except when made gently on that portion of the palpebræ which has been described as being free from redness, and then slowly and not suddenly so as to shake the whole, and provided it was in a direction upwards towards the roof of the orbit. The report then shows that there had been a severe attack of rheumatism : loss of blood from the temporal artery, with calomel and opium, cured the ocular and general disease.

In the second case, of which a mere outline will suffice, both eyes were consecutively affected. The right eye, the first attacked, protruded three-quarters of an inch, and looked bright in the midst of an amber-coloured chemosis, without vascularity. The upper eyelid was of the dusky colour and tawny appearance of that in the above case, and as in it, the orbital portion did not participate in the change—the two portions being separated by a very abrupt line of demarcation—pressure upon the upper was not followed by pain. The second eye was invaded in precisely the same manner. Both were cured by the iodide of potassium. Other parallel cases have been met with; and the following practical comment, which does not admit of condensation, is appended to Dr. O'Ferrall's valuable cases.

"Protrusion of the eyeball, which, when attempted to be explained by uncomplicated periostitis, requires some stretch of imagination, appears a very simple and inevitable result of inflammation of the tunica vaginalis oculi. There are here no soft parts to receive and divide the pressure or protect the globe. The tunic is supported by other fibrous layers on its outside, as well as by the muscles, of which they constitute the sheaths. Inflammation of this capsule must then be immediately followed by pressure; and when we recollect its conical form, and that, as happens in the case of inflammation of other fibrous tissues, effusion at once takes place into the cellular membrane connecting it to the ball of the eye, we perceive there is nothing to prevent the dislocation of the latter.

" This effusion into the cellular tissue will make itself evident in another way. The conjunctiva at the place where it forms the fold, in being reflected from the eyelid to the eye, closes up the tunica vaginalis in front. At this point it will not only receive the pressure of the effused serum, but will become separated from its connexion with the sclerotic coat, by the extension of the infiltration; hence the amber-coloured chemosis without vascularity of the conjunctiva. Chemosis originating in conjunctivitis, always presents, in addition to serous infiltration beneath, one or other of the forms of hyperemia. The chemosis of which we treat is, in uncomplicated cases, the consequence of effusion from a deeper source. I can easily imagine the extension of inflammation from the fibrous structures of the lid to its conjunctival surface, and thence to the sclerotic conjunctiva; but this complication did not occur in the cases which I have related.

" The limitation of the redness and swelling to the lower two-thirds of the superior palpebra, is also a symptom inconsistent with the notion of mere periostitis, but which admits of an easy and natural explanation when the anatomy of the parts is clearly understood. The fibrous tissues of the upper eyelid, which we have traced into the orbit, belong to that portion only of the lid which is below the fold in the skin, or to its inferior two-thirds. The inflammation of the internal parts, being propagated to those portions of the lid alone with which they are continuous, is, therefore, only manifested there, and thus becomes an additional aid to diagnosis. If the inflammation had possession of the general cellular tissues of the orbit, there is no reason to suppose that the upper third of the lid, which corresponds to the part of the cavity where fat and cellular tissue most abound, should not exhibit its effects. If the disease were confined to the periosteum alone, it is, in fact, this upper portion of the palpebra which ought principally, if not solely, to give evidence of its existence.

"When pressure on this uninflamed portion of the palpebra, directed upwards towards the roof of the orbit, is not productive of pain, there can be no hesitation in deciding that the periosteum of the parietes is free from the disease. Should this experiment increase the patient's suffering, it would be a reason for supposing that the mischief had extended in that direction.

"In distinguishing those cases, I would not be supposed to mean that inflammation of this tunic is disease apart and never combined with a similar condition of the periosteum or cellular tissue on the one hand, or inflammation of the eyeball itself on the other. I am aware they may exist together, for I have seen such cases. All I mean to assert is, that inflammation of the tunic described may be the primary affection, and the point of departure from which the diseased action may spread to the other fibrous layers in the orbit, and finally reach the periosteum; and that the attack may even be limited to the tunica vaginalis oculi—that it may here produce a train of symptoms of the most dangerous kind, and which have been hitherto supposed to reside in the periosteum, because the existence of other fibrous membranes in the cavity was not suspected. Presuming that there were no other tissues in the orbit to which to attribute the disease, practitioners naturally referred the majority of cases to one or other of those with which they were acquainted. The solution of such cases would have been less difficult if our clinical researches were based upon a more correct knowledge of the structures actually existing in the orbit."

This research and reasoning render lucid many of the heretofore anomalous cases given by authors, and several that have occurred to myself; some appearing after fever, or erysipelas, or other constitutional disturbance. An interesting girl of thirteen was brought to me with slight protrusion of one eye, with the single accompanying symptom of slight chemosis of the conjunctiva, which had a dirty white metallic-like aspect, without a trace of vascularity. I watched the case for months, scarcely adopting any treatment, for no particular plan was indicated; that there was effusion in the ocular sheath can scarcely be doubted. In another instance with protrusion, the lower half of the conjunctiva was chemosed without vascularity. In a third the globe of the eye projected, with a sudden elevation of the conjunctiva, by serum, on the outer side of the cornea.

Dr. O'Ferrall speaks of adhesion of the tunica vaginalis; by which is meant the adhesion of the ocular sheath to the globe of the eye, from inflammation, as a cause of prominence with immobility. Protrusion and violent inflammation of a motionless eyeball, with distracting pain; immoveable and dilated, but regular pupil; imperfect vision; a tumid and slightly œdematous upper eyelid; were the symptoms. The immobility remained after the other states had nearly passed away. He imagines that the real cause of such symptoms is adhesion of the sheath, as well as the consolidation of the several fibrous layers which envelope it and form the thecæ of the muscles. Moreover, that the adhesion may be supposed to be accompanied by abnormal union of the tendons of the muscles to the edges of the openings through which they pass, the ocular movements being thereby impeded in proportion as the usual gliding motion of the parts is destroyed. That he is correct in this case, I doubt not; but immobility is not always the effect of adhesion. Dr. Mackenzie met with prominence and a fixed state of the eyeball, which were due to mere effusion within the "ocular tunic," as was proved by evacuating the fluid, when the prominence disappeared and the movements returned. He remarks, too, in connexion with this, that when the eyeball is protruded, and its motions free, the cause of pressure is certainly without the ocular capsule.

ABSCESS.

An abscess may form within the ocular tunic, and the symptoms would be protrusion of the eyeball and pouting, or swelling externally between it and the eyelid. A lady had protrusion, with intense suffering and general symptoms of the formation of matter; several medical men were consulted, and more than once a puncture was made deep into the orbit, but ineffectually. The lancet seemed to have been directed away from the globe of the eye to avoid injury to it, or to the parts around. Her almost insupportable state, and the loss of sight, induced the medical advisers to talk of extirpation; but Dr. Farre, who was now consulted, directed that a lancet should be passed through the distended conjunctiva by the side of the globe. A large quantity of pus flowed out, and in a few weeks the eye was perfectly restored.

A case of precisely the same nature was brought to me by Dr. Sawyer, of Guildford Street. The eyeball projected three-quarters of an inch. The child was well a week after I evacuated the matter.

Pus may be deposited in the orbital cavity without the ocular tunic, and whether it be acute, subacute, or chronic suppuration, the physical characters will be the same; namely, the bulging of the orbital portion of the eyelid corresponding to the seat of the suppuration. The formation of pus is, according to my experience, a common orbital affection; and when, with protrusion, there are the usual constitutional symptoms attendant on abscess—the pain, with or without movement of the globe, the redness and puffiness of the eyelid, and the throbbing—we should early endeavour to discover fluctuation by an exploratory puncture, made, if practicable, within the eyelids, in the probable direction of the abscess.

In vol. ii. of the "Dublin Hospital Gazette," Dr. O'Ferrall gives a case of subacute orbital abscess, with depression of the globe of the eye, without any appreciable protrusion, which he deems dependent upon the limitation of the abscess posteriorly by adhesive inflammation.

ABSCESS AND HIGH INFLAMMATORY ACTION.

Mr. Tyrrell has narrated a case which illustrates a marked degree of vascular disturbance attendant on inflammation and abscess within the orbit.   Symptoms of acute inflammation, with great protrusion of the palpebræ and globe of the eye, induced preparation to be made for the evacuation of pus, when it was discovered that so strong a pulsation pervaded the whole swelling, even moving the eyeball, that the presence of an aneurism was suspected.   Reviewing the history of the case, a different opinion prevailed, and it was decided that a small puncture should be made between the globe and lower eyelid, which was done by Mr. Scott, and the result was an immediate escape of blood, of an arterial character, in jets corresponding to the pulsatory movement of the swelling, which was syn-chronous with the pulse.   Pressure stopped this, and when the compress was removed a day or two after from the pain it occasioned, there was a free discharge of matter, and all the symptoms were greatly mitigated.   A free incision is the proper treatment when phlegmonous disease is diagnosed; and, in this instance, would no doubt have at once evacuated the pent-up pus.

INFLAMMATION OF THE ORBITAL AREOLAR TISSUES.

Inflammation of the orbital areolar tissues may produce protrusion of the eyeball, with more or less chemosis.   This is a more common affection in various stages than is supposed.

FIG. 89.

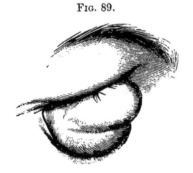

I had under my care a child of two years old, with a very marked example; the upper part of the orbit, to all appearance, alone suffering.   The above illustration was taken when I first saw her.

It gives the idea of chemosis of both eyelids, a state that I thought existed, till a careful examination proved that the upper only was affected. The groove in the swelling answers to the spot of reflection of the conjunctiva from the eyeball to the upper tarsal cartilage. The poor child being most rebellious, chloroform was administered in order to examine the disease carefully, and to adopt any surgical measure that might be deemed requisite. The eyeball was slightly prominent, and the lower eyelid only slightly inflamed. Attempts to reduce the tumour, and to keep the eyelid over it, were fruitless; and no surgical operation, beyond a few incisions, was considered justifiable. Excision of any part would probably have been followed by entropium.

It is not very uncommon to meet with protrusion from this cause, after severe blows about the temples, or on the margin of the orbit. Of course all the contents of this cavity are more or less involved. In one year I saw four examples; they were very much alike. In all, the injury was on the outer edge of the orbit. There was considerable prominence, and the eyeball was motionless. In all, too, vision was affected. I was able to learn the condition of one only, after the lapse of some months. I was called to see that patient by Mr. Coulson. Although the eyeball regained its position, the motions were not quite restored, and the state of vision was so imperfect, that the eye was useless. There were not any objective symptoms in the eyeball itself in any of these.

But a still more marked, although a very rare form of this kind, is hypertrophy of the areolar tissue, just as occurs in elephantiasis; whereby the eyeball is thrust out of its socket. Soon after the publication of this work, I recognised my first case, in a remarkably powerful man in the meridian of life. The eyeballs were prominent, but yet unhindered in motion. The conjunctivæ were highly injected, of a coarser structure than natural, and bolstered out around their ocular attachments, by the posterior swellings, which were dense and doughy. Vision was perfect; there was much pain; I saw my patient but a few times, and never learned his fate.

Another was in attendance at the Ophthalmic Hospital, with only one eye affected, as a patient of Mr. Taylor.

Mr. Lawrence met the affection in a more marked stage at Bartholomew's ; simple ocular protrusion, occurring first in the one eye and then in the other, ended in excessive prominence and collapse of the globes. Extirpation was resorted to, on account of the intense pain that existed. The details will be found in the "Medical Times and Gazette" for March, 1858.

In the same Journal, for November 17th, 1860, is related a very similar case. Like the above, the eyes were attacked consecutively, both corneæ gave way from exposure, and extirpations were done to relieve pain. In neither was there conjunctival purulent secretion, but a dry mucous surface. This person was a young woman. After the extirpation, there was yet too much of the hypertrophied tissue in the orbit to admit of a glass eye being worn. Mr. Lawrence's patient was a robust man.

PERIOSTITIS.

Inflammation of the periosteum of the orbit, which must, I presume, be always more or less combined with inflammation of the bones, may protrude the eyeball; and although such disease may follow traumatic injury, constitutional causes, such as struma, and syphilis in particular, generally produce it ; but whichever it may be, the diagnosis is seldom obscure, if proper investigations be instituted.

DISEASE OF THE OPTIC NERVE.

Disease of the optic nerve has been a cause of protrusion, as Böhm, of Berlin, observed in dissecting a young man who died of phthisis. Here a tumour on the optic nerve, of the size and shape of an olive, just a little behind the sclerotica, and consisting principally of thickened neurilemma, the nerve-tubes being unaltered, had displaced the eyeball upwards and outwards, and nearly destroyed vision.

PROTRUSION FROM CAUSES EXTERNAL TO THE ORBIT. MORBID CHANGES IN THE CRANIUM. ZYGOMATIC FOSSA. MAXILLARY SINUS. NASAL FOSSA. SPHENOIDAL SINUS.

Protrusion arising from pressure external to the orbit is apt to be overlooked, unless the surgeon be aware of the probability of the occurrence, and the sources from whence the pressure may arise. The position of the orbit exposes it to encroachment on all sides. Diseases of each of the cavities and sinuses around may reduce its capacity, and protrude the eye.

MORBID CHANGES IN THE CRANIUM.

The most common example from a cerebral origin is to be found in chronic hydrocephalus: the roof of the orbit is pressed down, and the depth of the cavity much lessened. The cause is here at once palpable, and so are most of the disturbing cranial influences. Cerebral tumours may protrude the eye. Other changes in the cranium may displace it, as the following example shows.

A black thief, jumping out of a window to escape detection, fractured his skull just above the left orbit; probably damaging the frontal sinus. A portion of the frontal bone which was loose, was removed; suppuration ensued, and there was a discharge of pus for a year. The eye protruded to about three-quarters of an inch beyond its fellow, and was in that state when I saw the man, six years after the accident. Vision was unaffected.

Where the physical causes, although cerebral, are less marked, and their seat is not perceptible, headache, loss of memory, fits, partial paralysis, or other indication of lesion in the great nervous mass, with the previous history of the case, will generally determine them.

I have met with an example of suppuration in the frontal sinus producing protrusion; distension with elasticity of the bone over the abscess declared its seat, and evacuation of the pus remedied all disturbance.

Writers speak of hydatid and encysted tumours, and polypi, being found in the above sinus; but such occurrences are remarkably rare.

ZYGOMATIC FOSSA.

I have seen an exostosis that appeared to have its origin in some part of the temporal or zygomatic fossa, throw the eye forwards; this is the only instance I know of disturbance from this quarter.

MAXILLARY SINUS.

The maxillary sinus or antrum of Highmore is the seat of the most frequent external cause of displacement, for it is frequently diseased, and a tumour of any magnitude, having its seat here, can scarcely fail to throw up the orbital floor sufficiently to affect the eye, and such a cause could rarely be occult. Distension in some other direction, and some collateral symptom, would coexist and determine it; and it matters not what may be the nature of the tumour, whether aneurism by anastomosis, polypus, or other soft growths of a mild, or of a cancerous nature, simple exostosis, or malignant affection of the bones; all of these have been met with. Suppuration, however, may greatly enlarge the maxillary sinus, which in the natural state is very small, without throwing up the orbital boundary. I have met with several examples of this, and the most remarkable was in a patient in private, submitted to me for an opinion by Mr. Coulson. The orbital, palatine, and nasal sides did not bulge, the expansion being externally, anteriorly, and posteriorly. An aperture was made through the distended bone in front, and so great was the cavity, that my forefinger could but just reach the back wall.

Simple accumulation of mucus has been known to distend the antrum and to displace the eye.

NASAL FOSSA.

Nasal tumours, and I allude especially to polypi, could not advance and injure the orbit without detection : a careful examination of the nose would always render the cause apparent. Obstruction of the lacrymal duct too would surely usher in such intrusion. In treating of obstruction of this conduit, I shall give an example of both nostrils being blocked up by polypus, and each lacrymal duct temporarily destroyed.

SPHENOIDAL SINUS.

Notwithstanding that I cannot advance any instance of protrusion of the eyeball from a distended sphenoidal sinus, I would wish to impress the possibility of the occurrence ; for the anatomical arrangement of the parts, I should say, would seem readily to admit of it.

POSITION OF THE EYEBALL A MEANS OF DETERMINING THE NATURE AND THE SITUATION OF THE CAUSE OF PROTRUSION.

In obscure cases of prominent eyeballs, where there is not any indication to be gathered from the state of the eyelids, the direction of the protrusion might somewhat assist in diagnosing the nature of the cause by localizing it more certainly. But such evidence may be wanting, and in no instance can it be solely relied on, because of the irregularity in form and unequal development of morbid growths. I have mentioned, in narrating the case of an enlarged lacrymal gland, that a posterior and smaller process went back far in the orbit, and would have pushed out the eye, but for an anterior portion which was still larger, and thrust it back.

In estimating the value of doubtful physical signs, the dissimilar axes of the eyeballs and of the orbits demand attention ; while the manner in which the globe is tied by the oblique muscles, and the anatomical relations of the optic nerve, will influence the direction it will assume from pressure posteriorly. Displacement inwards is more readily effected than in any other direction. When from the commencement the displacement is lateral to the axis of the eyeball, it is reasonable to presume that the force also is lateral. Direct protrusion will, in general, prove the most embarrassing; for with bony and other growths at the side of the orbit, within certain limits of size, and situated rather posteriorly, the eyeball may be pushed forwards without any lateral displacement; this, I presume, must be attributed to the mechanical properties of the fat in the orbit. Yet if the only symptom be direct protrusion, until further evidence to the contrary, the cause must be considered to be seated at the back of the orbit; I will not say the apex, for that is indeed a very rare position.

FOCAL RANGE SUBSERVIENT TO DIAGNOSIS OF THE POSITION OF
    AN ORBITAL TUMOUR.   STATE OF PUPIL IN PROTRUDED EYES.
    DISTINCTION BETWEEN MERE PROTRUSION AND ENLARGEMENT
    OF THE EYEBALL.

It has been supposed that attention to the focal range may assist in ascertaining the position of pressure on the globe of the eye, the theory being that, if behind, the antero-posterior diameter will be lessened, and the range be shortened; if at the side, it will, on the contrary, be lengthened. I question the practical application of this; the imperfection of sight has, in all the cases that I have seen, resulted from decided loss of power in the retina.

With the greatest protrusion the pupil may be natural; but it may be dilated and moveablé, dilated and fixed, or of its natural size and motionless. I am not aware that any practical indication can be gathered from any of its assumed states.

A protruded eyeball is frequently mistaken for an enlarged one, an error very excusable in the inexperienced. Congenital enlargement has been met with, but very rarely; and while the proportions of all parts remain the same, the greater absolute magnitude is very apparent. Enlargement from disease always carries the evidence of diseased action; if not in the altered form of the cornea, or in the increased size of the chambers of the eye from greater aqueous secretion, certainly in the bulging and altered colour of the sclerotica. With moderate knowledge of the subject, and a little care, a mistake is unlikely to occur.

Dr. J. O'Beirne, of Dublin, has written on the diagnosis of these two states in vol. xviii. of the " Dublin Journal," and the conclusion he arrives at is, that in mere protrusion of the eye without distinction of causes, the upper eyelid covers the eye, and hangs down lower than usual, is more or less paralytic and puffed, with its surface generally of a dusky red colour, and traversed by large veins. On the other hand, in actual enlargement, the eye is remarkably uncovered, and presents a staring appearance, while the upper eyelid is merely pushed forward and retained in that position, but is in other respects unchanged.

CASES NOT ADMITTING OF CLASSIFICATION.

The causes of protrusion heretofore mentioned do not embrace all that may protrude the eye ; at least this seems to be the legitimate conclusion when there is protrusion without the apparent presence of any of them. A healthy girl, twelve years old, applied at the Central London Ophthalmic Hospital, with her eyeball almost out of its orbit. In the following sketch, the eyelids are a little retracted, to give a more adequate idea of the distance between its front and the orbit.

The movements were in concert with those of its fellow, which was natural, and rather retracted than prominent. Great pains were taken to test her power of vision, which proved to be perfect. The most careful examination failed in detecting any other symptom than the prominence, which had commenced a year before, and gradually progressed. Mercury was tried, but in vain, and no success attended the use of iron and other tonics. Slight pressure was adopted for a time, and at first seemed beneficial, but ultimately proved to be inefficient; for in

a day or two after remitting it, the protrusion became as marked
as before.

FIG. 90.

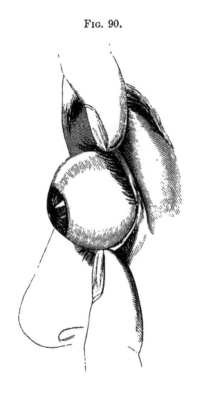

If there is any state justifying the suspicion of an increase
of the orbital fat, unattended with changes in the vascular,
nervous, and motor apparatus of the eye, surely this is it. Any
dense substance at the bottom of the orbit, large enough to
prótrude the eye, should, I presume, derange some of these
structures that are so blended in that situation, and produce
corresponding effects—pressure on the muscles and motor
nerves, influencing motion—and pressure on the optic nerve,
injuring vision.

Another remarkable, and perhaps unique, case of protrusion,
that does not admit of classification, is related by Dr.
Mackenzie. A man discovered that when he stooped forwards,
if only for a few minutes, he had a sensation as if something
was pressing above his right eye, which immediately began to

protrude, and when the head was raised the protrusion was very striking, and he then saw indistinctly. The eye soon began to retire, and in a few minutes was replaced. There was not any loss of muscular power when the eye was in the natural position, and even when displaced he could move it considerably. The iris acted naturally. He complained of considerable pain in the orbit, which was removed by bleeding and purging. The peculiarity had existed for five years, and commenced after carrying a heavy load on the back.

DISLOCATION OF THE EYEBALL BY ACCIDENT.

In the "Dublin Medical Journal" for January, 1853, is this Report. At a meeting of the Surgical Society of Ireland, Dr. Jameson detailed a case of dislocation of the eyeball that had lately come under his notice.

A powerful man, thirty years old, while staggering about in his room, drunk, struck his right eye against a small iron hook, or nail, which entered at the outer angle of the upper eyelid, and protruded the eyeball, rendering it firmly fixed, staring, and devoid of vision. When examined two hours and a half afterwards, the cornea was dry, cloudy, and rather opaque, and the pupil, moderately contracted, was uninfluenced by the light of a candle. Blood was not extravasated, nor was there any unnatural vascularity of the conjunctiva, although its upper sinus was partially torn through.

The margin of the upper eyelid, which was invisible, was elevated, and the eyeball pressed back to its place, which it entered with a distinct snap. Pains in the head and in the eye ensued, for which he was cupped and purged. Six days after the accident, all symptoms had disappeared, and vision was quite restored.

In the discussion which ensued, Dr. Jacob said that as far as he could recollect, an occurrence of exactly the same nature was scarcely to be found on record, and suggested the following solution of the accident:—Some persons possess very large eyes and shallow orbits; and often, while examining such eyes, he found that by pressing the eyelids above and below, he could with ease get a view of the back of the eye. It was not that he merely saw one half of the eyeball, but by a little manipulation he could obtain a view of its posterior part. Now, if by means of violence the lids were tucked in, they would grip the back of the eyeball, and produce a protrusion of the organ from the orbit. He could not conceive any other way in which the accident could have happened, because neither the muscles sustained injury, nor was the optic nerve ruptured. Another speaker considered that the snap produced by the reduction of the dislocation proved the fact of the muscles being uninjured.

Some years ago I was extracting an osseous cataract from a disorganized eye. I made the upper section, and had just got out the cataract with the curette, when, before the eyelids were released, the eyeball was forced out, actually dislocated; and as it appeared to me, by the action of the orbiculous muscle. The protrusion was evidently increasing, and I quickly put the spoon of the curette under the edge of the upper eyelid, and lifted it forwards, while I pressed the eyeball back and restored it to its place. The whole occurrence could not have occupied twenty seconds. Vitreous humour did not escape.

CHAPTER XIII

STAPHYLOMA OF THE CORNEA AND OF THE SCLEROTICA—GENERAL ENLARGEMENT
OF THE EYEBALL WITH DISORGANIZATION.

THE fanciful term staphyloma, derived from the Greek word
which signifies a grape, is unhappily chosen, for it is inadequate
to express pathologically the two states of the eye that it is
meant to include ; staphyloma of the cornea, and staphyloma of
the sclerotica, for they are dissimilarly constituted.

STAPHYLOMA OF THE CORNEA.

When the cornea is destroyed in part or entirely, and its place
supplied by an opaque projecting substance ; when after it has
been penetrated by a wound, or an ulcer, a like swelling
protrudes, there is said to be a staphyloma ; which is, in fact, a
natural repair of the injury.

It is only within a few years that the nature of staphyloma
has been understood.   We are indebted to Mr. J. W. Jones, for a
correct explanation of it.   This writer has clearly shown in a
memoir published in the "London Medical Gazette," vol. xxi.,
page 847, that staphyloma, or pseudo-cornea, as it is aptly
called, is not a mere bulging of the cornea.   He explains its
formation by pointing out that when the iris is partly exposed
by the loss of more or less of the cornea, it becomes covered by
an opaque firm tissue, the same as that of a cicatrix, which
is incorporated at the base with the cornea, constituting a partial

staphyloma, which consists of protruded iris covered by new tissue, intended to supply the loss of corneal substance; and he remarks that the formation of a total staphyloma is precisely the same, the degree only differing, and the form of the tumour depending on the extent to which the cornea has been destroyed: when the whole is lost, the new tissue becomes incorporated with the sclerotica.

This has been confirmed in a dissection by Mr. Bowman. The staphylomatous piece was unequal in thickness; the posterior surface to which the iris adhered, was irregularly pitted; the anterior surface was formed by a thickish coat of epithelium, somewhat resembling cuticle, being composed of eight or ten layers of cells, the deep ones globular, the superficial ones scaly, and more like epidermic cells than those of the healthy cornea. There was neither anterior nor posterior elastic lamina, and the entire remaining portion of structure consisted of a dense and most singular interweaving of white and yellow fibrous tissue, with imperfectly developed nuclei intermingled, and the meshes of the tissues, large, unequal, and open on all sides.

In consequence of pressure posteriorly, the new material grows and expands.

Staphyloma may form a long time after the receipt of an injury; that is, the process of growing may not be excited for long after. In a case that I took a note of, twenty years intervened between the wound and the effect.

Writers have described several forms, specifying particularly the globular and the conical, besides employing the expression staphyloma racemosum, when there are several projections, from their supposed resemblance to a bunch of black currants. The various colours also of staphylomata have been tediously detailed, but without any practical advantage, and only to the confusion of the subject, since nearly every individual case possesses peculiarities.

The physical characters of the affection are marked and unmistakeable. The following figure represents them well.

The individual in whom it occurred, aged sixty, had received a wound of the cornea. When she came to me, six months after the accident, there was but a small projection, the cornea itself was opaque and shrunken. I saw her again a year later, at which period the sketch was taken.

FIG. 91.

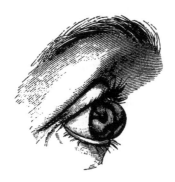

The greater opacity of some parts of the projection is well shown, and the ring around the base of the tumour represents a portion of the true cornea, which seemed to have been gradually pushed aside by the new growth.

Independently of the peculiar unsightliness of staphyloma corneæ, the irritation it may produce, or its sympathetic influence upon the other eye, as I have already fully described in the chapter on "Sympathetic Inflammation of the Eyeball," may demand its reduction. These consequences, however, are not always in proportion to the size, for some run their course, attain great magnitude, and burst, without having produced any uneasiness. Again, the pain of a staphyloma, which would seem to arise from mere distension, irrespective of bulk, may require operative treatment.

There are occasionally changes in the crystalline lens accompanying the staphylomatous state, whereby it is ossified or becomes cretaceous; and although it is not possible to know when it is so altered, or to be able to refer with precision any set of symptoms to either of those conditions, proof is not wanting of their occasionally producing prejudicial effects.

The following case occurred under Mr. Tyrrell, at Moorfields Ophthalmic Hospital, while I was acting house-surgeon.

A cook, thirty years old, was burnt in her eye by some boil-
ing lard; a moderate-sized staphyloma followed, and remained
for years without any inconvenience; then on a sudden, and
without any perceptible cause, intolerable pain ensued. The
staphyloma was removed; and the lens, which was black, very
hard, and apparently consisting of earthy matter, escaped: no
analysis was made of it, nor do I know the true nature of
its change; but I have little doubt that it had been suddenly
detached, or partially thrown from its position, in consequence
of which it acted as a foreign body.

When the staphyloma demands attention, from the deformity,
from irritation, or from sympathetic influence on the other eye,
the whole of it should be removed by " abscission."

Unless all be taken away, there is a chance of reproduction
to a greater or lesser degree. This is particularly likely in the
thick, small, and conical form, when only a slice is excised. But
only the true staphylomatous portion should be cut off, and
every part of the corneal structure that is sound should be
saved. Where the entire cornea has been lost, the excision
should still, as a rule, be in front of the sclerotica; because
there will be less bleeding, the proceeding less severe, and the
form of the eye more likely to be preserved; although in so
aggravated a case complete collapse is imminent.

The operation is best performed in this manner. The eyelids
having been retracted, I transfix the staphyloma with a
cataract needle, the curette, or better still, an ordinary
tenaculum, and cut it off with a long and narrow scalpel, gently
and rapidly. It may be requisite to make the amputation a
little behind the cornea, and then the iris, or whatever remains
of it, is excised. Should the lens be present, whether opaque or
not, it should be removed. If the vitreous humour be healthy,
I try to prevent its escape by gentle manipulation and rapid
closure of the eyelids; and sometimes none of it is lost. What
should follow is very important. There is no more necessary
step in the whole proceeding, and without it there may be
copious bleeding and suppuration in the stump. I place a
roll of cotton wool, or what is next best, a pledget of lint,

quickly on the closed eyelids; maintain it with a bandage, and keep it there for two or three days; and afterwards apply straps of plaster. Healing is effected by the cicatrizing of the cut surface, and its rapidity depends on the healthiness of the vitreous humor. It is not unusual to find the parts sealed up in a week.

The more the eye is diseased, the quicker and the more copious is the bleeding. It is this tendency to hæmorrhage that has induced some surgeons to speak disparagingly of this procedure, and to recommend instead, extirpation; but it is an operation far better adapted to the vast majority of these cases. Both are necessary, and the greatest benefits are conferred when each is assigned to its proper place.

When the bleeding is from the vessels in front of the eye that have been cut through in the operation, it can easily be restrained, and is never of any consequence. When it is internal, it may for the most part be stopped by the compress. I have long been convinced that the source of this internal or intra-ocular hæmorrhage is not the central artery of the retina, as generally supposed, but the choroid; and my opinion has been publicly stated for years. More extended observation has strengthened my views. There is always a previous escape of the unhealthy vitreous humour, and the removal of pressure or support from the diseased choroidal vessels causes rupture of them. I have seen the whole of the vitreous humour thrust out by clots; the retina hanging in shreds in the wound. Perhaps in some cases, by the removal of the front of the eye, so much support is taken from the diseased choroid, that the bleeding forces out the vitreous humour. Much internal hæmorrhage ends in total collapse of the eye, and necessarily the process of recovery is retarded.

Mr. Wilde recommends, in the removal of a conical staphy-loma, that we should pass a thread through the base of the cone, in order that, after the operation, the lips of the wound may be brought together, and the escape of the vitreous humour be prevented. Mr. Browne, of Belfast, also advises the same practice.

The operation once well performed, suffices. Some exuberant granulations may arise, but they are of no consequence ; for if they do not decline of themselves, the use of an astringent lotion, or the application of a mild escharotic, as the red oxide of mercury, will reduce them.

The sketch below was taken from a patient after the operation, and shows the eyeball just a little reduced, and well adapted for the application of an artificial eye.

FIG. 92.

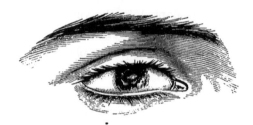

I advocate early operating because the general tendency of the disease is to increase; and the smaller the tumour that is removed, the more is the form of the eye preserved. The following case is an example.

A child lost an eye from purulent ophthalmia ; nine months after, a small and well-defined staphyloma stood out in bold relief from the centre of an opaque and somewhat irregular cornea. A month's watching assured me of its increase, and I shaved it off: the wound healed with a firm cicatrix, which was sound when I last saw the girl, eighteen months after, and the eyeball was but little reduced.

When, with slight partial staphyloma, the remaining cornea is clear enough for the transmission of light, although the pupil must always be displaced and irregular, and vision imperfect, it has been proposed to endeavour to prevent further increase of it, by applying escharotics, so as to induce a certain degree of inflammation, and thereby a thickening and contraction of the prominent mass. There should be a proper selection of the true staphylomata for this method; as it could not be expected to benefit an irregular prominence of the cornea from the yielding of its texture, consequent on pus having been deposited between its layers, or a partial slough from any cause. I have not myself witnessed any satisfactory results, and am acquainted with a few instances in which the treatment did harm in increasing the corneal opacity; but as Mr. Tyrrell, in his ophthalmic work, gives very decided testimony in its favour, I feel it incumbent to notice his remarks, which I do in his own words :—" I have succeeded, in several instances, in effecting a reduction of partial staphyloma, by the careful application of nitrate of silver, or hydrate of potash in substance ; and have applied the escharotic first, at the base of the projection, taking care not to injure the remaining sound portion of the cornea. The effect has been the separation of a small slough ;· but previously to such separation, a deposit of fibrin beneath, by which the deeper part has become more solid and strengthened. After the part has recovered from an application, I have made a second close to, but not upon the same spot, and nearer to the summit of the projection : again and again I have repeated this operation, acting upon the more prominent part, until a considerable or perfect reduction of the staphyloma has been accomplished; and this has enabled me, in a few cases, to form an artificial pupil, subsequently of much more utility to the patient. I prefer the hydrate of potash, unless the projection be very small, for its use is followed by a much larger deposit of fibrin than results from the nitrate of silver."

Some continental surgeons speak highly of the plan.

Singularly enough, an artificial pupil has been formed, by the increase of a partial staphyloma in connexion with healthy cornea ; the iris having been torn away from its ciliary connexion by the expanding growth. A notice of the case, with a drawing, is in Mr. Dalrymple's work on the " Pathology of the Human Eye." The pupil happened to be formed opposite to a transparent part of the cornea. Even a plurality of pupils have occurred.

STAPHYLOMA OF THE SCLEROTICA.

This signifies a distension of the sclerotica, sometimes

generally, but for the most part into a dark blue, or black-
ish tumour. The usual seat of enlargement is at a little
distance around the cornea, nearly in correspondence with the
circumference of the posterior chamber, and this is spoken of as
"staphyloma corporis ciliaris." The colour of the projection
renders it very conspicuous. Unlike staphyloma of the cornea,
several tumours generally exist ; the cause also, and mode of
production, are wholly different. Inflammation is developed in
the interior of the eyeball, the choroid being supposed to be
usually its primary seat. It is more frequently slowly and
insidiously developed, than actively. Ultimately the sclerotica is
involved in the morbid action, which destroys its intimate structure, and it becomes adherent to the choroid. Preternatural
vascularity of this coat is one of the changes attendant on the
process, and the large vessels are persistent. With much bulging
of the sclerotica, vision is, I believe, always lost. I never met
with a case in which it was not. The general invasion of disease
destroys the eye; the cornea being the tunic that suffers the
least. The fact of the staphylomata being so commonly in correspondence with the position of the posterior chamber, has
induced some pathologists to attribute their formation to an undue
secretion of the aqueous humour, but the theory is not tenable.

The following illustration of the affection was taken from a
young woman.

Fig. 93.

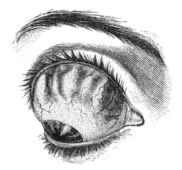

The eyeball is directed downwards, and the eyelid elevated,
to give the more extended view. The staphylomata were very

tense, and nearly confined to the upper portion. There was not any vision. The crystalline lens was absorbed, and its capsule floated in the posterior chamber. The iris was not thrown forward. The history of the case is, that when a child, a scratch on the cornea from the finger of an infant excited intense inflammation, on which the disease supervened.

Whatever be the call for treatment, whether pain from distension, irritation, deformity, or sympathetic influence, the course is, when practicable, to reduce the size of the eyeball, by letting out some of its contents, and to effect it with the least possible sacrifice of the ocular coats; for although the stump which is left never equals that which follows the removal of a staphyloma corneæ, still a sort of button may be preserved for the adaptation of an artificial eye.

It must be left to the judgment of the surgeon to determine, according to the severity of the case, whether this should be done by removing the cornea; or by mere incision; or by laying hold of the distended portion of the tunic, and, after having made it flaccid by letting out some of the fluid, cutting it off. But if there be complete disorganization of the interior of the eyeball, and the staphyloma be very large, or if there be several, " extirpation " may be preferable. The after-treatment is the same as for the operation of " staphyloma corneæ."

I have not had any personal experience of the efficacy of lunar caustic, combined with pressure, as recommended by some foreign authors.

Although the treatment of staphyloma does not fall within the province of this work till circumstances arising out of its size call for operation, yet I introduce an interesting fact mentioned by Mr. Tyrrell. A staphylomatous projection at the upper and outer part of the globe, near to the cornea, occurring in acute choroiditis, quite subsided, and left the sclerotica thin and slightly flaccid at the part where it had existed, under general treatment alone. The patient had distinct perception of light with that eye.

In the " Medical Times and Gazette " for May, 1855, is a

clinical lecture of mine, that contains the particulars of a case akin to the above. For the irritation, that was consequent on a fly getting under the eyelid, the solid nitrate of silver was used. Considerable inflammation of the eyeball ensued, and the sclerotica bulged in a distinct staphyloma, at the upper part, just posterior to the cornea. Complete recovery ensued, the vision not being in the least impaired. The only remains of the staphyloma were a few small stains of a sepia colour where it occurred.

Staphyloma of the cornea and of the sclerotica may coexist. " Extirpation " is for the most part needed, but " abscission " should be practised when it may.

ENLARGEMENT OF THE EYEBALL WITH DISORGANIZATION.

There may be an increase of the entire eyeball, attended with disorganization, that does not come strictly under the head of staphyloma, but which may, I presume, be most appropriately considered in this place.

In this affection the cornea is not lost, and the iris covered by a plastic material; it is enlarged, sometimes conical, and of a dark blue colour. The sclerotica does not generally yield in any one spot, but is uniformly distended in every part, with more or less loss of its whiteness, being dark blue or brown, or coloured in spots.

This state answers to what is called by systematic writers, dropsy of the globe or hydrophthalmia, and may be an idiopathic affection, in which case it is more frequently seen in strumous girls ; or it may result from unhealthy action consequent on wounds. It is more generally called " scleroticochoroiditis." The fact is, that there is general inflammation of the whole eyeball, not one of its parts escaping, and each exhibiting changes which arise out of its peculiar organization.

The cornea generally suffers the least, its circumference alone may be opaque; perhaps the whole only opaque; or both opaque and enlarged, or a part only may be thus changed, so that its implication is a matter of degree only. The demand for surgical aid may arise, as in true staphyloma of the cornea or sclerotica, from the great increase in the volume of the eye, and the consequent symptoms of irritation and sympathetic affection of the other eye; or what is more likely, from the mere pain, which is insupportable, and which seems to arise solely from distension: this result seems almost inevitable when the eye is much stretched, as is illustrated by the following example of the disease.

FIG. 94.

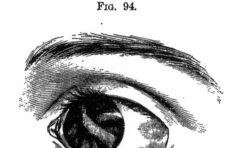

The young woman received, at three years of age, an accidental blow from a beef-bone thrown by her father, and sight was immediately lost. From the position and extent of the cicatrix on the cornea I conceive that it was burst. At fourteen the eyeball began to enlarge; it then became painful, and continued to increase and to ache for two years, since which it had been stationary and nearly devoid of uneasiness. The cornea was enlarged and blue, except at the cicatrix, and the sclerotica generally enlarged, with irregular dark blue protrusions. The other eye was becoming sympathetically affected. The long interval in this case, between the receipt of injury and the enlargement, is remarkable.

The treatment must be precisely after the principles laid down for the reduction of staphyloma of the sclerotica.

In the first volume of the "Lancet" for 1850, Mr. Dixon has recorded some excellent examples of this affection, occurring both from spontaneous inflammation, and as the result of wounds. A delicate boy, five years old, received a wound on the cornea; the iris prolapsed, and the lens and capsule became opaque. A little more than two years afterwards the whole globe was enlarged, and its forepart changed into a half-opaque, conical protuberance, of a dark bluish colour. Five years later the eye was considerably larger, the cornea more nearly hemispherical, and its surface uneven from hypertrophy and vesication of the epithelium. The sclerotica was thinned and bluish in several places, and unsightly; besides, there was much pain. The central third of the cornea was cut off, and after various symptoms and consequences, that need not be detailed, the eye ultimately dwindled to a little less than the bulk of the sound one. Mr. Dixon remarks that the morbid changes which took place in the cornea itself, and in the chambers of the aqueous humour, appear the more unaccountable as the lens had undergone complete absorption. I presume it is inferred, that by the removal of the lens the posterior chamber would be more or less destroyed, and the aqueous secretion arrested. He adds that the pain seems to have been entirely owing to distension of the forepart of the eye from over-secretion of aqueous humour, the vitreous body being apparently unchanged either in bulk or quality.

Another case is remarkable as showing the period over which the diseased action extended. An extensive wound of the cornea was followed by gradual enlargement and pain, occurring twenty-seven years later.

A female, thirty-seven years old, came under my care at the Central London Ophthalmic Hospital, with inflammation of the whole eyeball of five months' standing. The globe was enlarged, and the lens, which was opaque, was thrust against the hazy cornea which was just yielding at its circumference, where there was an ash-coloured ring. Three months later there was considerable expansion at the circumference, and the cornea stood out almost square and greatly enlarged, and the sclerotica was now distended to a prodigious size, and uniformly discoloured.

Tapping the eye, with a broad needle, every two or three days, either through the cornea or posteriorly, with pressure by compress and bandage, has been recommended as likely to be serviceable in this general enlargement, especially if done early; and its advantage is positively spoken of by some surgeons. Dr. Jacob is an advocate for the tapping merely, not only here, but in true staphyloma. In a clinical lecture in the "Medical Circular" for March 21st, 1860, he says,—"But I must premise that it is not a very showy proceeding, or one very likely to redound to your ophthalmological fame, for it is often tedious, and leaves the patient not much more improved in appearance than before, however he may be as to his comforts. I begin by a small puncture with the point of an extracting knife or a Saunders's needle; but you may be content with a lancet, or, as you have seen me in subsequent punctures, with a common needle; all you want is to let out all the aqueous humour that will flow, and to leave an opening likely to heal by first intention, until you see how your patient bears injury; mind that, for I can tell you that a very small matter sets up awful inflammation in some people. I have not seen either afford the least benefit, except temporary relief from pain. In a few days, or weeks, there has been a re-accumulation of fluid and a return of the symptoms. In one case, after the second tapping, acute inflammation with suppuration followed." In the case I have illustrated, this plan and pressure were fairly tried, and for a time were supposed to have been beneficial; but after the bandage had been left off for a few days, and the vessels of the orbit had re-filled, it was evident that there was no reduction. After this attempt I learned that another surgeon had tried pressure without tapping, for several weeks, without any benefit. Ultimately I performed "abscission." A large portion of the degenerate vitreous humour escaped, but there was not complete collapse, and, strange to say, no bleeding. A tolerable stump remained, to which a glass eye was fitted, and I never saw a nicer adaptation of this appliance. Dr. Mackenzie speaks very confidently of curing a case of dropsy of the vitreous body resulting from an injury, in which the lens was opaque and displaced, by tapping repeatedly through the cornea.

The removal of a portion of the staphyloma originated with Celsus, who also proposed the double ligature. The seton treatment, too, is very old. Even an issue at the margin of the tumour has been suggested by Richter.

Mr. Lawrence makes some very practical remarks concerning the nature of the distending medium in enlargement of the eyeball, expressing his inability, from the nature of the symptoms, to determine whether enlargement at the posterior part of the eye is caused by an effusion of watery fluid, or by an increase of the vitreous humour. In the only example of the increase of the vitreous body which he had seen, he did not discover the nature of the case till he had made a puncture behind the cornea for the purpose of lessening the size of the globe; in all the other instances of hydrophthalmia witnessed by him, the distension was by aqueous fluid. Hence he coincides with the following passage in Scarpa:—"The generality of surgeons teach, that the immediate cause of the dropsy of the eye is sometimes the increase of the vitreous, at other times of the aqueous humour. In all the cases of dropsy of the eye which I have operated upon, or have examined in the dead body, in different stages of the disease, I have constantly found the vitreous humour, accordingly as the disease was inveterate or recent, more or less disorganized, and in a state of dissolution; nor have I been able, in any instance, to distinguish, on account of the increased quantity, which of these two humours, vitreous or aqueous, had had the greater share in the formation of the disease." In two cases of enlargement of the globe after traumatic injury, in which I removed a part of the cornea, there was an increase of the vitreous humour; at least that seemed to be the state of the case, for vitreous fluid, apparently not in the least altered in consistence, filled the distended tunics.

CHAPTER XIV.

AFFECTIONS OF THE PUNCTA LACRYMALIA AND THE CANALICULI — DISPLACEMENT OF THE LOWER PUNCTUM — OBSTRUCTION OF THE LACRYMAL DUCT.

PROBE.

A SILVER, or a gilt steel instrument of this shape, is more manageable, and can be used with greater precision and effect, than the thin flexible piece of wire that the surgical instrument makers generally supply.

FIG. 95.

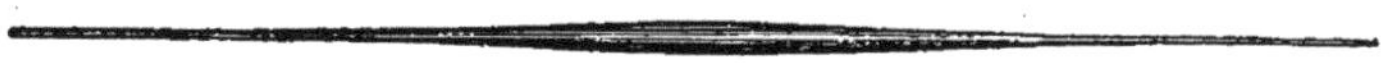

One extremity is larger than the other, and more conical. It is necessary to have a second probe, of larger dimensions.

OBSTRUCTION OF THE PUNCTA, AND OF THE CANALICULI.

These parts are not often the primary seats of disease, nor do they remain alone affected.

I ignore the idea that a patulous state of the puncta interrupts the passage of the secretions, and I must confess that I am not familiar with such a pathological change. Now and then large ones are met with, but I have not seen any defective action associated therewith. The watery eye of the aged is commonly assigned to this cause; but it would be more correct to attribute it to failure in those mechanical movements of the eyelids, that are so necessary to bring the puncta into proper play; and also, to the more or less displacement or loss of adaptation of other parts, from those alterations incidental to age. Senile lacrymation is, I suspect too, often due severally to an unhealthy condition of the lacrymal gland, and of the conjunctiva.

Contraction of the puncta, and thereby obstruction to the passage of the excretions, is really very uncommon. Mr. Tyrrell speaks of it as being rare; he had seen it only in persons naturally of an irritable temperament, and who had been rendered additionally so from debility. In a recent conversation I had with Mr. Lawrence, he confirmed this immunity.

As the result of ulceration of the eyelids, and of burns, it is often seen.

The puncta may be destroyed by accident. I know an instance in which, in consequence of this, and the co-existing adhesion of a large part of each eyelid to the eyeball, it was deemed prudent to remove the lacrymal gland from the annoyance that the overflowing of the tears produced.

The puncta may be congenitally absent, as many writers testify. In vol. xxvii. of the "Dublin Journal of Medical Science," Mr. Wilde alludes to a case mentioned by Morgagni in his "Epistolæ," in which all four were closed; and gives an instance, lately seen by himself, of a young girl without a punctum on the left upper eyelid, or the papilla, on which this little aperture is usually situated.

Obstruction of the canaliculi is more common than contraction of the puncta; and the narrowing is mostly at the inner side.

I have met with congenital deficiency. In one instance the lower canal was not developed in the inner half, while the remainder was remarkably fine, and the punctum so minute as scarcely to be recognised. I discovered this while making a dissection on a young man who had died of consumption. I ascertained that the defect produced no inconvenience, and was unknown to him. The upper one, with the punctum, were unusually developed.

In another instance, in an infant, the entire canaliculus was dilated, and looked like a cyst, without any external opening.

Congenital fistula is mentioned by Blasius.

The ordinary effect of stricture in these minute parts is a watery eye: a simple overflowing of tears, unassociated with chronic inflammation of the conjunctiva, except perhaps at a very late period; and no regurgitation of any kind of fluid when the lacrymal sac is pressed. Occasionally minute abscesses form in the eyelid, in the immediate vicinity of, or around the lower canaliculus, in connexion with stricture of it. I am describing simple obstruction, uncombined with any change of position of the angle of the eyelid; I have to show that displacement alone of this part will produce epiphora.

The evidence in the case of a closed punctum is palpable. In that of the canaliculus, exploration is needed to determine it. When the probe cannot be readily passed, and made to touch the lacrymal bone, in all probability there is disease, and a very careful survey should be made. Stoppage in the outer part is readily detected; not so, however, in the inner, and the following rule will be useful. When the outer wall of the lacrymal sac, with the skin over it, moves towards the nose, and an elastic resistance is felt, there is more or less occlusion.

The treatment is far more satisfactory than might be supposed. When a punctum is merely narrowed, the patency is readily re-established by careful use of the probe. When it is closed, provided there be no distortion of the parts around, the canaliculus may possibly be reached by a cross-cut, or by a careful dissection, then slit up, and the channel so established to the nose. It has been suggested by Mr. Bowman, supposing that no orifice can be found after the transverse section, to open the sac below the tendo oculi, and then slit up the canal near the obstruction on a probe run into it from the opening in the sac; the internal orifices of the canaliculi being so large that a skilful surgeon could readily accomplish this, if he had previously taken pains to acquaint himself with the anatomy of the parts. Mr. Streatfeild tells me that he has successfully passed a probe into the lower canaliculus by the route of the upper which had previously been slit up, and re-established an aperture in the position of the punctum by cutting on the end of it.

When the canaliculus is narrowed, the probes must be called into requisition, at first the smaller, then the larger, and repeated at intervals of a few days. As the punctum is of less size than any part of the canal, it may be required to slit it up, fully to carry out the treatment. When there is such obstruction as to produce resistance to the entrance of the probe, and all attempts at dilatation have failed, a passage may be made by pushing the lacrymal director into the sac, and dividing the perforated part along with the rest of the canal.

There are several details in so establishing a conduit by incision, and I shall give them when speaking of a displaced lower punctum in the next subdivision. For the treatment of the excretory lacrymal apparatus connected with division of these parts, we are indebted to Mr. Bowman.

I have met with congenital deficiency of the inner part of both canaliculi in one eye. The patient, a girl, was fourteen years old. In early childhood an unnatural flow of the tears was noticed. The persistence of this annoyance prevented her from entering on any employment. I operated, and established channels to the lacrymal duct. The treatment occupied two weeks.

Several authors make mention of obstruction of the canaliculi by polypi. Calculi have also been met with. Mr. Travers says, that in more than one instance he has turned out a considerable quantity of calcareous matter wedged in these tubes, like the calculi of the salivary ducts. M. Desmarres gives a most voluminous description of the chemical analysis of one removed by himself from the lower punctum: many parallel instances are on record.

Mr. T. C. Jackson brought me a patient who had been troubled with a watery eye, and afterwards a purulent discharge from the lower punctum. I found swelling of the integuments over the lacrymal sac, and a tumour in the course of the canaliculus, by which the corresponding portion of the eyelid was everted. I at once mentioned my suspicion of a calculus. I made an incision over the swelling ; first a chalky-like material, which proved to be epithelium, was removed, and then a phosphate of lime calculus, just the size of a No. 4 shot. Perfect recovery ensued.

Epithelium alone may choke up the canaliculi.

DISSECTION SHOWING THE PUNCTA, THE CANALICULI, AND THE LACRYMAL SAC.

All the parts covering the corner of the eye have been dissected away, and the course of the canaliculi and the head of the lacrymal duct, the " sac, " above the bony channel, made apparent. A part of the tendo oculi is left attached to the bone.

The canaliculi opened in this instance into the sac separately; sometimes they communicate by a common aperture. Their irregular course is altered by the bristles that were inserted, and they are made to assume a straight line; whereas, to reach

FIG. 96.

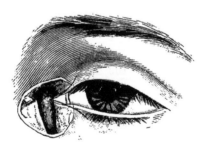

the surface, each bends almost at a right angle, forming an elbow, and then turns a little inwards,—a beautiful provision, whereby the puncta are the more certainly adapted to their office. This bend should be remembered while using a probe, and this little impediment thereby overcome, by drawing the eyelid out, and straightening the canal, or merely everting the tarsal edge a little, and passing the probe vertically for about half a line, and then inwards.

z 2

Irrecoverable injury is caused by rough and violent probing. I advise the student to practise on the dead body before he tries on the living.

LACRYMAL DIRECTOR.

FIG. 97.

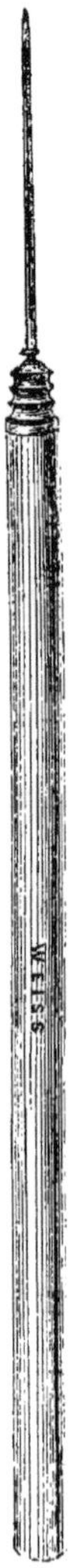

This instrument is more readily used when attached to a handle. The stem is fine-pointed, not actually sharp, and grooved in its entire length, so that the knife may run out without impediment. On the handle, corresponding to the groove, is a dot which may be useful to indicate the side that is channelled. I have many times seen the want of this little index when blood is about the instrument. The artist has not depicted it.

DISPLACEMENT OF THE LOWER PUNCTUM.

Considerable disturbance of the functions of the lacrymal apparatus comes from a displaced lower punctum. The dislocation occurs under two states : simple eversion from a variety of causes ; and malposition associated with some structural changes in the tarsal edge, and in the punctum. Mr. Bowman has pointed out that the prominence on which the punctum is placed may have disappeared, the orifice lying on a flattened, rounded, cutaneous surface, at a little distance from the mucous lining of the eyelid ; much reduced in size, and not wetted by the tears, but dry.

In every instance of watery eye, therefore, the lower punctum should be carefully surveyed, and its integrity scrutinised. But any deviation from its position, or any slight morbid change, cannot be appreciated, except by one who has studied the part in health. The beautiful manner in which it is brought into play by muscular action in winking, and applied against the eyeball, must be inspected in different individuals. It would be useless for me to say more. It is enough to direct how to observe, as it is only by observation here that the subject can be learned.

When there is displacement, and that only, the removal of this partial ectropium will generally suffice to bring the punctum into play. It has been all-sufficient in many cases that I have thus treated. So far as I know, the practice originated with myself. My plan is to dissect off the palpebral conjunctiva from a spot just posterior to the canaliculus, and to regulate the amount removed by the degree of the eversion; for as it is by the ensuing contraction that the eyelid is traced to its place, a proper proportion is required. For the most part, I have not applied sutures, but my present impression is in their favour.

This operation is far more generally applicable than I suspected when I first applied it. Indeed, it is a very rare thing not to find some eversion of the eyelids, whenever the punctum is inactive; and the physical change that I have mentioned as occurring in and around this capillary aperture, is due to chronic inflammation of the palpebral conjunctiva, the most common cause of ectropium.

When, however, with displacement of the punctum, the tarsal edge has been rounded, or so changed by chronic inflammation that perfect re-adaptation of parts, or at least restoration of function, is impossible, the tears may yet be directed in the proper course by slitting up the punctum and the canaliculus. A director is introduced, and the canal opened with a knife, in its entire length. Some care is required to do this effectually, as a part near the sac hangs, and is apt to escape division. This cannot be thoroughly done without opening the sac to some extent. I do not say that in every case it is absolutely requisite to divide the entire canal, as here directed, but nearly always it had better be done.

As might be suspected, there is primary union in a few hours after this little operation, and the new channel should be re-opened with the director or probe each day, for two, three, or more days, till no longer required. This is, I think, the best of all the suggestions that have been thrown out for effecting the object.

I often combine the above methods, and there are these advantages: ectropium of the lower eyelid from chronic inflammation of the conjunctiva is a progressive affection, and early treatment by operation, as I recommend, is all-effectual. Then, if there be much displacement of the punctum, the division of it and of the canaliculus does not altogether obviate the overflow of the tears; but by adopting the two, the greatest procurable benefit is commanded, and a degree of perfection often ensured, that could not be attained by any other known measures.

I have found, in a few instances, that enlargement of the caruncle has been an impediment to the completion of re-establishing the tear channel. I have removed it, partially and entirely, with benefit.

FIG. 98.

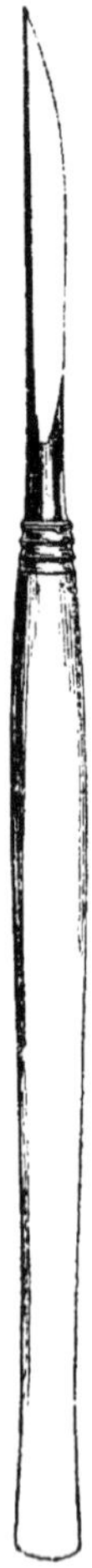

KNIFE FOR THE LACRYMAL DUCT.

The requisites here are sufficient narrowness, length, and strength of blade. It is better for the trustworthiness of so slight an instrument that it be without a shoulder, a spot at which delicate knives frequently break. The upper part of the blade is quite round, the next oval, and the point nearly flat.

OBSTRUCTION OF THE LACRYMAL DUCT.

I regard this disease as generally of scrofulous origin; for not only does the state of the patient's health frequently declare the fact, but the local manifestations of struma are very often coexistent. The common occurrence of symmetrical development of it, is likewise significant of this. Prostration of the system may induce it; and in children, the severer exanthemata are occasionally precursors. I believe that, in severe cases, the entire tract of the mucous surface is more or less invaded by the morbid action, the consequence of which is obstruction.

Stricture of the canaliculi, especially of the lower, is frequently associated.

The encasement of the greater portion of the duct by bone

precludes the exhibition of those results that are manifested in its upper and free end, the lacrymal sac; and hence the idea that this part alone is generally diseased.

Very slight narrowing would, I imagine, be attended with interruption to the functions; as it is probable that the means of escape is not much greater than that required. In the healthy condition any augmentation of the excretions produces an overflow; and, with the slightest stricture, the ordinary amount must be too much for the transit.

The obstruction usually begins imperceptibly, and increases insensibly, till a watery eye, and distension of the sac by tears and by mucous secretion, disclose its existence. The common history of these cases is, that for an indefinite period there has been a watery eye, sometimes particularly troublesome, united perhaps with the occasional escape of mucus or pus through the puncta, and perhaps dryness of the nostril; attacks of inflammation supervene, and not unfrequently an abscess forms and bursts externally; the position of the opening is determined by accidental circumstances, and may be at some distance, even on the cheek: the common situation is over the sac, as portrayed in the following sketch.

FIG. 99.

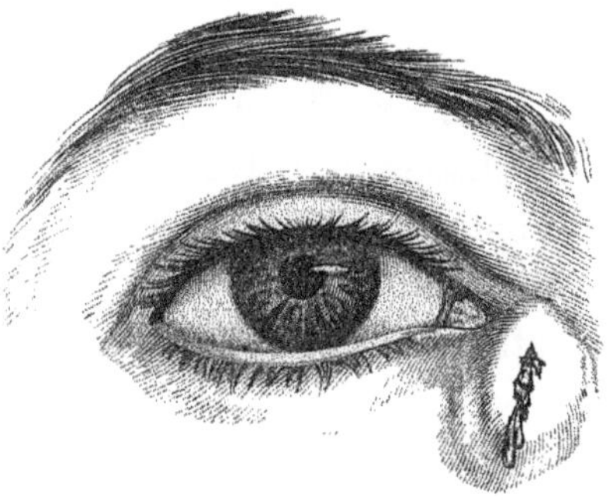

According to the extent of the suppuration, and the degree of accompanying inflammation, will be the size of the fistula; should the maxillary bone become carious, it may be very large. A lad, thirteen years of age, with suppurating cervical glands, had lost from ulceration the greater portion of the bone in front of the duct.

Although these stages are usually spread over months, sometimes even years, there may be such rapid succession of them, as to induce the belief that the attack is due to acute primary inflammation in the duct; an occurrence which I suspect to be of great rarity.

With the suspicion of stricture I invariably press on the sac, and if tears alone, or mingled with any morbid secretion, or tinged with blood, escape through the puncta, I consider that more or less obstruction exists. The quantity of fluid that may accumulate is surprising : on one occasion, when both ducts were stopped, at least a drachm of thick humour escaped from each. I have known distension from mucus produce inflammation that bordered on sloughing, and probably in a few hours the vitality of the integument would have been lost had not a bistoury, used under the suspicion of an abscess being present, given vent to the glairy fluid. During the accession of acute inflammation, there is seldom any discharge through the puncta, even when the sac is pressed on. This is the case so long as tumefaction exists.

Except for the severer paroxysms, which disclose the severity of the affection, a person does not generally seek advice, unless perhaps the conjunctiva is secondarily involved, and the Meibomian secretion is vitiated; and these derangements, which are so frequent, are often considered to be the cause of the obstruction. But the disease is not an ordinary termination of strumous or other kinds of inflammation of the conjunctiva; indeed, it is remarkably seldom seen as such. I strongly suspect extension of inflammation from the interior of the nose to be rather common.

The treatment of obstructed duct is threefold. Constitutional means are required to conquer the cause of the disease, local treatment is needed, and, in a late stage, some mechanical measure is demanded, to dilate the narrowed channel, or to open it when completely occluded. We should at once, therefore, seek for the general disarrangements, and direct means to improve them, medically and dietetically.

Among the poor, undoubtedly, sufficient clothing, especially flannel to the skin of the delicate, proper food, and ventilation to dwellings, are the things that are mostly needed. Without improving mal-nutrition, we shall attend to the ophthalmic symptoms in vain. In cases where the indication is apparent, the change of residence from this country to a tropical climate produces wonderful benefit. I have seen complete recovery from advanced stages of obstruction. By my recommendation, patients have found voyages to Australia and to India very curative.

With any evidence of acute inflammation, I apply leeches over the sac—one, two, or more—and resort to them as many times as may seem necessary. When chronic inflammation, rather than acute, prevails, I apply a succession of small blisters on the same part: I generally employ a blistering fluid. Besides this, I teach the patient how to empty the sac, and direct him to do it several times a day; and in the night, should he awake.

I avoid entering into a consideration of the many phases that a diseased lacrymal sac may pass through, and which have been described as mucocele, relaxation of the sac, and so forth; as it tends to no practical end, and only mystifies and puzzles. These are all merely more or less aggravated symptoms of an unhealthy mucous membrane, of which the prejudicial effect is more exercised below, where the rest of the tube—the lacrymal duct—is encased by bone, causing stricture in that part.

But the disease may not cease under any measures short of dilatation; and when this should be undertaken, is a nice practical part to decide. For many years I have sought for the indication, and I now rely on two simple facts as the most sure and unerring guides. These are the state of the canaliculi, and the condition of the parts about the lacrymal sac, as conveyed to the touch.

When one of the canaliculi is choked at the inner end, especially the lower one, there is, as far as I have observed, almost invariably stricture of some part of the duct as well. Again, when there is decided thickening of the parts over and about the lacrymal sac, so that the edges of the bones cannot be felt as in health, there is that condition that needs dilatation. These rules have fewer exceptions than any that I know of. A profuse discharge, even of purulent matter, through the puncta, although frequently associated with stricture, is not in itself, as I have frequently ascertained by actual exploration, an unerring sign of obstruction. Again, all degrees of narrowing of the duct, and even complete occlusion, may exist, without the escape of pus, and but little of any secretion.

The age of the patient gives no guidance, and I fear that surgeons are often tempted to postpone mechanical treatment on account of tender years. I have often been obliged to resort to it in children, and once in an infant three months old, who was brought to me with a lacrymal fistula. Nine days after the birth, an abscess over the duct was opened, and a fistula ensued. It cannot be doubted that the disease commenced *in utero*.

Fig. 100.

Being satisfied, from any circumstance, that dilatation is necessary, we must proceed to effect it by the natural channel: this is done by getting at the duct through the lower canaliculus. The first thing therefore is to slit it up, and to maintain it open. How to do this has already been told. Mr. Bowman, to whom we owe the plan, is, so far as I can gather, an advocate for gradual dilatation with probes of different sizes. The process is, however, as I find, tedious; and so disagreeable that but few persons, in public or in private, will submit to it sufficiently long. Many patients have left other surgeons and come to me, solely because they would not submit to it; and I know that some have left me on the same account. My practice in general, therefore, is to dilate for a short time only, using in the first instance the smaller probe, and afterwards the larger one; and then to introduce a style. Almost every surgeon has a particular fancy about probes. Any of the large London surgical instrument makers keep different kinds and sets of them, some of which are straight and others curved, as in fig. 100.

I am thoroughly convinced that where there is really that degree of change in this conduit, which imperatively calls for instrumental treatment, the wearing of a style is the less irksome, the more beneficial, and the quicker plan.

In some instances, when my patient's time was short, I have introduced the style at once. In a lady, who visited England to be treated by me, I applied two styles at the same time that I divided the canaliculi; and kept them in so long as she could remain, nearly two months; and, as I hear, a better result could not be. On other occasions, when I could not see my patient more than once or twice, as also in highly nervous persons, who required chloroform, I have acted likewise.

Styles of different calibre and of pure silver should be kept, because it may be advisable at first to use but a small one.

FIG. 101.

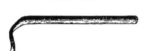

That here shown is of full size. The form was given by Mr. Taylor, when ten or more years ago, at the suggestion of Mr. Shaw, of the Indian Army, he attempted dilatation through the sac inside the eyelids, and with marked success. It was a more perfect plan than had yet been adopted. The little tail prevents the instrument from getting out of sight, and should be worn just outside the lower eyelid.

From time to time the style should be removed and cleaned, and if its pressure have been uncomfortable, the cessation of wear for a day or more generally suffices to make it tolerated afterwards. Some patients have worn it at night only.

When the stricture is so dense that it cannot be penetrated

by the probe, it should be divided by the style-knife, which ought to be passed down till resistance is overcome, and, if needs be, to the end of the duct. Many times I have met with that degree of obstruction, and sometimes too when I have not expected it, that required an incredible amount of pressure to overcome, a degree indeed that one would hardly have courage to exert on a first occasion.

An operator should be certain that he has really made a proper channel into the duct, and is working within it, and not outside, or through the lacrymal bone; and the only sure test is to feel the palatine process of the superior maxillary bone with the probe. I know of no more common mistake in Ophthalmic Surgery than for a false passage to be made here, in the attempts to introduce probes and styles.

Patients are ever naturally anxious to know how long the style should be worn. I generally tell them till inflammatory action has been subdued, which is indicated by an absence of any purulent or other secretion from the canal of an unhealthy nature. And this is what I act by.

Among the several advantages of dilating an obstructed duct through the natural passages is this, that there is no after trace of treatment, no marks on the face, no stains, no fistula to heal up, no sinuses to destroy. Besides, it has a more extended application than any method yet devised. There is hardly a complication beyond its reach. Although I have purposely refrained from giving the details of any cases, I shall briefly allude to an instance in which I was able to effect marvels.

A boy was kicked on the face by a horse, and the inner corner of the eye, together with the nasal bones, much injured. When I saw him four years after the accident, the internal commissure was drawn inwards by a cicatrix on the nose, the inner portion of the lower eyelid inverted, and the lacrymal sac distended with thick mucus, which was always overflowing through the upper punctum, and producing much distress. It was a long time before I could discover the lower punctum, from being out of the usual position, no doubt from having been injured, and withal hidden by the folded lid. When found and penetrated, I learned that the inner portion of the canaliculus was imperfect, and the sac could not be reached. I first established an opening to the sac by pushing the director through the occluded canaliculus, dividing the canal in the entire length, and using the probe each day till the edges no longer united. Then I operated for the entropium with success. After that I proceeded to dilate the duct; and as it was almost impervious, I introduced the style at once, preparing the way with the style-knife, and allowed it to remain till no longer needed. There yet lacked a little practical surgery. The caruncle was enlarged to a degree that interfered with the passage of the tears, and I removed it. With these four operations the channel from the eye to the nose was efficiently established, the misery of an obstructed duct abolished, and the boy's personal appearance materially improved.

But a few years ago such an example could only have been half-treated. Although the duct might have been made pervious, disease would have yet lingered in the sac, because of stricture in the lower punctum. This condition has for years been a source of anxiety to me.

I have not taken notice of that condition of an obstructed duct in which an acute inflammatory attack is grafted on chronic disease. The symptoms are unmistakeable. They are— considerable swelling of the integuments at the corner of the eye; perhaps even closure of the eyelids, with more or less tumefaction of the cheek, and intense pain. A deposit of pus is the usual climax. In the early stage a few punctures, or leeches, with hot or cold applications, as the indications may be, and attention to the accompanying state of the system, will often stop the severity of the attack. But it must never be forgotten that such treatment, however judicious for the time, is only after all palliative. There must be recurrence, if the stricture be not systematically attended to, and this ought to be done at the time, or soon after, as may be thought fit. We should not wait till the abscess bursts, as that necessarily prolongs the patient's suffering, and risks a fistulous aperture.

When there is the suspicion even of pus, a search should be made for it. Pus may form at some distance from the lacrymal apparatus, even low on the cheek. I have not come to any definite conclusions as to the relative frequency of the abscess being within any part of the lacrymal canal, or external to it; and practically the question matters little, as the lacrymal sac should always be opened, and the knife pushed into the duct, and through any obstruction. At least, this is my practice, because I think it the most effectual. If there be suppuration of the sac, it must then be discovered. Very frequently the pus does not escape till the duct is penetrated. The following directions may be useful in this procedure, for the usual rule that is given to find the position of the sac by pulling the eyelids outwards, and making tense the tendo oculi, is not applicable when disease exists. Indeed, with very much swelling and induration, there is not any landmark absolutely trustworthy; but so long as the lower and internal angle of the orbit can be felt, it may form an unerring guide. The correct place for the puncture corresponds externally, to a spot a little

FIG. 102.

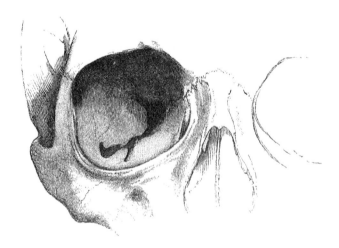

below, and internal to the inferior punctum. With the forefinger of the left hand placed on that part of the edge of the orbit that stands in front of the bony canal, to get the level, and to give an idea of the distance of the sac from the surface; the knife, with the edge outwards, should be entered below and internal to the punctum, carried a little inwards behind the ridge of bone, and then downwards, inclining slightly outwards and backwards, to the required extent. A reference to the sketch of the orbit, which is for the purpose of showing the relations of the bony canal, the ductus ad nasum, may be useful.

It is needless to attempt to pass the knife while the point is in contact with bone, for the right course has been missed. When the instrument is adroitly used, a bony surface is not touched.

The inclination of the facial angle influencing the direction of the nasal duct should be remembered. In the Ethiopian variety of our race it inclines very much forward; in our own or the Caucasian, it inclines backwards.

I have not had to attend to fistula lacrymalis associated with much loss of the soft parts since I have been practising the modern treatment of dilating an obstructed duct, and I cannot therefore say whether the old method of introducing the style externally, can here, too, be always dispensed with. I venture, therefore, to notice that practice, till very lately our only resource. It is a common custom when any new plan of treatment or any practical suggestion is brought out, to decry all or much of what has gone before on the subject. Through this many good things are laid aside, and the place taken by inferior. We should select our measures and adapt them from, all the sources at our command.

Fig. 103 shows the style which is required for an adult. The measurements are an inch and a quarter in length, and the thirteenth of an inch in diameter. For children the dimensions should be reduced. The bend causes it to sit better, and prevents the head, which should be thick with obtuse edges, from resting on and irritating the skin. Styles are sometimes fluted or per-forated in a part of their extent, under the supposition that the tears will pass more readily; but that form of construction, a modification of the metallic tube of Wathen, which used to be placed within the palpebral aperture, is decidedly objectionable;

FIG. 103.

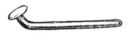

the secretions will flow readily between the smooth metal and the walls of the duct.

I have found in these severe cases of fistula, especially where the bone also was diseased, that a globular head was preferable, as not being so likely to irritate the healing surfaces. I have also found it requisite to have the stem sufficiently long to rest on the palatine process of the maxillary bone, and thus to prevent any pressure whatever above, even from the weight of the instrument. Besides the advantages of this in a curative point of view, there is prevented the inconvenience of the style dropping into the canal, and so becoming hidden. The plan usually adopted to prevent this is to apply a string, which is really very insufficient, as it only facilitates the removal when sunken, but does not prevent the act. I have often been called on to raise many that have dropped in deeply. I have never been unsuccessful but once, and as in that case it could not be effected except by cutting away some of the maxillary bone, I advised the surgeon who brought me the patient, to wait for symptoms before he urged interference.

With fistulæ there may coexist sinuses, which should be divided and made to heal from the bottom. Fungous granulations are not uncommon, and may be readily removed by a mild escharotic, or a stimulant, such as the powder of the red oxide of mercury.

When there is caries of the maxillary bone, the gouge should be used at the proper time, and the unhealthy surface cut away. Necrosed bone should not be allowed to remain. I beg to refer to the chapter on " Caries of the Orbit."

The silver style may become tarnished, or even receive a

deposit and corrode, during the ulceration stage of the soft parts or of the bones. The decomposition of the tears may affect it. I met with an unusually marked example of this in a youth from whom it had not been withdrawn and cleaned; and when I saw him after the lapse of two years, the instrument could hardly be pulled out, from the enormous mass of accumulation, especially on the end. Suspecting that the incrustation was something rather unusual, for my patient had during the last year taken great quantities of mercury for syphilis, I sent the style with it to Dr. Garrod for analysis. His answer was, " The style I examined, and find to be coated to a considerable depth with sulphuret of silver, which rendered it exceedingly brittle. The sulphuret is doubtless formed from the sulphur compounds contained in the lacrymal secretions acting gradually on the metal." This is a sketch after the deposit had been burned off.

FIG. 104.

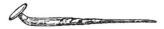

It will be seen that the neck was nearly corroded through.

Syringing the lacrymal sac and duct through the style-hole may be useful; indeed, I may say almost requisite, if there have been disease of the bone, or copious suppuration, when some astringent, or other preparation, may be added. I subjoin a sketch of the syringe that I use, reduced a third less than the

FIG. 105.

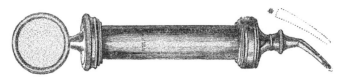

original. The lesser figure, marked with a star, gives the real size of the nozzle, and it is well to have these of various sizes and lengths, for different cases.

Patients naturally desirous of disguising all blemishes, ask how the head of the style may be best concealed. White metal is certainly conspicuous, and a bit of black or coloured wax, melted smoothly on the roughened head, tends to render it less apparent. Instrument-makers usually put on paint or enamel; but neither wears well, and as any one can apply the wax, a clean unbroken surface can always be commanded. Gold is less conspicuous; and if the head of a gold style be reduced, as it may with safety after a few weeks' wearing, nearly to the diameter of the body, very little unsightliness remains.

Without any internal disease of the lacrymal duct, the function may be arrested by external causes : as pressure from tumours in any of the neighbouring cavities; the orbit; the antrum; and especially those of the nose; a single example of which will be enough to illustrate the whole of this class of obstructions. A girl, eighteen years old, came to the Ophthalmic Hospital, with a large lacrymal fistula on each side, of several months' duration. Till there were these free apertures, she had frequent abscesses, attended with much discharge of pus through the puncta. The bridge of the nose was enlarged, and the integuments very red. Both nostrils contained polypi, and on the right side part of one protruded. The treatment was very apparent—to remove the obstructions, wait the result, and in case the fistulæ did not heal, to pass styles. Strangely enough she indignantly refused to have the nose touched, but was not the least unwilling for the fistulæ to be treated. I do not know what became of her.

More than once a polypus has been removed from the duct itself.

Actual bony deposit may occlude a part of the nasal duct, and several instances have been met with. Mr. Travers says, " I have often found the canal completely obliterated by ossific inflammation at its upper orifice in skulls, and I know cases of enlargement of the ossa nasi, and of periosteal inflammation and thickening, marked by habitual overflowing of the tears, and occasionally by erysipelatous inflammation of the surface, in which the canal is evidently destroyed."

A young man applied to me with the tertiary form of syphilis, having large nodes on several places. There was a deposit of bone on the orbital ridge that quite obstructed the nasal duct. I here adopted that course which should always be followed if practicable, whatever be the cause of the deposit, whether specific as in this instance, or arising from simple exostosis. I carried the style through the obstruction, a practice which is preferable to perforating the lacrymal bone; an expedient that should be resorted to only in cases of the greatest emergency. A small hydrocele trochar was used, and after a short penetration, the duct was reached. He was able to dispense with the style.

On two other occasions I have re-established the channel through bone, but I have lost sight of the patients.

An instance of supposed congenital fistula lacrymalis is mentioned by Mr. Lawrence. It occurred in a boy at school, in whom it seemed to be a natural peculiarity, as no inflammation or any other affection of the part had been noticed. A small drop of clear fluid appeared frequently on the surface of the skin, just below the tendon of the orbicularis. Mr. Middlemore appears to have seen this defect several times, for he speaks of it as the most frequent congenital deficiency of the lacrymal apparatus he has witnessed; in all the cases both ducts were affected, and the tears flowed over the cheeks. I have met with one example. The question of treatment must depend on the inconvenience that is produced. It would be well in all instances to examine the duct from the nose.

A more remarkable defect is that of absence of the nasal duct. A man, twenty-one years of age, was admitted into the Hospital Necker, on account of congenital fistula lacrymalis, which discharged a limpid transparent fluid: there was constant epiphora. When the angle of the eye was pressed in the morning, a muco-purulent fluid flowed from the fistulous orifice and the puncta. An artificial nasal duct was made by piercing the os unguis after the manner of Woodhouse. The inferior border of the internal portion of the tendon of the orbicularis was laid bare by incision, and a trochar directed downwards, backwards, and inwards, perforating the inner wall of the orbit. A silver canula, half an inch long, and enlarged at both its extremities, was introduced. Three days after the operation the small wound had cicatrized. In two months, the patient having neglected the directions of the surgeons—what they were is not stated—returned with epiphora; the canula was changed, and the case is said to have done well. ("British and Foreign Medical Review," vol. xii., quoted from the "Bulletin Général de Thérapeutique.")

I find in the work of M. Desmarres, in connexion with this subject, the following remarkable passage, which is placed under the head of "occlusion of the natural passages :"—"This method appears to me likely to prove serviceable in some cases of obstinate fistula. It is founded upon this observation, that if the lacrymal conduits do not exist congenitally, as has been observed by many surgeons, or if they have been destroyed accidentally, which is certainly still more frequent, the patients are not on that account afflicted with epiphora. I have seen many fistulæ, dressed with Scarpa's nail for several years, cured by obliteration of the upper part of the sac. This method encouraged me in some difficult cases to imitate Nannoni, the inventor of this method, and I have had every reason to be satisfied that I did so. Among other examples the following especially seems to deserve attention :—A lady of Rheims had for many years suffered from a lacrymal fistula, and had been several times operated on, but unsuccessfully. I also operated and used Scarpa's nail, but I effected nothing more than those who had preceded me. Taught by former facts the difficulty of closing the lacrymal passages by introducing a piece of nitrate of silver, I now proposed to destroy them by Vienna caustic, and in presence of my colleague who had sent me the patient, I deposited a certain quantity in the upper part of the sac, where I left it a few moments. Cauterization was deep, extensive, and followed by so free a suppuration, that for some days I feared there would be no other result than a deformity towards the great angle; but, on the contrary, the wound cicatrized perfectly, and the disease was cured. This lady is now free from fistula, as also from the epiphora, which has completely disappeared. Frequently since, I have employed cauterization of the lacrymal sac with Vienna caustic, but with greater precaution, and I have had good reason to be satisfied. Nevertheless, however good may be the results obtained by Delpech, Bosche, M. Caffort de Narbonne, many other surgeons, and myself, I think one ought not to have recourse to the closing of the nasal canal except as a last resource, and that, if it can be cured by any other means, they should be preferred."

FIG. 106.

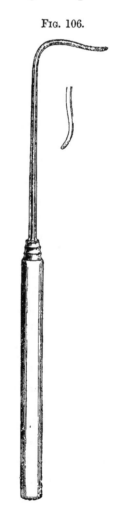

This practice has been imitated in England, and even the actual cautery has been employed to destroy the duct. In my opinion, it cannot be too strongly condemned. It is founded on fallacy.

PROBE OR SOUND FOR THE LACRYMAL DUCT.

I introduce this instrument to condemn it as a means of treatment, rather than to recommend it. Indeed, I should have dismissed it with but a very few words, but for the possibility of being of use in affording some information as a sound, relative to the degree and position of a stricture, in connexion with morbid growths that encroach on the duct.

It is about the average size for an adult; and the form is that
I find to be the best, after many trials on the dead body.   Each
nostril requires one for itself, and this belongs to the left.   The
metal should be soft, or virgin silver, admitting of easy adaptation by the fingers, or a pair of pliers, to any figure, for the
individual peculiarities of a patient.   The round and delicate
handle almost ensures gentle usage, and is an improvement on
a broad flat one, which affords considerable leverage, and is
besides awkward.

The lesser figure is a front view of the end, or bent
portion.

Nasal probing of the duct has many times been abandoned
and revived; and to the late Mr. Morgan is due the last resuscitation in England.   The difficulty of the proceeding from the
anatomical intricacies of the part, the necessary tortuosity of
the instrument, and the injury to the duct that is inseparable
from the operation, are more than sufficient to banish it from
practice.

It must not be supposed that, because a sound can be
forced into the passage in the dead body, a similar proceeding can with impunity be done on the living.   I was not a
little amused to read of a recommendation from an advocate of
the practice, that it should form part of the morning toilet.
To use the probe, the point should be introduced into the nose
horizontally, and carried along its floor to a distance that will
ensure the position of the duct being reached, when it should
be turned upwards and outwards under the turbinated bone,
against the wall of the antrum, and moved about till it is
engaged in the aperture.   The usual cause of failure in its
entrance consists in not carrying the instrument sufficiently
low to ensure its being in the proper chamber of the nose, and
in attempting to find the orifice before it has been carried
enough back.   It is to be feared that the membranous wall of
the duct is more often entered than its orifice.   When the
sound is passed, the end may be felt at the angle of the orbit in
the sac.   The entire proceeding, the introduction and the withdrawal, requires much delicacy of touch.   I have introduced it

a few times in the living body. There has always been much bleeding, and an expression, as well there might be, on the part of the patient, of considerable dissatisfaction, and of a strong determination not to submit to it again.

The subjoined sketch of a dissection of the nasal duct, from an adult female, may prove useful.

FIG. 107.

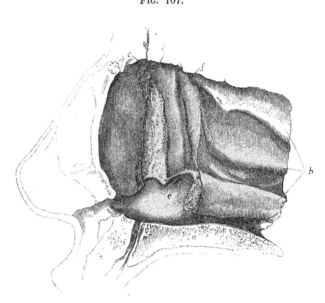

a, The palatine process of the superior maxillary bone.

b, The turbinated bones: the anterior half of the lowest one has been cut away to show the opening of the tube (*e*) in the lowest chamber of the nose.

c, The surface left after a part of the nasal process of the superior maxillary bone has been cut away to exhibit more clearly the duct (*d*), the entire surface of which is bared of its bony parietes.

f, The point at which two bristles, that were passed through the puncta, met.

In many examinations that I have made of the nasal opening of the duct, the aperture has not been discoverable, as might be imagined, after the inferior turbinated bone had been cut away ; but has always required to be searched for with a probe.

It is, in fact, but a minute slit. Indeed, to make it apparent for the sketch, it was a little ruptured and opened. There is variation in its position, perpendicularly and horizontally. Sometimes, too, it is on a depression in the wall of the antrum, or on a projection.

CHAPTER XV

THE first indication of the conical change is short sight; imperfect vision follows, bodies are multipled, or have zones around them, and the best sight is got by looking side-ways, because nothing can be clearly seen through the apex of the cornea, but at the circumference only. As the affection advances, the eye becomes quite useless.

A few words in explanation of the symptoms. Instead of the rays of light being concentrated, as by the natural cornea, and the images of objects formed and directed through the pupil, they are bent and thrown off, and otherwise influenced by the mechanical changes in the part.

All this is very puzzling to the patient, who cannot discover any external alteration in his eye.

Surgeons not engaged in ophthalmic practice often fail to detect the disease. Unless the eye be examined in profile, in the early stages mere increase of the lustre is the only objective symptom; but when looked at sideways, it seems as though a drop of water was placed on the cornea. In exaggerated examples the apex of the cone may become opaque at the summit, or dotted with opacities, or be ulcerated. The anterior chamber always looks large in proportion to the corneal projection, and the iris may be slightly tremulous. Soon after the ophthalmoscope was introduced, I examined a young woman whose defective sight could not be accounted for. She seemed near-sighted, but then concave glasses scarcely gave benefit. I now learned for the first time that this instrument could detect the conical change, the true cause of the impaired vision, in a degree so incipient that in the first instance I had failed to notice it. I pointed this out to some of my colleagues. When the reflection from the instrument was made to play about the cornea at different angles, a darkened circle was seen on the sides not in the focus.

Further experience has convinced me that the ophthalmoscope may be made subservient to the diagnosis of the early stage of the affection.

FIG. 108.

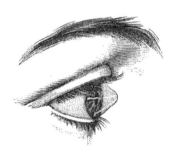

The above sketch was taken from an eye that was in an advanced stage; the cornea had not, however, lost any of its transparency.

The cone varies in prominence, size, and pointedness.

It was long since pointed out by Sir David Brewster that the cone is not quite regular, but more or less undulated : this is best shown by means of a lens. The multiplying effect is due to this inequality.

The affection has been seen at birth, and has also occurred hereditarily: it usually appears at the time of puberty. The slowness of its progress is striking, especially if bursting of the cornea be regarded as the necessary termination, for that may not happen in a long life, even when the disease commenees in youth; yet I have more than once known it occur before the fortieth year.

Both eyes are nearly always implicated, and the second is

usually attacked after the abnormal change is well developed in the first, so that generally a long period intervenes.

The ratio of increase is uncertain, and there may be an arrest at any stage.

It appears to me that we are in ignorance of any predisposing causes of this peculiar ocular change; it cannot be said that debility induces it, for it appears in the strong and robust; indeed, I have scarcely seen it except in healthy persons.

Regarding the direct cause, not anything has been proved, and the opinions are very various and contradictory. I have not been able to satisfy myself of any immediate preceding influence, in any instance of genuine conical cornea, in which there is nothing but the transparent cone. Bulging of a part of the cornea, after partial ulceration or slough, should not be considered identical with the disease; neither should general increase in the convexity of the cornea, so common after long-continued inflammation of this part, and often, I suspect, regarded as conical cornea; whence the supposed inflammatory origin. The form, however, is not quite pyramidal; there is mere increase in dimensions of the whole cornea. That there may sometimes be an approach to the pyramidal form I well know; indeed there may be, after corneitis with ulceration, a decided cone, but then there is more or less the appearance of staphyloma. While I thus advance my own opinions, I do not ignore those of others to the contrary, attributing conical cornea to inflammation, and I willingly quote the following passage from Dr. Jacob's work on Inflammation of the Eyeball :—

"The alteration in form is not always of the same shape. The surface is sometimes apparently spherical, sometimes an irregular spheroid, and sometimes projecting at one side more than another; but the most remarkable deviation is that wherein it becomes conical and acquires the peculiar form which in the sequel constitutes the very remarkable and singular result of disease called staphyloma pellucidum. I am prepared for a denial of the correctness of this statement, that the staphyloma pellucidum, or conical cornea, is owing to the disease under discussion; but I nevertheless venture to insist upon it, because I have seen and traced the change from its commencement to its termination more than once. That there should be doubt and difference of opinion on the subject is not surprising, because true corneitis is not a very common disease, and the change in shape to the conical is not a frequent consequence of it. The alteration takes place in childhood, for the disease generally occurs at that period of life; and after the inflammation has disappeared and the opacity has been dissipated, no defect, except this conical state, remains, which is not perceived until the young person is called on to apply the eyes to books, or to work requiring good sight. Then it is that the surgeon's attention is directed to the case, and he for the first time sees it, and, perhaps naturally enough, thinks that it is a disease in progress, and only recently commenced. Hence the difference of opinion respecting its nature, and the various speculations as to its origin. That I have seen the cornea become opaque from corneitis, then conical, and finally perfectly transparent, retaining its conical form, I am quite positive; but not only have I seen this, but also have I seen it become distinctly conical in a case of common idiopathic inflammation of the eyeball in a man of middle age, although not transparent or resembling the true staphyloma pellucidum."

I now approach the important topic of surgical treatment, and the discrepancy among authors as to the results of similar methods is certainly astonishing. Frequent evacuation of the aqueous humour has been tried more than any other operation, but the general testimony is against it. Desmarres, when speaking of tapping, says that if surgeons had joined to it a methodical, immediate, and long-continued compression, as he daily practises in opaque staphyloma, and as he has done with great advantage in two cases of transparent staphyloma, this method would perhaps have been followed with better results. He continues, that he, like Demours, has found, after long practice, compression (which is thought by some practitioners to be dangerous and inefficacious) to be of the greatest use in numerous cases. He has reason to think that those who blame it have never tried it, or if sometimes they have had recourse to it, have done so neither with perseverance nor method. For eighteen months he treated a little girl of eight years of age, whose right eye was lost in consequence of purulent ophthalmia, and in whose left there was an opaque staphyloma in the internal half; the cicatrix hardened daily, and the pupil, kept dilated by belladonna, was available on the outer side. Puncture of the cornea, followed by immediate compression, appears to him the best means actually known of treating this disease; but the compression ought to be light, accurately made, and kept up for a long period, and from time to time the centre of the tumour should be cauterized with nitrate of silver, and laudanum should be dropped into the eye.

The late Mr. Tyrrell tells us, in his practical work on the Eye, that within the last six years he has succeeded in giving relief to a considerable extent, by a plan so simple that he was surprised it had not been previously tried. It consists in altering the shape and position of the pupil, and removing it from beneath the centre of the cornea, or that part which has its figure most changed, to near the margin, where the least change has occurred, sometimes cutting off a bit of the iris, sometimes leaving it strangulated in the corneal wound. He performed this operation seven or eight times; in each case it benefited the vision, and in two cases considerably. No one that I am aware of, besides Mr. Tyrrell, has met with like success. I saw two cases that he operated on after the publication of his work, not only without the least benefit, but unfortunately with the disadvantage of adding to the confusion of vision, perhaps, on account of the large portion of iris that was excised. Many surgeons, encouraged by Mr. Tyrrell's writings, have followed his practice and failed.

The late Mr. Dalrymple, Mr. Tyrrell's colleague, in his "Pathology of the Human Eye," gives his opinion on all operations for the disease in these words:—"Various have been the surgical measures for remedying this deformity, and all with so little success as not to warrant us in the attempt to interfere by surgical means."

It is a physical impossibility that the removal of the lens can confer any benefit; on the contrary, it makes the vision worse.

It is with much pleasure I refer to a communication by Mr Bowman, in the "Ophthalmic Hospital Reports" for October, 1859, "On Conical Cornea, and its Treatment by Operation," wherein it is stated that, by making a slit-like figure of the pupil, by which this aperture is limited in size, while it is changed in position, very material improvement in sight has ensued. He applies the operation "iriddesis," and by operating on both sides of the eye, is enabled to obtain the desired form and size. He prefers seizing the iris with the blunt hook, rather than the canula forceps, as being simpler and less likely to produce injury, while it affords greater precision in fixing the pupillary edge to the wound, from which he finds no disadvantage, as the pupil acts as well afterwards as when the natural pupil is still entirely within the chamber.. He likes the interval of a week between the operations. In not any of the six cases so treated, had he reason to regret having operated; not one had been made worse; all with one exception had been improved, and not any had caused anxiety by subsequent inflammatory threatening.

He continues, "It has been a matter of great interest with me to ascertain, as far as the limited number of cases presenting themselves enabled me, how far the second iriddesis was useful; in other words, whether an elliptical or slit-like pupil gave better sight than one of a balloon-shape; and again, whether the vertical direction was better than the horizontal, or the reverse; also whether other modifications in the direction of the altered pupil were desirable.

"Of course, this is a subject which must be worked out in detail by surgeons, and the following remarks are but hints for future experimental inquiries.

"The slit-like figure of the pupil suggested itself to me as the most feasible method of much limiting the size of the pupil while changing its situation. If the thing be well considered, it will be found difficult to conceive any plan of rendering the pupil very small by operation; it is much more easy to enlarge it. While the pupillary margin is free, any displacement of the iris is most likely to enlarge the pupil, for I despaired of being able to seize the iris at one side of the pupil, and draw and fix it over towards the other side. Any excision of the iris must, of course, enlarge the pupil, and so must any marginal iriddesis; but by a double iriddesis in opposite directions the central region becomes slit-like. · By making this slit horizontal the light is admitted from each side, as well as through the centre, and the range of the field would probably be expanded, while the precision of the image would be impaired by the inequality of refraction through the central and marginal regions respectively. The appearance of the horizontal pupil was, besides, not agreeable. The vertical position of the slit offered the prospect of its virtual reduction in size, by the overlapping of its angles by the lids in ordinary vision; and I hoped that the patient would learn to use the lids for this purpose, so as to clarify the image. I cannot say that this expectation has been borne out in any marked degree; but, nevertheless, the vertical slit is much more sightly than the horizontal, and certainly equally good for vision, so that at present I prefer it.

" The improvement of vision from a first iriddesis downwards has been in almost every case decided, the patients being delighted with the result. In some the second iriddesis upwards has not seemed further to increase the precision of view, in others it has certainly done so, and in the present state of the inquiry I am disposed to continue to practise it in cases of considerable conicity. The improvment, however, consequent on the second operation, is never so marked as that which follows the first, and it can only operate by narrowing that part of the pupil which lies behind the bulge. Its more or less influence in different cases may perhaps depend on varieties in the curvature of the apex of the cone."

This remarkable and startling announcement follows,—that the operation proposed by Graefe, of removing a bit of the iris for certain internal diseases of the eye, elsewhere noticed by me, is applicable in conical cornea. Graefe, he says, "has within the last three or four years discovered the important fact that the excision of a portion of iris diminishes the intra-ocular pressure, a fact of frequent interest in many diseases of the eye, and which he has applied with consummate skill to the treatment of glaucoma, of certain staphylomata, and last autumn to that of conical cornea."

The subject is concluded in these words: "The influence of these operations in lessening the corneal bulge has been very remarkable. It is not easy to give in any case the exact amount of this result; but that the bulge diminishes speedily, and continues to do so for a considerable time subsequent to the operation, admits of no doubt, and I attribute it to the moderation of the ocular tension. Further experience will show whether I am right; but at present I am for operating quite early in slight cases in a downward direction only, if only to arrest the progress of the conicity; and certainly to obtain this result in almost any degree will make it worth while to perform so safe an operation in a disease otherwise so intractable, and, in its advance, so destructive of all useful sight."

Two ideal sections are given of a girl's cornea before and after the operation; and, as it is stated that the improvement has been little exaggerated by the draughtsman, one's wonder is much increased.

Very likely it has occurred to the reader that the operation of Graefe, and that of withdrawing a portion of the iris, are not exactly identical, and that they differ, besides, in the quantity of the iris taken away. By the German method, two or three times as much is removed from the eye; and yet the latter process seems equally efficacious in diminishing " intra-ocular pressure."

A valuable part of the paper relates to the morbid anatomy of conical cornea. The examination was made by Mr. Hulke on an eye that had been extirpated by Mr. Bowman, in consequence of a tumour in the orbit. It is as follows :—

"The cone is a very prominent one, and is confined to the central region. The apex is nebulous, but elsewhere the cornea is quite transparent. Its surface is polished, and not facetted. The aqueous humour, iris, and lens are normal.

"A section was carried through the line of the ora serrata, so as to remove the anterior ring of the sclerotic, with the ciliary processes, the iris and cornea entire; this portion was then pinned out flat on a piece of wood, with the iris downwards, and dried. Various sections were then made, and moistened with water or acetic acid.

" The central conical nebulous portion was much thinner than the transparent periphery of the cornea where the curve was natural. This thinning began at the base of the cone and progressively increased towards the apex, where it reached its maximum. At this point the mean depth of several vertical sections was only one-third of that of the peripheral region. The continuity of the anterior elastic lamina was perfect; but upon the cone this structure was much thinner than elsewhere, and wrinkled; it was underlaid by a stratum of crowded, elongated, club-like nuclei, and beneath these the normal lamellar tissue was replaced by a web of candate and nuclear fibres, amongst the meshes of which clusters of large oval and fusiform cells were packed. The structure of the transparent peripheral region was perfectly normal, and at the base of the cone there was a gradual transition from the healthy to the diseased tissue, the inter-lamellar corpuscles becoming more plentiful, branched and drawn out into fibres, which in many instances coalesced with those from neighbouring corpuscles. The posterior elastic lamina and the epithelium, both on the front and on the back of the cornea, were unchanged.

" The changes I have described were confined to the laminated tissue of the cornea and the anterior elastic lamina. The substitution of a web of nuclear fibres and cells for the regular lamination of the cornea, explains the nebulosity of the cone and the liability to bulge."

I had not omitted to try the effect of displacing the pupil, after the manner of Tyrrell; but without decided effect. I am, however, now able to testify to the value of the linear form. I suspect that Tyrrell's success was when he made such an aperture,—an accidental circumstance, no doubt, as he had not quite discovered the secret. It is well known that, in operating with his hook, the form of the pupil depends on the amount of the iris hooked up. This will also explain the failure in the hands of other operators, many of whom, no doubt, like myself, tried to make a large opening.

A well-grown and robust farmer's daughter, twenty-four years old, was brought to me by Dr. Forester, with conical cornea in both eyes. In the left the disease was less advanced, and she could yet read and use her needle. The cone in the right was so prominent that the apex was slightly opaque, and all useful vision extinct. She could not count my fingers. I made a linear pupil directly downwards by "iriddesis." A fortnight later I operated above in the same manner, with perfect success. I tested the vision directly that the irritability of the eye had passed away, and had the pleasure of finding that some sight had been restored; but the greatest effect was when a deep concave glass was used: she could now read the large words in title pages. Heretofore this appliance was useless. She determined to return to town and have the other eye operated on in like manner, should it get more defective. This sketch of the pupil was taken at her last visit.

FIG. 109.

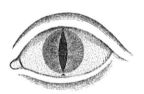

Various appliances of art, optical and mechanical, have been tested, and sometimes beneficially.

Dilatation of the pupil I have known to confer benefit, but the advantage was lost when the cornea grew more prominent.

I was not a little pleased when, some years ago, I read this paragraph on conical cornea in the late Dr. Hull's work on the " Morbid Eye." " In as bad a case as ever I saw I have known most benefit received through an instrument made by a Mr. Abraham, an optician, in Bartlett Street, Bath. It is formed of two lenses, with an adjustment. The farthest and largest lens is convex. The lens near the eye is smaller and doubly concave." I immediately wrote to Mr. Abraham, but he had long been dead; his son, who has left Bath and carries on the same trade in Clifton, never heard of his father's ingenuity. Very deep concave glasses will sometimes, especially in the incipient stage, afford relief: this I have witnessed several times. I met with a gentleman who discovered, that by having his spectacle-frame so bent at the bridge that the glasses were at a certain angle to the eyes, he could see better.

The fact of a person so afflicted generally seeing better and further through a pin-hole, from the reduction of the rays of light entering the eye, while the narrow aperture directs those that do enter through the centre of the cornea, suggested the use of those diaphragms with small round apertures or with slits of different forms and sizes, with which every optician of any repute is now acquainted. The diaphragm is affixed to a spectacle-frame, and an aperture is made in correspondence with that which has been found to suit best. Some opticians keep a kind of tryer in which the apertures may be graduated.

I believe that the adaptation of a concave glass behind one of these diaphragms, is rather of modern date, and I understand that several cases of conical cornea, no doubt incipient ones, have been benefited by the contrivance; although many of my own patients with very large cones, who have tried every variety of aperture, behind which was placed each number of both concave and convex glasses, have obtained no relief. The experiment is simple, and should always be adopted and conducted with great care and patience.

I have said nothing respecting the use of local applications, simply because nothing has been of use. There has been no lack of experiments with every description of local astringent and stimulant. General treatment, too, has been unavailing.

Dr. Pickford's plan of emetics and purgatives ought not, perhaps, to be passed over; though I do not introduce it because

I can speak as to its results, for with them personally I am unacquainted; I mention it from the originality of his pathological theory, and on account of the success he declares he has met with. I have heard of patients who have commenced, but could not possibly continue it; few persons, I am sure, would put sufficient faith in the remedy to submit to be vomited and purged daily for months in succession; most would discontinue the process before many weeks had passed over.

The following extract, which embodies his opinions and all his theory, is taken from his pamphlet on the subject:—

"In conclusion, I may repeat that I believe conical cornea to depend upon some disturbance in the function of the great sympathetic, spinal nerves, and par vagum; producing, through the medium of the lenticular ganglion and fifth pair of nerves, faulty action of the nutrient capillaries and absorbent vessels of the cornea itself: that emetics and purgatives, by the powerful influence they induce upon the gastric, associate, and consensual nerves, restore the healthy function of the weakened nutrient and absorbent vessels, the result of which is a slow but progressive retraction of the diseased corneal growth, and a consequent restoration of vision."

The treatment in one case was twenty-five grains of the sulphate of zinc early in the morning twice a week; afterwards repeated every morning. It is said that in six months the case was much relieved. In subsequent instances purgatives were united. In one, the treatment was used daily for a year, and succeeded; however, the conical cornea returned, and a second cure was effected by the same means!!!

CHAPTER XVI.

STRABISMUS, OR SQUINT.

SCISSORS.

THE obtuseness of the
points of these scissors
effectually prevents in-
jury to the eyeball, while
it interferes in no degree
with their powers of cut-
ting.

Large bows facilitate
the use of the instrument
by allowing it to be held
easily, and in a line with
the fingers; and short
handles ensure greater
steadiness in directing it.

All kinds of curved
scissors are unnecessary,
as being unsuited to the
operation.

BLUNT HOOK.

The curvature ought
not to be greater than
will allow of ready pas-
sage of the instrument
under the muscle, while

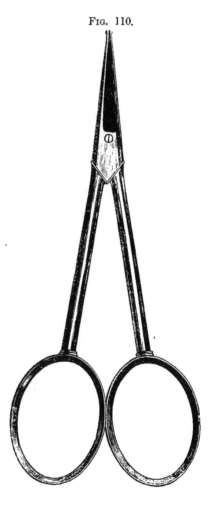

FIG. 110.

FIG. 111.   it should be sufficient to be used as a hook. The point should be round and smooth.

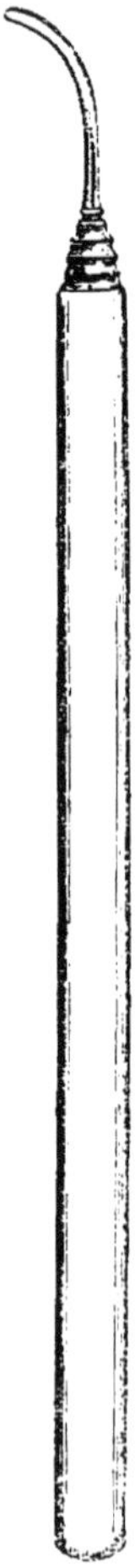

It is more than a hundred years ago, that our countryman, Taylor, operated for squint; for, according to the "Bibliothèque du Médecin Practicien" for 1849, there is in the " Mercury of France" for June, 1737, the following announcement :—" Dr. Taylor, oculist to the King of Great Britain, has just arrived at Paris, at the London Hotel, rue Dauphine, where he proposes remaining till the beginning of July, after which he will leave for Spain. He requests us to publish the discoveries he has made, of straightening squinting eyes by a slight and almost painless operation, and without fear of accident."

It was suspected that he operated only on the inferior oblique muscle ; but being a charlatan, he kept his secret, miracle as it was called, to himself, and it is most probable that the lateral recti were divided. Heuermann, who wrote at Leipsic, in 1756, on the newest surgical operations, criticises Taylor's practice, declaring that it was attended with only temporary benefit, and that patients would scarcely submit to it, on account of the pain and uncertain results. In 1738, Taylor published a pamphlet, entitled " De Verâ Causâ Strabismi." ;

In the first supplement of the "Annales d'Oculistique," p. 258, the following sentence, relative to the treatment of squint in England by an operation, occurs in the " Dissertation" of Verkeyden, 1767 :—" Strabones, permultos ferro sanatos apud Anglicos vidi."

It is well known that Mr. Anthony White, of the Westminster Hospital, suggested, thirty years ago, the division of the recti muscles. Stromeyer, in the year 1838, appears to have been the next to propose it ; and Pauli, of Landau, operated on a girl, but failed. The first successful case was by Dieffenbach, on the 26th of October, 1839. Many aspirants for the honour of the practice have appeared; but it is universally conceded that we are indebted for its introduction to Dieffenbach.

The new operation was quickly adopted and zealously advocated in London, and has long since been recognised as belonging to legitimate surgery. It is singularly successful, equalling in its permanent effect that of any other operation, and surpassing most of those which are practised for the removal of deformity; yet many professional men still speak of it very disparagingly, and would even deny its utility. When I consider the discredit into which it fell after its introduction, from indiscriminate application and ineffectual execution, and reflect. for a moment on the many cases of failure from faulty operating that are to be seen, I am not surprised that it holds no very favourable place in professional or popular regard.

The literature of the subject is enormous; and most dissimilar principles and results fill the pages of authors.

INTERNAL, OR CONVERGENT SQUINT.

From early infancy the eyes may lose their parallelism, and turn inwards. Squint may even exist at birth. But the age at which the deformity generally appears is between the fifth and ninth years; thus agreeing with the period of the diseases of early life, to which it would seem to be frequently due, although the immediate association can seldom be satisfactorily traced.

Derangement in the visual apparatus; opacity of the cornea, of the lens, and affections of the encephalon, comprise the circumstances that induce it; but really, in the majority of cases, it cannot be accounted for. It frequently occurs in the healthiest of children.

It would seem that the balance of antagonistic power in the orbital muscles is remarkably nice, and peculiarly susceptible of disturbance from causes within and without. It may be, too, that the individual muscles are more likely to be influenced, in consequence of the different sources of nervous power. Some persons squint a little, it may be inwards or outwards, if very much fatigued, or where vital force is reduced from any cause. A common example is in the drunken.

Of the treatment of squint by general means I have little to say, because the result is so miserably barren. Squint is the most persistent of all deformities produced by muscular action. There are many instances of its contemporaneous appearance with deformities in other parts of the body, all of which have passed away while it remained.

I question whether a squint, attended with any degree of impaired vision, and not produced by paralysis, is ever removed except by practical surgery; I have never met with an authentic case. I shall show, as I proceed, that paralytic squint in the adult may right itself; at least four examples have come under my notice. Even without any defect in sight, after the persistence of the distortion of a few months, recovery must be an exceedingly rare event—a unit in thousands— so rare as practically to be out of all therapeutical calculations.

Cases are published of persons who, having squinted from resting the head in a certain attitude, recovered when the position was changed; but these are not veritable instances of diseased action of the muscles of either eye, but simply that of an acquired habit of looking sideways in the one or other direction, and which endures only while the necessity for such remains.

The attempts at cure by goggles, side glasses, side reading, by binding up one eye, by patches of black sticking-plaster on the outer edge of the orbit, and by prismatic spectacles, which are even theoretically wrong, are unavailing and worse than useless if they cause delay of the proper, only certainly effectual, and perfectly safe remedy,—an operation.

With this full and candid expression of my opinion, as the result of my own observation, I wish to state that I do not deprecate general treatment, nor deny its influence in the early stage of squint, when the disorders directly inducing it are present and palpable, and to which the measure must be directed; yet I say that much issue must not be expected, and that such treatment should have its bounds.

VARIETIES OF INTERNAL SQUINT.

There are several well-marked conditions of the deformity that admit of classification, with reference to the treatment by operation; and perhaps the most practical division, that which I shall use, has been adopted by Mr. Holthouse,—"Holthouse on Squinting," wherein five varieties are recognised. It affords an easy analysis. But it must be borne in mind after all, it is but an artificial division, and, like all arbitrary tabling of disease, is necessarily imperfect, as only the more marked examples, among which even there are exceptions, can be classified; and that the gradations must be left out.

The first is the fixed squint of one eye. There are degrees of this fixedness,—that is, more or less power of straightening the eye under strong volition; but there may be total absence of lateral movements. The inversion may be excessive, the greater part of the cornea being hidden.

Except in rare instances, where an orbital tumour interferes, or the squint is manifestly due to direct mechanical injury or lesion, paralysis of the external rectus, in some degree, is probably the cause. Paralytic seizures, and marked cerebral derangements, are sometimes associated. The disease may be said to be more frequent after youth.

It is the only form of decidedly confirmed internal squint in which I have seen spontaneous recovery. A well-known member of our profession overtaxed his brain at sixty-five years of age; and with other evidence of muscular paralysis, internal squint appeared in one eye, and the vision became very presbyopic. I saw him after he had been dosed with mercury and rendered more feeble. In a year the squint no longer existed. havin~

passed away gradually as the health improved. Vision remained
affected. The other paralytic symptoms were lost.

I have been told of a parallel case in a middle-aged man.
Perfect recovery ensued, and there was almost restoration of the
sight, which had been very imperfect.

It has been ascertained from actual observation, that for
months or even years, the internal rectus may be but passively
contracted; that ultimately hypertrophy ensues, and to this
may be added shortening and degeneration; and, according to
Messrs. Elliott and Lucas, complete atrophy. I have long
been well aware of the hypertrophied state, from observation in
operating. The eye has been so tightly bound that, although
the patients have been chloroformed, I have been scarcely able
to move it; and, as might be expected, I encountered almost
insurmountable difficulty in securing and dividing the swollen
muscle.

True paralytic squint is most unfavourable for surgical treatment. But it is not altogether irremediable. There will be
degrees of improvement when the internal rectus is divided,
in proportion to the power that yet exists in the external.
An operation is not positively contra-indicated merely from
the great degree of adduction, because it is impossible to tell
how much of it is due to deficiency in the external rectus, or
acquired over-power in the internal. It is therefore a practical
test not to be disregarded, except on strong grounds. A
successful result has occurred to me when least expected.

In the second, there is also single deformity; the one eye is
ordinarily inverted, but there is ability to bring it parallel with
its fellow, and often to evert it.

This is, perhaps, the rarest form of all. Like the first, there
can be no doubt as to the affected eye. It is impossible with
the least care in examination to make a mistake. Under strong
volition the parallelism is maintained for a few seconds, or
longer, and then the inversion gradually returns.

Sometimes the squint exists only when a near focus is
required, and not when distant bodies are looked at. The

distortion may be only occasional; hence this is often called periodic squint. It has occurred to me to be disappointed so often after an operation, that I suspected the influence of some peculiarity which I have not been able to detect.

In the third, the squint always affects the same eye, and does not appear to shift to the other. But when the eye is straightened, the fellow turns in.

When the squint is but slight, or when the abducting power is but little impaired, it may be no easy matter to say which really is the defective eye. As a rule, the state of the vision will materially assist in the diagnosis, for nearly always, more or less, defective sight is present. But there are exceptions; besides, there may be such very slight difference in the visual power, that a mistake might occur unless the test which I have employed and relied on for many years be used.

In the "Medical Times and Gazette" for October, 1856, I published the particulars of a case on which I had operated, with remarks showing that the squinting eye may be the better seeing of the two. Since then, and as my attention has been directed to the point, I have met with many examples, several of which I have pointed out to my colleagues and to my pupils.

I place the patient in front of me, at the distance of four or five yards, or further; tell him to cover one eye, say the left, to look at me with the other, and to keep his head straight. The right eye will then be in the centre of the orbit. I direct him to uncover the left. Now, if the right, which has been open, be normal, it will keep its central position, while the left is turned inwards; but if it be deformed it will turn in, while the left will become straight. The experiment should be reversed. In the case of a child, I place an adult behind, and make him cover and uncover the eyes as required.

When there is any doubt, the patient's attention should be directed from a fixed gaze, and volition interrupted, by causing him to wink a few times. He should also be made to close the eyes for a few seconds, then to open them, and quickly to look at an object. Cases are met with in which the greatest nicety is required to detect the faulty eye. Some are even scarcely embraced in the test.

I venture this explanation of the matter. The eye which may be called sound, in which there is no individual loss of antagonistic force among its muscles, is actually affected, as I believe, through the influence of the associated movements of the lateral recti, and partakes of the greater amount of volition which is required for the play of the muscles of the deformed eye. For instance, the right eye squints: to look to the right with that eye, much greater volition is needed, and more muscular power called into action, than if it were straight; and that extra-exercise of power is, by the associated movement of the eye, transferred or directed to the associate muscles of the other eye, the left, and especially to its internal rectus, overmatching the antagonising muscles, and turning it unduly inwards. This must hold good whether the squint arises from a defect of power in the external rectus, or an excess of it in the internal muscle. To avoid intricacy and minute detail, the lateral recti alone are here taken into consideration, although the other orbital muscles are more or less involved.

It might with sufficient plausibility be assumed that the exaggerated associated action of the internal rectus of the sound eye, or that functionally affected only, will in time pass into a new and independent sphere of contraction, whereby it is rendered an undue antagonist for the external muscle, causing in fact a confirmed squint. Indeed, I am sure this often happens; and that one squint thus produces another. But I am also aware that exceptions are met with,—that one eye may squint for very many years without the other eye becoming affected. I have operated on patients who have squinted in one eye for years, in whom were those conditions favourable for the implication of the other eye; namely, good abducting power and good sight, enabling the squinting organ to be used freely, and consequently the internal rectus of the other eye to be unduly acted upon, and yet the second eye has escaped deformity.

In this variety, then, although at the commencement one only is affected, ultimately both may be implicated. I often point to the circumstance as one of the strong reasons for an early operation, when only one eye need be treated; for when the two squint, the double operation is necessary.

Next to the ineffectual division of the contracted muscle, nothing has so tended to bring the surgical treatment of squint into contempt, as not operating on the second eye when it needed it; and not to do so is certain failure on the part of the surgeon. Certainly the operator is often deterred from finishing his work, because he thinks the deformity is slight, that it may get better of itself—a great delusion; or because he has not courage to demand that it shall be done against the objections of the patient, or his ignorant friends. Except parallelism be restored in the first instance, the second eye should always be operated on.

Now, it is not always possible to say till the one eye is done, whether the second squints. I assure my reader that after many years of practical acquaintance with the subject, and many hundred operations, I cannot be certain. When it has seemed that two operations would be necessary, one has sufficed; but still more commonly, when it appeared that one only was needed, two have been imperative. It is, therefore, well not to commit oneself in any unnecessary communication or discussion on the subject. I undertake to set the eyes straight, but this only, if full sanction be given me to act as may seem necessary.

I do not think, therefore, that the two eyes should ever be done as a matter of course. Putting aside the argument against an unnecessary operation, I am sure that eversion is often caused by operating on the second eye, when there is no permanent contraction of its internal rectus; and more certainly when with this immunity there is any very marked defect in the vision of the squinting eye. Such caution necessarily requires, when chloroform is given, that the patient

should sufficiently recover to be able to use the eyes, so
that they may be examined. All the necessary information
may be got even before consciousness is completely restored.
A single glance of the eyes, as they roll from side to side,
is enough for one accustomed to the examination. No
certain information can be obtained so long as the patient is
in the anæsthetic sleep: I have been often deceived. My
conclusion then is, that one operation may suffice where both
eyes have appeared to be implicated, and that the double
operation is not always requisite; that therefore there should
be a selection, and the more implicated eye first attended to,
and the effect ascertained, before the other is touched.

Here must be noticed a matter of much importance, of which
the explanation is obscure. I examine a case, and suspect only
single squint. I operate; the power of abduction is improved,
or even quite restored, when the eye is used singly, but with
the other open there is yet squint; it may be as bad as before,
and the deformity seems still confined to that eye alone. I
operate on the other, and parallelism is restored.

Hence, if after being satisfied that the muscle of the one eye
has been thoroughly divided I ascertain that the abducting power
is good; whether this has been so originally or restored by the
operation matters not; I invariably operate on the other. This
rule should apply with equal force to internal and external
squint, and to every variety of both.

The fourth kind is that in which the squint seems to pass
from the one eye to the other, alternating readily, so that either
might for the time be regarded as the squinting one. This is
undoubtedly the most common of all, and it is nearly always
double squint, and so requires the double operation.

It is very seldom, as proved by a careful examination, that
each eye is equally affected, although to a casual observer there
is no difference. When my test is applied, it is often discovered
that the one differs in its movements from the other, being more
adducted, and having a greater tendency to remain distorted.
Moreover, that the power of abduction varies.

Generally, there is very little, or even no disparity in vision. The exceptions are rare.

Although I am convinced that this form is often only an advanced stage of the last, I am equally sure that it is more frequently an original condition.

When there is no disparity in vision, nor in the muscular movements of the eye, the two may be operated on at the same time. When there is any marked difference in the latter, I do the worst first, as in the last variety, and look for the effect.

In the fifth and last, both eyes are always more or less inverted, although the one is generally the more turned in; but not always the same eye: so that there is even here a tendency, although a very limited one, to alternation. It is seldom either can be fully everted, and any degree of eversion is attended by remarkable inversion of the other. This is, for the most part, the squint of the adult and the aged. It is merely a more advanced stage of the ordinary double squint of early life, treated of in the last division; and sometimes two, of the third variety. Next to the paralytic squint it is least amenable to treatment.

The deviations from the horizontal position, in an upward or downward direction, occasionally existing in internal squint, require no more notice, besides mentioning the fact, and adding that they cannot be considered a complication since they do not, according to my frequent and special observation, at all sensibly affect the result of an operation.

EXTERNAL, OR DIVERGENT SQUINT.

This form of the distortion is very much less frequent than the other.

It seldom appears before puberty, except in connexion with a diseased brain, and commonly occurs in advanced age. It may be induced by loss of vision from any cause. It is a fact difficult to be explained, that the circumstance which at one time determines an internal squint, shall at another be followed by the outward deviation of the eyeball. An eye is rendered useless, the vision being destroyed by a blow, or by disease, and it may become misdirected on either side. I cannot call to mind any instance of the production of internal squint in the aged from cataract, although a slight outward deflection is not very uncommon.

The varieties are few and easily recognised. They may be arranged as follows :—

First, disease of the motor oculi, or third cerebral nerve, whereby the muscles that turn the eye inwards are paralysed and eversion follows.

The internal rectus alone may be paralysed, and there may be degrees of this impaired power.

There is generally disparity of vision, and so far impairment, when the eyes are used together, due to loss of the adjusting power, through the influence of the ciliary muscle and the recti. An irregular or much dilated pupil has, too, its effect on the sight. But there may be confusion, arising solely from the mal-position, or loss of parallelism of the eyes ; in which case, the single vision of the disturbed eye is not impaired. Ptosis is the usual accompaniment.

But the early stage of the affection in its full development does not strictly belong to my subject. For as recovery from the paralysis is so frequent and so perfect, it would of course be highly imprudent to think of an operation, till its perma-nency has been proved by well-instituted and long-sustained treatment. I have seen complete restoration of all the ocular movements after the most marked abduction, although the total loss of vision, which occurred from the commencement, yet continued. Then there are degrees of recovery. The ptosis also may disappear entirely or in part.

Here, as in internal paralytic squint, the prognosis is neces-sarily unencouraging ; but most certainly operating is not contra-indicated. It would be useless to meddle with a fixed eye, or when there is but very slight restoration of the movements ; but even with tolerable recovery, especially if there be ability to bring the eye centrally, considerable improvement or actual restoration may ensue. The result, therefore, depends on whether the squint have become confirmed in consequence of the tonic contraction of the external rectus already alluded to, as the consequence of the loss of power in an antagonist; or in persistence of the paralysis. When all the recti muscles supplied by the third nerve have been paralysed, the recovery of the upper and the lower, so far as can be ascertained, would be strong presumptive evidence of the persistence of squint being owing to change in the external muscle; but there can be no certainty, as it is well known that the internal rectus alone may remain paralytic. I am not in the possession of any practical test whereby to determine the question, but that of operating; and the majority of persons will submit to it when the circumstances are intelligibly stated to them, and the absence of all risk explained. At least this is the result of my own experience.

A few weeks ago I saw a lady, aged thirty, who had severe cerebral disturbance, four years ago, which produced ptosis and external squint. The squint was now much improved, and so far as it was possible for the action of the upper and lower recti to be scrutinised, they seemed healthy. The ptosis was half removed. The vision was not perfect, but there was no confusion. I was requested to do my best in attempting to straighten the eye, and to enable it to be opened. I pointed out that the squint would be still more apparent, if the ptosis alone were removed, and effecting the latter should therefore be made contingent on that of the former. I divided the external rectus, but no benefit ensued.

I suspect that single squint bears a far less proportion to the double in the divergent kind than in the convergent. I think that the deviation of the second eye from the proper position is, as in the latter, at first merely functional, only it is a more common occurrence. Subsequently a material change takes place in the abductor muscle.

The second form is very similar to the second of internal squint, but more common in its kind. The eye can be brought to the centre of the orbit by strong will, and it often becomes parallel when only near objects are looked at. Sometimes it can be inverted.

When I began to operate on external squint, I was so distressed with the result, from not sufficiently discriminating my cases, that I almost ceased to treat it. It was, however, first by success in this single variety that I got assurance, for in it, is to be obtained the best results. For years I have taught that if the eye could be brought to the centre of the orbit, and maintained there for a few seconds, the operation may be undertaken with the fullest assurance of success. I scarcely meet with an exception. It has been suggested in explanation that there is no structural change in the abductor muscle, but that the eye simply takes the direction of the axis of the orbit, since volition is no longer directed to it, because of impaired vision. I question the correctness of this, because in some cases I have found the sight to be perfect, and in a few it was the better seeing eye.

The third, the commonest variety, is the double squint,—that, it would seem, into which all the single squints have a tendency to pass. According to my observation, except produced by paralysis, it rarely exists from the beginning; in this it differs from internal squint, in which the double affection from the first is common. In the very marked cases the mutual convergence is very striking, and the diagnosis therefore unmistakeable. In the lesser degree there is rather a deceptive appearance, the deformity seeming to alternate. But implication of the two eyes can generally be made out, although there is nearly always a difference in the degree of the eversion; and not so much by individual examination as together. Taken separately, either may be brought to the centre of the orbit, and even more or less inverted. But they cannot be made to converge, nor even to become parallel.

The influence of the associated movements of the recti muscles is, no doubt, exerted also in this kind of squint, and causes the better eye to be turned unduly outwards, when an attempt is made to bring the more squinting one to the centre of the orbit.

The double operation is absolutely necessary in all degrees of the double deformity whenever it is prudent to operate; and in unequivocal abduction of both eyes, the operations may be done at once, and before the patient has recovered from the effect of the chloroform. If doubt exist, there should be a careful inspection before the second is undertaken.

While writing this chapter, a girl, fifteen years old, was brought to me with an external squint of four years' duration. To all appearance the left eye alone was affected; but as with it she saw the better, and used it for minute vision, holding her book or her work to the left side of her face; I suspected the existence of some peculiarity. The adducting power was good, and the features of the case therefore promising. I operated on this eye, and as chloroform was not used, it was quickly apparent that, although there was considerable improvement, the eyes were not quite parallel. I now, for the first time, detected very slight divergence in the other eye. I operated on it and obtained a perfect result.

Respecting the pure pathology of squint, not very much has been made out. No one seems to have looked more fully into the subject than Mr. Holthouse, who says, "It is one of those difficult subjects that few have cared or dared to discuss." He ends an analysis of 378 cases, 83, or about 22 per cent. of which were of uncertain origin, with conclusions from which, as well as from the context, I take the following.

That the most frequent exciting cause of squint is lesion of the nervous centres or nerves, producing spasm of the distorting muscle, and subsequently structural shortening, without appreciable alteration in the muscular tissue.

Next in frequency are inflammatory affections of the eyeball, during which the eye is turned in to get relief, as in ulceration of the cornea, or in fact any state in which the acquired position gives ease; and when so placed exudation probably takes place, if the inflammation persist, and glues together conjunctiva, sclerotica, and muscle, the latter ultimately getting

shorter; this change being in consonance with what is observed
in other parts of the body, as noticed by Mr. Adams.

That the essential or immediate cause of confirmed non-
paralytic squint is shortening of the muscle, with or without
hypertrophy, or simple hypertrophy.

That muscular alterations may be associated with thickening
and contraction of the conjunctiva, and the areolar tissue
beneath, and adhesion of these to the sclerotic coat of the eye.

OPERATION FOR SQUINT.

There are certain local conditions positively contra-indicating
an operation, and these are among the chief :—Inflammation
of the eyeball, or its appendages; opacity of the cornea, producing obliquity, thereby enabling the person to see, the other
eye being lost; tumours; cicatrices from wounds; contractions
after abscess; or indeed any accidental mechanical means that
pushes, or draws the eye from its axis.

When I am satisfied that a squint has settled into a permanent deformity, there not being apparent any symptoms
of the disease to which it seemed due, or at least accompanied
it; when general treatment has proved · unavailing; when,
on first seeing my patient, I learn that the squint has existed
for years, or even many months; or when it is congenital,
I advise an immediate operation.

There are many disadvantages in delay. Vision gets worse
when its impairment is due to the squint; the contracted
muscle undergoes pathological changes, and we have evidence,
too, of its antagonist becoming abnormal; the other recti, in
all probability, acquire a different sphere of action; during
the years of growth the distorted position favours the irregular
development of all the displaced parts, so that success must
be imperfect in proportion to the postponement. These are
of course, the reasons why the treatment in manhood is so very
seldom beneficial.

A late surgeon did much harm by strongly advising that
a squint, occurring in infancy, or in childhood, should not be
submitted to the operation till after the period of puberty.

In consequence of his extensive ophthalmic practice, this opinion was disseminated in public, as well as among the profession. I know that he did not regard the proceeding at any age with much favour, and that he never operated extensively. It would be as reasonable to delay the treatment of congenital club-foot till the sufferer was fourteen or fifteen years old, or of any deformity or defect of infancy, till the same period of life. Much, therefore, is to be gained by the early treatment; and double squint may frequently be prevented by timely removal of the single affection. I cannot mention a single fact in favour of the delay, while half-a-dozen may be given against it. I have operated as early as the seventh month on a double congenital squint, with success.

The several operations for squint with which I have any personal acquaintance, or have seen performed, may be classed into those executed with the knife, and those with the hook and scissors.

According to my knowledge, the first is objectionable on account of the extent of the wound inflicted, as in that practised by the late Messrs. Guthrie; or the uncertainty of dividing the muscle, as in the sub-conjunctival plan of Guérin; or the great danger to the eyeball when the knife is the only instrument used, and therefore made so sharp as to enable it to penetrate the conjunctiva, to say nothing of the general inapplicability of the proceeding.

The second comprises the hook and scissors method; and includes Guérin's, executed with these instruments after the manner of Mr. Critchett; and the better known and old plan of cutting through the conjunctiva, over where the muscle is divided.

I advocate and practise the latter, with modifications of my own, adopting the application of sutures, as first devised by M. Cunier; because I find it the most sure, the easiest in execution, the least detrimental, the most generally applicable, and, as I fully believe, that which gives the best result, and leaves the least trace of performance.

OPERATION FOR INTERNAL SQUINT.

There is less disturbance to the surrounding parts by dividing the muscle close to its attachment, and therefore internal to the ocular tunic. I ask my reader to refer to the description of the sheath. This, too, secures the new attachment of the muscle to the eyeball not far from the natural one. A probe passed vertically under the internal rectus muscle of an adult, and pressed against its attachment to the sclerotica, will reach to within nearly three-eighths of an inch of the cornea. Just a little external to this, then, I would make the preliminary incision, were I about to operate on a full-grown person ; therefore, to be accurate, the distance should be regulated according to the period of life of the individual, but in reality it matters not whether it be a trifle the one way or the other ; and I merely endeavour to leave enough of the conjunctiva on the corneal side to hold the sutures. The eyelids are best retracted with the spring wire retractor. Should the eye not be sufficiently straight for commencing, I draw it to the required position with a pair of forceps applied to the outside. Taking up a fold of the conjunctiva horizontally, I cut it through vertically opposite the lower edge of the muscle, which generally corresponds to the inferior edge of the pupil, to about a couple of lines, and then incise the sub-conjunctival tissue to an equal extent. The latter is sometimes divided along with the conjunctiva, but it may be thick and very dense, and need special attention ; and it can never be certain that the division is effected except the sclerotica be exposed. I now introduce the hook, secure the muscle, make it prominent, and, if the upper part be covered by the conjunctiva, as in all probability it will be, I push this off with the forceps, while I make the hook-point more prominent, and, keeping the muscle very tense, divide its tendinous expansion between the hook and the eyeball with the blunt-pointed scissors. I would rather advise a beginner to incise the conjunctiva more freely, as he will thereby take up the muscle the more readily, and there can be no particular objection against the extended incision. I often do it when I expect any little difficulty. At any rate, scarcely more need be cut through than actually covers the muscle. The hook should always be passed a second time, to ascertain whether the operation has been completed. Besides muscular tissue, portions of condensed areolar might escape division in the first instance.

It is a very common error to attempt to secure the muscle before cutting through the sub-conjunctival tissue. When the tissue is thin and natural, the hook may readily be pushed through it; not so when thickened, as is often the case in squint of some standing, or where there has been inflammation of the conjunctiva; indeed when so changed, I have seen it mistaken for muscle, and treated as such. Sponging is seldom required. I conclude by applying one or two sutures, using such a needle as that depicted in the chapter on instruments, but one carefully adapted generally suffices. This is very readily done by raising the corneal portion of the membrane with the forceps, transfixing it close to the margin, and dealing with the other edge in the same manner. I am particular about the exact position of the suture, lest there be any tension of the conjunctiva, and because when so placed, the thread is thrown off in three or four days, which is better than having to remove it. Not the least irritation ensues, and the patient is rarely ever aware that he has a stitch in his eye.

In the sub-conjunctival operation, the conjunctiva is divided horizontally at the lower part of the eyeball, and the hook and scissors are employed beneath the membrane. A larger aperture is required than I find necessary for the above. I have seen it done very readily in prominent eyes. My objections to it are, in the first place, as regards the uncertainty of thoroughly dividing the muscle where the eye is sunken; when there is fixed inversion of the eyeball; when the muscle is shortened; in the small eyes of children and infants; when the conjunctiva is thickened and thrown into folds, and especially when the sub-tissue is likewise altered. Then, as regards the peculiar consequences, the parts are very much disturbed, the conjunctiva freely separated, and blood is extravasated. It is a common practice to make a counter puncture to attempt to let the blood out; but, in fact, little can be got away in this manner because of the coagulation. I have seen very extensive chemosis and ecchymosis thus produced even in the hands of the best operators. I have read of the effusion being so considerable that the eyelids closed with difficulty. The uncertainty of dividing any condensed tissue about the muscle that should be severed, or of any posterior adhesions, must be self-evident, and need not be dwelt on.

The following quotation from the writings of Mr. Critchett, advocating the operation, will show that I have not made over-statements. In his " Practical Remarks on Strabismus, with some Novel Suggestions respecting the Operation," he says, " But it may be asked, if there are any objections to this operation, and any cases in which the old operation is preferable. It must be admitted that it is rather more difficult to perform, that there is a greater liability to leave some portion undivided, and sometimes some inversion remains, in consequence of the attachment of the muscle to the fascia after it is divided from the sclerotic. This will often rectify itself afterwards, and where this is not the case, it is better either to operate on the other eye, or, if the cast is slight, be content to leave the ease in that state, rather than risk eversion by further interference. It is only in cases of long standing, and where the strabismus is very extreme, and where the eye is small and deep set, and where the sub-conjunctival operation produces but very little effect, that the old operation is justifiable."

Guérin devised his principle to obviate the vacancy produced at the inner corner of the eye, by the interference with the caruncle and plica semilunaris, inseparable from the dissections that were practised in the early operations, when it was thought necessary to cut through the body of the muscle far back. That it was an improvement in this respect there can be no doubt; but that neither it, nor any other method, always completely obviates this, I shall show as I proceed; and I am convinced that it is very much less effectual than the course I pursue.

The use of the suture must set at rest all the objections about dividing the conjunctiva in a line with the caruncle, as rapid primary adhesion is thereby produced. It is the rare, the very rare exception, not to have this. I cannot therefore conceive a more efficient and perfect manner of operating. The little ecchymosis, the slight redness, and the rapid removal of all trace of the operation, point to this. There is no fungus growth from the edges of the wound, a likely occurrence whenever the conjunctiva does not heal at once, and no irritation, which is common with the process of granulation. A comparative trial was made on a patient, between a gentleman who practises exclusively the sub-conjunctival plan with the scissors and hook, and myself. On my side, the thread was cast off on the fourth day, the conjunctiva being quite healed; and on the eighth there was scarcely any trace of surgical interference. On his, at the end of two weeks, there was so much conjunctival inflammation that treatment for it was considered necessary, and the conjunctival wound was yet open.

No particular course of after-treatment is ordinarily required. Nothing more is demanded than the general attention necessary for a wound of the ocular appendages. I prefer that the eye be not bandaged up, as I suspect that it is better for the muscles to be used, if only, as in the case of a weak abduction, to prevent the divided tendon from uniting too anteriorly. Prior to the introduction of this valuable operation, any like injury to the eye, either accidentally or surgically inflicted, and followed by an equal amount of action in the process of repair, would have been treated most rigorously; and even yet there are surgeons who cannot watch the natural course in the most circumscribed limits, without applying leeches, and irritating the eye with lotions.

A well-executed operation is, as a rule, immediately followed by success. Any suspension of the restoration of parallelism

is a rare event, but it does happen. The first case of this
deferred success that occurred to me, was in a private patient
thirteen years old, who had squinted from infancy. Both
eyes were adducted, the right, in which the vision was the more
impaired, to a greater degree than the left; either could be
abducted as far as the centre of the orbit. I performed the
double operation at a sitting, assisted by Dr. Alleyne, of
Gloucester Road, Hyde Park. The left was slightly improved,
the right not at all. Diligent search was made in vain for any·
remaining muscular or cellular connexion. The case was considered a failure. On my visit next day, both eyes were
straight. There was inability to turn them simultaneously,
or singly, towards the nose; but they could be moved freely
in other directions. The second happened in the practice
of Mr. Lawrence, whom I assisted at the operation. The
patient, a male adult, squinted in one eye. The operation
produced no improvement. I saw him two months after, and
the squint was gone. Nearly a week elapsed before the eye
was straight.

Of later examples that have occurred to me, I have not
kept any notes.

Failure depends on more or less paralysis of the antagonist
muscle; adhesions; variety in, or abnormal position of the
muscles. Before I consider any of these, I venture to say that
a long and familiar acquaintance with the subject has convinced
me, that to the operator is to be attributed the odium of failure
in most of the unsuccessful cases occurring in early life. Over
and over I have seen patients dismissed under the supposition
that it was impossible to put their eyes right, when I have been
certain that the muscle had not been divided. That there is a
great liability to take up a portion only, any one may convince
himself by operating on the dead subject, when he will find
that, unless there be great precision, this will occur. A partial
separation will frequently lessen the squint; but for its entire
removal not a portion must remain intact, and to this there is
no exception. After the muscle has been divided, the patient
has not the power to adduct the eye in concert with the other.

It is often erroneously supposed, in consequence of an imperfect examination, that the eyes are parallel. The inability, or often the unwillingness of the patient to open the eye, prevents a satisfactory inspection. These obstacles must be overcome by gently raising both eyelids at the same time, and comparing the positions of the eyeballs.

Paralysis of the external rectus muscle, is undoubtedly the commonest cause of impediment to success.

My own experience of the existence of adhesions interfering with the eye assuming a central position, is limited to what I have supposed to be condensation of areolar tissue, around and about the muscle. In order to divide any such adventitious connexions, it has generally been necessary to make the conjunctival incision rather longer than ordinary.

I know nothing of the attachments said to exist between the body of the muscle and the sclerotica; nor can I quite comprehend how they exist, as the "ocular tunic" intervenes. This sheath, I suspect, is often mistaken for adhesions. Mr. Duffin remarks, in his papers on squint in the "London Medical Gazette," that bands of fibro-cellular connexion, passing between the sclerotica and the under surface of the muscle and its sheath, frequently retain the eye in an abnormal position after the tendon has been divided, and render many cases only partially successful; that he has met with them very far back, even beyond the greatest diameter of the globe of the eye; and in two cases they were almost cartilaginous, and so unyielding, that the patients were wholly unable to move the pupil out of the inner canthus.

Another surgeon records finding in two cases a strong fibrous band, closely united to the sclerotica, beyond the vertical axis of the eye; and in a third, numerous short, strong ones, situated likewise as posteriorly, retaining the organ in the inverted position after the muscle and the conjunctiva had been freely divided. I can well understand that the "ocular tunic" might adhere to the eyeball, and the possible occurrence should be remembered when the eye is not righted after the muscle has been severed.

The following quotation from Mr. Wilde's ophthalmic report, in vol. xxvii. of the "Dublin Journal of Medical Science," expresses nearly all that is known of the irregularity in the muscles: "Since the adoption of the operation for strabismus, much attention has been paid to the pathological condition of the muscles in the orbit; but few of the abnormal appearances described by authors appear to have been original and not acquired defects after birth. And those attachments of one to another, or the blending of two muscles with one, as the levator palpebræ with the superior rectus, the trochleator with the internal rectus, and the trochleator itself with the trochlea, &c., appear to be also acquired pathological conditions (Morgagni and Wrisberg); but instances have recently been recorded, by good authorities, of decided false insertion, and also bifurcation of the internal rectus at its sclerotic extremity (Dieffenbach); of the external rectus being double (Zagorsky), and also the superior oblique (Albinus); while Caldani saw, more than once, an additional muscle, which, from its insertion and use, he has denominated m. detractor palpebræ inferioris; and both recti and both obliques have been found wanting, in cases of monstrosities, by Seiler and Colomb."

I may add that Ammon has seen bundles of fibres inserted behind the tendon of the muscle.

It is supposed by some that thickening of the conjunctiva, and the subjacent tissue, may retain the eye inverted. It would seem that for this effect, there must be more or less of contraction of these tissues.

The practical lesson to be gathered from the foregoing considerations is, that an operator should be careful to divide the muscle, to be certain of which he should always ascertain, by the re-application of the hook, that no muscular fibres have escaped; that, after the efficient performance of this part of the operation, should the eye be still adducted, he must seek for adhesions, and separate any that may be found.

OPERATION FOR EXTERNAL SQUINT.

There is no difference in the details between the operations for internal and external squint, beyond that the attachment of the external rectus muscle being a little more posterior than the internal, the conjunctiva should be divided a little further from the cornea. The hook should be passed just below the muscle, and close to its attachment to the sclerotica, or the inferior oblique muscle is liable to be taken up. The operator must be prepared to find the conjunctiva and the subjacent tissue looser and thicker on this side of the eye, and that the tendon of the muscle does not admit of being so indefinitely raised and exposed as in the internal operation, in consequence of being broader : it appears more like fascia than tendon. The operation may, therefore, be said to be the less easy of the two ; and there can be no doubt that it is far more likely to be ineffectually performed. I always apply sutures, for, although less important here, still they are very serviceable.

I understand that some of the warmest advocates for the sub-conjunctival operation, do not apply it to external squint. I have not seen it adopted.

Of course all that has been said above, respecting care in dividing the muscle and seeking for adhesions, must be understood with reference to this ; and so too as regards after treatment.

Several accessory operations have been practised when the division of the one or the other of the recti has not been followed by the removal of the squint.

The internal edge of the upper and that of the lower rectus, has been divided simultaneously and singly. I have no personal knowledge of the proceeding.

In the Ophthalmic Hospital Reports for October, 1858, this is stated : " In a case of congenital extreme internal strabismus, aged fourteen, with congenital cataracts, both internal recti and the neighbouring fasciæ were divided; but the eyes being still turned in, Mr. Poland passed the hook beneath the superior and inferior rectus; encircling that edge of the muscles nearest the internal rectus.   This was done sub-conjunctivally through the same opening by which the internal rectus had been divided.   Both eyes now remain straight."

The following plan, applicable to both kinds of squint, appears, from all I can learn, to have originated with Dieffenbach.   Mr. Wilde, who seems to have applied it first in divergent squint, was not, he says, at the time (1841) aware of Dieffenbach's use of it in the convergent.   I take my description from his "Monograph on Entropium and Trichiasis," extracted from the "Dublin Journal of Medical Science" for March, 1844, to which is appended the description of "a case of severe trichiasis and convergent squint of both eyes successfully treated by operation, and the application of ligatures on the recti muscles."   The patient, a female, was thirty years old.   The right eye was first operated upon, and a primary difficulty was to bring any portion of the sclerotica internal to the cornea into view.   Having satisfied himself that every fibre of the muscle was fairly divided, he examined both eyes together, and found that while the position of the left eye continued unmoved, considerable convergence still remained in that on which he had operated.   Again examining carefully and with the blunt hook, and receiving further assurance that the operation was not at fault, he laid hold of the sclerotic extremity of the muscle with a pair of forceps, and passed a fine curved sewing needle, armed with a single silk ligature, through it in two places.   Having obtained a direct purchase, he drew the eyeball towards the external angle, till the cornea was rather inclined outwards, and secured the ends of the ligature over the malar bone by adhesive plaster.   This was done on the fourth of the month; on the morning of the seventh, the thread had cut its way through the end of the tendon, but the eye retained its new straight position.   Nine days after, the other eye was similarly treated.   On the evening of the second day the ligature was withdrawn, and both eyes were now in a natural position.   There was temporary double vision.   The woman was last seen after an interval of nine months, and her favourable state continued.

Other instances of the adoption of this method in double convergent and in divergent squint, are alluded to by Mr. Wilde, who states that he has employed these means with perfect success in seventeen cases of divergent squint, and thirteen of convergent; and in nine of the latter the ligature had been applied to both eyes. The length of time the ligature is allowed to remain varies according to circumstances; but, as a rule, it should never be removed till the eye has righted itself. Luscitas, or fixture of the eye, in the straight position, has followed, especially in cases of divergence, where he had reason to believe that paralysis and atrophy of the internal rectus had previously existed.

Injunctions are given that in fixing the ligature care should be taken to fasten it securely; for if any play be allowed, it will cut through before the effect is secured. Also when its necessity is suspected, to divide the muscle far back, and not to let the eye be encroached on by the crossing of the ligature, but to carry it without the lower eyelid, notwithstanding the eyeball is turned a little downwards.

The defects of the operation for squint need a careful review. More or less of eversion is the inevitable consequence of bad operating, and this together with the almost invariable accompaniment of considerable prominence, were the chief causes that brought the operation into disrepute. For a time, the great mass of the profession was against it. The same may be said of the educated classes of the community. It did not escape even the burlesque of the pantomimes. All operators were at fault, but in different degrees. They had not yet learned how to operate. A great surgeon from the north, who did more in his short time to improve the practice of surgery than any of his contemporaries, turned out the worst examples that I have seen. His very free dissection, by which he exposed the greater part of the inner side of the eyeball, and his manner of cutting through the body of the muscle, were the causes of it. Besides this, he in common with others, thought it well to thrust back the proximal end of the muscle with a probe.

It is almost incredible the distortion that might be thus produced.

I believe that no one earlier than myself, as my writings will show, endeavoured to remedy this by a more limited operation; although at the time the *rationale* was not apparent, it has since been revealed by actual dissection. We now know that the divided muscle requires an attachment to the sclerotica, either directly, or by cellular connexion, or through the intervention of the conjunctiva, or it adheres to the ocular tunic, or the ends may unite with more or less intervening new material, or lie far apart between the sclerotica and the conjunctiva, or become joined to the conjunctiva alone. Herr Böhn, of Berlin, as mentioned in the " Dublin Journal of Medical Science " for 1847, gives us much of this information. Now, in exact proportion as the influence of the muscle is lost by being dissected away and completely displaced, or by a piece being cut out as I have seen done many times, will there be eversion, with the existence of a healthy abductor. Our aim and object, therefore, should be to provide for the occurrence of re-adhesion with as little displacement as possible. Retraction to some degree is certain, but it will be less when the tendon only is cut through, and if done as I advise and practise, there is secured the minimum of displacement. The reader will remember what stress I have laid on not unnecessarily disturbing the ocular tunic.

It should be understood, however, that some eversion may follow the best-executed operation. It is not possible to interfere with the beautiful and accurate adaptation of the ocular appendages, without generally causing some corresponding and palpable alterations in the contour of the eye, but this may be too slight to be apparent without much scrutiny; sometimes it is wholly absent, and I may say positively and undeniably, that when the double operation is done, and the eyes are made alike, the exceptions are so rare as almost to be beyond consideration, and that I no more expect any very marked or objectionable eversion, than I do the still less probable condition of the excess of it to which I have alluded.

Some degree of eversion may ensue on one side, months after the eyes have been parallel. In all the cases of which I have made many notes, this has seemed to arise from the very impaired state of the vision. As there has been an inability to use the eye, and to bring it under the influence of volition, abduction has followed. I am always, therefore, guarded in giving any prognosis when the sight is very defective.

The treatment of eversion has not been overlooked. The first was that of dividing the antagonist muscle. It was done to a great extent at one time in London. In several of the persons who came under my notice, considerable prominence of the eyeball ensued, although the defect was more or less remedied. In one instance, it was so excessive that the eyelids could not be closed without great effort. This deterred me for a long time from interfering, but I ventured at last to divide the muscle, in the same careful and limited manner that I advocate, in two of my own cases—not, however, of excessive abduction,—that I had operated on some years before. I was certainly well satisfied with the success. This led to the fearless adoption of the measure several times, although I have never applied it where there has been besides a great degree of protrusion. I should not, therefore, hesitate to execute it wherever from failure of attachment of the internal rectus to the desired spot, or any other cause, an objectionable degree of eversion existed.

It may truly be said, that no degree of this eversion is beyond removal or amelioration by a more extended operation, and Dieffenbach was the first to improve the practice. He cut away a certain amount of the conjunctiva and sub-conjunctival tissue from the inner side of the eye, then divided the external rectus, attached thread to the anterior part, and fastened it to the nose with plaster for eight days. The effect is derived from the contraction consequent on the first proceeding, and the attachment of the muscle in a posterior position. I have done it twice with decided benefit, but the detail was altered by applying sutures where I excised.

Still considerably more ingenuity was displayed by M. Guérin, an account of which is published by M. Desmarres, who says,

in the first edition of his work on the eye, that he had practised
it, and could testify to the magnificent result. I append the
case which he gives:—

"A young woman, eighteen years old, was operated on for
double squint; both eyes became prominent and turned outwards. The external rectus was separated three times without
benefit. The particular eye is not specified. After certain
adhesions at the external angle were destroyed, the muscle was
searched for, discovered far back adherent to the sclerotica, and
detached. The position of the internal rectus was in like
manner sought for through dense cicatrices of 'consecutive
vegetations;' and after a dissection, which is described as something desperate, it was found drawn within its sheath, and the
orifice obstructed. The sheath was opened, the muscle was
drawn out, and applied against the sclerotica. Now was fulfilled the important indication of maintaining the eye inwards,
to favour the insertion of the muscle and the fascia, at a point
sufficiently anterior to prevent the former evil. A waxed thread
was passed with a sewing needle through the fascia near to
the cornea, and the eye thus secured was turned inwards about
a centimetre, and so maintained, by attaching both ends of the
thread to the nose by plaster. In the afternoon of the next day
the thread became loose, and, says the author, almost incredible
to relate, the inward movement of the eye was re-established,
but not the outer. The globe still turned in a little. In proportion as the wound at the external angle healed, the outward
movement was restored, and in less than eight days the eye was
in a correct position, and almost acquired its normal motions.
The fate of the other eye is undeclared."

Guérin's plan has been carried out in a more systematic
manner by Mr. Critchett, and published in the pamphlet already
quoted. He had applied it five times with a satisfactory result.
This is his description —:

"Having freely exposed the globe by means of the wire
speculum, the parts covering the inner part of the globe,
including conjunctiva, sub-conjunctival fascia, old cicatrix and
muscle, with condensed tissue around it, must be all carefully

dissected off the sclerotic, commencing about two lines from the inner margin of the cornea, and extending upwards and downwards and then inwards, so as to expose the inner third of the surface of the globe. This dissection must be carefully made, so as to preserve the flap thus made entire : it can most readily be done with a pair of scissors. When this stage of the operation is completed, the external rectus muscle must be divided. It is better to defer this part of the operation until now, because the action of the external rectus is useful in keeping the globe well fixed outwards during the first stage of the operation. The next part of the operation is the most difficult and the most important. It consists in passing the sutures. For this purpose small semicircular needles must be used, armed with a piece of fine silk; the flap that has been raised from the eyeball must be firmly held with a pair of forceps, and drawn forward so as to make it tense; the needle must then be passed through it, as low down—that is, as near the inner corner—as possible. Two or three sutures may be passed in this way, at intervals of about two lines. The corresponding part of each suture must then be passed through that portion of conjunctiva which has been left attached to the sclerotic near the cornea. This constitutes another difficulty, because the membrane is here so thin that the fine silk is apt to cut through; this I found a serious difficulty, in my first operation, and one that materially interfered with success. In order to obviate this, I adopt now the following expedients :— I first separate this portion a little upwards towards the cornea; the needle must then be passed through it, and then back again, so as to include a portion, which must be tied tightly, so as to prevent it from tearing out. The next point is to cut away all that portion of the lower flap that can be spared beyond the part where the suture has entered, merely leaving a sufficient margin to hold it. The silks may be now drawn tightly, and tied to the end that is already fixed near the cornea. The immediate effect of this proceeding ought to be to procure some inversion, if the various steps of the operation have been properly performed. The hope and intention are, to get the parts to unite to the globe in their new position, and thus retain the eye. This, however, is only partially the case; there is always some tendency to relapse, and in two cases I had to repeat the operation, but with ultimate success. The sutures may be allowed to remain until they ulcerate through; the subsequent inflammation is usually slight. The amount of mobility in the eye is very limited, but so long as it occupies a central position this circumstance is not found practically to occasion the deformity, and is an immense improvement upon the facial discord resulting from extreme eversion."

The vacancy or depression at the inner corner of the eye, as the effect of the loss of the semilunar fold of the conjunctiva, and the destruction or displacement of the caruncle, has been already noticed in the description of the operation, and the means of preventing any marked degree of it fully given. As, however, I have stated that it is not possible always altogether to obviate it, I shall explain the inability. This is evidently due to the unavoidable disturbance of the adaptation of the parts beneath, and especially to the alteration in the position of the rectus muscle. The defect is more apparent in some cases than in others, owing perhaps to the natural formation or setting of the eye. I have seen it after every method of operating that I have mentioned. Apart from mere disfigurement, any very decided disarrangement of this nature is a positive evil, if the proper use of the caruncle be to throw the tears into a little pool above, where they may be taken up by the puncta : the lower punctum glides above it in the act of winking.

Protrusion of the eyeball in some degree is common, but oftentimes so slight, that very close inspection is required to discover it. Naturally prominent eyes will display it more than those that are deeper set. In eyes that are popularly called small, it never constitutes a deformity. It is always less noticeable when both eyes have been operated on. Like the above, it is unavoidable in a slight degree, but an exaggerated amount can never occur with judicious operating. It is often combined with eversion. Indeed it cannot be very marked without it. Whether remediable or not by Guérin's operation, I cannot say.

It should be remembered respecting all these incidental blemishes, that as there is often a disparity in the eyes, so will they be the more palpable when the more prominent, apparently the larger, is operated on; and that they will still be visible even when the two have been done.

Another unpleasant result is double vision. For the most part it exists only when the eyes are directed to a body in some particular direction. It is not uncommon a day or two after the operation, whether one eye have been done or both; but generally it quickly disappears. Like the double sight which is an early effect of squint, it soon passes away. In proportion as the parallelism is restored is it absent. It is, therefore, common in eversion, but not a necessary concomitant with it. I know only of a single instance of its permanency among my own patients. I operated on a young man, slight eversion ensued, and very troublesome double vision followed. For years he continued to call on me, ever telling the same distressing tale, and always refusing to allow the external rectus to be divided. Eventually he assented to submit to any treatment that I advised, but never submitted to it.

Relapses are commonly talked of, but I am aware of only three instances in my practice, and all within six months from the operation. Two were in medical students, of the respective ages of twenty-one and twenty-two; one of which was a single squint, the other a double, one eye of which relapsed. In both the second operation was successful. The third was in a male, thirty years of age, and, like the others, was ultimately set right. There can be little doubt that, in many of the supposed cases of the recurrence, the operation has never been completely done. I have verified this when operating on them. M. Malgaine has noticed the occurrence a year after the eye has been straight.

In repeating the operation, far more nicety is needed than in the first instance, as conjunctival cicatrix must be cut through, and the muscle is not so readily found, nor so easily divided.

STATE OF THE VISION IN SQUINT.

This may be practically considered under two heads: impaired vision the cause of the squint, and impaired vision the consequence of it.

I suspect that bad sight is very frequently productive of the deformity, through pathological changes at the fundus of the eye; in the optic disc, the retina, the choroid coat, singly or together, and unaccompanied by any objective symptoms. My opinion is gathered from ophthalmoscopic examinations. So early in childhood are morbid conditions of these parts discovered, that I am tolerably sure of their congenital origin. As such changes are found to exist in the earliest degrees of convergent squint in children, who to all appearance are otherwise healthy, surely they may be associated as cause and effect.

So far, therefore, as I can ascertain, the squint is not the effect of any specific disease of the eyeball, but merely the consequence of impaired sight. It is in this class of cases that the restoration of parallelism is followed by slight improvement to sight, or not any, accordingly as there is much or little ocular structural lesion.

That impaired vision is a consequence of squint is a well-recognised fact, not only from restoration of sight when the deformity is removed by an operation, and which is generally immediate, the exceptions being rare, but because the defect is of one kind and peculiar. It much resembles presbyossia, or far-sightedness, being relieved by convex glasses, but differs from it in the focal range being short. There is often, too, a want of definition for objects in general. It may exist in a marked degree without any appreciable structural change in the eye, but that it is never associated with such I cannot say, for I have not investigated the subject ophthalmoscopically, extensively enough to enable me to give a definite opinion. In search of a cause, one naturally turns to the mechanical influence that the contracted muscle may exercise on the eye, for an explanation can hardly be found in any other direction.

It would therefore seem to be the result of pressure. Mr. Holthouse takes the same view, and in addition attributes the effect to the external rectus as well as the internal, and ascribes, too, the degree of the impairment to the amount of the pressure. He argues, that if the internal rectus be very slightly shortened or hypertrophied, but little force will be necessary on the part of its antagonists to straighten the eye, which will merely be submitted to slight pressure in the antero-posterior direction, and the focus thereby lengthened; but if a greater amount of shortening or hypertrophy exist, a corresponding effort must be made by the external rectus to maintain the eye straight, and the pressure thus exerted is such as not only to alter the focus, but possibly also to diminish the sensibility of the retina.

In the above consideration we have, perhaps, a solution, in some cases at least, of the hitherto unexplained occurrence of but slight improvement of sight occasionally, after the most successful operations with regard to the removal of the obliquity of the eye. There has existed impaired vision, both irrespective of the diseased muscles, and as a consequence of it; the effect of the latter of which only was capable of restoration by the removal of perverted muscular action. It is probable enough that simple duration of the muscular pressure may render the impairment of the retina irremediable: I mean the duration of squint for many years.

It only remains for me to notice the favourable effect of the operation. It surpasses the issue of any other surgical measure which is done for the removal of deformity. All that is desired is accomplished at once. No appliance is needed; no mechanical after-treatment wanted. There is really no risk, if the commonest care be·observed, and therefore absolutely none in the hands of a good operator. The removal of the distortion may be but a small portion of the benefit when impaired sight is ameliorated or restored; and the preservation of this function should be duly considered when the admissibility of the operation is discussed.

CHAPTER XVII.

MALIGNANT AFFECTIONS OF THE EYE.

GENERAL CONSIDERATIONS — DIVISION OF CANCER — MEDULLARY CANCER ;
VARIETIES—ENCEPHALOID CANCER OF THE EYEBALL—QUESTION OF PRIMARY
SEAT—DIAGNOSIS—MELANOSIS—SCIRRHUS—MALIGNANT TUMOURS OF THE
ORBIT : ENCEPHALOID AND MELANOSIS ; SCIRRHOUS ; SCIRRHOUS ENCANTHIS
—RECURRENT FIBROID ; EPITHELIAL—MALIGNANT AFFECTIONS OF EYELIDS :
SCIRRHUS AND EPITHELIAL CANCER—QUESTION AS TO THE PROPRIETY OF
OPERATING.

THE eye itself, or the orbit, may be the seat of nearly all the forms of cancer. The frequency of the occurrence of malignant disease, however, in these situations, is a point upon which very erroneous ideas are prevalent among those who have not devoted particular attention to the subject. These misconceptions I believe to arise in part from the many specimens which are to be found in pathological museums, and in part also from the publication of a large proportion of the cases met with : facts illustrating merely the interest they excite, which would not be so strongly felt were they more common. The only conclusive method of proving what I believe to be the fact, that cancerous disease of the eye is a rare occurrence, would be by accurate and extensive statistics—a desideratum which unfortunately cannot at present be supplied, owing to the imperfect manner in which the pathological records of many of our large hospitals are kept. I draw my conclusions partly from the results of my own experience, and partly from the unanimous answers to inquiries on the subject, with which I have been favoured by several gentlemen who have had extensive opportunities of witnessing ophthalmic disease. These are still further confirmed by all that has hitherto been made out, with regard to the statistics of cancerous disease generally.

It is unnecessary to pursue this part of the subject farther; enough has been said to show that the affection is not one of common occurrence, and much more extensive investigations than have as yet been made would be required before we could, with any certainty, state its relative frequency as compared with other morbid changes to which the eye is liable. I shall therefore proceed at once to consider the varieties of cancer, giving such particulars of the intimate structure and pathological history of each as may seem necessary for the purposes of diagnosis, or as indications for treatment.

DIVISION OF CANCER.

Cancer is divided into four great varieties: medullary, or encephaloid (under which are included melanoid and hæmatoid); scirrhus; colloid; and epithelial. With these may be considered as malignant diseases, though not possessing all the characteristics of well-marked cancer, recurrent fibroid, and myeloid tumours.

These forms do not occur in or around the eye with equal frequency. Colloid cancer has never yet been found in the eye or orbit, and will therefore require no further notice. Scirrhus is exceedingly rare, as an affection either of the eyeball or its appendages. Epithelial cancer attacks only the eyelids or conjunctiva. Recurrent fibroid disease has been met with as intra-orbital tumour in one instance only that has come to my knowledge. Myeloid tumour is here mentioned chiefly because of the occasional implication of the orbit in its extension from other parts. Medullary cancer, in the form of encephaloid, or melanosis, may attack either eye or orbit; and it is the one or the other variety, more particularly the former, which is present in the great majority of cases.

MEDULLARY CANCER.

Before entering upon a description of the special appearances presented by medullary cancer in the eyeball, it will be necessary briefly to review the general character of the disease, and in doing this I shall make free use of the labours of those who have directed special attention to malignant affections. One of the names given to it, encephaloid, is derived from the close resemblance which its section frequently bears to the human brain; but this, though in common use and designating well some of the forms, is likely to give place to the older and more general term, medullary, selected by Mr. Paget as being the more appropriate. It occurs most frequently in infants, and young persons below the age of puberty. No period of life, however, is exempt from its attacks, and it is seen occasionally, though comparatively rarely, in those far advanced in years. It attains a greater size, runs a more rapid course, and appears to indicate a greater degree of malignancy, than any of the other varieties. In some situations in the body, it frequently acquires the bulk of a man's head, or may even be larger : it has been known to fill the abdomen. It is not unusual to see a mass, in connexion with the eye, as large as half of the head on which it rests. Though it may occasionally lie dormant for a considerable period, it more usually runs its course with great rapidity ; a few months, or even a few weeks, may carry the case from the commencement to a fatal termination. Like all forms of cancer, the medullary consists of a stromal or containing, and an intra-stromal or contained substance ; the former a fibrous structure, and the latter being chiefly nucleated cells of various shapes and sizes, and free nuclei. According to the preponderance of the one or the other element, the tumour varies in consistence ; in the harder and more slowly developed species, the fibrous structure being in excess, and in the softer and more rapidly developed, the cellular or nuclear. The intra-stromal substance may be pressed out usually in great abundance, constituting the highly characteristic cancer juice, and in many instances may be separated from the stroma by gentle washing ; the latter being left in the form of a delicate filamentous web: but in the harder varieties, considerable manipulation and pressure may be necessary to effect the separation.

The section of medullary cancer, as already hinted, sometimes presents a striking likeness to brain, being white and soft, mottled here and there with spots of grey or pink, the latter colour depending on the presence of blood-vessels, with which this variety of cancer is largely supplied. The coats of these blood-vessels are of great delicacy; and from the small degree of support they receive from the structure in which they ramify, they are very liable to rupture, giving rise to hæmorrhage, more or less copious, into the substance of the tumour. To this is due the dark and bloody appearance which was formerly thought to indicate a distinct variety of cancer, distinguished by the name of fungus hæmatodes. Hæmorrhage is peculiarly liable to occur as the tumour begins to soften and decay, and numerous shades of colour are then seen, partly from the presence of blood in different stages of disintegration, and partly from the changes which the cancerous matter itself undergoes. The tumour varies in consistence in different parts, and in the different stages of its development. Here and there the fibrous structure will be found collected in masses, little inferior in density and hardness to what is seen in scirrhus, into which in fact it frequently merges; while at other parts, where the cellular element predominates, it is soft and almost diffluent. Medullary cancer occurs either infiltrated into the structure of organs, or in separate masses enclosed in an investing membrane, which was formerly described as a true cyst, secreting from its walls the contained matter. This opinion, however, is not now generally received; most pathologists agreeing with Dr. Walshe, that the investing capsule is formed by the condensation of the surrounding cellular membrane. When medullary tumours approach the surface, as invariably happens with those with which we are more immediately concerned, they involve the investing skin or conjunctiva, which undergoes changes, not merely from distension, but also from becoming infiltrated with the cancerous matter; the skin assumes a dusky and livid colour, and large blue veins ramify over its surface. In either case, but more speedily when the disease is sub-conjunctival, ulceration finally takes place, and the tumour, released from pressure, bursts into luxuriant fungous growths, which rapidly increase in bulk, and by their profuse discharge, and frequent hæmorrhage, bring the case to a fatal termination.

MELANOSIS.

This is considered by Müller, and several other distinguished pathologists, to constitute a distinct variety of cancer. The accuracy of this opinion, however, is now disputed, and, I think, upon good grounds. The blackness is dependent solely upon the presence of pigmentary matter, different in no respect from that of the choroid, for the most part free, or when associated with a morbid growth, partly infiltrated into the peculiar cells, or among the elementary structures, of which it is composed. The black matter cannot of itself be considered as cancerous; it is never met with in the human subject associated with any stroma peculiar to itself; it has been found colouring tumours not of a malignant character, and it is asserted that it in no way modifies the growth or progress of the structure in which it occurs, though I am inclined to think that this latter assertion has been made on insufficient grounds, and that the subject has not as yet met with that careful consideration which its importance deserves. I shall revert to this question when describing the progress of melanoid disease as it appears in the eyeball, and shall state my reasons for adopting the above opinion.

In applying also these general considerations to the case of soft cancer affecting the eyeball, the two forms—encephaloid and melanoid—on account of the different appearances to which they give rise, will be separately described; the use of the term "encephaloid" being here resumed as a contradistinction to melanosis.

ENCEPHALOID CANCER OF THE EYEBALL.

Encephaloid cancer of the eyeball has been occasionally met with in middle life and in elderly persons, though so rarely that the fact has been questioned by some writers. Several instances, however, are on record, which prove the possibility of its occurrence : one in particular is mentioned by Mr. Saunders, where the examination of the eye after extirpation, and still more, the formation of secondary tumours in various parts of the body, leave no room for doubt as to the nature of the disease. Besides this, specimens of the disease in the Museum of the Royal College of Surgeons, render the fact unquestionable. It is equally certain that in the vast majority of instances the period of its appearance is in early childhood, generally before the fifth year, and rarely after the tenth. Mr. Travers gives a drawing of a child eight months old, in whom the disease was congenital, the tumour having acquired the bulk of a walnut at the time of birth ; and Dr. Mackenzie has seen it in an infant of nine weeks, in whom, as it had been observed six weeks previously, it also was probably congenital. Instances are not unfrequent in which it has been seen in an advanced stage of development before the completion of the first year ; but the mass of cases will be found to have occurred in children from two to four years of age. It is usually confined to one eye, but occasionally attacks both, either consecutively or simultaneously. I shall, to facilitate description, divide the affection into three stages.

First Stage.—The earliest symptom that generally attracts attention is a shining, yellowish, and deep-seated reflection at the bottom of the eye, as if from a piece of metal; this is best seen in particular lights, and somewhat resembles the appearance of a cat's eye in a darkened room. At the same time the iris will be found to have changed in colour, being rather darker than that of the other eye ; the pupil is dilated and sluggish, and vision, even now, is nearly or altogether lost. Slight external inflammation, lacrymation, and intoler-ance of light occur in some instances ; but these are by no means necessarily, or even frequently, present; more usually there are no indications of pain, and there is every appearance of perfect general health. As the disease advances, the cause of the metallic reflection becomes evident. It is now seen to be owing to a tumour springing up apparently from the fundus of the eye, of an irregularly rounded form, generally divided superficially into two or three lobes, and traversed by one or two small blood-vessels, which ramify on its surface. In colour it varies from a deep orange hue to nearly white, the most usual being, perhaps, a bright canary yellow. The growth gradually increases in size, approaches the front of the eye, causing absorption of the vitreous humour, and affects the lens, which becomes opaque, and in most instances is ultimately absorbed; previous to which it is pressed on the iris, which loses whatever brilliancy it may have retained, changes to a greyish brown colour, and is thrust forwards against the cornea; both the anterior and posterior chambers of the eye being completely abolished. Towards the conclusion of this stage, there is considerable tension from the internal pressure; the eyeball feels hard, its motions are limited, there are attacks of external inflammation with epiphora, and frequent and severe paroxysms of pain, restlessness, fever, and emaciation.

Second Stage.—The external parts of the eye now undergo a change. The cornea expands and becomes opaque. The sclerotica, thinned by absorption, allows the choroid to appear through it, is irregular in outline, rising into small dark-coloured knobs where the pressure has been most severe, or the absorption most rapid. In many instances it is so densely covered with large varicose vessels, that no alteration in colour is perceptible. The eyelids now become œdematous, and the eyeball prominent, and, apparently, greatly enlarged in size. I say apparently; for though I admit that enlargement takes place to a considerable extent, I cannot conceive the possibility of the dense fibrous structure of the sclerotica expanding to two or three times its normal dimensions, as some authors have asserted. I agree rather with Dr. Argyll Robertson, that "it is probable that, in most instances, these writers have been deceived by an unnatural prominence being given to the eye by the infiltration of the cellular tissue of the orbit projecting the eyeball forward, thus giving it the appearance of being augmented in bulk." Rupture of the eyeball next ensues; and this may take place either in front or laterally. In the former case, the cornea becomes more and more attenuated, pus or lymph is effused into its structure, and ulceration or sloughing ensues. These changes are not witnessed in the sclerotica, the fibres of which, previously thinned and opened up by long-continued distension, finally give way in a small rent, through which the morbid mass, still covered by the conjunctiva, protrudes. During the latter part of this stage the sufferings of the patient are acute, the pain extending over the whole side of the head, and even down the neck, and is accompanied with the usual symptoms of febrile excitement. Great relief is experienced when the fungus escapes and the distension is removed.

Third Stage.—The tumour, now released from pressure, rapidly increases in bulk, so as in a short time to distend the orbit and eyelids, and efface all appearance of the eye. When it has escaped through the sclerotica, at some little distance from the cornea, it is at first covered by the conjunctiva, but this is finally destroyed by ulceration and sloughing. In other cases of less frequent occurrence, the sclerotica gives way at the back part of the eye, so that the fungus escapes directly into the orbit. Under such circumstances the eyeball will be displaced in various directions, according to the position of the protruded mass, until finally this latter has acquired sufficient bulk to extend beyond the margin of the orbit, when it overlaps and conceals any remains of the eyeball that may have been visible.

The fungus, on its first escape, is soft, and generally of a light red or yellowish colour. This appearance, however, is rapidly changed as it increases in bulk; the surface becomes irregular and covered with ulcerations, which discharge profusely; large, livid, and fungoid granulations form, which bleed freely on the slightest touch; interstitial hæmorrhage takes place, forming clots in the interior of the growth, while large masses are detached from its surface by sloughing, giving rise to fresh bleeding, in some instances so profuse as to prove the immediate cause of death. No diminution of the size of the tumour ensues from the separation of the sloughs; on the contrary, the growth seems to take place with increased vigour, and is limited only by the length of time that the patient survives. I have already spoken of the enormous magnitude to which encephaloid sometimes attains. The skin of the distended eyelids, and of the adjoining parts of the face, assumes a dark livid hue, and is traversed by large varicose veins. The glands in the neck and under the lower jaw enlarge, and, in exceptional cases, proceed to ulceration. Death finally ensues, in some instances from extension of the disease to the brain, when it is preceded by coma or convulsions; in others from constitutional irritation, and the exhausting effects of pain, hæmorrhage, and discharge.

A *post-mortem* examination discloses that the contents of the orbit have undergone great changes. In cases of long standing, all means of distinction between the various textures is lost by their disorganization; the bony structures are softened and expanded, and frequently partially removed by absorption, so that the diseased mass is in direct contact with the brain. In many instances, I believe in most, the optic nerve will be found to be involved in the disease; thickened by the deposit of cancerous matter, except where it is constricted by the foramen opticum during its passage to the brain, and frequently again expanded so as to form a tumour immediately on its entrance within the skull. This change may take place at the earliest as well as at the most advanced stages of the disease; a pathological fact of much importance, and one to which I shall again refer, as bearing strongly on the question as to the propriety of operating in these cases. In pursuing our examination to the other regions of the body, we may find secondary cancerous deposits in various situations; for, in this respect, encephaloid obeys the same laws as when it commences primarily in any other organ. The brain seems to be very liable to these deposits, but in many instances, when in this situation, they can scarcely be called secondary, as they are the consequence rather of direct extension along the tract of the optic nerve. The uterus and the testicles, and the various thoracic and abdominal viscera, are the seats of what is strictly called secondary deposit, and will be found to be attacked in the usual order of their liability.

Much discussion has arisen as to the particular tissue of the eye which is the primary seat of the cancerous deposit. This is a question which it is very difficult to determine by *post-mortem* examination, as we seldom have an opportunity of making a dissection till the disease has so progressed as to involve all the tunics, and in an especial manner the retina; which, from the delicacy and great vascularity of its structure, is peculiarly unfitted to withstand either the extension of the disease, or the effect of pressure. The uniform manner in which the tumour appears to spring from the fundus of the · eye, and the constancy with which the nervous structures have been found on dissection to be to a greater or less extent involved, have led to the opinion that the disease has its origin in the optic nerve, just as it begins to expand into the retina, or in the latter tunic, close to the nerve. Lebert, however, and Paget concur in stating, that the retina is not in all, or even in the majority of cases, the point of origin; and Mr. Travers held the opinion " that this is not a disease of this or that texture, as writers would insinuate, but of all the textures, the crystalline lens and cornea excepted, which yield to its progress, but never exhibit a specific change of texture."

Examples are not wanting in support of these conclusions, as will be seen. Dr. Mackenzie describes a case in which the entire space of the vitreous humour and lens was occupied by a tumour springing by a pedicle from the optic nerve; the retina, though damaged by pressure, was not involved, and the optic nerve beyond the sclerotic had no appearance of disease. The tumour resembled brain substance, and was enclosed in a delicate membrane. Within a few months the child died, the entire orbit being occupied by a medullary tumour growing from the stump of the optic nerve, which was greatly enlarged. Constricted by the optic foramen, it again enlarged within the cranium, and between the foramen and commissure was as thick as the middle finger. The same author also mentions a case in which an encephaloid tumour sprouted from the junction of the cornea and sclerotic on the exterior of the eye. In No. VI. of the "Ophthalmic Hospital Reports," among the diseases for which extirpation was performed, is enumerated medullary cancer, growing from the upper and outer part of the cornea itself. Several instructive specimens may be seen in the Museum of the College of Surgeons. Among them are two eyes from the same child, in one of which is a medullary tumour originating between the sclerotic and choroid coats near the posterior part of the globe; in the other, a similar growth in the vitreous humour, without apparent attachment to the optic nerve or any of the tunics. But while these examples are sufficient to show that soft cancer may originate in any of the tissues of the eye, not even excepting the cornea, a careful examination of the preparations in the same Museum, together with my own dissections, has led me to the conclusion, that for the most part the retina is its primary seat; and the implication of the optic nerve, even within the cranium, which is constantly present in advanced stages of the disease, or in recurrence after extirpation, is evidence of a special determination to the nervous structures.

From the striking appearances exhibited by encephaloid from the very commencement, its diagnosis might be thought to be an easy matter. Such, however, is not the case. There is no disease as to the nature of which mistakes are more constantly made; and I shall endeavour to show that a positive diagnosis is in the present state of our knowledge totally impracticable, until the fungus has protruded through the external coats of the eye. I shall first mention one or two of the complaints with which it may be confounded by a superficial or unpractised observer, but from which it may be readily distinguished by a little attention.

The opacity of the lens occasioned by the pressure of the

tumour has been mistaken for idiopathic cataract, and attempts have even been made to perform the operation for depression. I need scarcely say that such an error ought not to occur. The condition of the lens may for a time conceal the true nature of the affection, but the history of the case, the discoloured and bulging iris, and the general symptoms of internal disorganization, which are invariably present, will be sufficient to deter any surgeon of ordinary intelligence from operative interference.

The colour of the vitreous humour may be altered in various ways, giving a dull red or yellowish appearance to the pupil, which might at first sight cause some embarrassment. The most ordinary cause of this discoloration is effusion of blood into the hyaloid cells: this may be almost invariably traced to the effect of a blow, or of some violent muscular exertion; it occurs suddenly, the blood is readily absorbed, and it seldom produces any very serious symptoms. A deposit of lymph on the surface of the retina from traumatic inflammation, occasions a yellowish reflection through the pupil; but the history of the case will sufficiently indicate the nature of the disease, while the indefinite and unchanging appearance of the discoloration, and the absence of anything like a tumour gradually advancing to the front of the eye, will assist still farther in forming a correct diagnosis. Attentive observation of the progress of these affections, and careful inquiry into their history, will seldom leave much doubt as to their real nature. It is far otherwise, however, with deposit of inflammatory exudation or scrofulous matter in the interior of the eye, occurring either spontaneously or as the result of injury, which may assume an appearance so exactly similar to that which was formerly considered as peculiar to malignant disase, as to render the diagnosis, in most instances of its occurrence, absolutely impracticable.

The true nature of these cases seems to have been first clearly pointed out by Mr. Travers. In several instances of what appeared to be malignant disease, as indicated by permanently dilated pupil, with a deep-seated opacity of a splendid yellow tint, the healthy appearance of the children induced him to abstain from operating, when he found, to his surprise, that the disease remained stationary for years, unaccompanied by any disorder of the health. Subsequent observation induced him to express the opinion that the "peculiar tint and splendour of the opaque substance is not to be depended on as a sign of malignity;" and he remarks further, in a paper read before the Medico-Chirurgical Society, "That the appearance I allude to is very analogous to that of the medullary tumour, will be inferred, when I inform the Society that (in the case of a lady who several years since recovered with the loss of sight, but is still in perfect health), at a consultation, including some eminent members of the profession, the extirpation of the organ was overruled by one dissentient, although I had sat down to perform it on two several occasions." Another instance came under his observation, in which a wound of the eyeball with a fine-pointed pair of scissors was followed by a deep-seated, fawn-coloured, resplendent surface, with red vessels branching over it, presenting exactly the appearance of malignant disease. In this case vision was lost, and the eye gradually shrank. The accuracy of these views has since been confirmed by numerous observers. Mr. Lawrence has frequently witnessed similar instances at the London Ophthalmic Infirmary, and details the case of a boy, ten years of age, in whom a wound of the cornea was succeeded by a bright yellow deposit, which gradually extended over the whole fundus of the eye, was accompanied by change of colour in the iris and extinction of vision, and led to softening and atrophy of the globe. Dr. Mackenzie, in illustrating the same subject, details an interesting case in which the same appearances were produced by suppuration of the globe. The patient, a boy eleven years of age, was admitted into the Glasgow Eye Infirmary on account of an attack of inflammation of the eye, which had followed exposure to a thunder-storm, by which he had been much frightened. Vision was extinct, the pupil was dilated and fixed, the iris changed in colour, and symptoms of general inflammation of the eyeball were present. "On examining the bottom of the eye, a tawny appearance presented itself, exactly similar to that which attends the incipient stage of medullary fungus." These changes were considered by Dr. Mackenzie and his colleagues to indicate the presence of malignant disease, and extirpation was proposed; but as the friends would not consent, calomel and opium were administered. The eye continued to enlarge, the tawny appearance became still more distinct, the lens was forced forwards in contact with the cornea, and the sclerotica finally yielded towards the inner canthus, giving exit to a quantity of thick purulent matter, after which the globe shrank and became atrophic.

Mr. Tyrrell relates cases which he has witnessed, both in children and in adults, in which prominent yellow tumours, with red vessels ramifying over their surface, have gradually disappeared under a steady and well-directed course of treatment. In one of these cases, extirpation had been determined on, and postponed only on account of the condition of the patient's general health. Mr. Dalrymple, in his "Illustrations of the Pathology of the Human Eye," observes: "The metallic lustrous appearance of the pupil may be caused by a deposit of simple exudation-cells, in fibrinous dropsy of the eye, in acute or chronic choroiditis, or in scrofulous inflammation;" and he concludes that the diagnosis in the early stages is therefore impossible. It is unnecessary farther to multiply authorities. The frequent occurrence of such cases is now admitted by all ophthalmic surgeons, and the difficulty of diagnosis is acknowledged. It has been asserted that in the non-malignant disease, the metallic lustre is not so brilliant, and the colour not so deep; that the iris and lens remain unchanged; that the globe becomes atrophic without previous enlargement; that the tumour never proceeds so far as to rupture the coats of the eye and escape externally. These, and all other attempts which have hitherto been made to establish diagnostic marks, have failed; their accuracy having been disproved by an appeal to recorded cases. The occurrence, in a scrofulous subject, of the peculiar symptoms soon after the receipt of an injury, or, on the other hand, an hereditary predisposition to cancer, would be sufficient reason for forming a strong opinion as to the scrofulous or malignant nature of the disease; but in the present state of our knowledge the only sure grounds upon which we can pronounce authoritatively as to its character, are, the atrophy of the globe, or the progress of the growth after it has escaped from the interior of the eye.

I am not aware that ophthalmoscopic investigation affords assistance by dispelling doubt. At all events, there has scarcely been time enough for investigations that may be depended on.

I may just allude to the proposal of Mr. Travers to make a deep incision across the globe in doubtful cases. This proposal was made at a period when the pathology of these affections was very imperfectly understood; and the advances that have been made since that time, render such a proceeding inadmissible. When the deposit is scrofulous, any operative interference is unnecessary: when it is malignant, an incision would only hasten the fatal termination.

I am not convinced that encephaloid cancer attacks the surface of the globe primarily. In the " Northern Journal of Medicine," for December, 1844, Dr. Argyll Robertson relates a case in which he believes this to have taken place. The patient, a woman sixty-two years of age, had been subject from childhood to attacks of inflammation of the left eye. Three years before she came under Dr. Robertson's notice, one of these was followed by the formation of a fleshy, elevated ring round the cornea, which after remaining stationary for a year and a half, began to increase, and was accompanied by severe lancinating pain, darting through the temple and head; the growth appeared to proceed from before backwards, projecting the eyeball from the socket till it could no longer be covered by the lids. Excision was followed by rapid recovery, and the patient survived the operation for twelve years, when she died from general decay, without any marked disease. The coats and the contents of the eyeball were perfectly healthy; " exterior to the sclerotic, and under the conjunctiva, it was surrounded by a dense mass of medullary sarcoma, which, when subjected to the microscope, presented spherical cells." While I do not mean to deny that this may have been a genuine case of encephaloid disease commencing on the surface of the eye, I think that the proof adduced is far from sufficient.   We can draw no conclusion from the bare announcement of the presence of spherical cells; besides, cure of encephaloid cancer by operation is very questionable; and all the appearances above described are produced by chronic inflammatory deposit in the orbital tissues.

Fungus-looking growths of various kinds occasionally spring from the conjunctiva, near the margin of the cornea; these, when neglected, may attain a very large size, completely concealing the eye, and projecting between the lids in the form of a livid tumour, which bleeds readily when handled.   There can be little difficulty, in most cases, in ascertaining the external origin of such; and this, so far as we yet know, must be taken as sufficient proof of their non-malignant nature.   Where they have proceeded so far as to destroy the eyeball and to fill up the orbit, as we are informed by Dr. Mackenzie that they occasionally do, the diagnosis will be difficult, and must depend chiefly upon the history and progress of the case, and the absence or presence of the cancerous cachexia.   This subject has been already considered in the chapter on Tumours, under the subdivision "Polypi and Warts," p. 247.

MELANOSIS.

I have stated that it is the general opinion of modern pathologists, that deposits of melanic pigment do not occur in the human subject, except in association with some other structure; that no growth contains it so frequently as cancer; that encephaloid is the variety of cancer with which it is most frequently combined; and·that, as it occurs in the eye, it is invariably associated with this growth, which, moreover, is not modified in any respect by its presence.   That these opinions are, in the main, correct, I readily admit, but I have seen reason to doubt their universal applicability; and I think it can be shown that in some respects the peculiarities of encephaloid do undergo modification, or what is equally probable, that these melanotic growths are more frequently of a non-malignant nature than is commonly supposed.

I have shown that encephaloid cancer of the eye is a disease almost peculiar to early life, and that instances of its occurrence after the age of puberty are comparatively rare. Such is not the case with melanosis of this organ, which is unknown in infancy. The earliest age at which I have seen it occur has been twenty-three; the patient, a female, was under the care of Mr. Lawrence, at St. Bartholomew's Hospital, during my house-surgeoncy. Mr. Lawrence met with it in one instance at the age of twenty-two, but confirms the general statement that it rarely occurs before the middle period of life.

In other respects it does not differ materially in its progress from uncomplicated encephaloid. At the commencement, extinction of vision is the only objective symptom; the shining reflection from the fundus of the eye is wanting, and there is seldom any way of distinguishing it from amaurosis, though, in exceptional cases, a dusky, slate-coloured tumour may be seen deep in the eye. As the disease advances, however, the symptoms of distension become evident; the eyeball is gradually enlarged; the lens becomes opaque, and, with the iris, is thrust forward against the cornea; the sclerotica assumes a dusky hue, is traversed by numerous large, tortuous vessels, and is elevated into dark-coloured prominences, which eventually give way, and permit the escape of the dark-coloured tumour. This increases in size; there is occasional bleeding and sloughing, and copious discharge of thin inky fluid; death takes place, either from the exhaustion produced by the local disease, or from the formation of secondary deposits, of a similar nature, in various parts of the body. When the eye is examined after death or after extirpation, the tumour is found to be soft in consistence, and of a deep sooty black colour, streaked here and there with various shades of brown or grey. This appearance is well illustrated by a preparation in the Museum of the Royal College of Surgeons. In Mr. Lawrence's experience, melanosis has always appeared to originate in the choroid; he states that where it is deposited, the choroid cannot be distinguished, while, in those parts of the eye to which the disease has not extended, this tunic has not undergone any alteration.

At the period of its growth before the sclerotica is ruptured, it is liable to be confounded with sub-choroid dropsy. Dr. Robertson has witnessed two instances of the latter disease in which the mistake had been made, and in which he saved the eyes from excision. He agrees with Mr. Lawrence in considering the state of the iris as the best means of diagnosing between them : in melanosis, the iris is thrust forwards by the opaque lens, in contact with the cornea, and though the pupil is generally dilated, it is not irregular, or only to a very slight degree ; in sub-choroid dropsy, there is no protrusion of the iris, but it is dragged in the direction of the tumour of the sclerotica, so as frequently to be altogether invisible on that side of the eye.

Melanotic growths occasionally take their origin from the outer surface of the globe. In his " Illustrations of the Pathology of the Human Eye," Mr. Dalrymple relates and figures a case of this nature which exactly resembled another that had been under his own care. The patient was a lady, sixty-two years of age. After many attacks of superficial inflammation, a tumour, pyriform in shape, and of a dark bluish-brown colour, sprang from the junction of the sclerotica and cornea, and gradually increased till it covered half of the latter tunic. It was dissected off without opening the anterior chamber ; and seven years after the operation, the cornea still remained clear, and there had been no return of the disease. Microscopic examination was made immediately after its removal, and the following description is given of its appearance:—" Its structure was soft, dark brown, and made up of nucleated cells, of a discoid elliptical figure ; flattened and varying in size, some transparent, others filled with dark-brown sepia-like material. In some of the cells the nuclei were numerous, in others, few ; in certain points there appeared congeries of minute cells aggregated together, while in others a few large cells were connected one to the other ; the long diameter of the largest

426 MALIGNANT AFFECTIONS OF THE EYE.

measuring 1-2200th of an inch. The parietes of the cavities
in which the cells were contained were composed of fibres,
which here and there were also collected into bundles. The
tumour seems to have had its origin in the development of these
cells in the interspaces of the fibrous tissue at the junction of
the sclerotica and cornea."

A growth, apparently of a similar nature, was removed from
the eye of a gentleman aged sixty, by Dr. Hibbert Taylor, of
Liverpool. It had commenced four years previously with vascularity and a dark appearance of the outer part of the sclerotica, and increased slowly and without pain till the time of its
removal, when it had attained the size of a sewing thimble. It
was attached by a narrow neck to the outer part of the right
cornea at its junction with the sclerotica : was of a dark bluish-
black colour, and soft consistence, and bled when handled ; the
pupil, and the eye generally, retained their natural appearance,
and the patient could distinguish one person from another with
this eye. The tumour was removed by ligature in June, 1849 :
it soon reappeared, and in January, 1850, it had attained nearly
its original bulk ; the pupil was sluggish, and vision was
limited to the perception of light and shadow, but the eyeball
retained its natural size and form. It was on this occasion
excised with scissors, and has not again returned.

Mr. Travers describes a tumour which he removed from the
eye of an elderly lady, and which was in his experience unique ;
a careful examination of the illustrations which accompany his
description induces me to think that it was a case of melanotic
deposit in the structure of the cornea. It was of a dark-purple
colour, lobulated, so as somewhat to resemble a bunch of
currants, and of sufficient size to project between the lids, and
cause great inconvenience. When examined after removal, it
was found to have its origin in the cornea, and to a certain
extent also in the sclerotica; its section was of a dark colour
and varied consistence, being soft and pulpy in some places,
firm in others.

I am at present unable to say how far the ophthalmoscope
may assist here in diagnosis. I have had but one patient in

whom an internal examination of the eye was made. An adult female, with very impaired vision in one eye, was inspected by myself and some of my colleagues. On the outer side and nearer the front than the back, was a tumour, apparently black, about the size of a horse-bean, and evidently covered by the retina. After it had been so discovered, it could also be made out, when the pupil was dilated, in a favourable light, with the naked eye. There were no other objective symptoms. The patient attended the hospital but a few times.

· SCIRRHUS.

Scirrhus of the eyeball, as a primary affection, is a very rare disease. Doubts as to its existence are expressed by Mr. Wardrop, who had never witnessed or obtained a correct account of a single case. Mr. Tyrrell does not even allude to it, nor does Mr. Paget mention any instance of it. Mr. Lawrence, in the last edition of his work on " Diseases of the Eye," expresses himself nearly to the same effect as Mr. Wardrop; since then, however, a case has come under his observation, of which he has given a brief description in the "Medical Gazette," July 2, 1847. Mr. Middlemore appears to have seen more of the disease than any other English author, and his description of its origin and progress is the fullest that we possess; though, unfortunately, he does not illustrate his general statements by any detailed cases. Little reliance can be placed upon what is said on this subject by the French authors, on account of the indiscriminate manner in which they apply the term "Squirrhe" to any affection of which pain and hardness are prominent symptoms.

Scirrhus is rarely met with in any part of the body till after the middle period of life, and the few cases in which it has been known to attack the eyeball have not been exceptions to this rule. This disease is best known as afflicting the female breast; and ninety-five out of every hundred cases of scirrhus, are computed by Mr. Paget to occur in this organ. It is from the appearances it here assumes that the descriptions of this form of cancer are most commonly taken, but the characters which it presents in this situation are not by any means universally met with elsewhere. The most characteristic features of scirrhus are its hardness and toughness, which are so marked as often to cause it to creak under the knife. The cut surface is often cupped, and on firm pressure more or less milky juice commonly exudes, in which may be found the characteristic cancer cells; it may be of uniform appearance, or it may present fibrous bands radiating in various directions. Under the microscope, scirrhus is found to consist of fibres, often described as a peculiar stroma, but by Mr. Paget regarded as remains of the tissues in which the morbid growth is deposited; and in the meshes of this fibrous tissue are cells of irregular and varied form, containing one or more large, well-defined nuclei. It is never enclosed in a cyst, but extends into the surrounding structures, infiltrating them in various directions, in such a way as to appear to send out long roots into them; a fact of much practical import, and one which should never be forgotten in operating. Scirrhous tumours are rarely of large size, and are generally of slow growth, usually causing atrophy of the part in which they are developed: thus in the breast the nipple is retracted, and in the eye, instead of the phenomena of distension met with in medullary cancer, there is often shrinking of the globe. As I have not myself witnessed a genuine instance of this disease affecting the eyeball, my description must be entirely borrowed.

As before stated, scirrhus does not attack the eyeball until middle or advanced life; the most common age is between forty and fifty, and it has been more frequently observed in females than in males. It has been seen to follow a blow or other injury, but more commonly is preceded by numerous attacks of inflammation, generally of an intractable nature, and is attended with more or less pain. After one of these attacks, there is dimness of vision, and this gradually increases until the sight is totally lost; the cornea becomes flattened and hazy; the sclerotica assumes a dirty yellow hue, is traversed by enlarged vessels, and losing its regular rounded shape, becomes puckered, contracted, and nodulated. As the disease advances, the eyeball generally shrinks, though in some instances it is said to enlarge slightly; the different tunics are gradually invaded, and all distinction of texture is lost; there is constant severe, lancinating, or burning pain, generally with nocturnal exacerbations; profuse lachrymation and spasmodic closure of the lids are also common, as well as extension of the pain to the whole side of the head. The disease is usually long in passing the limits of the eyeball, but eventually extends to the surrounding parts; the eye becomes fixed and immovable, and the whole contents of the orbit are converted into a scirrhous mass, firmly adherent to the bone, which, in some instances, is also involved in the disease. This condition of parts may continue for a long period, and the patient may succumb, worn out by pain, constitutional irritation, and want of rest, without the appearance of ulceration; Mr. Middlemore asserts that he has never witnessed this termination of the disease; ulceration has been observed, however, by other authors, who describe it as commencing in the conjunctiva, and gradually extending to the whole diseased mass, involving the lymphatic glands, and producing frightful destruction of the face.

In the case which was observed by Mr. Lawrence, the patient was a middle-aged man: "The tissues of the anterior and inferior third of the right eye were occupied by an irregular growth of firm and very vascular substance, with a granular, warty, and very vascular surface. The posterior segment of the eye, and the lacrymal appendages, were sound." The eye was extirpated by Mr. Wormald, and the patient died two years afterwards, with medullary tumours in the heart and various other organs. There was no return of the disease in the orbit. This is the only case of primary scirrhus of the interior of the eyeball which I can find recorded; further details are very much wanted.

Mr. Butcher, of Dublin, in his "Reports on Operative Surgery," Series the Sixth, 1861, page 12, relates an exceedingly interesting case of true scirrhus of the eyeball, occurring as a primary affection. The following is a very short abstract of the case:—The patient, Elizabeth Doran, aged sixty-nine, was suddenly attacked with severe pain in the eye, which remained unabated for some days; gradually the sight became dim, until at last vision was lost. Five months after the attack, a "red, fleshy pimple" appeared in the cornea, which increased up to the time of her admission into the hospital, in November, 1859. The tumour then was as large as the section of a walnut, projecting between the eyelids, but not occupying more than the base of the cornea; it was mammillated, dense, flesh-coloured; to the touch it was as hard as cartilage; it did not bleed on being handled; a thin, watery secretion was passed from its surface; pressure did not cause suffering, but a wearying, lancinating pain never ceased, accompanied with an aggravated hemicrania during the night.

It was clearly demonstrable that the morbid product was limited to the cornea, the lacrymal apparatus being unimplicated in the disease. Mr. Butcher operated, on November 11, 1859. The contents of the orbit, with the lacrymal gland, were accordingly removed, and the patient made a good recovery from the operation, leaving the hospital on December 5. Examination of the parts after removal disclosed its true scirrhous nature, and this was further confirmed by the microscope. A point of very considerable interest exists in the fact of the growth itself being entirely confined to the cornea; the muscular, fatty, and areolar tissues of the orbit being healthy. The eyeball was very carefully examined, after having been five weeks in spirit. Not the least morbid change could be found in any of its tissues. The iris rested on the capsule of the lens, but did not adhere.

I may perhaps mention here a curious case which is given by Mr. Lawrence in the same paper, and considered by him to be unique. By a less experienced observer it might readily have been mistaken for scirrhus. A soldier of the Guards, twenty-four years of age, was seized suddenly with pain and inflammation of the eye, and vision was soon afterwards lost; notwithstanding a variety of treatment, no improvement was effected, and the patient was brought to Mr. Lawrence four months after the first attack. The globe was unnaturally prominent, distending and protruding the eyelids; on the nasal side, behind the cornea, was a dark, undefined prominence. The conjunctiva, which was uniformly red and thickened, covered it. The crystalline lens was opaque, and pushed forwards against the cornea. The patient had all along suffered severe pain, and his general health was impaired. Some time afterwards the globe was still further protruded, so that the lids could not be closed. There was now a red, fleshy mass, in the centre of which there was an ulcer the size of a sixpence, in the situation of the cornea, which it evidently penetrated. The eye was extirpated—I was present at the operation. The patient made a rapid recovery, and in a few weeks was again fit for duty. "The globe was filled with a diseased growth, moderately firm, partly yellowish, partly reddish, of considerable vascularity, without any trace of the normal structures; it was very much like what is frequently observed in a scrofulous testicle. If it had been seen detached, no one would have supposed that it had formed part of an eye. Upon careful examination, it was found that this diseased mass was choroid and iris, both of them much thickened, entirely altered in structure, and in great part deprived of their normal coating of pigment-cells. In the middle of the eye there was a small cavity, with smooth and darkish surface, containing a little dark fluid. This cavity was filled with a mass consisting of the reflected iris; it had pushed forwards against the posterior surface of the cornea, and had been from thence reflected towards the centre of the globe. The sclerotica was much thickened, in some parts to the extent of a quarter of an inch, its texture being softer than usual. The cornea was extended and thin. At the extremity of the optic nerve, there was a small shred of the retina. The ulcerated spot upon the anterior surface of the globe penetrated the cornea, and opened into the anterior chamber. There was no trace of crystalline lens or ciliary processes." It was also examined microscopically. "The sclerotic coat, 4-5 lines in thickness, was composed as usual of white fibrous tissue. The choroid was thickened by the deposit of numerous small granular corpuscles (cytoblasts), and a few nucleated cells, in a dense fibrous stroma. The pigment-cells of the choroid were in a great measure deprived of their colouring matter."

MALIGNANT TUMOURS OF THE ORBIT.

Malignant tumours originating deeply in the orbit exhibit no peculiarity in the physical changes which they produce in the orbit, orbital appendages, or eye, by which they can be at first distinguished from simple tumours in the same situation; and in my chapter on "Tumours," I have already fully dwelt on the symptoms to which these give rise. In some instances, the rate of progress, or other peculiarities of any given case, may, however, produce the suspicion of malignancy at an early period; and when the tumour has approached the surface, or when the constitutional effects of the disease have become developed, the diagnosis is easy. On the other hand, we may have a tumour which neither in its progress, early or late, nor in its appearance after extirpation, resembles any of the ordinary forms of cancer, but which recurs repeatedly; assuming, at each recurrence, a more decidedly malignant character till it destroys life: this is the recurrent fibroid.

I shall make but brief mention of the different forms in which malignant disease has been observed in the orbit, merely relating a few well-marked cases in illustration of the subject.

ENCEPHALOID AND MELANOSIS.

Encephaloid and Melanosis occasionally have their primary seat in the orbital tissues, forming tumours which protrude or displace the eye in various ways, according to their situation and the direction of their growth, and one or other of these forms of cancer almost invariably spring up in this situation, after extirpation of an eye affected with medullary cancer. Cases are recorded by Mr. Lawrence, Dr. Mackenzie, and others, in which these diseases appear to have been consecutive to local violence, and there is no doubt that injury occasionally produces them, though in perhaps the majority of cases no directly exciting cause can be assigned. The seat of the deposit may be either the cellular or the adipose tissue; in some instances, growths of considerable size have been found to spring from the optic nerve, while the eye was still sound. It is important to recollect that when these growths attain a large size, their pressure is very liable to cause absorption of the bony walls of the orbit; hence, should any attempt be made to remove them, the greatest caution will be necessary to avoid injuring the brain. That this is not an imaginary danger, we have the authority of Dr. Argyll Robertson, who, on one occasion, while extirpating an enlarged eyeball, had his finger in contact with the membranes of the brain, the greater part of the orbital plate of the frontal bone having been removed by absorption.

Malignant growths, originating in the immediate neighbourhood of the eye, as for instance in the frontal cells, the Antrum Highmorianum, &c., frequently make their first appearance in the orbit, after having given rise to symptoms the nature of which was, for the time, misunderstood. I am indebted to Mr. Solly for the details of the case to which the annexed illustration refers.

The first symptom that called for surgical interference was epiphora, caused apparently by obliteration of the ductus ad nasum; at this time there could have been no external indication of the true nature of the disease, as Mr. Travers, under whose care the patient then was, introduced a silk seton through the lacrymal duct, and allowed it to remain for two months. The tumour subsequently appeared at the inner angle of the eye, and its true nature was recognised. When it had increased to about the size of a walnut, an attempt was made to remove it, which was only partially successful, owing to its soft and friable consistence. During the operation, the finger passed freely into the nostril, the bones having been absorbed. The fungous mass was repressed by pure nitric acid, and the man left the hospital considerably relieved, but returned in about a year with active disease in both orbits. The growth pressed downwards into the nostrils, and at the same time upwards so as to cause absorption of the orbital parietes, and death by pressure on the brain.

Fig. 112.

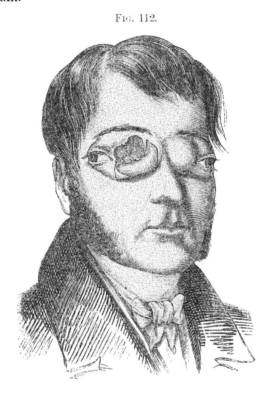

With a single exception, all the cases of encephaloid that I have met with, have made their external appearance at the inner side of the orbit. The eyeball has been more or less pushed aside, and sometimes thrust forwards. The characteristic of malignancy has been chiefly manifested in the immobility of the tumour. Indeed, this fixedness is more to be relied on for the nature of the disease, when the growth admits of examination, than any other symptom. If it be disregarded, the absence of pain, and the apparent health of a patient, are apt to lead to a wrong diagnosis. It holds good, whether the cancer be dense to the touch, or of less firmness. Only when there is a degree of softness that causes a feeling of what is called fluctuation, may the intimate attachment be more or less masked, or not easily made out, and the nature of the affection rendered very obscure. The following case exemplifies this:—

A girl, fourteen years old, whose general appearance, bright complexion, and high spirits conveyed the idea of excellent health, was a patient of mine, at St. Mary's Hospital, on account of a tumour in the orbit. The morbid mass occupied the inner side of the orbit, bulged the eyelids about three-quarters of an inch, keeping them open, and thrust the eyeball upwards, outwards, and forwards, although less in the last position, as the cornea was concealed by the outer commissure. The superimposed conjunctiva had a healthy look, and except a few enlarged veins in the skin of the lower eyelid, next the tarsal border, no preternatural vascularity was present. To the touch, it conveyed a sense of fluctuation, and might readily have been taken for a cystic formation; indeed, it was considered to be composed of hydatid cysts by more than one surgeon. The lacrymal apparatus at the inner corner of the eye was not interfered with. Vision was imperfect. The disease was discovered a year before, and had seemed stationary for nine months. The greatest ratio of increase was within the last three weeks, when for the first time pain was felt. The great probability of malignancy did not escape my attention, but I had some doubt, as there was a degree of fluidity that I had never witnessed in any malignant affections of the orbit. There was no appearance of any adhesion to the surrounding parts.

It was determined in consultation to make an exploration. The conjunctiva was incised to a small extent, and the growth exposed, when the brain-like aspect dispelled all idea of anything except encephaloma. A portion submitted to the microscope corroborated the malignant character.

SCIRRHUS IN THE ORBIT.

Scirrhus rarely selects the orbit as its seat, but it has been met with infiltrating the cellular tissue both behind and in front of the eyeball, or forming small hard, circumscribed tumours in different parts of the orbit. Its appearance in this situation seems generally to have been determined by some previous injury or attack of inflammation. It is slow in growth and not attended with much pain, so that it is especially difficult to distinguish it from simple tumours.

Dr. Mackenzie relates two cases, in one of which the disease followed an injury to the outer edge of the orbit, and assumed the form of a small tumour so hard and so firmly adherent to the edge of the orbit as to be taken for an exostosis: in the second, the entire areolar tissue of the orbit and conjunctiva was converted into a scirrhous mass.

The only example I ever saw, was in an old man at St. Bartholomew's while I was house-surgeon. There was no trace of the eyeball; the orbit, half emptied, was in a state of scirrhous ulceration, which extended externally all around, but more at the temporal side. Of the history of the case, nothing of pathological interest could be gathered; for four or five years the disease had existed. There was not much pain, nor were the absorbent glands affected. I lost sight of the patient, as he was dismissed as incurable.

SCIRRHOUS ENCANTHIS.

The caruncula lacrymalis is said to be the occasional seat of scirrhous enlargement. It must be a disease of very rare occurrence, as it has never been observed by Messrs. Wardrop, Travers, Lawrence, Guthrie, or myself; it is described, however, by Dr. Mackenzie, and Mr. Middlemore has removed a tumour which he believes to have been of this nature.

Authors speak of it as forming a hard, irregular swelling, mottled with spots of a pale colour, traversed by varicose vessels, and liable to bleed when touched. If left to run its course, it eventually ulcerates; the discharge is acrid and excoriating, and the ulceration extends to the surrounding textures, after the manner of scirrhous sores generally.

RECURRENT FIBROID TUMOUR IN THE ORBIT.

Several cases are on record of return of tumours removed from the orbit which at the time of extirpation were regarded as fibrous, but I have not met with any account distinctly indicating that the tumour had the characters of recurrent fibroid. The following case, kindly supplied to me by Mr. Edward Cock of Guy's Hospital, seems, however, to be clearly of this nature. " A boy ten years of age had for six months gradually increasing swelling and protrusion in the left orbit; when admitted into the Hospital the upper eyelid projected, the eyeball protruded, and vision was nearly lost. It was evident that a tumour existed in the upper part of the orbit, and an attempt had recently been made to remove it. On September 12th, 1855, it was completely removed, coming out of its bed much in the same way as a fatty tumour sometimes does, being only loosely connected with the surrounding cellular tissues. The character of the tumour was that usually denominated fibro-plastic, as ascertained by the microscope. The wound rapidly healed, the eye receded into the orbit, vision was completely restored, and he left the Hospital quite well three weeks after the operation.

" He was re-admitted on December 18th of the same year, with the orbit filled up by a diseased mass which had made its appearance only a fortnight before, and which had caused great exophthalmia, with complete disorganization of the eye ; the entire contents of the orbit were removed, the tumour had the same structure as the one first extirpated, but it was much larger, and had contracted more extensive adhesions to neighbouring parts. The boy made a good recovery, and there had been no return in the March following."

EPITHELIAL CANCER.

Epithelial cancer occasionally appears in the orbit in the form of a subcutaneous or sub-conjunctival tumour, which may acquire considerable bulk before it ulcerates, or shows any indication of malignity. Two of the cases of this description, which I have witnessed, I shall give in detail, as they present several points of great interest.

Fig 113.

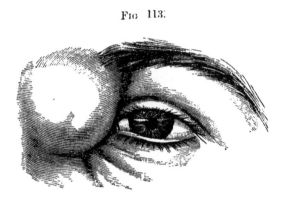

A man, sixty years of age, applied to my colleague, Mr. Taylor, at the Ophthalmic Hospital, on account of a tumour at the upper and inner angle of the orbit, which he had first observed several months previously, and which was gradually increasing and displacing the eye downwards and outwards. It was about the size of a nutmeg, smooth and regular on the surface, firm, elastic, and immovable, but apparently not attached to the skin (fig. 113). There was occasional slight pain in the situation of the frontal nerve, which was pressed upon by the growth. Vision was not impaired, though the eye was considerably displaced; and the protrusion gradually increasing, he was anxious to have the disease extirpated. There appeared to be nothing to contra-indicate the operation, and his wish was complied with. The tumour, which was found to be pretty firmly adherent at one point to the bone, was removed, apparently entirely, partly by evulsion, and partly by dissection, and the spot to which it had adhered was carefully scraped. The wound healed by the first intention, but the eye only partially recovered its proper position. A few weeks afterwards it was evident that the disease was again growing; the same situation was re-occupied by a firm, elastic growth, and the displacement of the eye became greater and greater. A second attempt was therefore made to effect its complete removal, and the operation on this occasion was attended with considerable difficulties, as the morbid growth had extended deep into the orbit, adhered firmly to the bone and the upper tarsal cartilage, and was thoroughly matted between the muscles and other surrounding textures. The wound was carefully washed, every portion that presented a suspicious appearance dissected out, and the edges brought together by sutures. The relief afforded by the operation was only temporary, as the disease soon re-appeared. After an interval of six months, the eye was much displaced and compressed. The tumour had increased to the size of a hen's egg, and had involved the skin, which was of a dark purple colour, studded here and there with small tubercular elevations. An ulcer, the size of a sixpence, occupied the seat of the wound; the discharge was scanty, but contained nume-rous characteristic cells. The patient suffered occasional severe pain, and his general health was much impaired.

Immediately after the last operation, the tumour was sub-mitted to microscopical examination by Mr. Quekett, who pro-nounced it to be a well-marked specimen of epithelial cancer. While making the examination he received for inspection another tumour, which had just been removed from the orbit of a young man aged twenty-two, by Mr. Guthrie, and which proved to be of an exactly similar nature. The patient had been for some time annoyed by lacrymation and irritation of the left eye, when he discovered a small swelling along the lower margin of the orbit. This was treated by leeches, poul-tices, and lotions, but it continued to increase in size, and produced partial exophthalmia. Mr. Guthrie being now con-sulted, recommended and effected the removal of the growth. The operation was succeeded by severe inflammation and rapid extension of the cancer. I had an opportunity of seeing the patient about four months after the first appearance of the disease, and six weeks after the operation. Both eyelids were then involved, forming a tumour about the size of an orange, which completely concealed the eyeball, was of a dark livid colour, traversed by large veins, ulcerated in many places, and bled profusely when touched. He was worn out with pain, discharge, and hæmorrhage, and was evidently fast sinking under their exhausting influence.

MALIGNANT AFFECTIONS OF THE EYELIDS.

Encephaloid and melanosis occasionally, though rarely, have their primary seat in the eyelids. In this situation, they present no peculiarities which merit separate consideration.

Scirrhus and epithelial cancer are the varieties of malignant disease to which these parts are especially liable, and in the majority of cases, the under eyelid is the one that is attacked; a fact of which no satisfactory explanation has hitherto been given.

Occurring here, these two varieties of cancer present, in many respects, a close resemblance to each other; so close, indeed, that it is to their history and mode of progress, rather than to their external appearance, that we must look for marks by which to distinguish the one from the other. Dr. Jacob, and after him Mr. Middlemore, were the first to draw attention to the fact that malignant ulceration of the eyelids occurs under two forms; and the general accuracy of the distinctions which they drew has been confirmed by subsequent observers, who have placed it beyond a doubt that the " Peculiar Ulcer," which they described, was that which is now named, epithelial cancer. Both forms of the disease are unknown in childhood; they occasionally attack young adults, but are much more common in those somewhat advanced in years.

In scirrhus, the attention of the patient is generally first attracted by a feeling of stiffness in the lid, by which its free motion is impeded; and on farther examination, this is found to be due to an undefined thickening and hardening of the subcutaneous cellular tissue. As the disease advances, adhesions are contracted to the bone, and the eyelid may appear as if somewhat retracted within the orbit; the skin also gradually becomes involved, and assumes a dusky, livid hue, from the presence of numerous small veins which ramify upon its surface. In some instances, severe lancinating pain is an early and prominent symptom; in others, there is merely a sense of uneasiness or itching, which induces the patient to rub or scratch the part, and this, by breaking the skin, leads to the commencement of ulceration. This process having once begun, follows the same destructive course as in other parts of the body, and produces the most frightful deformity. The bones as well as the soft parts are destroyed by ulceration, and the nose, mouth, and orbit have been seen to be thrown into one large cavity. As is the case with fibrous structures generally, the sclerotica long resists the attacks of the disease; and though all the other contents of the orbit should be destroyed, the eyeball may be seen lying in the cavity, almost as completely detached as if it had been dissected. In other cases, the irritation to which it is exposed leads to inflammation and sloughing of the cornea, the humours escape, and collapse ensues. Death takes place from the contamination of the system, and the formation of secondary deposits, or from the exhausting influence of pain and constitutional irritation.

Epithelial cancer commences by the formation of small white elevations or tubercles, generally towards the inner canthus; they are hard to the touch, and appear to be situated in the texture of the skin. They slowly enlarge and increase in number, producing, as Mr. Middlemore says, the appearance that would be caused " by introducing a knotted thread, or a minute white bead, or a series of them, beneath the skin of the eyelid." In process of time these tubercles coalesce into a mass; itching or uneasiness is felt; the surface is irritated or scratched, and ulceration commences. This proceeds gradually, but irregularly; at one part of its circumference it may be extending, while at another, cicatrization may be going on. Ultimately, the destruction of the face which takes place is equal to that which is seen in scirrhus; the soft parts of the orbit and cheeks being destroyed, and the cavities of the mouth, nose, and orbit thrown into one, by the ulceration of their bony parietes. One of the most striking peculiarities of this form of cancer is the remarkable slowness with which it progresses. If the general health of the patient be unimpaired, and the local affection shielded from irritation, six or seven years may elapse before ulceration supervenes. Its progress after the commencement of ulceration may be equally slow; ten, fifteen, or even twenty years may elapse, without any advance having been made; in other instances, however, and especially when by any means the general health of the patient is depressed, or the sore is injudiciously treated by irritating applications, the disease may advance with the most destructive rapidity. Another striking peculiarity is the tendency to partial reparation in one part of the sore, while ulceration is in active progress in others; smooth, shining cicatrices, of a pale bluish colour, are formed, but are seldom of long duration; they are again involved in ulceration, while the same process is repeated in another part. Pain is not a prominent symptom of epithelial cancer; in some cases, even where the disease has committed the most extensive ravages, it may be almost entirely absent. At other times it is acute, but this seems to be owing rather to incidental complications, such as the exposure of the nerves by ulceration, &c., than to be an essential feature of the disease. Ultimately, the cancerous cachexia is induced, and the patient dies, most frequently from exhausting irritation.

In those in whom the constitutional conditions necessary for the development of cancer are present, the spot at which the epithelial growth makes its appearance is frequently determined by local irritation; in the neighbourhood of the eye, for instance, it may be induced by the repeated friction of optical instruments, as has been witnessed more than once by Mr. Simon.

From the above description it will be seen that the distinction between scirrhus and epithelial cancer is to be drawn rather from their history than from their appearance. In the early stage, when alone the diagnosis is of any practical importance, it will be found that in scirrhus the skin is movable over the indurated mass, whereas the epithelial growth appears to be deposited in its texture. The tubercles of scirrhus are less prominent, more speedily become adherent to the subjacent textures, are of a more decided colour, and are more frequently attended with pain, than those which usher in epithelial cancer. The progress of the former, too, is in general more rapid; the constitutional cachexia is more speedily and decidedly developed, and the lymphatic glands are in general implicated; a complication which is rarely seen in epithelial cancer. Such are some of the distinguishing features by which it is stated that the two forms of the disease may be recognised in their early stages; in many cases they are so slightly marked as to be scarcely perceptible, and the diagnosis becomes exceedingly difficult; it should, however, be always attempted, and every effort should be made to add to the number of diagnostic marks upon which dependence can be placed, as experience has shown that a correct appreciation of the nature of the disease may materially influence our prognosis.

I have not hitherto given any account of the structure of epithelial cancer, though I have referred to several of the characters which distinguish it; its superficial origin; its slow progress; and to the fact that extension to the lymphatic glands, and dissemination throughout the system, are comparatively rare. It is made up entirely of epithelial cells, varying somewhat in form, but for the most part resembling the flattened scales of the superficial cutaneous epithelium. They are not, however, in the normal situation of epithelium, on a free surface; but are disseminated among the tissues of the part affected; and it is this peculiarity of relation to other structures, and not the form of the cells themselves, which constitutes the characters of malignancy. Here and there these cells exhibit a characteristic arrangement in "nests," as they have been termed, or "laminated capsules," in which the cells are concentrically arranged so as to form a spherule often large enough to be visible to the naked eye. A section of these bodies may give rise to the appearance of fibres, or fibres may be seen belonging to the structures among which the cells are infiltrated, but none are formed as elements of the disease; there being, in fact, no stroma. It has been described by Lebert and Bennett as a cancroid growth; that is, resembling cancer in progress and in external appearance, but in minute structure presenting marked differences; it is often also termed semi-malignant. These names have had great influence on the ideas with which this affection has been regarded, and on the treatment adopted for it; they are now, however, almost abandoned, and the term epithelial cancer is intended to express not only its external similarity to the other forms of cancer, but its relation to them in nature. The cells, though as a rule individually undistinguishable from those of normal epithelium, do yet, when formed interstitially and infiltrated into the tissues of a part, constitute a true heterologous growth.

QUESTION AS TO THE PROPRIETY OF OPERATING.

There is, probably, not any subject in the whole range of surgery, upon which more discordant opinions have been expressed than upon the question as to the propriety of extirpating malignant growths. This is attributable to various causes, one of the chief of which I believe to be, the careless and indiscriminate way in which the term cancer is applied. In a Lecture published in the " Medical Gazette " for February, 1844, Sir Benjamin Brodie relates, that, having been requested by a surgeon to examine a scirrhous mamma which he was about to amputate, he found the so-called scirrhus to be a chronic abscess; the same surgeon informed him that he had excised ten cancers with success. For the credit of the profession, I should be disposed to consider this as an extreme case; but there can be no question that fibrous and other non-malignant growths are constantly confounded with cancerous affections, and, next to the mamma, this mistake probably occurs more frequently in the eye than in any other organ, from the exact similarity which exists between scrofulous and encephaloid diseases of the eyeball in their early stages. Although the researches of modern pathologists have made us acquainted with many distinguishing marks by which the recognition of malignant growths may be facilitated, yet in numerous instances the diagnosis is still extremely difficult;

and the most careful and well-informed observers are liable to be mistaken, until they have an opportunity of examining the disease after its removal from the body. Another, and very common source of fallacy in examining this important question, is the prevalent custom of reporting cases as cured within a very short period after the operation. Were recovery from the immediate consequences of the operation to be considered as a true test of success, we might look upon cancer as equally amenable to surgical treatment with almost any other form of disease : to do so, however, would be to overlook one of its most distinctive and deadly characteristics, its liability to return, as well in its original seat as in the form of secondary deposits in the internal organs. If instead of losing sight of patients as soon as the wound is healed, their future history could be carefully traced, it would be found, I believe nearly always, that a recurrence of the disease had proved fatal within two years. Such a result cannot be termed a cure ; I shall inquire presently whether it can be regarded as a prolongation of life.

All that we have hitherto ascertained as to the origin and nature of cancer, leads to the conclusion that it is a constitutional, not a local disease ; that the tumour or sore is merely the evidence of the poison that is at work within; the outlet, so to speak, at which the *materies morbi* endeavours to escape from the system. If this be true, it is evident that any attempt to arrest the disease by the removal of its local manifestation, can be attended only with disappointment. I do not mean to assert that cancer in general, when left to run its course, is inevitably fatal; or that an operation for its removal is invariably followed by its recurrence ; cases occur from time to time in which it disappears spontaneously from the system, by processes which it is not necessary here to describe. Some well-authenticated instances are on record, in which the extirpation of malignant growths, even under the most discouraging circumstances, has been followed by complete and permanent recovery. Such exceptional cases, however, are so rare, and the conditions under which they occur are so little understood, that it would not be safe to make them the basis of any practical conclusion. But more than all, the many circumstances arising out of the peculiar position—the local peculiarities—of the eye and its appendages, place it beyond these considerations. It is but fair, however, to mention, that one of our most eminent authorities, Dr. Bennett, has drawn a different inference from the same facts. At page 242 of his work on "Cancer and Cancroid Growths" he remarks :—"It seems to me that a cancerous may supervene upon a cancroid growth, and that both for a time may be local," a statement which I am at a loss to reconcile with his observations upon the origin of cancer, in which he endeavours to trace it still farther than has been done by other pathologists, to disorder of the primary and secondary digestions; and at page 245 he proceeds to say,—"So long as a cancer remains fixed in a part which is capable of being removed, and the strength of the patient is not too much reduced, so long is the surgeon warranted in operating." To this proposition I can by no means agree ; and, therefore, while I concur with him in thinking that these exceptional cases of recovery should prompt us to increased diligence in investigating the conditions under which they occur, I am of opinion, that in the present state of our knowledge, the unfavourable views expressed by Dr. Walshe as to the results of surgical interference, are more in consonance with sound pathological reasoning. Dr. Walshe's conclusions are founded partly upon physiological grounds, and partly upon an extensive statistical survey, from which every source of fallacy has been carefully excluded. My space will not permit me to do more than to state the results at which he arrives ; for details I must refer to his admirable monograph upon Cancer. At page 236 he thus sums up his argument as to the operation as a means of cure :—"First, inasmuch as the number of permanent recoveries is infinitely small, and as no combination of circumstances, however favourable, protects the patient from relapse, the operation cannot, in any individual case, be recommended as likely to cure the disease. Secondly, inasmuch as no operation by excision is performed without the chance of some of the diseased structure being left behind, an accident which hastens the progress of the malady;—inasmuch as absolute certainty of the freedom of internal organs from the disease is unattainable;—inasmuch as the dormant cancerous diathesis is sometimes roused into activity by the removal of a tumour;—inasmuch as cancers in a state of active growth acquire increased energy of vegetation, if reproduced after extirpation;—and lastly, inasmuch as the operation itself has not very unfrequently proved both the occasion and the cause of death; excision cannot be undertaken without imminent risk of placing the patient in a worse condition than he or she was previously to the use of the knife."

Dr. Walshe next examines into the truth of two opinions which are almost universally prevalent among the profession; namely, that the best chance of success is afforded by operating at an early stage of the disease; and again, that though not curative, the operation may be undertaken as a means of prolonging life. Upon both those questions, he arrives at the most unexpected conclusions; upon the first, he asserts,—"Of a given number of cancerous individuals, a considerably larger proportion will be saved from untimely death under the influence of well-devised and judiciously-sustained treatment, aided, if this become necessary, by extirpation, performed at a comparatively late period, than will recover under the influence of the operation (unpreceded by methodised treatment) effected at the very earliest stage of local development;" and, upon the second, his researches lead him to infer that "the use of the knife decreases by more than half the chances of surviving the sixth year of a cancerous affection."

Mr. Paget, in his admirable Lectures upon Cancer, delivered at the Royal College of Surgeons, has added the weight of his testimony to the conclusions of Dr. Walshe. His opinions are founded upon extensive and independent research, and appear to be amply established by the evidence which he has adduced.

The above observations are intended to apply to the operation as undertaken with a view to the *cure* of cancer, and especially of the two varieties, encephaloid and scirrhus. In certain cases of melanosis and epithelial cancer, I believe that an operation may be performed with some prospect of permanent success; and even in encephaloid and scirrhus, circumstances may occur which will render their removal not only permissible, but even necessary. I shall be better able to state my views upon this subject, by passing under brief review the different forms of malignant disease of the eye with which we have to contend.

ENCEPHALOID.

In the encephaloid disease of the eyeball which occurs in children, I can scarcely conceive any combination of circumstances that would warrant us in extirpating the organ. In support of this opinion it is needless to cite authorities; every author of experience coincides in denouncing surgical interference in terms more or less strong; even the older writers, who may fairly be supposed to have frequently removed eyes affected merely with scrofulous disease, found the general results of the operation so unfavourable as to have almost abandoned it. I should scarcely consider it necessary to do more than allude to this subject, did we not from time to time see instances recorded in the journals, in which, in defiance of the lessons of ample experience, this operation has been repeated; while Desmarres, and other French ophthalmic surgeons, inculcate and practise it in every case. The invariable result of such attempts has been recurrence of the disease, as well locally as in the form of secondary tumours of the brain or other vital organs; and from all that I have seen, and most certainly when the optic nerve is involved, I fully believe that the fatal event has occurred sooner than if the disease had been left to run its course. I would fain give many cases in support of this, but it is hardly necessary. I am not aware that there is a single unequivocal ease of success on record; while numerous instances might be quoted in which death has taken place within a few months or even weeks after the operation. The impossibility of forming a correct diagnosis of the nature of the deposit during the early stage of the disease, appears to be of itself sufficient ground against interference; "but so far," says Mr. Dalrymple, "from that circumstance being to the disadvantage of the patient, I am inclined to rejoice that it offers another bar to the performance of the operation of extirpation of the eyeball." He further shows that even at the earliest stage of the ocular disease, and while to external appearance the eye may be in a favourable state for operation, there may be extensive latent disease of the brain; and illustrates his remarks by drawings from preparations taken from children dying of extensive fungoid tumours within the cranium, while as yet the ocular deposit was confined to the back of the eye, and the globe had undergone no alteration in form or size. In short, every fact, practical as well as pathological, with which we are acquainted, tends to show that, in the words of Mr. Syme, "It would be better, both for the interests of humanity and the credit of surgery, if the operation were entirely abandoned." Mr. Liston, in speaking of excision of the cancerous mamma, while the neighbouring glands are involved in the disease, expresses himself as follows:—"The practitioner who would advise interference with the original tumour, must be grossly ignorant, atrociously unprincipled, or of unsound mind." I consider that this language, though strongly expressed, would be equally applicable to the surgeon who, in the present state of our knowledge, would indiscriminately sanction or perform extirpation of the eyeball for the encephaloid cancer of childhood.

The same observations apply to the rarer instances in which the disease appears in the adult; for though it may not always be so rapid in its progress, it has hitherto been found to be equally fatal in its results, and beyond the control of operative surgery. In either case, careful and well-regulated treatment has frequently been found to effect much towards the alleviation of the more distressing symptoms, and the prolongation of life; and instances have occurred to Mr. Dalrymple, in which it has

G G

even appeared to induce a pause in the progress of the malady:
on the other hand, it cannot be too carefully kept in mind, that
irritating applications by which the afflux of blood to the part
is increased, as well as every debilitating cause which tends to
impair the general health of the patient, adds renewed energy
to the vegetative force of the morbid mass, and accelerates
death.

SCIRRHUS.

With regard to scirrhus of the eyeball, our experience is as
yet too limited to warrant us in forming any ópinion as to the
propriety of extirpation, except from our observation of its
results when applied to other organs similarly affected. I have
already stated that these have hitherto proved highly unfavourable. Dr. Mackenzie, however, recommends operation in these
cases.

MELANOSIS.

Whatever be the true nature of melanosis, whether, when it
occurs in the eye, it invariably present the characters of encephaloid, as is supposed by some, or whether it be occasionally
associated with tumours of a non-malignant character, it is the
opinion of some of the most experienced surgeons that it differs
materially from uncomplicated cancer, in the result of operations
for its removal. Mr. Dalrymple says, "There seems, if one
may use the term, less malignancy in it, and its extirpation
by operation is unquestionably less liable to be followed by
reappearance of the disease, than that of either medullary
sarcoma or carcinoma." In support of this view, he details a
case, to which I have already referred, in which the removal of
a melanotic tumour from the exterior of the eyeball of an
elderly lady was followed by what may be considered a permanent cure, as there had been no return of the disease seven
years after the operation. In the "Medical Gazette" for
October, 1845, and again for July, 1847, Mr. Lawrence reports
several cases in which the operation was followed by various

results. One of these cases I had an opportunity of witnessing during my house-surgeoncy at St. Bartholomew's Hospital. It occurred in a young woman, twenty-three years of age, who was admitted into the hospital on account of some trifling venereal affection, during recovery from which she called attention to the state of her eye, which was the seat of great pain. There was considerable conjunctival and sclerotic injection; the pupil was dilated and motionless; and the lens, dull and dingy in appearance, was, with the iris, thrust forward in contact with the cornea: there were also three dark staphylomatous projections of the sclerotica, close to the margin of the cornea. The eye was extirpated in 1841. Towards the end of 1844, having previously enjoyed good health, she began to complain of pain and swelling of the abdomen; her symptoms rapidly increased in severity, and the case terminated fatally nearly four years after the extirpation. On *post-mortem* examination, melanotic tumours were found in nearly every organ of the body. In this instance, judging from what we know of the usual progress of the disease, I think we are warranted in asserting that life was prolonged and much suffering averted by the performance of the operation.

Another case, reported in the same paper, is worthy of notice, and not the less on account of the eccentric means adopted by a surgeon who was consulted, in order to stop the progress of the tumour.' The patient was a robust man, forty-four years of age, who had lost one of his eyes twelve years previously from inflammation. When he applied to Mr. Lawrence, the melanotic growth was of eight months' duration; it had sprung from the shrunken eyeball, and had rapidly increased in size so as to fill the orbit and partly project from it. To check this growth, the surgeon sewed the lids firmly together, by strong sutures, which, in spite of the distension occasioned by the increasing bulk of the mass, still performed their office when the patient presented himself to Mr. Lawrence. The disease was removed at the man's urgent request, with the effect of affording immediate relief; and there had been no return of it a considerable time after the operation. The conclusion at which Mr. Lawrence arrives, as well from his own experience as from that of others, is, that though it is probable that melanosis will always be found to terminate fatally sooner or later, yet that life may be prolonged by the early performance of an operation ; and that surgical interference should be limited to those cases in which protrusion and ulceration of the melanotic growth has not yet taken place.

Dr. Argyll Robertson, in an interesting paper in the "Northern Journal of Medicine" for November, 1844, relates six cases in which he had extirpated the eyeball on account of melanotic growths, and the results of which lead him to form a very favourable opinion of the operation. One of his patients, a man fifty-two years of age, was in good health two years afterwards, and a small melanotic deposit above the cornea of the other eye had existed for nine years unchanged.

Less favourable views are entertained by some other surgeons, whose operations have been succeeded by a rapid development of the disease in various parts of the body, and consequently, by speedy death. The question is as yet far from being decided. Much more satisfactory evidence and accurate statistical research are necessary, before any trustworthy conclusion can be arrived at, either for or against the propriety of operating; but I think that, as the matter at present stands, we are warranted in hoping that an early operation will be followed by prolonged life, and relief from suffering. When protrusion and ulceration of the tumour have taken place, and still more, when there is any reason to suspect that the internal organs are affected, surgical interference will almost certainly precipitate the fatal termination.

MALIGNANT TUMOURS OF THE ORBIT.

When we have satisfied ourselves as to the malignant nature of a tumour of the orbit, experience shows, that as in the case of the disease in other situations, surgical interference is, as a general rule, injudicious. I have already mentioned two cases that fell under my own observation, in which the removal of epithelial tumours pressing upon the eye, was followed by unfavourable results; and we have abundant evidence that there is nothing in their position which exempts them from the laws by which our treatment of malignant disease in general, should be regulated. I am often earnestly entreated to operate after I have declined to interfere.

In all the cases of encephaloid cancer in which I have operated, or been present during the performance of an operation, it has either been impossible to clear the orbit without scraping the bones, or a portion of the cancer has passed out of reach through some of the orbital apertures. In neither case, therefore, could the disease be said to be removed.

Under certain circumstances, however, an operation may be not only permissible, but necessary. When, either from their original position, or from the direction of their growth, such tumours are in close contact with the roof of the orbit, they are liable, as they increase in size, to cause absorption of the bone, and death from pressure on the brain. In such cases, after having made the patient fully aware of the danger of his position, and having explained that our interference is not with the hope of effecting a permanent cure, but merely with the view of averting impending death, it will be proper to deviate from the general principle, and to excise the tumour, removing at the same time the whole of the contents of the orbit, should it be judged expedient to do so. In the " Dublin Hospital Gazette " for February, 1846, Dr. O'Ferrall relates a case in which he removed an encephaloid tumour from the orbit of a girl twelve years of age, with this object in view. The immediate result was satisfactory, but the child's subsequent history is unknown.

LACRYMAL GLAND.

Were we to place implicit confidence in the statements generally repeated in books, we should arrive at the conclusion that scirrhus of the lacrymal gland was a disease of by no means unfrequent occurrence. I have already (p. 295) expressed

my dissent from this opinion, and my belief that the term
" scirrhus" has been indiscriminately applied to affections of
this organ, which possess no single character of malignancy.
Everything in the history of these growths appears to me to
prove the accuracy of this opinion. The large size to which
they attain ; the absence of ulceration ; of adhesion to or implication of the surrounding parts ; of disease of the neighbouring
lymphatics, and of constitutional cachexia ; and, finally, the
invariable success which attends their extirpation, are characters which are unknown in connexion with scirrhus in any
other situation, but which are universally recognised as features
iṇ the chronic inflammatory induration and hypertrophy of
other glandular organs. I by no means intend to assert that
the disease never occurs, or that there is anything in the structure of the lacrymal gland which should exempt it from liability
to scirrhous infiltration ; we have the authority of Dr. Mackenzie, Mr. Dalrymple, and other competent observers, for
believing in its existence ; and their descriptions lead us to
suppose that the stage of induration is, as in other situations,
succeeded. by softening and ulceration, which involve the surrounding textures. This, however, is certain, that it is an
affection of very rare occurrence. Mr. Lawrence doubts the
correctness of the opinion that the enlargement and induration
of the gland which is occasionally observed is due to scirrhus,
" never having seen any evidences of malignity in such cases ;"
and I have failed in discovering a detailed account of any case
at all resembling the general descriptions of the disease which
are given by some authors.

The symptoms are represented as being the same as those
which indicate enlargement of the gland of a non-malignant
nature ; but the pain is said to be much more severe, and of a
lancinating character. I am not aware of any means by which
its cancerous nature could be ascertained, previous to the
occurrence of softening and ulceration.

MALIGNANT ULCERATION OF THE EYELIDS.

The same unfavourable results have been found to follow the excision of scirrhous growths and ulcerations from the eyelids, as from other parts of the body; in such cases, therefore, reliance should be placed rather upon judicious and well-sustained general treatment than upon operative interference.

In epithelial cancer, however, we have more encouragement to hope for success. "It is in this form of cancer," says Mr. Simon, "that the development of true cancer-growth appears to be at its minimum; it is in this form that the bulk of the morbid mass consists of elements seemingly not foreign to the normal structure of the part; it is in this form that cancer most nearly ceases to be what is called heteromorphous, and is least remote from the signification of a simple hypertrophy." On these grounds he advocates, under certain circumstances, the removal of epithelial ulcerations, even of considerable magnitude; and supports his views by the details of several cases in which such operations were followed by success. In remarking on these cases he observes,—" I considered, from the pathological affinities of each case, that the constitutional tendency to cancer could not be of extreme strength; and that accordingly, if I removed the existing masses of disease, a long period, perhaps even the remaining years of life, might elapse, without the cachexia having sufficient intensity to reproduce them anew."

I believe that by acting upon the views thus expressed, by excluding cases of scirrhus, and by limiting our operations to those of epithelial cancer in which there is no suspicion of secondary deposit, and in which every particle of the diseased structure can be removed, we should find that in some instances the operation was followed by a permanent cure, and in many by prolonged life, and relief from present suffering. It is now seven years since I removed two small cancers of this nature, one from the edge of the upper eyelid of a youth, in whom it had existed for a few months, and the other from the lower eyelid of an adult, of two years' duration; without, as yet, any return of either. Too much care cannot be taken, however, in forming a correct diagnosis—a matter, in many cases, of extreme difficulty; a considerable number, even of a non-malignant nature, occasionally assume an appearance which it is impossible to discriminate by their naked-eye characteristics from genuine cancer. It is a wise precaution, therefore, never to operate without previously submitting our patient to treatment, which will in some instances clear up the real nature of the case, and will in all increase the chances of a successful result.

It will frequently happen that the disease is of such an extent, that to be removed it is necessary to sacrifice the whole eyelid in order to effect its complete extirpation. In such cases the eye will almost inevitably be lost, from the irritation produced by exposure, and the contact of dust and other extraneous matters. It will therefore be well, in every instance in which it is practicable, to conclude the operation by the formation of a new lid, which must be taken from any of the healthy skin in the neighbourhood that may be available. This proceeding, the filling up of the wound by a piece of healthy skin, was at one time thought to exert a powerful influence in preventing the reproduction of the disease; more extended experience, however, has shown that this opinion is erroneous.

There is one rule which applies with equal force to every case in which the removal of cancer is attempted; a rule of such importance, that, at the risk of repetition, I must again endeavour to impress it on the minds of my readers; it is this: that every particle of the diseased structure must be thoroughly eradicated, and that the healthy parts in the neighbourhood be freely included in the incisions. Without this can be done, an operation should on no account be entertained. Every stroke of the knife through the diseased part opens up channels by which the cancerous germs are conveyed directly into the circulation, and the condition of the patient, from whom the disease has been only in part extirpated, is thus rendered infinitely worse than if nothing had been attempted. When circumstances permit, the edges of the excised part should be carefully examined by the microscope; and that this is no useless precaution we learn from a case related by Dr. Bennett, in which the apparently healthy structures thus examined were found to be loaded with cancerous germs. Under such circumstances the knife should be resumed, and the operation should not be considered as complete till every trace of the disease has been eradicated.

In the above observations, I have made no mention of the use of escharotics, which are strongly advocated by some for the removal of superficial cancerous sores; and I have avoided speaking of them, because I believe that the instances are rare indeed in which the knife is not to be preferred, as at once more rapid and effectual, and much less painful. Escharoties undoubtedly sometimes effect the removal of the disease, but they frequently require to be several times repeated; their use is attended with intense pain, and in the event of their not succeeding, the irritation which they produce cannot fail to be followed by the most injurious effects.

In concluding this chapter, I shall briefly allude to those melancholy cases in which excessive and incessant pain induces the sufferer to implore the removal of his disease, at any hazard. For such cases it is impossible to lay down any general rule; each must be investigated on its own merits, and the surgeon must form his own judgment on the expedience of operating. For my own part, if after having fully explained all the circumstances, the patient should still persist in his request, I should feel disposed to comply with his wish, if it were possible that by so doing I could relieve him. Severe and protracted agony, besides incapacitating the sufferer from devoting his attention to those subjects which his situation so urgently demands, may of itself, from the exhausting nature of its influence, prove the immediate cause of death. In such cases we might be justified in performing an operation which, under other circumstances, would be altogether inadmissible; the result of even partial removal of the disease might not only cause great relief from present suffering, but, in all probability, prolong life.

I have determined to add some remarks of Mr. Paget, as conclusions of his respecting the question of operating; for although they were not written with reference to ophthalmic disease, they apply to it.

With respect to scirrhus, he says,—"In deciding for or against the removal of a cancerous breast, in any single case we may, I think, dismiss all hope that the operation will be a final remedy for the disease.

"The question then is, whether the operation will add to the length, or to the happiness of life. The conclusion, from the statistics cited, might be that the length of life would be the same, whether the local disease were removed or not. We have to ask, therefore, whether it is probable that the operation will add to the length or comfort of life,—enough to justify the incurring the risk from its own consequences; and I cannot doubt that the answer may often be affirmative.

"1. In cases of acute hard cancer; 2. When the local disease is destroying life by pain, or profuse discharge, or mental anguish; 3. In all the cases in which it is not probable that the operation will shorten life;—a motive for its performance is afforded by the expectation that part of the remainder of the patient's life will be spent with less suffering, and in hope, instead of despair.

"Respecting the propriety of removing a medullary cancer in any single case, much that was said respecting the operation for scirrhous cancer of the breast might be repeated here. The hope of finally curing the disease by operation should not be entertained. The question is, in each case, whether life may be so prolonged, or its suffering so diminished, as to justify the risks of the operation. In general, I think, the answer must be affirmative, wherever the disease can be wholly removed, and the cachexia is not so manifest as to make it probable that the operation will of itself prove fatal.

"1. The number of cases in which the patient survives the operation for a longer time than that in which, on the average, the disease runs its course, is sufficient to justify the hope of considerable advantage from the removal of the disease.

"2. The hope that the removal of the cancer will secure a considerable addition (two years or more, for example) to the length of life, will be more often disappointed than fulfilled. But even when we do not entertain this hope, the operation may be justified by the belief that it will avert or postpone great suffering.

"3. A motive for operation, in cases of supposed medullary cancers, may often be drawn from the uncertainty of the diagnosis. This is especially the case with those of the large bones. All doubts respecting diagnosis are here to be reckoned in favour of operations."—*Lectures on Tumours.*

As to epithelial cancer, he continues:—"1. Though the instances of operations followed by complete recovery, or by very long immunity from the disease, are very rare; yet, in certain cases, these results may be hoped for.

"2. In the majority of cases, the removal of the disease may give great comfort for a time, and in general the greater part of the time that intervenes between the recovery from the operation and the recurrence of the disease, may be reckoned as so much added to life, as it is by the progress and consequences of the local disease that in the majority of cases the time of death is determined.

"3. Extension to lymphatic glands is not an insuperable objection."—*Ibid.*, p. 410.

CHAPTER XVIII.

EXTIRPATION OF THE EYEBALL.

REMOVAL OF THE ENTIRE CONTENTS OF THE ORBIT — REMOVAL OF THE
EYEBALL ALONE.

WHEN extirpation of the eyeball is undertaken on account of malignant disease, the whole of the contents of the orbit should be removed. Unless this be done, the important rule —always to endeavour to eradicate every part of the diseased structure by cutting beyond it, or by removing along with it some of the healthy tissues—could not be carried out. As this topic has been particularly dwelt on in the chapter on " Malignant Affections of the Eye," more need not be said.

Should the extirpation be required from disorganization arising out of a scrofulous affection, in which exhausting pain or profuse discharge are the urgent symptoms, the parts around may be so diseased, that their removal would be advisable. But it is very seldom, however, that such a case is met with.

In the Museum of the Royal College of Surgeons, is an eyeball that has undergone much pathological change, and was removed by Mr. Liston under the following circumstances. A man received a kick from a horse on the supra-orbital region, destroying vision in the corresponding eye. From that time he had frequent attacks of ocular pain, and twelve years afterwards, fistulous openings formed in several places around the eyeball, from which a constant discharge issued. After this had continued for ten years, and his health had begun to fail through the irritation, discharge, and occasional hæmorrhage, the eye was extirpated. The whole of the orbital plate of the frontal bone had been destroyed, so that the finger could rest on the dura mater beneath the anterior cerebral lobe. The patient completely recovered, and lived long after the operation.

The preparation is referred to in the catalogue, from which the above is taken, as "an eye extirpated after twenty-two years' disease, from a man sixty-five years old."

REMOVAL OF THE ENTIRE CONTENTS OF THE ORBIT.

It is a prevalent custom to place the patient on his back, but I prefer that he should lie on his side, to allow of the escape of the blood, whereby the operator sees what he is about, and is enabled to proceed safely and quickly.

Except circumstances demand it, there need be no external incisions, but if room be wanted on account of the size of the eyeball, or otherwise, the external commissure of the eyelids, including the conjunctiva, should be divided to the extent of half an inch, or more; and it may even be required to dissect up the divided integuments for more space. The eyelids should be retracted in whichever way may seem best,—by the fingers of an assistant, by the spring-wire retractor, or by bent spatulas.

When the eyeball cannot be laid hold of with the fingers, and it is seldom with enlargement that it may not, a large pair of tenaculum forceps must be substituted, because they can be readily shifted from place to place, and quickly laid aside when the fingers may be applied; some operators use a hook, others pass a few threads through it by a curved needle for the same purpose. With a small scalpel the reflections of the conjunctiva should be cut through,—whether first above, or first below, or in any other direction, must depend on circumstances; that should be done which is most likely to facilitate the subsequent steps of the operation. While dissecting at the upper edge of the orbit, the levator palpebræ should be divided as close to the tarsus as possible. The inferior oblique muscle should be severed close to its bony attachment; the trochlea of the superior oblique cut from the bone, and the eyeball turned from side to side, while the knife is swept around the orbital walls to divide the cellular connexions and the small vessels and nerves. The muscles, the optic and other nerves, and the ophthalmic vessels, are now to be divided at the apex of the orbit; to effect which the eyeball should be pulled forwards and inwards, and the scalpel or scissors used on the outer side, the slant of this wall of the orbit affording more room for the instruments. Lastly, the lacrymal gland is to be dissected away, together with whatever fat and areolar tissue may have been left.

I have not found that crooked instruments at all facilitate any steps of the operation, but that they rather constitute an impediment. Their introduction must have arisen from the assumption that they were superior, and never from a comparative trial of their merits on the dead or the living body. Besides sponging, syringing the orbit may be advantageous in cleaning away the blood and exposing surfaces.

The parts in the orbit in cases of melanosis are sometimes so altered from condensation, that the several structures can scarcely be recognised, and a tedious dissection with a scalpel and a pair of forceps may be required for the complete clearance.

The bleeding from the ophthalmic and other arteries, although very smart at first, readily ceases. Should it continue rather long, or after the application of cold water, a compress must be used. A tendency to oozing from the cavity may be checked by applying cotton wool or lint, wetted with a saturated solution of alum. Some surgeons invariably fill the orbit with lint; this is, I think, objectionable, and very likely to keep up suppuration.

The divided commissure should be united by suture, and water-dressing applied.

A patient demands much attention and careful watching

after the operation : several deaths have ensued. In one instance, I nearly lost a case from a consecutive attack of phlegmonous inflammation of the face and head.

REMOVAL OF THE EYEBALL ALONE.

The removal of the eyeball alone, by dissecting it from the "ocular tunic," was proposed almost simultaneously by Dr. O'Ferrall and M. Bonnet. Dr. O'Ferrall's suggestion is published in the "Dublin Journal of Medical Science" for March, 1841. M. Bonnet's recommendation was publicly announced just a year after.

When this may be done, it is certainly no small advantage; for, as its proposers have pointed out, hæmorrhage of any consequence may be avoided, and the parietes of the orbit not being stripped, there is less chance of dangerous inflammation. It is particularly applicable in non-malignant affections; whenever, indeed, it becomes necessary to get rid of the eyeball, and it alone.

The operation is remarkably simple. The effects are so slight that convalescence is generally established in a few days. I much fear that these circumstances have caused it to be abused; indeed, I am aware from personal knowledge that very many eyes have been sacrificed. Several times I have interfered successfully. However, I am happy to say that the *furore* is much reduced, and I hope that shortly this very valuable addition to ophthalmic surgery will be only legitimately employed.

The operation may be done thus, which is O'Ferrall's plan —: The eyelids having been retracted, the conjunctiva is dissected off, with forceps and scissors, close to its ocular attachment; the recti and oblique muscles taken up with a hook, as in the operation for strabismus, and divided at their insertions; the tunic detached by a probe or hook from the eyeball, which should now be turned aside, and the optic nerve cut through. I have usually adopted this.

It is recommended by Mr. Dixon as a more expeditious

method, after dividing the conjunctiva, to cut through with forceps and scissors the external rectus, the tendon of which an assistant seizes, and by it pulls the eyeball inwards; then to divide with scissors alone, in the following order, the superior rectus, superior oblique, inferior rectus, then the optic nerve, and subsequently the internal rectus, and whatever vascular or other attachments might exist. This is less applicable when the eyeball is enlarged. Moreover, it demands an assistant.

It is a material point that as much conjunctiva be left as possible, the reasons for which are given in the chapter on "Artificial Eye." Some surgeons approximate the edges of this membrane, or adapt them when they admit of it, by one or two sutures.

Usually there is so little bleeding from the central artery of the retina, when the optic nerve is divided, that attention to it is not needed; but I have seen very acute hæmorrhage, on a few occasions, requiring well-adjusted pressure to control. Except, then, a compress be at once applied, a patient ought not to be left alone, but watched.

A description of the ocular tunic, accompanied by the sketch of a dissection, will be found in the chapter on "Tumours."

CHAPTER XIX.

ARTIFICIAL EYE.

CONDITIONS MOST SUITED—ADVANTAGES—PREPARATIONS—MODE OF
APPLICATION—THE WEARING NOT ATTENDED WITH PAIN.

THE improvements which have of late been effected by the
principal artists of London and Paris in the manufacture of
artificial eyes, especially in the method of colouring them,
render the imitation so perfect that not only may the casual
observer be deceived, but even the professional man who is
conversant with ophthalmic practice may not detect the substitute readily.

An artificial eye is but a very light, almost hemispherical
shell, made to represent the front of the living feature. The

FIG. 114.

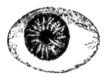

shape and the size must vary to suit different cases, and this
adaptation and correspondence demand much more nicety than
is necessary merely to match the colour. The entire surface,
including the edges, should be enamelled; but it is a common
practice among agents for sale who are not makers, to grind
the shell to the required size without afterwards restoring
the desired smoothness, for which the action of fire is required.

H H

There are not more than three or four houses in Europe that have attained high proficiency in the art. Among these are Messrs. Grossmith and Desjardins, and Messrs. Gray and Halford, of No. 7, Goswell-road, Clerkenwell. The latter firm has supplied many of my patients to my entire satisfaction.

All, however, does not rest with the mechanic: the best mechanism will fail in fullest effect, unless the globe of the eye retain sufficient fulness to be moved by the muscles, and so to act in concert with its fellow. Those eyes, then, that are just a little below the natural size, are best adapted to receive the enamel : an enlarged one must therefore be reduced by operation, and staphylomatous projections must be excised. With very little more than a mere button of collapsed tissues, I have seen artificial eyes that few persons would have detected, except from their imperfect movement. Some degree of motion is obtained through the conjunctival reflections by the influence of the recti muscles; and the eyelids themselves also impart some vertical action.

When the eyeball has been removed by dissecting it from its cellular sheath, a limited degree of motion is sometimes got, especially for a few months after the operation, through the conjunctiva and the pad that remain; a fact which points to the importance of saving the conjunctiva. But when the swelling and infiltration have passed away, and especially when the natural wasting of the tissues ensues, this is greatly reduced and often lost. But an artificial eye that is motionless, is certainly very much less objectionable than the distressing vacancy of an empty orbit, or the disfiguring patch that is worn to conceal it.

When the entire contents of the orbit are taken away, we have the worst condition for adaptation.

With collapse of the eye before adult age, the orbit seldom attains full growth, and the eyelids are similarly influenced. The earlier in life that this has occurred, the less will be the development, and the case will be proportionally less adapted for the assistance of art. This points to the advantage of preventing such an occurrence in staphyloma by the timely reduction of the enlargement, and thereby the saving of healthy parts; and it is one of the many reasons against indiscriminate extirpation of diseased eyes.

The false eye may be of essential service in keeping the eyelids in their natural position, and preventing the cilia from turning in and irritating the parts that they may touch; in placing the puncta in a more natural position for conveying away the tears; in acting as a defence against intruding bodies, which are apt to be retained, and produce irritation, and may thereby sympathetically affect the other eye; and as a means of keeping the orbital cavity free from collections of lacrymal secretions.

Some preliminary surgical measures may be required, such as the removal of bands and bridles, or of thickened conjunctiva, or of ectropium: I have prepared a squinting stump by setting it straight. But extensive adhesion between the eyelids, or of the eyelids to the eyeball, may render the application inadmissible.

By the bursting of a gun a man lost the right eyeball, a part of the outer wall of the orbit, and some of the skin of the cheek. The cicatrisation on the face produced a well-marked ectropium of the outer portion of the lower eyelid, and, besides, pulled the upper eyelid considerably downwards, and threw its cilia on the conjunctiva lining the floor of the orbit. The deformity was necessarily very great. I was applied to for relief from the annoyance occasioned by the constant discharge of tears over the cheek, and the irritation produced by the cilia. An artificial eye was placed as well as could be, so as to give an indication of the kind of operation required to restore the eyelids to their proper places, and to allow the full benefits that such an eye, well fitted, might afford. This having been ascertained, I left it to my patient to decide whether that description of operation should be done which would enable him to wear the false eye, by which, most probably, the lacrymal secretion would be carried away through the natural channel (this, of course, depending on the degree of accuracy with which the edges of the lids could be brought to bear on the surface of the enamel), and his countenance also improved; or whether the lacrymation alone should be attended to, by the removal of the lacrymal gland. He was also given to understand that in case the first operation failed to arrest the discharge over the cheek, the lacrymal gland might then be extirpated. The first proposition was preferred. I removed a wedge-shaped piece, including skin, muscle, cartilage, and conjunctiva, from the most everted.portion of the lower eyelid, and dissected the skin of the cheek from its attachment sufficiently to admit of being drawn up. I applied sutures, raised and supported the cheek with strips of plaster. By this the ectropium was entirely removed, and the edge of the tarsus brought nearly to a straight line. The upper eyelid being released, the levator palpebræ acted, and the cilia were righted. In a few days the sutures and the plasters were taken away. Three weeks later, the false eye was applied, and my expectations were realized, for the tears passed by the natural conduits; and although the stump of the eyeball was small, and the movement of the artificial eye necessarily limited, my patient and his friends were agreed as to the improvement effected in personal appearance.

The eye is to be inserted in the following manner:—It is to be wetted, and the broad or outer end first passed under the upper eyelid, slid as far as it will readily go, and kept there with the forefinger of the one hand, while the under eyelid is drawn down with the other hand till the lower part slips in. For removal, the lower eyelid must be depressed, and the finger-nail, a toothpick, the head of a hair-pin, a little hook, or any small blunt instrument (Mr. Halford supplies a neat little spatula for the purpose), passed under the edge of the eye, and made to lift it forwards, when the whole will slip out. Care should be taken to receive it in the hand, or on a handkerchief, or on a bed, as a fall on the ground would fracture it. A person soon learns to do this for himself, after a few lessons quietly, and slowly, and encouragingly given, and children acquire the knack quickly. Occasionally it is necessary, in the first instance, to allow it to remain in for a few hours only; and it may even be requisite to begin with one of a smaller size, or to use several in gradation. When deemed necessary at the first introduction not to remove it for several days, the lower eyelid should be depressed, and the lower edge lifted forwards with something, at least once in the twenty-four hours, to allow the tears that are apt to collect behind, to escape.

An artificial eye requires great cleanliness, and should be removed every night. This cessation of use is further necessary to prevent ulceration of those parts on which its edges rest. If the eyeball be much reduced, the interior of the eyelids should, if possible, be syringed with tepid water every morning. Should there be an habitual unnatural conjunctival secretion, or should that be excited by the pressure of the enamel, a weak astringent lotion used night and morning may remove or lessen it.

Patients always couple the idea of pain with this appliance, and from its supposed size, and the belief that the sensitiveness which belongs to the eye only in its integrity is still retained. With the destruction of the cornea, the greater portion of the sensibility is destroyed. Instances have, however, occurred in my own practice, where the false eye caused too much uneasiness to be worn. I know of two cases in which suppuration of the reduced stump occurred in consequence of continuing to wear the eye when it produced irritation. When the eyeball is merely atrophied, in which case some of the true corneal tissue yet remains, irritation is apt to occur, except there be a sufficient hollow to prevent the cornea from being touched. When this provision cannot be secured, the cornea must be excised.

After the gloss is lost and the surface roughened, a new eye is needed; for if the damaged one be still used, irritation of the eyelids is set up. The average period of wear is about twelve months.

CHAPTER XX.

ENTOZOA WITHIN THE EYEBALL, AND ABOUT THE OCULAR APPENDAGES—CYSTS
WITHIN THE CHAMBERS OF THE EYEBALL — CONDITION RESEMBLING A
CYST.

ENTOZOA WITHIN THE EYEBALL, AND ABOUT THE OCULAR
APPENDAGES.

THE cysticercus cellulosæ, well known as the so-called
measles in pigs, has been found in many parts of the human
frame, especially in the cellular tissue of muscles, generally of
the Glutei, Iliacus internus, Psoæ, and Quadriceps extensor
cruris : it sometimes also takes its habitat about the eye.

It may not be uninteresting to delineate this parasite, and
I have for the purpose borrowed the annexed illustrations from
the article " Entozoa," by Professor Owen, in the " Cyclopædia
of Anatomy and Physiology."

FIG. 115.   FIG. 116.

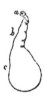 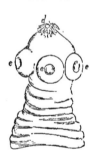

The smaller figure shows a full-sized entozoon in its cyst :
a indicates the head, *b* the neck or body, and *c* the dilated

vesicular tail. The larger one exhibits the head sufficiently magnified to display the uncinated rostellum, or proboscis *d*, for irritation and adhesion, and the suctorious discs, *e e e*, for imbibing the surrounding nutriment.

While it is confined to the eyelids, or to the external part of the eye, danger does not impend, but should it exist in the interior of the eyeball, the organ is endangered, and, as far as records allow me to speak, would be sacrificed, unless the cysticercus were removed.

A child, two years and seven months old, whose vision was perfect, was brought to Mr. Canton at the Westminister Ophthalmic Hospital, with a small yellowish tumour of the consistence of soft jelly, near the inner canthus of the eye, lying between the conjunctiva and the sclerotica. A snip of the conjunctiva gave exit to serum and a Cysticercus. At the end of two or three days the edges of the wound were united.

The entozoon was about the size of a garden-pea, and presented at one part of its circumference a circular opaque body, projecting into the interior of the vesicle; the retracted head and neck. I copy these illustrations of the animalcule deprived of its cyst, from Mr. Canton's publication in the "Lancet" for July, 1848.

Fig. 117.   Fig. 118.

The natural size is observed. In the first sketch, *a* shows the head, *b* the neck or body, *c* the tail vesicle. In the second, the head and body are retracted within the tail vesicle.

A very analogous case occurred in the practice of M. Baum of Dantzig, and is reported in the "Annales d'Oculistique,"

t. 11, p. 69.   The patient, a female, was twenty-three years old; the tumour, which had been noticed for six months, was at the internal angle of the eye, in the sclerotica; the conjunctiva covering it was thickened. A depression remained in the sclerotica after its removal. Vision was unimpaired.

In the same journal is the record of another case by Hoering, in a girl seven years old; the cyst adhered to the sclerotica, towards the external angle of the eye. Sight was saved.

Mr. Estlin of Bristol, published in vol. xxii. of the "London Medical Gazette," a similar instance that occurred in a girl six years old.

The Cysticercus has also been found in the subcutaneous cellular tissue of the upper eyelid, as recorded by Sichel, in the "Revue Medico-Chirurgicale," April, 1847; as well as in the neighbourhood of the palpebræ.

Great interest attached to the internal implication of the eye, from the attendant risk, and till lately, the forlorn hope of recovery. A man, forty-five years old, applied to me at the Ophthalmic Hospital in consequence of frequent pain that had existed in his right eye for six weeks; the sight had been quite lost a year previously, from a sudden attack of inflammation. The conjunctiva was much inflamed, the cornea, vascular and semi-opaque. At his next attendance I saw in the anterior chamber what I took for an opaque capsule, which slipped into the posterior chamber when I commenced to examine the eye, and could not be got to its former place by any change of position or shaking of the head. The man, who was quite aware of this shifting, which he said occurred many times in the day, was directed to apply when the body was visible. The following sketch of it expresses all that a woodcut can convey. The cornea is supposed to be semi-opaque. In the original the pupil was not by any means so visible.

To relieve the pain the body was extracted, and proved to be a Cysticercus. The cornea healed readily, and cleared very considerably; the pain was removed, but of course vision was

not restored. The crystalline lens must have been absorbed,
or the Cysticercus could not have passed so readily through
the pupil. The opacity of the cornea obscured the only means

FIG. 119.

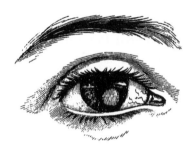

of diagnosis—the alteration in the form of the vesicle, by the
descent and retraction of the tail.

Mr. Logan's remarkable case, originally published by him
in a pamphlet, and afterwards recorded in the "Medical
Gazette," vol. xii. p. 110, by Dr. Mackenzie, possesses many points
of value. A girl seven years old was the subject of it. From
August to January there had been several inflammatory attacks
in the left eye, producing slight opacity of the lower part
of the cornea. Then a semi-transparent body, from which
hung a slender process, with a slightly bulbous extremity like
the proboscis of the common house-fly, sometimes retracted,
sometimes protruded, was seen loose in the anterior chamber.
When floating, the vesicle is uppermost. Objects placed above
the level of the eye could be distinctly seen, but not when
placed below, or directly in front, showing that in the latter
positions, the rays of light were merely obstructed, and that
the eye was not damaged. Increase of size was not observed
by Mr. Logan, and he trusted that its natural period of
existence coming to a close would free the eye from the
danger of disorganization. Various means were suggested
for killing the insect in its situation, that it might be afterwards removed or left, according to circumstances ; such as
electric or galvanic shocks passed through the eye, oil of

turpentine rubbed round the orbital region, and given internally, or the administration of some vegetable bitter known
to be inimical to the life of parasitical animals. The sequel
is given in Dr. Mackenzie's work. Several weeks afterwards,
extraction was attempted by Dr. Robertson, of Edinburgh.
The child struggled so much that the cornea was opened,
the lens was forced out, and the hydatid ruptured. After a
long interval she was induced to open the eye, and the Cysticercus was brought away in shreds; a portion of the iris
remained in the wound, but nothing would induce her to
allow Dr. Robertson to attempt to return it. The eye healed,
and the cornea remained clear, except at the cicatrix: there
it was only semi-transparent. The pupil was elliptical in
consequence of adhesion of the iris to the cicatrix, and was
occupied by opaque capsule. The power of recognizing the
presence of light remained.

There cannot be a doubt as to the propriety of extracting
any entozoon from the eye that can be readily got at, on the
earliest recognition of its existence. The cornea should be
opened to an extent equal to the size of the mass which is
to be removed.

Directly that the knife is withdrawn, the blunt canula
forceps, the cross-spring, or any other appropriate ones, should
be used, without letting the eyelids free. In other respects
the proceeding is to be conducted as for the extraction of a
cataract. In Mr. Logan's operation, the unfortunate issue
arose from the perversity of the patient; chloroform should
therefore be given whenever a Cysticercus is to be removed
from within the eye of a child, or any irresolute individual.

In Dr. W. Sœmmerring's case, which has been often quoted
by writers, from having been one of the earliest, if not the
first ever recorded, the parasite was extracted alive; it moved
about in lukewarm water for half an hour, and then gradually
turned opaque, and white. In the original, given in the " Isis
Von Oken" for 1830, the result of the operation is not mentioned; the record seems more with a view of illustrating
a point in natural history than for the advancement of

medicine. As in Mr. Logan's case, the Cysticercus was observed after active inflammation, which subsequently subsided, and it scarcely produced inconvenience, except when moving about. In seven months it had doubled its volume, and when extracted was as big as a pea. The subject was a girl aged eighteen.

In a case which Rosas quotes of a lad fourteen years old, who was under Neumann, the eye was otherwise healthy, and dilatation of the pupil caused the Cysticercus to quit the anterior chamber and lie across this aperture, from which the further use of belladonna could not free it; the new position caused much pain. The animalcule was depressed and the pain was comparatively removed, but suppuration of the eyeball ensued.

The most satisfactory case of extraction of a Cysticercus from within the eye, on record, is to be found in a communication to the Medico-Chirurgical Society by Dr. Mackenzie, and is published in vol. xxxii. of the "Transactions." The girl, who was sixteen years old, applied at the Glasgow Eye Infirmary. Inflammation of the eye was the first symptom. Vision would have been perfect but for the partial obstruction by the Cysticercus to the rays of light. Eighteen days after recognition of the animalcule, the cornea was opened to the extent of three-twentieths of an inch, and it was removed, and received into a tea-spoonful of warm blood-serum; but its movements were not so lively as when transferred to tepid water. Next day the patient felt quite well, the eye appeared natural, and she said she saw as well with it as with the other. No reaction followed. The author thinks that the attack of ophthalmia immediately preceding the appearance of the hydatid, was owing to the development of its ovum in one of the blood-vessels of the iris or choroid; and that the inflammation ceased suddenly as soon as it dropped into the anterior chamber, where it lived at its ease, amply furnished with sustenance from the aqueous humour, and unrestrained by any external cyst, such as that which surrounds the same entozoon when lodged among the muscles. The truth of this theory would seem to be confirmed by the presence of inflammation in the majority of the other cases prior to the full development of the insect, and it might have existed in each instance for any proof that we have to the contrary

After a Cysticercus cellulosæ has destroyed the eye, mischief is not certainly over, even though its extraction has been accomplished, as the morbid action excited by its presence may continue. Mr. Canton watched one for several months previous to its removal; the symptoms were gradual diminution of vision, consequent upon an increasing nebulous state of the cornea, with slight inflammation of the conjunctiva and the sclerotica. By degrees the central part of the cornea became more opaque than the circumference. Almost constant darting pain in and around the eye was unrelieved by the various modes of treatment that were resorted to. An opening was made by Mr. Guthrie, through the most prominent part of the cornea, and a Cysticercus in a perfect state escaped. Relief ensued. The circumstances of the case, six or seven months after, appearing to require a similar procedure, the cornea was again opened, and what was supposed to be a Cysticercus removed, but this most likely was the crystalline lens, a close examination of the body not having been made. Three years afterwards there was constant pain about the eye, and such symptoms as induced Mr. Guthrie to suspect the presence of another Cysticercus. The cornea was again divided, and vitreous humour alone escaped. The operation removed the pain.

The following case, narrated by Dr. Mende, is copied into the " Medical Times and Gazette" for March 23rd, 1861, from " Gräfe's Archiv für Ophthalmologie," vol. vii. p. 122.

" The wife of a shoemaker, 25 years of age, of healthy appearance, and far gone with her first child, applied to the author on account of an obscurity of vision. On inspection a Cysticercus was perceived with the utmost distinctness in the anterior chamber of the right eye. The worm was of a delicate white, the bladder being so transparent that the brownish iris could be seen through it. It was of the size and shape of a small pea, and below was a process which was somewhat whiter and less transparent than the rest of the worm; and from this, projected a white untransparent neck, about a quarter of a . line in length, having at its extremity a small round head, which, examined by a lens, exhibited lateral swellings, and resembled the head of tænia. The bladder of the worm covered the lower part of the pupil, leaving this free for two-thirds of its circumference, while in appearance it did not differ from that of the other eye. The worm was motionless, and movements were not induced when the patient moved her head, or when a strong light was directed on the eye. At different examinations during the next three days, the worm was found to have assumed different positions, and various shapes. It was very interesting to observe through a lens how it thrust its head here and there, just as a leech, before it fixed on a spot to commence sucking from. When it attached to the anterior of the iris its neck was bent backwards, and the bladder almost completely obstructed the pupil; a slight quivering movement, like that seen in a sucking leech, being imparted to the tube-like process of the animal, while the bladder remained motionless. Sometimes the process was distended into a bladder much smaller than the other, below which it was placed, and from which it was separated as if by a ligature. The woman was confined on the third day after being seen, and continued under observation for about three weeks before an operation was performed, the animal frequently changing its position, attaching itself to the various surrounding parts, without seeming to inflict any injury on them by its sucking process. The pupil at last became narrower than the opposite one, while its form was converted into an oval, and vision got more and more impaired. Fearing the production of iritis, a linear incision was made, and the worm, discharged with the aqueous humour, was carefully captured. It was placed in tepid water, but exhibited no movement. The wound in the cornea soon healed under the employment of ice, and the eye has regained its perfect powers. The worm, three months after its extraction, has contracted from eight to five millimètres in length."

The Cysticercus is also found in the vitreous humour, and in the retina. In these situations it appears to occur more frequently in Germany than elsewhere; at all events the best descriptions of it are given by German authors. Seen by the ophthalmoscope, it appears as a roundish tumour, of a blue, green, or gray hue, bearing different relations to the retinal vessels, according as it is situated in front or in the substance of the retina. It is covered by a very fine transparent membrane, to which a certain diagnostic value is attached. In the " Archiv für Ophthalmologie," band iv. abt. 2, are the details of a case in which Professor Gräfe removed a Cysticercus from the vitreous humour. The method adopted was as follows. He first performed iridectomy; at a subsequent period he extracted the lens, which was clear and transparent; and finally he succeeded in removing the Cysticercus; the patient recovering from the three operations with a fair amount of vision.

Mr. Gulliver has given a good general account of the Cysticercus cellulosæ, with illustrations, in vol. xxiv. of the " Medico-Chirurgical Transactions." Dr. Knox also has written on it in the " Lancet " for June 16th, 1838.

Other entozoa have been discovered in the human eye, but from their rarity and diminutiveness, being mostly microscopic, few persons have detected them, and they possess scarcely any surgical interest.

The Filaria oculi humani, was so called by Dr. Nordmann of Odessa, who discovered two of them in the fluid of a degenerated cataract which was extracted from an elderly woman. With a microscope their true nature was determined, and in one which was uninjured, its organization was clearly discernible. Specimens of the genus monostoma and distoma have also been discovered in the lens by the same observer, and by Drs. Gescheidt and Ammon.

The Filaria Medinensis, or Guinea worm, may infest the eye. According to Rhind, this worm was known at a very early period, the first mention of it having been by Agatharchides, four or five hundred years before Christ.   He mentions also that Plutarch described it very accurately.   It has been extracted from under the conjunctiva of a negress, and from its frequently infesting the inhabitants of the tropics, and occurring in numbers in the same individual, it is not unlikely that it takes its resting-place more frequently about the eye than the rare mention of it by authors would lead us to infer.   I saw an example in King's College Hospital, in the leg of a lad who had just returned from the coast of Africa.   It generally lies in a coil, producing much itching, and afterwards abscesses form.   When the head protrudes, it should be secured with strong thread, and the process of extraction commenced by coiling the worm around some small substance by gentle turns daily, and continued till the whole is removed.   Without great care it will be broken.   When the head does not protrude, the worm must be reached by incision, secured, and wound out.

Many other observers have verified the existence of these and of other living bodies in the eye, some even between the layers of the cornea.   The Echinococcus oculi humani has been discovered between the choroid and the retina.   " Notes sur les Helminthes des Yeux, dans les Archives de Médecine comparée," par P. Rayer : Paris 1843, p. 67-154.

In the chapter on tumours, an instance has been given of the occurrence of hydatids in the orbit, p. 277.

An entozoon that infests the Meibomian glands remains to be mentioned; but its presence, like that of some just described, is not of any surgical interest, and I allude to it merely to complete the number of those that have been found about the eye.   It is the " Steatozoon folliculorum " of Mr. Erasmus Wilson,—an animalcule formed in the oil-tubes whenever there exists any disposition to the unnatural accumulation of their contents.   It is very minute, being the forty-fifth of an inch in length.   In form and shape, in the perfect state, it is like a caterpillar, having a distinct head with feelers, a chest with four pairs of legs, and a long tail.   In Mr. Wilson's work on the " Healthy Skin," all relating to the history of this little insect is narrated.   It appears that Dr. Simon discovered it; but his descriptions and figures were imperfect; several points of entomological importance were overlooked, and Mr. Wilson has completed our knowledge of the subject, and changed the name of the insect to that it now bears.

CYSTS WITHIN THE CHAMBERS OF THE EYEBALL.

A cyst in these situations is liable to be mistaken for a dislocated lens, or for the Cysticercus cellulosæ, both of which it much resembles; the chief characteristic distinction being that the cyst is attached. Should there be slight opacity of the cornea, it might not be possible to distinguish between them, except from the history of the case.

Unless it exist at birth, a cyst generally has a traumatic origin; a wound or a blow on the eye inducing it. Either of the chambers may be the seat of the growth, the iris being generally the part involved. The increase of a cyst, although slow, is, I believe, almost certain, and as it enlarges, unless it be destroyed, the disorganization of the eye from pressure or irritation is inevitable. We have abundant evidence that the mere early evacuation of the cyst contents by an incision, will generally suffice; the disease will be conquered, and the eye will recover its integrity. Successful cases from my own practice have been published in the medical periodicals. I think that the incision should be as extensive as can be accomplished, in order to afford free contact of the aqueous fluid. I have always used the smallest iris knife. A second incision has been successful when the first has failed. Even a third has been required. This practice, therefore, should be fairly tried, and not prematurely abandoned.

The following very instructive case is recorded in the "Mirror" of the "Lancet" for June 12th, 1852. A child, five years old, thrust the point of a fork into his eye, from which accident he speedily recovered. About a year and a half after, uneasiness and inflammation induced the parents to apply for advice: there was now in the anterior chamber a large transparent body, at first supposed to be a dislocated lens, but ultimately recognised as a very delicate, watery cyst protruding from the posterior chamber into the anterior; the lower part of the iris having been detached from its ciliary connexion, and pressed upwards. The cyst was punctured; a considerable quantity of fluid escaped, and it collapsed. The pupil lost much of its irregularity, and the interval formed by the separation of the iris became less. Soon afterwards the cyst refilled, and in two months it was re-punctured through the cornea by Mr. Jones, who had not seen the case before. After a few days inflammation followed, and according to the report, " There was, at the bottom of the collapsed cyst, a small quantity of yellow matter or lymph, with a minute vascular ramification upon its anterior wall." The eye became worse, from some indiscretion on the part of the child's mother. Leeches were applied, and calomel and Dover's powder were given. Some of " the matter of the cyst worked its way outwards at the junction of the cornea and sclerotica by a narrow passage." The mercury was discontinued after all the matter was absorbed. The cyst shrank in a manner that left little trace of it, and sight was quite restored.

A somewhat similar case is recorded by Dr. Mackenzie:— A lady was affected with considerable pain in one of her eyes, which presented the appearance of a small vesicle pushing into the anterior chamber from under the ciliary margin of the iris, behind the lower edge of the cornea. The vesicle gradually increased, separating the iris more and more from the choroid, and as it caused severe pain he punctured it through the cornea, with an iris knife. A minute quantity of fluid was discharged, and it immediately contracted so much that it was no longer visible, and the pain was removed. It refilled and appeared in its former situation, but was larger than before. He punctured it a second and a third time, at the respective intervals of six and eight weeks. After this it did not fill again, the iris returned to its natural place, and vision was preserved.

Mr. Dalrymple gives the following particulars of one in a

I I

girl twenty-five years old. A semi-transparent cyst attached to the iris and to the posterior surface of the cornea, partly hid the pupil. It was punctured and evacuated of its pellucid fluid, without the aqueous humour being lost. In a few days it refilled, was again punctured, and now collapsed completely. Its walls were very thin, and through them could be seen an apparent aperture in the iris, which led Mr. Dalrymple to believe that the cyst originated in the iris, or from behind it, and elevated its serous covering into a watery cyst. " I am aware," he writes, " a serous covering to the iris is denied by modern anatomists, but in that opinion I cannot yet acquiesce." To admit this explanation we must suppose that two cysts were present.

When a cyst is too large or too dense to be reduced by the above treatment, the only chance of saving the eye is by removing it; but this is fraught with danger directly and remotely. Except the base be very small,. and attached near the pupillary margin of the iris, separation of this membrane from the ciliary connexion is apt to ensue during the attempt. At all times opacity of the lens and its capsule is likely to be produced.

Mr. Tyrrell gives an example of a cyst growing in the anterior chamber, in consequence of injury from the beard of an ear of corn, that well illustrates the danger of inflammation from extraction.

The patient was a girl : the cyst was about the size of a pea, glistening, and attached near the margin of the pupil, with the motions of which it somewhat interfered, but vision was good. As it increased and excited inflammation, Mr. Tyrrell was induced to operate. The cornea was opened, the cyst drawn out, and the portion of iris to which it was attached cut off. The wound in the cornea healed readily. Active inflammation of the eyeball ensued, in consequence, it is said, of imprudent exposure; the other eye sympathised, and was similarly affected, but to a slighter degree, " exhibiting inflammation of the iris and aqueous membrane." After many weeks passed in treatment, the pupil became very much contracted, and the iris adhered to the capsule of the lens ; however, large bodies could be discerned. The eye sympathetically affected recovered perfectly.

I saw an eye lost by suppuration in an attempt to remove a cyst, which in all probability could have been destroyed by puncturing.

Mr. Dalrymple mentions that the late Mr. Scott removed from the anterior chamber a cyst from which was growing a hair that resembled an abortive eyelash.

In the following case, extraction of the cyst was demanded, from urgent symptoms ; often puncturing it had been inefficient.

A girl, six years of age, wounded the right eyeball with a pair of scissors, and destroyed vision for all practical purposes. At eighteen years of age, she became one of my hospital patients, with the following symptoms. The eyeball was a little shrunken and inflamed ; a cicatrix on the upper part of the cornea, passing from the inner margin nearly to the opposite side, indicated the position of the injury. The iris had not prolapsed. The upper half of the anterior chamber, to the very circumference, was occupied by a semi-opaque cyst, which seemed to be connected with the cicatrix in the cornea, and certainly had an attachment to the margin of the pupil, which was much contracted and partly covered.

The cornea was not pressed forward, but the increased space required for the morbid growth was obtained at the expense of the iris, which was thrown back, and the portion of which corresponding to the centre and greatest convexity of the cyst was rendered very concave, and attenuated. It could not be ascertained if the crystalline lens were present. Pain about the eye and orbit had induced relief to be sought. I punctured the cyst through the cornea with the iris knife, and fluid escaped, it was supposed from the cyst alone. A decided reduction followed this treatment, but the effect was temporary. Repetitions of it on two other occasions, at intervals of about a month, were not more effectual; indeed, they seemed to have been rather prejudicial in exciting the growth of the part, for it increased in all its dimensions, and the pupil was covered. The eyeball became very vascular, there was constant pain in the eye, and occasionally headache. I recommended extraction, but this was not assented to till the symptoms were worse. Sympathetic irritation soon set in, involving the sight, the symptoms being intolerance of light to a slight degree, and then excessive irritability of the retina which prevented the eye from being used at all, with paroxysmal pain. I feared that partial excision of the tumour would not be sufficient, and I determined to remove every part of it. The extents of the attachments could not be clearly ascertained, and it was probable that to effect my object, such external damage might be inflicted as would risk suppuration of the eyeball. Rather than do this, therefore, I resolved to remove the front of the eye, if any difficulty should supervene. I made the upper section of the cornea, as for cataract, passing the knife through the body of the cyst. Along with the aqueous humour, which was small in quantity, there escaped a transparent jelly-like substance, that was evidently the cyst contents. The flap of the cornea was held down by an assistant, and the cyst seized with a pair of tenaculum forceps, and after a little trial drawn away without any difficulty. The iris rent, at the part where it was rendered thin by distension. No vitreous humour was lost. The crystalline lens was supposed to be absent. The cut surfaces of the cornea were adjusted, and the eyelids retained together by adhesive plaster.

The cyst wall was composed of delicate fibrous tissue. It seemed to spring from a minute whitish cicatrix on the iris.   .

The corneal wound healed in a week. Vision had, of course, been destroyed. There was no trace of pupil. Already had the woman received benefit, for she could use the left eye without discomfort, and the third day after the operation she had not any pain in the right, only a sense of soreness.

Closely allied to a cyst in appearance is a condition of the eye arising from a wound at the margin of the cornea. The corneal tissue does not heal, and the aqueous humour is retained by a sac or cyst under the conjunctiva, probably formed by a condensation of the sub-conjunctival tissue, which forms a boundary of the anterior chamber.

A girl received a cut at the outside of the eye, and several years after she was brought to town for my opinion. I saw what I supposed to be a cystic tumour on the eye, which was so large as to interfere with the movements of the eyelids, and produced all the irritating effects of a large staphyloma, even to involving the other eye in sympathetic ophthalmitis. I was induced to perform the operation of "extirpation." The vitreous humour was healthy, and so were the posterior parts; "abscission" might, therefore, have been done, but this pathological state of the eye was new to me, and I did what appeared to me to be the more safe treatment.

It is, I think, a formation of this kind, to which Mr. Dalrymple alluded in speaking of a cyst that was produced at the point of puncture of the cornea, after the use of the needle for cataract.

CHAPTER XXI.

REMOVAL OF OPACITIES OF THE CORNEA BY SURGICAL OPERATION. —
TRANSPLANTATION OF THE CORNEA.

THE ingenious proposal of restoring transparency to the
cornea by removing that portion of its texture in which the
opacity resides, is far from being of recent date. "The vulgar,"
writes Dr. Mackenzie, "have a notion that specks can be
removed by operation, but by medical men that has generally
been regarded as impossible. Mead, indeed (who wrote in
1762), speaks of paring specks every day with a knife; and
Darwin (who wrote in 1801) of trephining them; while
Dieffenbach has actually cut out a leucoma from the centre
of the cornea, and brought the edges of the incision together
with sutures. Notwithstanding such high authority, we may
safely regard as generally impracticable any attempt to operate
on specks of the cornea, except when the opacity is merely
a crust of oxide or carbonate of lead deposited on the surface
of an ulcer of the cornea, in consequence of a solution of Acetas
plumbi having been employed as a collyrium. It sometimes
happens that such a crust remains after the ulcer is cicatrized;
and I have repeatedly succeeded in lifting it off with a sharp
point of a probe, leaving the cornea beneath nebulous merely,
and susceptible of clearing completely under the continued
application of Vinum opii."

Within a late period this operation of paring the cornea has
been somewhat revived, and there has been even a controversy
in the French capital concerning the priority of the claims
to its introduction.

In the "London and Edinburgh Monthly Journal of Medical Science," for March, 1844, is a memoir by Dr. R. Hamilton, in which it is stated that in the session 1833-4, Professor Rosas operated on two cases; in the one, the greater number of the layers of the cornea was taken away, and failure ensued; in the other, the external and opaque layers only were removed: the wound healed without opacity, and after six months the cornea was transparent. It appears, too, that in subsequent years the operation was performed without marked success. In 1841-2 Dr. Gulz drew public attention to the following case.

A tailor, twenty-eight years of age, presented himself at the Vienna Clinic under the care of Dr. Gulz, in the session of 1841-2, having been two years previously attacked with purulent ophthalmia. The left eye was staphylomatous. In the right, the external layers of the cornea had been more or less inflamed, ulcerated, or destroyed, and a whitish and opaque deposit was substituted in their place. There was ready discrimination between light and darkness. It was thought that the opacity did not extend through the whole depth of the cornea, and that the case was a fair one for slicing off the opaque portions. The operation was performed by Dr. Gulz, under the direction of M. Von Rosas, the instruments employed being the cataract knife of Rosas, with a double-cutting edge, and the pyramidal knife of Beer, together with a small-toothed forceps, and a delicate pair of scissors. The eyelids of the patient were fixed by the fingers of an assistant, and the knife, frequently introduced, was made to pass through the external layers, and gradually to the internal parts of the cornea, the hand following the motion of the eyeball. The manœuvre required to be repeatedly and adroitly performed, until the transparent part of the cornea was at length reached; when, by the help of the different instruments, it was bared to the extent of a line and a half in diameter. The innermost layers of the cornea being fortunately uninjured throughout, the anterior chamber was not opened. The operation occupied about a quarter of an hour, and after its completion vision was improved to such an extent that the patient could perceive different shades of colours, and small objects, such as the hands of a watch, with facility. The subsequent treatment consisted in the application of plasters over the eyelids, to prevent their motion, and the application of cold and iced water. At the end of eight days the plasters were removed, and a collyrium first of a solution of hydrochlorate of potash (gr. 1 to the ounce), and subsequently of a solution of muriate of ammonia, was used. All went on promisingly for the first four weeks, after which the eye was attacked by ophthalmia, which was soon subdued, and in a few days, to the great joy of all parties, vision was found to be uninjured. Near-sightedness was the result.

I learn from the same number of the "London and Edinburgh Journal" that Malgaigne has published a long and learned paper on the subject, in the "Journal de Chirurgie," in which he states, on the authority of Blandin, that a couple of travelling oculists in France have for fourteen years been in the habit of performing this operation with varying success, putting forth no claims to invention, but affirming that they only followed a practice which had been successful before their days. Two memoirs are alluded to, one by M. Rognetta, in "Les Annales de Thérapeutique," and one by M. Desmarres, in "Les Annales d'Oculistique." To Saint Ives is ascribed the first notice of the operation in medical records, and opinions laudatory and condemnatory of the practice are quoted. Baron Larry thought it worth a trial, and believed that, in opacities of the cornea of a certain degree of thickness, the membrane may be thinned down by repeated strokes of a long bistoury. He had performed the operation upon a young lady at Toulon, removing an old opacity which covered the whole extent of the cornea, and the patient ever after saw fairly.

I must warn those who are unaware of the almost incredible manner in which the cornea is capable of clearing by the natural process, not to attempt the removal of an opaque surface, so long as there is evidence of inflammation still remaining; for, with few exceptions, so long as minute vessels traverse its substance, the power of nature may remove, or greatly reduce the opacity. I may say even more: there is no better established fact in ophthalmic medicine, than that an opacity will become less, or may be entirely removed, long after all trace of redness of the cornea has passed away. Sufficient time should, therefore, always be allowed for natural restorative power, and the application of those measures, generally and locally, which are known to aid it. This applies still more particularly to early life.

Two excellent examples of the removal of earthy deposit from the cornea have been published by Mr. Bowman, in his "Anatomy of the Parts concerned in the Operations on the Eye." One was under his own care, the other under that of Mr. Dixon, and there is so close a similarity between the two, that I shall give only the first, which is headed, "Symmetrical opacity of both corneæ, extending horizontally over the central region, and obstructing vision; consisting of an earthy deposit limited to the anterior elastic lamina." "On each cornea was a horizontal band, of brownish opacity, extending from side to side, and so much broader opposite the pupil as completely to hide it from view, unless the pupil was dilated, or was examined either from above or below, through the still transparent cornea. Both the iris and the pupil could then be seen to be perfectly natural and active. When the pupils were considerably dilated, he obtained some useful vision, especially with the left eye, where the opacity was not quite so extensive as on the right. The opaque part was very finely mottled with dark dots, some of which were only to be seen with a lens; its margins were shaded off rather abruptly, and the cornea beyond them was perfectly clear. The opacity had the appearance of occupying a superficial position, and of being very slightly raised, but the surface reflected the light as brilliantly as other parts. The shape of the opaque tract was peculiar in being slightly inclined downwards from the inner side, so that its lower edge in each eye corresponded exactly with the margin of the lower lid, when the eyes were directed to a near object. The inner end of the opacity in the left eye was traversed by a narrow line, in which the cornea was as transparent as ever.

" The singularity of these opacities led me to inquire into the man's history. He had had an ophthalmia ten years before, lasting only a fortnight, and leaving no blemish. After a period of about three years, his wife noticed that he had a speck on each eye, but as his sight was perfect, he doubted it. After two or three years more, the specks were more evident to others, and he began to find that in a strong light his sight was clouded, so that he applied for relief at the Ophthalmic Hospital, and remained a patient there for about two years, during which he was treated with drops and lotions, but rather got worse than better; in fact, the opacity seemed confirmed and incurable, and was steadily encroaching over the front of the pupil. Within the last year he has been quite thrown out of work, able to see only in an obscure light, and then only objects on one side.

" Like those who had previously seen him, I regarded these opacities as indelible, but as he came from time to time, it occurred to me to make an attempt to shave off a portion of one of them, in order to examine its nature more completely. I accordingly made the patient come from the hospital to my house, where I could at once place any particle I might be able to detach under the microscope. The first scratch with the point of the lancet on the right eye (Jan. 20th) detached the epithelium, which seemed healthy, and brought me down upon the opacity, which felt hard to the instrument, and had a smooth surface. In scraping and trying to slice off a thin film of it, a thin flake cracked off and separated, leaving what seemed a hole through the cornea, but the aqueous humour did not escape, and I then saw that the pupil was visible through the perfectly transparent lamellated texture, behind the opacity. It was now easy to chip off the opaque film over a space corresponding to the pupil, and when this was done he could see large letters plainly, for the exposed surface was nearly smooth.

"The pain attending this little operation was great, and the poor fellow fainted; but the subsequent inflammation was slight, and in a few days the epithelium was restored, without any return of opacity, and he could see very much better.

"The fragments which had been removed became of an opaque white when dry, and when examined under a sufficient magnifying power presented the appearance of an aggregation of rounded, highly refracting grains, disposed in a sort of network. They all lay nearly in one plane, and the epithelium which had covered them was perfectly healthy." The deposit, submitted to chemical analysis by Prof. Miller, consisted of phosphates of lime and magnesia, with a considerable portion of carbonate of lime.

"On the 22nd of February, the area exposed by the operation on the right eye remaining clear, I performed the same operation on the left, and with precisely corresponding results, so that in a few days afterwards he could see almost as well as eight years before. With this eye he could, in fact, with some care, read the type called pearl type."

I have not myself met with such favourable instances for operation as the foregoing. On two occasions in which I attempted the removal of what I considered to be earthy deposit, the entire texture of the cornea proved to be pervaded, and I desisted when that was discovered. I have twice attempted to shave off circumscribed central opacities, apparently of the nature of deposits, that were just large enough to interfere with vision, but found that their depth would not admit of it; in each case, however, the opacity was lessened by the slight subsequent inflammation.

The fact of secondary inflammation, under certain circumstances, especially in cases of interstitial deposits, having the power to remove or reduce an opacity which seemed indelible, was long since known. Scratching the cornea with a needle, or any instrument, so as to excite inflammation, is certainly of benefit, in chronic cases, when the opacity is superficial. I have done it many times with marked success, and there has never been any ill result. I believe that very often, so long as there is any trace of vascularity about the cornea, provided there be no staphyloma, the extent or the intensity of the opacity may be reduced. It would of course be useless to interfere with cicatrices.

Acupuncture, with partial or complete penetration of the cornea, has been practised for opacities, and it has even been recommended to charge the point of the needle with irritating substances.

The practice of purulent inoculation, for the same purpose, has not found many advocates in this country. Of late, some cases have been treated by the application of gonorrhœal matter to the conjunctiva. I have seen two of them. One was avowedly the worse, the cornea being more opaque, and moreover ulcerated, after the eye had recovered from the severity of the excited inflammation. The other was not any better. Both the patients were under puberty, and so far as I could learn from their history, had not been long afflicted with strumous corneitis, the disease for which they were inoculated.

If any treatment can be proved to be more beneficial than another for the removal of corneal opacities, it should most undoubtedly be adopted. But assuredly there has not been established anything, so far as I can make out, in favour of this method. That it is directly accompanied with danger is apparent, for its first object is to produce inflammation of the eye of a dangerous character, the ordinary secondary consequences of which are generally fatal to sight. I consider it so dangerous as to be unjustifiable when there is any useful sight.

There is a disgusting loathsomeness about procuring the pus from a venereal source, that, to my mind, is in itself condemnatory of the measure.

TRANSPLANTATION OF THE CORNEA.

I have determined not to give any of the many experiments that have been made in this operation, which, as might be expected, have never succeeded. In my last edition the subject is fully noticed.

Among the novel German suggestions is that of wearing a glass stud, in shape like a shirt-stud, in an opaque cornea, for restoring sight.

CHAPTER XXII.

Fig. 120. INCISION OF THE CONJUNCTIVA IN PURULENT

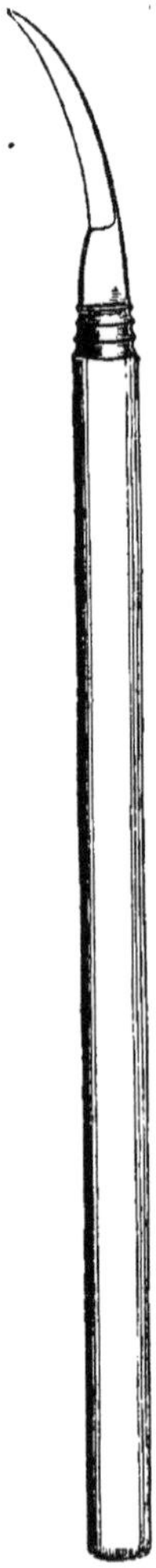

OPHTHALMIA OF ADULTS.

KNIFE FOR DIVIDING CHEMOSIS.

A CURVED blade is more efficient, and is safer than a straight one.

The distinctive characters of purulent ophthalmia in the adult are, externally; swelling and dusky redness of the eyelids with more or less inability to open them, purulent discharge which collects on the eyelashes; internally conjunctival redness and infiltration, and swelling that causes it to overlap the cornea in a fleshy looking mass, producing what is called chemosis.

The cornea quickly loses some degree of its polish, but the first bad symptom generally is ulceration, which often begins partially at the margin beneath the chemosis; but it may be quite within it and nearer the centre. The ulceration may proceed to penetration, and produce prolapse of the iris, or more generally cause the surrounded part to lose its vitality, become hazy, although it might still shine a little, and ultimately die by ulceration, infiltration of pus, or sloughing. Sometimes the sloughing stage is more quickly reached, and grayness rapidly passes into brownness, to be followed by ash colour, which indicates total loss of vitality. The whole cornea is rarely destroyed, and the ulceration, or slough, does not always penetrate its entire thickness. Pain and constitutional disturbance are always present.

The rapid destructiveness causes it to be greatly dreaded. I have seen cases where in twenty-four hours all chance of recovery has been lost. The danger, therefore, does not so much depend on the whole globe of the eye being involved in inflammation, that produces disorganization and atrophy, although this may happen, as upon the direct effects on the cornea—ulceration, sloughing, deposit of pus between its layers,—the termination being penetration with prolapse of the iris, and opacity of a part or the whole of what remains.

The gonorrhœal—fortunately not a common disease—is the most terrible of all the purulent ophthalmiæ.

A young practitioner will, doubtless, be at a loss to know how gonorrhœal ophthalmia is to be distinguished from the other purulent discharges of the eye, and in what respect it differs. In the absence of any proof to the contrary, and from its resemblance, it would seem that it is one and the same kind of disease, notwithstanding the mode of origin, differing only in degree or intensity ; there being no determinable pathological difference. It is closely allied to the purulent ophthalmia from other causes ; and the diagnosis must rest on the history of the case ; no set of symptoms that can be strictly relied upon are proper to either, especially at a late period. But a diagnosis, if it can be made, is valuable, for we are then more on our guard, and it is important to be able to tell the friends of a patient when his disease is such as to excite apprehensions. The co-existence of a gonorrhœa with a severe purulent ophthalmia is most unquestionably one of the strongest confirmations of the specific nature. It is commonly stated that the ordinary purulent ophthalmia of adults commences with inflammation of the conjunctiva of the eyelids, and then spreads to that of the eyeball ; and in the gonorrhœal form, the reverse is the case—an opinion which seems to be generally correct : and hence, perhaps, the greater amount of chemosis in the latter, and therefore, the greater probability of sloughing, or ulceration of the cornea; hence, also, the eyelids in gonorrhœal ophthalmia are generally not so very much swollen. But this diagnostic sign is lost when the disease has advanced.

It is a fact fully confirmed, that gonorrhœal matter, when applied to the conjunctiva, may produce violent inflammation of that membrane, with purulent discharge, whether the matter be from the same individual or from another.

That accidental inoculation is very frequently the cause of the disease, there can be no doubt, but it is often impossible to prove the infection.

The period between the first evidence of inflammation and the stage which immediately precedes destruction is uncertain : in one of my patients it was so long as seventeen days. Dr. Mackenzie mentions an instance that came under his care thirteen days after inoculation, where partial recovery ensued. When he saw the patient the left eye was violently inflamed and chemosed, there was a great discharge of purulent fluid, and the cornea was totally opaque; under treatment the cornea cleared beyond expectation, and a considerable share of vision was preserved.

Since the treatment is better understood, the termination of purulent ophthalmia in the adult has been more favourable. It is not now considered necessary to reduce a patient to death's door by depletion, in order to endeavour to cure his complaint. For this, and indeed, for much that is valuable in the treatment of diseases of the eye, we are greatly indebted to Mr. Tyrrell. It is surprising, however, with what tenacity the strict antiphlogistic system of treatment, of which blood-letting is the principal means, is still adhered to by some. The late Mr. Morgan used to tell his pupils that to control this disease, it was necessary to produce a degree of depression very little short of that occasioned by profuse and continued hæmorrhage.

I employ hot or cold applications and opiates to assuage pain, as mentioned in the treatment of inflammation of the eyeball. The local astringent I generally use is a solution of alum, of three or four grains to the ounce of water, and when nitrate of silver is employed, the strength is one grain or half, to the same quantity of water. I believe that these substances are most effective when so used. All applications to the conjunctiva, that produce severe or prolonged pain, are injurious. The secretions, as far as practicable, should be previously removed with warm water, the eyelids being well separated during the washing. I usually direct a syringe to be used for these purposes, and enjoin the frequent repetition—that is, once or twice in the hour, or even more, according to circumstances. In the intervals, the edges of the eyelids should be kept greased, to prevent partial adhesion, and cleanliness will be best ensured by cutting off the cilia.

Marked debility, sometimes apparent from the first, is generally developed as the disease advances, and must be well attended to. I never saw a severe case unaccompanied by great prostration, irrespective of the termination. In a late instance of undoubted gonorrhœal ophthalmia in private, in a young man in high life, alarming depression appeared on the fourth day from the time I saw him, and the seventh of the disease. Large quantities of direct and diffusible stimuli were given, and later, quinine and other tonics. The eye was saved, the only remains of the attack being slight opacity of the circumference of the cornea, where there had been deep ulceration, but no penetration.

The feverish excitement and accelerated circulation must not be considered as indications for employing depressing agents —and, above all, for taking blood,—but for the appropriate remedies of modern therapeutics. Local bleeding must be but sparingly employed, and chiefly, if not entirely reserved for assuaging pain, either in consequence of its high degree— the evidence of very acute disease,—or when it does not give way to any other measure.

The special part of my subject—that relating to the surgical treatment of the chemosis—must now be considered.

Incision of the swollen, inflamed, infiltrated conjunctiva, and the subjacent cellular tissue, " to relieve the strangulation of the vessels by which the cornea is nourished," was strongly insisted upon by the late Mr. Tyrrell, and its benefits highly lauded. Whether the manner of making the incisions by dividing the conjunctiva longitudinally, and not circularly, originated with him, is uncertain. Mr. Middlemore had advocated the same principle in his work several years before Mr. Tyrrell's opinions were publicly expressed; and the only difference in their views is, that Mr. Tyrrell put implicit faith in the direction and locality of the incisions, believing it essential to make them between the attachments of the recti muscles, "avoiding immediately the transverse and perpendicular diameters of the globe, that the larger vessels, passing to the cornea, might not be injured;" whereas Mr. Middlemore directs the incisions to be distant half a line from each other.

The supposed discovery produced considerable excitement, and was hailed by the profession as the most important one that had been added to ophthalmic treatment for many years. Mr. Tyrrell made it the sole subject of several very long lectures at the Royal College of Surgeons. He believed, and convinced the majority of surgeons, for a time, that it was a sure and certain method for preventing the cornea from sloughing, and he produced evidence in corroboration of it. Censure was thrown on any one who ventured to doubt the infallibility of the remedy. However, Mr. W. Jones undertook to show that " the cornea was not nourished entirely by vessels prolonged into it from the conjunctiva," as stated by Mr. Tyrrell, and that it did not, therefore, perish because its means of vitality were so cut off. This met with violent opposition. Mr. Jones's views are published in the " Medical Gazette " for 1839, vol. i.

A dispassionate examination of the practice, irrespective of the wrong theory, afforded by the lapse of time, and after the personal influence of the propounder has passed away, leaves no doubt that Mr. Tyrrell had deceived himself, and was wrong as to the complete remedial agency of the method. This has led to complete reaction, and incisions are too generally given up. Purulent ophthalmia is often fatal to the eye, in spite of all the means at our disposal; but that freely incising the chemosis—it matters not as to the form or the position of the cuts—is a valuable adjunct to treatment, I have no doubt.

I regard it as important as incising the skin in phlegmonous erysipelas. I believe that by it I have saved many eyes that would otherwise have been lost. It is unattended with the slightest disadvantage. I resort to it whenever the chemosis is well marked,—which is quivalent to saying, whenever the disease is intense.

The operation may be readily performed by standing behind the patient, who should be seated on a low chair, raising the upper eyelid with the retractor, while an assistant depresses the lower, introducing the point of the knife, nearly vertically, at the reflection of the chemosis on the lower part of the cornea, and carrying it along the sclerotica to the sinus; then depressing the handle, and including within the curve of the blade the swollen palpebral conjunctiva. I generally endeavour to make four such incisions at equal intervals. The division of the upper part of the chemosis is not so readily effected as that of the lower; but it may be done by applying the retractor first on one side of the eyelid, to make room for the knife, and then shifting it to the other. A sponge should be used, and the place for the entrance of the knife made apparent. With common care, the sclerotica will be uninjured. It is so imperative to make these incisions thoroughly, that, unless there be a certainty of the patient being submissive, chloroform should be administered.

Should a case retrograde, and chemosis recur, secondary incisions must be practised; and, as the progress of the disease will probably be under surveillance, they may be done early, and a less number of them will then suffice.

The case of a young man, twenty-one years old, a portmanteau maker, furnishes a marked example of very severe purulent ophthalmia without specific origin:—at least there was no gonorrhœa, nor was there any evidence of gonorrhœal origin; and, therefore, I attributed the disease to debility occasioned by overwork, and the sudden change from the pure air of Cheltenham to the emanations of a narrow back street, near Maiden Lane, King's Cross. It well illustrates, too, the effect of treatment.

For two nights previous to the attack the poor fellow had not gone to bed—his employer, to meet an order, demanding a certain amount of work in a given time. The right eye was first attacked : on the third day there was considerable chemosis, and superficial sloughs in two spots on the cornea; and he then applied to Mr. Taylor, who divided the chemosis. He would not on any account come into the hospital, and did not reapply as an out-patient. On the sixth day I visited him at his miserable lodgings, and induced him to become an in-patient. At this time the right iris was prolapsed ; the cornea of the left eye hazy and surrounded by chemosis, having become so on the morning of the previous day. His prostration, mental and physical, was very great : he was unable even to walk. I divided the chemosis in the left eye freely, and for the second time that in the right, which, however, seemed destroyed. Alum lotion was used as I have specified; quinine, porter, ammonia, and strong. broths were prescribed, and any nutritious article of diet that he might fancy. On the third day of his hospital residence, the chemosis in the left eye had subsided sufficiently to expose the margin of the cornea, which was furrowed at the upper part for about a third of its circumference, and penetrated apparently by ulceration, sufficiently to allow of a slight prolapse of the iris. The haziness still remained. The eye progressed satisfactorily; the patient improved daily, and was soon able to take solid food, but continued so weak that on the first time he left his bed he fainted. He quitted the hospital at the end of a fortnight, and could then see his way about. Three months afterwards he came to town and called on Mr. Taylor, who furnished me with the following note of his state:—

" The left pupil is slightly displaced upwards, and shaded towards the sclerotic margin by a faint superficial opacity of the cornea, which becomes gradually more dense towards the point of penetration. Vision is almost perfect, and is daily becoming stronger. The cornea of the right eye is replaced by a dense cicatrix, and vision is completely lost."

CHAPTER XXIII.

CATARACT.

VARIETIES OF CATARACT.

THIS disease is generally divided into the spurious and the true. By the spurious is meant various morbid deposits, for the most part the result of inflammatory action on the capsule of the lens; hence, we hear of the sanguineous, purulent, pigmentous, and many other kinds of cataract; but these terms do not convey the true pathological states of the eye which they are meant to express, and it is more intelligible, as well as more correct, to say that there exists a deposit of lymph on the capsule of the lens, with more or less adhesion of the iris, &c., as the case may be. Besides, such a division makes so much confusion, by blending general diseases of the eye with what should be regarded as distinct and peculiar changes in certain textures, that it should be rejected, and the term cataract confined to those alterations in the crystalline lens and its capsule whereby their transparency is destroyed. It is certainly true that some of the changes alluded to, obstruct vision, demand an operation, and are even sometimes themselves impediments to certain operations for cataract: these will all be treated of in their proper places.

I shall describe, then, only two kinds of cataract—the lenticular and the capsular. The lenticular frequently exists alone. Whether the capsule is ever singly affected, is not positively known; the received opinion, however, is, that the perfection of the lens depends on the integrity of the capsule, and that when the capsule has lost its transparency, the lens must be similarly affected. To the double affection the appellation of capsulo-lenticular cataract is applied.

But the existence of capsular cataract is now questioned by Stellwag, who says, that having examined about fifty cataracts with opaque capsules, obtained at *post-mortem* examinations in the General Hospital at Vienna, he found in every instance that the opacity was due to earthy and fatty substances adhering to the lenticular surface of the capsule, and not to changes in the capsular tissue itself. He found, too, that the deposit was capable of removal by mechanical or chemical means. If these observations be correct, they increase our pathological knowledge respecting cataract, but do not alter or add to what was before understood respecting diagnosis. Besides, they cannot, I suspect, apply always to what is wont to be called opaque capsule, because the opacity often ensues after the lens has been removed by extraction, or by violence. To prevent confusion, I shall employ the old term, " opaque capsule."

Several very peculiar states may be associated with this loss of transparency: the opaque lens may be reduced; may degenerate into fluidity; or become stony, from earthy deposit; and the opaque capsule may lose all its delicacy of structure, becoming thickened, and even cretaceous.

CAUSE OF CATARACT.

Although cataract may exist at all periods of life, no age being exempt, from the fœtus in utero to that beyond the natural limit of man's existence, it appears to belong, as an idiopathic affection, more properly to infancy—when it is mostly capsulo-lenticular; and to advanced years—when it is usually lenticular. Of the exact nature of the change that produces the opacity, and the processes that regulate it, we know little; experience teaches that cataract may follow certain states or circumstances which may be regarded as causes: thus, a wound of the capsule may in a few hours cause both capsule and lens to be opaque ; and inflammation of the eye may produce the same effect. Idiopathic lenticular cataract cannot be accounted for; pathology and physiology do not yet afford any elucidation; and all the theories that have been advanced concerning it are untenable. It must be remarked, however, that we meet with it less frequently in an uncomplicated state —that is, as an affection by itself—than coexisting with other disease in the eye, either of an active type or of a low: the complication is more frequent in one variety—the soft; yet we are not thereby enlightened as to its cause.

That a connexion exists between lenticular opacity and diabetes is fully proved. It was known and taught many years ago by Dr. Craigie, of Edinburgh ; and among other Germans who have investigated the subject is Von Gräfe, who found that one-fourth of the diabetic patients have cataracts. I recommend to my readers a *brochure* on " The Synthesis of Cataract," by a great English physiologist, Dr. Benjamin W. Richardson, who has conducted a very valuable series of experiments, in which it is shown that saccharine and saline matters injected under the skin of some of the lower animals produce cataract. This opens a new field for the student in ophthalmic medicine.

Opacity of the capsule, also, often cannot be accounted for; yet it would seem, more commonly than that of the lens, to be owing to inflammation, from the changes of thickness and density that it frequently undergoes, which alterations bear an analogy to certain effects in other parts of the body, usually considered to have this origin. Besides, in traumatic cataract, the capsule is nearly always opaque ; and although the opacity may follow the injury in a few hours, that is quite time enough for its production by inflammation, which, to a greater or lesser degree, is always excited. Even when the cataract results from mere concussion, without any wound, inflammation might still be the cause. Furthermore, except in congenital cataract, the capsule is rarely found opaque, without there being evidence of some degree of inflammation in the eyeball, and the capsular changes are generally in proportion to the severity of the accompanying vascular action. Moreover, it is seldom altered in the uncomplicated cataract of the aged; or if changed, it is merely by the loss of transparency, which is often partial.

Whether these parts are ever the primary seat of inflammation which induces the disease under consideration is a question that has been often mooted. Dr. Jacob, who discusses it in a most masterly manner in his work on " Inflammations of the Eyeball," says that he cannot, as he has done in the case of the cornea, show that red vessels make their appearance in the body of the lens, or that purulent matter is formed in its texture in consequence of inflammation originating in and restricted to it. He sums up the discussion by expressing his belief that no insulated inflammation of the lens, originating in the part, and confined to it, so as to constitute a distinct variety or species— to be enumerated in a nosological arrangement, under the title of Lentitis,—ever takes place; and alluding to Dr. Walther's description of such isolated inflammation, remarks, that what Walther refers to, appears to him to be not an unusual effect of general inflammation of the contents of the eyeball, described, perhaps, with a little colouring, and such accuracy of detail as the establishment of a new species of disease seems to demand. "That the capsule of the lens, and in many cases, ultimately, the lens itself, becomes implicated in the general inflammation of the eye, commonly called iritis, there can be no doubt; and this I am of opinion it is that Dr. Walther has been describing. Dr. Mackenzie says : 'Inflammation of the anterior hemisphere of the capsule is always accompanied by a slight change in the colour of the iris and form of the pupil, the iris becoming a little darker and the pupil irregular, while the motions become sluggish and very limited.' Surely this is to say that the disease is accompanied by iritis, or coexists with it. He also says, that 'red vessels appear in the pupil itself;' and that 'other vessels seem to extend from the delicate membrane, retaining the pigment of the iris in its place;'

adding that, according to Professor Walther, 'vessels seem to be prolonged rather from the capsule into the posterior surface of the iris;'—all which proves that the inflammation described extends from the iris in protracted or chronic inflammation of the eye, and especially in persons of rheumatic or scrofulous habit, where there have been frequent relapses; the margin of the pupil almost always forms extensive adhesions to the capsule of the lens, in which adhesions red vessels, visible to the naked eye, are often observed; but these red vessels are not derived in the first instance from an inflamed lenticular capsule, but from an inflamed iris. Of the 'much rarer' 'inflammation of the *posterior hemisphere* of the crystalline capsule,' I do not venture to give a very decided opinion, not having been fortunate enough to see many cases presenting appearances resembling those described. I will not deny that 'ramifications of the central artery of the vitreous humour' may not 'spread out upon the posterior capsule;' but I cannot say that I have seen them; and as to the 'little knots of a whitish-grey semi-transparent substance, evidently coagulable lymph,' I am equally uninformed from my own observation. I may venture to add that it appears to me remarkable that, with all this inflammatory disorganization of the posterior hemisphere of the capsule, the lens should remain so transparent as to admit of a perfect view of them, and I am almost inclined to suspect that in some cases at least the appearances described are owing to certain curiously-formed opacities which are sometimes to be seen in this structure or in the back of the capsule, constituting a peculiar form of cataract."

What are usually assigned as the remote, or predisposing, causes of cataract are so vague—I may almost say so absurd—as to forbid any notice of them, with the exception of hereditary tendency, the effect of which may be very palpable in the congenital form of the affection. A young female came under the care with congenital lenticular cataract in each eye; the three sisters, maternal aunt and uncle, and maternal grandfather had all been similarly affected. All ophthalmic writers who have seen much practice, adduce similar instances from their own observation. We have not, however, parallel examples of the cataract of the aged being induced by consanguinity.

A cursory sketch of the natural structure of the crystalline lens, and of the alterations it undergoes at different periods of life, will assist in the elucidation of some of the pathological conditions of lenticular cataract, and add to the means of understanding and diagnosing its varieties. The external part —that in contact with the capsule—consists of a layer of extremely transparent nucleated cells, and is the softest portion. The next is the peculiar lens tissue, tubular fibres containing a clear viscid substance, constituting what is generally called the soft exterior. Interior to this, is the centre, the densest, spoken of as the nucleus. In infancy it is most convex, and softer than at any subsequent period; with maturing age its consistency increases, its form also undergoing change, becoming flatter; in the adult we find it less convex before than behind, and still more dense than in youth. About the thirtieth year, sooner or later, it ceases to be colourless, its nucleus then acquiring a light yellow tint; after that period the colour becomes more marked, and pervades the whole. At a very advanced age, it resembles a piece of amber. Both surfaces have now become less curved, and with the diminished bulk and maximum hardness, the specific gravity is greater. On these changes, when disease invades the lens, essentially is founded the division of lenticular cataract into hard and soft.

In youth the pupil is black. In the aged there is instead a yellowish tint, which seems to penetrate deeply, owing to the lens colour. It is often mistaken for disease.

HARD CATARACT.

Hard lenticular cataract is merely grayness or opacity,

appearing in an already discoloured and somewhat dense lens, and the greater the discoloration of the lens the less will be the amount of grayness required to obstruct vision. Hence hard cataract cannot occur before that time of life at which the lens begins to increase in density.

It has long been known that the most common structural changes in a cataract of this class are preternatural softness of the exterior with hardness and dryness of the centre. To break through the latter requires as much pressure as a modern cataract needle will bear. Mr. R. Taylor has examined these states minutely. The result of his researches, which are recorded in the "Pathological Transactions," vol. vii., is briefly this:—The nucleus becomes hard and dry, to a degree far exceeding what is ever seen in the healthy lens; while the superficial layers are softened, frequently to the state of a semi-fluid pulp. The nuclear lens-tubes are hard, atrophied, and brittle, and are rendered more or less opaque by fine molecular deposit, as well as by little cracks and fissures. Those of the superficies are softened and more or less disintegrated; they also are dotted over with fine molecular matter, which is also found floating free in masses, and filling up and rendering opaque many of the superficial lens-cells. This molecular matter is probably the result of the coagulation of the albuminous blastema, by which the whole of the lens-textures are pervaded. I saw many of the microscopic preparations from which the description is made.

Having given an idea of what hard cataract is, I must show how it is to be distinguished—what are its characteristics.

As it cannot occur under the middle period of life, the age of the patient will be a very material guide in diagnosis. Arising from a disorganizing process, the appearances differ at the several stages of the disease, till the whole body is rendered opaque; and as the destruction to tissue may not end there, but be progressive, even then the physical signs vary. Besides this, as the same part of the lens is not always first attacked, the early aspects are dissimilar. The appearance then of ordinary fully-formed cataract is a mixture of dark-gray and amber,

more deeply shaded in the centre, owing to the natural
anatomical arrangement, or mottling of gray and amber, or
amber colour only.

In an earlier state, when sight begins to fail, scattered opaque
streaks, or radii, of different lengths—bundles of opaque lens-
fibres,—or spots or patches may be visible. They may not,
however, be apparent, except the pupil be fully dilated, being
mostly situated at the circumference, the most usual place,
when they are generally very regularly disposed. Sometimes
they are more in the front, when their position is readily
recognised; or decidedly posterior, when they seem so deep as
even to be behind the lens. These last used to be supposed to
be opacity of the capsule. Or the change may be in the centre
of the lens only, when it is most difficult to distinguish. Still
more rarely, general diffused opacity may invade the entire
lens from the beginning. In the course of progress the striæ
or the patches increase and run together, while the rest of the
lens-tissue gets hazy; and merely the opaque anterior being
seen, the aspects above described, of the well-formed cataract,
appear.

I have said that the destructive process may not end after
opacity has invaded the entire lens. When it continues, the
circumference, already softened, breaks down into a semi-fluid
pulp, and may even, although rarely, pass into fluidity. This
further stage is apt to interfere with diagnosis, on account of
the whiteness, more or less patchy, of the surface, caused by the
addition of fatty or earthy and molecular matters. Long ago I
pointed out the fact that it is very common for cataract in
an advanced degree in an old person not to exhibit any amber
colour, but appear whitish, or whitish-gray, like the soft variety;
and after extraction to prove light-coloured on the surface
merely, there being a hard amber-coloured nucleus beneath,
sometimes with striæ still apparent. I am not aware that there
are any diagnostic distinctions between a hard lens, so altered,
and full-formed soft cataract occurring in early life, except that
the former is more uniformly of a whitish colour, and devoid of
cloudiness, never exhibiting radiating or other streaks; that the

capsule is rarely if ever opaque; and such as the size of the chambers may indicate. In hard cataract there is nearly always a posterior chamber, in correspondence with the age of the person. In soft cataract, the posterior chamber is very frequently reduced, and may be obliterated, the iris being pushed forwards, its movements impaired, and the anterior chamber reduced: the cataract may even protrude through the pupil. But the age of the individual helps out of the difficulty more than anything. In course of time the nucleus of the lens may get more or less broken down. This takes place sometimes by a more rapid process.

In the instances in which the cataract does not get whitish on the surface, from the causes explained, the darkness is apt to increase. A deep-mahogany colour therefore is not very uncommon in hard cataract, when the disease is apt to be unnoticed, and the hue may be so deep that very close inspection and much care are needed to detect any alteration from the natural state. There may, in fact, be black cataract. I brought before the Royal Medico-Chirurgical Society the particulars of a case in which a cataract was so black that it could not be detected by any one till the eye was examined with the ophthalmoscope, or the concentrated light of a powerful lens. The details are in the "Medical Circular" for December 5, 1855. A friend assures me that he witnessed the extraction of a perfectly black cataract. I have seen a lens quite black, escape from a disorganized eye after the removal of a large staphyloma corneæ. In the Dublin "Medical Press" for January the 19th, 1853, is the report of the extraction of a black cataract, copied from the "Bulletino delle Science Médiche." The fragments of capsule that escaped are said to have been darker than the lens, which was reddish-black. Sight was restored. It is not stated whether both eyes were similarly affected. I suspect that many cases of this kind are overlooked, and the loss of sight attributed to other causes.

It has long occurred to me whether the lenticular coloration of age is, in itself, ever intense enough to produce opacity of the lens—in fact, a cataract: I really think that it is. A strong

.suspici:on of this is to be gathered from the absence of the ordinary morbid changes in the cataract, especially of the central part, as observed by the naked eye. It is a point that I shall investigate. The coloration is often so marked in life, and especially in dark races of men, that it may not at first sight be possible to say when cataract does or does not exist. I have seen the amber change so apparent in mulattos, and I am told it is still more marked in negroes, that the most experienced surgeon might be deceived, and pronounce cataract to be present, if any of these persons had complained of defective sight. In the case of a woman of colour, an operation for what was supposed to be a cataract was proposed by one to whom, both as an author and as a practitioner, ophthalmic surgery in this country owes much of its advancement : the coloration was so intense as to deceive him, the defect of sight being due merely to presbyopia, and vitiated secretion from the Meibomian glands, in consequence of chronic ophthalmia.

SOFT CATARACT.

Soft cataract may be considered under two heads. In the one, as opacity invading a lens that has not become amber-coloured and denser by age, and existing in children and young persons; or, in which the coloration is still slight, occurring in young adults. In the other, as disintegration of the lenticular tissue, happening at any period of life.

Respecting the first, the remarks that I have made about the appearances of hard cataract varying at different stages of the disease, apply equally here. When well formed, it is of a light gray colour, or grayish-white; and in proportion as the cataract occurs earlier in life is the gray more apparent. Sometimes there is a bluish whiteness, resembling milk and water. The colour is generally deeper in the centre, but the contrast is not so marked as in the hard variety, from the greater aggregation of opaque particles.

In the earlier state, radii and streaks, or opaque patches, may be seen. These are more common here than in the old lens, and are brighter sometimes—even glistening. A very common appearance is that of fractured spermaceti. These points of opacities may occupy the margin of the lens, the surfaces, or the centre, and are owing, as before expressed, to the greater opacity of certain bundles of fibres. As the cataract proceeds, the other parts, which, till now, have been transparent, or but merely hazy, become opaque, and at last only the front surface is seen.

There is a last stage precisely analogous to that which I have described, in hard cataract, when new products are developed from the breaking up of the surface, and produce whiteness.

It has been supposed that soft cataracts increase in size; and indication of it is afforded in smallness of the posterior chamber. This is really no proof, as changes in the posterior part of the eye, especially preternatural vascularity of the ciliary apparatus, may throw the cataract forward, and even more or less destroy the anterior chamber: besides, this could not take place except the capsule enlarge—a very unlikely occurrence.

Fluid degeneration, the second head, under which I place soft cataract, is certainly a rare condition. The entire lens undergoes that kind of alteration which I have described as sometimes taking place on the surface of any form of lenticular cataract. Soft cataract, then, as such, may exist at any age; but when it occurs after the middle period of life, it is either the *débris* or remains of a hard cataract, or rapid degeneration of the lens, the opacity being in the latter case merely the inseparable consequence of that destruction. Hence it is that soft cataract in an elderly person is never like the cataract of early life, where the consistence of the lens is unchanged. The milk-and-water look, in which a bluish cast is apparent, is here the commonest appearance. Sometimes there is a dirty-gray, sometimes a yellowish tinge. The colour, of whatever hue, may be uniform, or it may be somewhat mottled or curdled. In some cases, when the eye has been at rest, the lower part of the cataract is manifestly the denser, from the thicker portions gravitating; and the general colour is restored by moving it about, or rubbing the eyeball. More rarely, but not very uncommonly, the fluid degeneration is dark, or very brown, chocolate, or even sepia-coloured ; and when this is most marked there is not, so far as I know, any decidedly distinguishing mark that can be pointed out between it and the hard, very coloured, or deep-mahogany cataract, and I have seen a mistake occur under the treatment of two surgeons. On one occasion, during extraction, when I proceeded to rupture the capsule, a dark fluid escaped, and for a time interrupted my progress by obscuring the iris. In another case, a lady seventy-seven years old, with double cataracts, consulted all the present men of ophthalmic eminence in London, and, without an exception, extraction was recommended. I saw her, took the same view, and was selected as the operator. The capsule did not contain a particle of lens, but was filled with material like coffee-grounds. I operated only on one eye: sight was restored. There is always an absence of all striæ or markings that can exist only so long as the lens-fibres remain. Among the fluid oil-globules abound, and often plates of cholesterine.

In all the above descriptions of cataract I have taken no notice of opacity of the capsule, because it is not necessarily associated with any of those changes; but here it is common in some degree, and accordingly obscures the changes that the lens has undergone. Sometimes it is quite opaque.

Should my reader have at all looked into ophthalmic subjects, he must have heard of the so-called Morgagnian cataract, named after the distinguished man from whom, through several generations, the error has descended. It is fluid degeneration of the lens in part, or in whole, that has given rise to the term defined as opacity of the fluid, which was supposed by Morgagni to exist naturally between the lens and its capsule. Now, such a fluid does not exist, as the superficies of the lens is, as I have said, in contact with the capsule, the nucleated cells forming an organized connecting medium, there being no interspace. After death the cells become loaded with water, which is probably absorbed from the aqueous humour, and constitutes the aqua Morgagnii that has been supposed to exist naturally.

With this pathological change the capsule is apt to quit its attachments; on some occasions, while I have been extracting, it has escaped entire, and was, in each instance, semi-opaque; the fluid was light brown; the nucleus of the lense hard, and of a deep amber colour.

This division of lenticular cataract, with the accompanying minuteness of description, is solely with reference to treatment, in order that each kind may have the appropriate operation. I may just premise here, therefore, that for the hard, "extraction" is that best adapted; for the soft, "solution."

As the natural changes in the crystalline lens are gradual, the density increasing by slow degrees, it cannot always be determined when a cataract should be classed as hard or soft, especially as there is such very great variation in different individuals in the arrival of those several changes of structure incidental to age. Authors tell us that hard cataract does not occur under the forty-fifth year; and this is, perhaps, true, if we require as the proof of hardness a well-marked amber colour, or amber-gray.

The following anecdote illustrates the practical bearing of the matter. Some years since, a clergyman, forty years of age, consulted the late Mr. Tyrrell for cataract. Mr. Tyrrell, who never used the knife when he could employ the needle for solution, determined in this instance to extract; his sudden death, however, prevented the operation. The patient applied to the late Mr. Alexander, who always extracted when it was admissible, and whose success has probably never been surpassed, and we may fairly infer that he thought the cataract not hard enough to demand extraction, for he operated by solution. Here were two highly practical men, both in most extensive ophthalmic practice, differing on the question of consistence, and preferring different operations.

A very marked difference in consistence may occur in the opaque lenses of the same individual. I performed double extraction in a female sixty-nine years old : one lens had a hard amber-coloured nucleus, surrounded by soft whitish-brown matter; the other did not exhibit the slightest amber tint, but was gray throughout, and softer. Another difference was, that with the former the posterior chamber was natural, with the latter it was lost by the iris being pressed forwards.

CAPSULAR CATARACT.

Capsular cataract, or opacity of the capsule of the lens, has almost invariably the appearance of a dead chalky whiteness, rarely ever shining, and always showing the same opacity in whatever position it is viewed. It may be partial, occurring in one or many patches; as such it may be easily recognised by its definite outline, anterior position, and whiteness; and these characteristics are rendered more manifest by raising the upper eyelid, desiring the patient to look to the ground, and making the inspection sideways.

Whether complete capsular cataract encloses a lens is judged of principally by its volume : when the lens is absent, the symptoms are flatness of the capsule, greater size of the posterior chamber, with more or less retraction of the iris; and, if the capsule have been long empty, shrinking at the sides from partial or entire separation from its circumferential connexions. The more or less ragged and irregular capsule that remains after operation, is readily recognised as such. Although it scarcely involves a practical point, I may mention that when partial opacity of the capsule occurs, in conjunction with partial or complete opacity of the lens, the colour of the two may so resemble each other, that without looking into the pupil obliquely, in the manner I have described, an inexperienced observer will be deceived. The definite outline of the capsule is well contrasted with the posterior, hazy, and diffused lenticular opacity.

The posterior part of the capsule, differing in structure from the anterior, in being much thinner, has not the same tendency to become opaque; indeed the possibility of such an occurrence, without the lens being also opaque, has occasioned much controversy. The question scarcely possesses any surgical interest, for with deep-seated opacity in the pupil the lens is sure, sooner or later, to become opaque. I have already stated that the posterior opacity usually supposed to be capsular is, in fact, lenticular.

The capsule is rarely so densely opaque throughout as to conceal the cataractous state of the lens unless the opacity be caused by injury, or be congenital. Some little spots, less altered than the rest, generally afford the information; and the age of the individual does not seem to influence its changes, as in lenticular cataract, for precisely the same conditions may be observed at any period of life. A slight degree of opacity, whether in part or in whole, is attended with but little loss of other physical properties, and does not interfere to any extent with operations on the lens.

Very partial capsular opacity is not uncommon with a healthy lens, and does not seem to interfere with it. Complete opacity is always coincident with lenticular cataract.

Respecting traumatic cataract, little need be said, beyond that it is always capsulo-lenticular. Its aspect is generally cloudy, and in proportion as the capsule is thickened, so will it be the whiter. There can be no error of diagnosis, as the history of a case is a safeguard against this. Whenever the aqueous humour has been admitted to the lens, the process of absorption commences. Even when the cataract ensues from a blow on the eye, without rupture of its coats, or even displacement of the lens, I suspect that absorption, however slow, is the rule.

CONGENITAL CATARACT.

This scarcely requires to be spoken of apart from opacity of the lens and that of the capsule occurring at other periods of life, so far as diagnosis is concerned, for the same rules are applicable, but certain modifications of the disease demand a separate notice.

It is one of the peculiarities, and perhaps the chief one, that the cataract so frequently exists only partially, it may be but in the most limited degree—only just enough to be recognised, to an extent almost entirely invading the lens, and may so remain throughout life.

In the slightest state it is a spot of whiteness, sometimes a mere dot in the very centre of the anterior part of the lens; being degeneration of the lens-tissue to that extent. The capsule may be affected to the same extent, or even less, but it may not be implicated. In many persons the cataract is not detected till years after birth; sometimes not till adult life. A state nearly allied to this is produced by infantile purulent ophthalmia. The dot then is always very small. A minute spot on the corresponding part of the cornea often coexists.

In a more extended form, the centre of the lens seems to have received a deposit—an abnormal deposition; for a white opaque excrescence stands out more or less pyramidically, with a base that may occupy the space corresponding to the pupil. This is the pyramidal cataract of the older authors. In the first case I ever saw, pointed out to me by Mr. Lawrence, while his house-surgeon, the apex extended to the cornea, and the base occupied the entire area of the undilated pupil. There happened here what is so common, that, while the lens was in the course of absorption, under operation, the pyramid fell off. It remained in the anterior chamber so long as the boy continued to attend. The excrescence is said to be a cretaceous mass within the capsule. The rest of the lens is frequently transparent; but it may be cloudy or quite opaque. The capsule is also prone to be affected.

The commonest condition of all is central lenticular opacity with grayish-white striæ passing to the entire circumference. This may look like a little cataract surrounded by a black zone. Indeed the usual description of it is opacity of the lens, with arrest of development. The striæ were supposed by Mr. Dalrymple to be fibres attaching the capsule to the vitreous body, or to the anterior layer of the zonule of Zinn. But the lens is not deficient in volume. The modern perfect mode of examining the eye dispels all doubt. Before we had such means at our disposal, I disproved the fallacy, and showed that in the operation for solution, the black zone was lost by the entire lens getting opaque.

Congenital cataract is almost invariably a double affection. I have not met with an exception, but a few single instances of it have been recorded. It has also been noticed as another rare exception, that the disease may appear as spots, or patches, on either surface of the lens.

The capsule may be more or less affected, and I should omit a great characteristic, did I not notice the morbid change that it may undergo in regard to thickness and opacity. The greatest alterations I have observed in these respects have been here.

Mr. Dalrymple says in his Pathology of the Human Eye, "In some cases of congenital cataract, the capsule is covered by dense opaque patches, which more rarely present a hard, bony, or earthy surface. In figure 1, plate xxviii., a case is given of one eye of a youth, aged nineteen, born with imperfect cataract, and in whom a dense earthy spot surrounded by a circle or ring of earthy deposit existed; while in the other eye, and in those of a brother two years younger, were scattered several similar deposits, of irregular shape and size. The lens in each case was but semi-opaque."

With complete capsular opacity, which involves capsulo-lenticular cataract, the last stage of lenticular change consequent on opacity, fluid degeneration, to which absorption succeeds, would seem to be more common here than in the other forms of lenticular disease. I suspect that the absorption is always greater the thicker the capsule. This is no more than might be expected, if, as is probable, that with much thickness, the lens undergoes rapid pathological changes. This is why I suspect capsule only is met with when the disease, originally capsulo-lenticular, is not early operated on.

Whether there is ever an arrest of lenticular development here I cannot say. I strongly suspect that when both capsule and lens are affected, there is not unfrequently, besides, other congenital abnormal conditions in the eye.

CATARACT.

DISTINCTION BETWEEN CATARACT AND OTHER DISEASES.

This subject used to demand many pages of detail, but the modern means of diagnosis dispenses with all but a very short description, whereby there is great gain to the student, and no small relief to an author. Many false theories that had accumulated through a long list of writers, were at once and for ever overthrown by the use of the ophthalmoscope, and truth and simplicity placed in their stead.

The early subjective symptom of cataract is merely mistiness of sight. Objects look as though they were viewed through a mist, or a bit of glass that had been breathed on.

There is, too, impairment of the adjusting power, a natural consequence, as the lens has much to do with the focussing, by actual changes in its form. Distant things are not so well seen as near ones. This has been very erroneously mistaken for ordinary short-sightedness, and as such considered a precursor of cataract.

As the disease forms slowly, vision declines in proportion. A dull, or subdued light is preferred, because with the expanded pupil more rays enter the eye, and there is more vision. As the transmission of light is interfered with according to the several centres of opacity that may exist, so is the effect on sight, and luminous objects are seen in fantastic forms, and often multiplied. A late elderly patient of mine, who had well-formed cataract in one eye, and incipient cataract in the other, was in the habit, when in London, of going out at night to be amused with the multiplication and refraction of the street lights: the pyrotechnic effect was beautiful. Looking at the long train of lamps in Piccadilly was his greatest treat. A perfectly successful operation on each eye proved that this peculiarity was due to the cataract alone.

Muscæ volitantes, frequently in great abundance, almost invariably accompany cataract.

Any other defect or deficiency of sight, or other symptom, such as pain, is due to disease in another part of the eye.

But the uninitiated must be warned that these rules alone,

especially in the early stage of cataract, might not, in consequence of complications, avail him much in forming a definite opinion. Doubts and difficulties may arise and sadly puzzle him. When thus, with failing sight, supposed to be characteristic of the disease, cataract is not apparent in the natural state of the eye, neither with the ordinary light, nor light condensed by a lens, the pupil should be dilated and search made.

In case of doubt the ophthalmoscope should be brought into requisition. I may say that with this most valuable and sure mode of examining the eye, cataract sufficiently advanced to induce a person to seek assistance, in consequence of the interruption to vision that it produces, can always be detected. It may readily be detected when as yet beyond recognition by any other means. The student of to-day, who knows nothing practically of the difficulties that formerly surrounded the matter, must with even his highest appreciation of the instrument have an estimate of it far inferior to the surgeon who used to practise without it.

I must here ask my reader to turn to a few pages in advance, to the chapter on the Ophthalmoscope ; and among the changes noticed as occurring in the crystalline lens, read the continuation of this subject.

Purkinge's candle, or catoptrical test, so much vaunted as the means of distinguishing incipient cataract, is really valueless. I pointed this out in the first edition of this work. But as the ingenious method enables us to pronounce with certainty whether the lens be absent or present, a matter frequently of no small importance, I introduce it here. The test is founded on the optical law that, if a lighted candle or taper be held a few inches in front of, and on a level with, the pupil of a healthy eye, three images appear each behind the other; the anterior erect, the middle inverted, and the posterior erect. The anterior, the most distinct, is formed by the cornea ; the inverted or middle, the smallest and often most difficult to see, by the posterior surface of the lens ; and the posterior, the least sharp, by the anterior surface of the same.

The examination should be made in a dark room, the patient's pupil being well dilated.

The observer should look rather down into the eye than up, shade his own eye from the candle flame, which should be bright and well defined, and move the candle about during the investigation, and especially laterally when he seeks the middle image, which will then seem to move to the opposite side. When, however, the lens is absent, only the anterior or most distinct image, that formed by the cornea, is seen. Opacity of the lens or its capsule from any cause, to a degree that interferes with the transmission of light, obliterates all but the anterior image, which will remain as long as the cornea is clear.

COMPLICATIONS OF CATARACT.

It may facilitate description to make this a subdivision.

Opacity of the lens and its capsule is often associated with disease of the eyeball, and is sometimes the consequence of it; so that it becomes a matter of surgical importance to know how to detect the complication.

The ophthalmoscope may be most advantageously used here also. But when the lens is too opaque to allow the interior of the eye to be satisfactorily seen, perhaps the most generally applicable criterion for our guidance is afforded by the state of the iris, and through it the pupillary movements; for whenever an eye is materially injured, this part does not escape implication—it loses colour and lustre, ceases to be a freely acting diaphragm, and as such is a certain index that the globe of the eye is unsound. A dark-coloured iris may undergo changes of structure that are not readily visible, certainly not as readily to be detected as in one of a light colour. Cataract itself undoubtedly causes some modification of the pupillary functions, for it acts as a veil to the retina, rendering it less sensitive to light. It is possible for a capsulo-lenticular cataract, especially if the capsule be very much thickened, or the lens much degenerated, to efface external impressions sufficiently to render the pupil nearly motionless under considerable variations of light and shade; but such instances are rather uncommon. If, after covering the eye and then exposing it to a moderately bright light, the pupil be motionless, suspicion is justly entertained of the unsoundness of the retina. The eye not experimented on should, of course, be covered all the while.

As a rule, there should be contraction and dilatation according to the opacity of a cataract, whether capsulo-lenticular, or lenticular only; for except the cataract, while incipient, press on the iris, and so impair its movements, there should be a marked action of the iris, scarcely, if at all, differing from that of a healthy eye. In certain forms of complete amaurosis the pupil may act freely, but this complication cannot lead to error, as the total loss of the perception of any degree of light, which can never occur from cataract, would alone declare the disease.

The ordinary habitual size of the pupil in different individuals must not be lost sight of in these examinations. There is a relation, I do not say invariable, but sufficiently constant to be recognised, between its accustomed dimensions and certain temperaments—a fact too often overlooked; hence our guide should rather be the relative, or proportionate, changes under different degrees of light, than the actual capacity; generally, the smaller the natural size, the more limited will be its movements. The various degrees of activity of the iris in different persons must be remembered, as well as the influence of age, it being more lively in the young. I examined the eyes of a lady, eighty-one years of age, with full-formed lenticular cataracts, at the window, on an autumnal day, when the pupils were contracted to a degree that at first induced suspicion of some coexistent ocular affection; but further examination with different degrees of light, showed a variation in them that removed all doubt. She herself was well aware of the activity of her irides, and the disadvantage accruing from the pupillary contraction had induced her, since the commencement of the cataracts, to wear a large shade to shut out bright light.

When only one eye has cataract, unless some other disease exist in it, or the other eye be defective, there is not any disparity in the pupils.

Variation in the pupillary apertures may arise from imperfect development of the iris, but this will be readily recognised as a congenital defect.

A dilated and motionless pupil is a pretty sure indication of ocular disease; and if with the dilatation there be irregularity, all doubt is removed. The opposite condition, contraction, may proceed from a like cause, but it is very rare.

I believe that the use of belladonna may be made subservient to diagnosis; and the very slow, as well as imperfect dilatation taken as an unhealthy index. Moreover, it might discover adhesions, and so show the true nature of the case, which might otherwise, perhaps, be overlooked.

It is not always possible, in particular cases, to say with certainty whether the faintness of the perception of light be owing to the opacity of the cataract, or to a diseased retina. Soft capsulo-lenticular cataract, especially with fluid degeneration of the lens, obstructs the light the most. Still, generally speaking, the degree of vision is in proportion to the opacity in the pupil, and its amount affords a pretty sure index of the health of the retina. Cataract alone never entirely shuts out the light.

Something, such as a penknife, or the finger, should be passed between the patient's eye and the light, as a test of sight: if he perceive the shadow, the retina may be considered sound, but unhealthy, in proportion as only larger bodies can be discerned. An operation undertaken when the membrane evinces decided feebleness, must ever be attended with doubtful results; with total loss of power, any practical surgical proceeding is inadmissible.

Certain conditions of the globe of the eye, indicative of pathological changes in the vitreous humour, go so far towards rendering operations abortive, that their detection is very essential. These are softness or flaccidity, or the opposite state, unnatural hardness. Tremulousness of the iris is frequently seen in connexion with an unhealthy condition of this humour.

Discoloration, or unusual vascularity of the sclerotica, especially if the anterior vessels be large and tortuous; diminution of the eyeball, and a diminished cornea, are all unfavourable prognostics for operating, and any one of these may be sufficient to contraindicate it. Without proceeding further in detail, it may be stated that any deviation whatever from what would be considered a state of health, in any of the textures composing the globe of the eye, except the lens, is a complication rendering, according to its kind and degree, an eye more or less unfit for any operation for cataract.

Inflammatory affections of the ocular appendages, and mechanical changes in the eyelids, that may in any way interfere with their proper motions, or produce irritation of the cornea, fall within the same category of objections to operating.

I am quite aware that, with all my detail and carefulness of description, a student may not be able to apply the above rules in detecting the symptoms that prove the existence of such a diseased state of the eyeball, or complication with cataract, as to militate against operating. It is impossible for a writer to lay down unerring marks that any one may apply. Only when an observer has acquired some knowledge of ophthalmic diseases, can the description be appreciated. Although I might be well satisfied that enough has been said on the diseased states severally, for all guidance, yet perhaps I ought to speak directly and especially of a condition of the eye that embodies all the changes alluded to; not only to explain the term then generally applied, " Glaucoma," but because opacity of the lens is a common and last result of the morbid phenomena. Without going here into the minute changes which the several tissues undergo, a description of which will be found in the chapter on "Iridectomy," I may define what is called " Glaucoma " as disorganization of the interior of the eyeball, with more or less marks of a diseased state on the exterior.

Glaucoma is common in elderly persons, seldom, if ever,

existing before the middle period of life, and for the most part affecting both eyes, although not simultaneously. In a case in an advanced stage, with all the usual symptoms well marked, the eyeball is hard, and not elastic, as in health ; the sclerotic coat discoloured, with, perhaps, dark patches, and large tortuous dark-coloured veins, ramifying about, and passing to within a short distance of the cornea, the spot where the blood is returned from the anterior part of the eye. The cornea loses its lustre, and always, more or less, its transparency ; looks uneven or rough, of a ground-glass-like appearance. The iris is in part or entirely discoloured, being dark and convex, apparently in contact with the cornea. The motionless pupil is dilated, perhaps, to a degree that shows only a mere ring of iris, and it may be round, or irregular, frequently transversely oval. The lens is opaque, and striæ may be seen, but it never exhibits the characteristics of uncomplicated hard cataract, nor those of soft, except when there is breaking-down of the superficies, or actual fluid degeneration. It rather presents hues peculiar to this general invasion of disease. A sea-green state of pupil, which, in fact, means a green lens, is so commonly described as the chief feature in glaucoma, that surgeons are apt to disregard all other evidence of the disorganization if this be wanting. Any actual shade of green is really very rare. The common appearances, which cannot be well expressed in words, are nearest represented by the expressions—dirty-white, dirty-yellow, copper-brown, greenish-drab. They often resemble the darker shades that are seen during the decline of a cutaneous ecchymosis.

If it were possible for anything more to be wanting to confirm the existence of glaucoma, it may be gathered from the subjective symptoms : flashes, coruscations, and bright colours are seen. Intense pain and loss of sight complete the catalogue. Added to these, the history of a case must afford the fullest conclusion ; for whether acute, and with such intensity of action that blindness ensues in a few days, or chronic, that weeks or months, or years, are required to extinguish sight, opacity of the lens is the last result.

It is a cardinal point in ophthalmic surgery not to operate on an eye for the removal of cataract so long as it may be rendered available for ordinary purposes by optical appliances or otherwise, except at the request of a patient, after he is aware of all the circumstances of the case. The advantage to vision to be derived from dilating the pupil with belladonna is remarkable. But it is impossible to tell, till it is tried, how far this may serve, in consequence of the arrangement of the opacity. Sometimes the dilatation confuses. The benefits are greatest in central cataract, and usually more lasting because the partial affection may be stationary. I saw a housemaid, eighteen years old, with partial capsulo-lenticular cataract that almost blinded her when the pupil was in the natural state, but when dilated by a solution of belladonna, applied three times a week, she executed her work so efficiently that her employer was unaware of her defect. The belladonna had been used since childhood.

I might mention other cases, in which, under the same assistance, the most minute work—as engraving and watch finishing—has been most efficiently executed. In the case of a young lady, the sight might be called microscopic. But generally the objects must be brought very close to the eye. The effects of the belladonna do not wear out, the same quantity always producing the same result at any interval, or for any prolonged period.

I may also add that an operation ought not to be undertaken in anticipation, because the ratio of increase in the cataract is very uncertain. It is often remarkably slow, especially in the hard variety; years may pass away with but little progress.

OPERATIONS FOR CATARACT.

The several conditions of lenticular cataract, as before expressed, require different operations, and the choice of any one should rest solely on the circumstances of the case.

The hard cataract must as a rule be extracted, that is, removed from the eye; or displaced, by being pressed into the vitreous humour. To attempt to produce absorption would be to incur very great risk of destruction to the eye, from inflammation.

Soft cataract, while allowed to remain in place, should be lacerated, or so broken, as to admit of the process of absorption, to which its softer texture readily yields; for, with this simple operation, the natural powers are quite capable of causing its complete dissipation.

Capsular cataract must be removed from the eye, or be cut, or torn through, to enable it to contract.

There are several circumstances that regulate the choice of either of the operations for hard cataract. Subsequent to the middle period of life, from the changes incidental to age, the anterior chamber may be so reduced in size that the cataract-knife cannot be used without wounding the iris to a considerable extent. The same may be said of diminished capacity of the chamber from a bulging iris, resulting from pressure behind the cataract. A preternaturally small palpebral aperture, by preventing sufficient exposure of the eyeball, or a very deep-set eye, may each be a hindrance to extraction. But not one of these is a decided objection, as all may be overcome by tact and management, as I shall show. Entire adhesion of the pupillary margin to the capsule of the lens forbids it. But this condition of the eye is necessarily associated with several morbid changes, and requires special treatment according to circumstances. The subject, however, elicits the question, With what amount of attachment may extraction be undertaken with prospect of success? It is difficult to answer hypothetically. The more the iris is damaged in texture, the less is its expansive power, and it may.be generally stated, that when so much of the pupil is involved that this aperture cannot open sufficiently to allow the cataract to pass, the simple operation of extraction is inadmissible. Adhesion of the iris to the cornea may forbid extraction, either from the extent of the connexion, or the part of the iris implicated. All these impediments and drawbacks will be fully discussed according to the importance of each, after the operation has been described.

The white ring sometimes existing around the cornea, known

as the arcus senilis, and discovered by Mr. Canton to be fatty degeneration, is no impediment to extraction; an incision in it heals as readily as in a transparent part.

The operation for displacement is essentially a very bad one, because the cataract is rendered a foreign body within the eye. It is only admissible when extraction would be dangerous, or is positively unsuitable, and ought to be regarded merely as a proceeding of expediency. Chronic cough and unhealthiness of the vitreous humour are often spoken of as states in which displacement is most suited. As regards the first, I can say with reference to extraction that I have never seen an instance in which it has not been so subdued as to be harmless. Respecting the second, although there would be danger of the loss of that body when diseased if the eyeball be opened, the condition is also very unfavourable for displacement, from the impossibility of keeping the cataract in the desired position.

The lesser degree of manual dexterity demanded for this operation, which is really very easy, has induced many surgeons to assign to extraction quite a secondary place, but I cannot allow that such a standard should regulate the decision. Cataract is not a disease of emergency, in which one is suddenly called on to operate, and I hold it to be the imperative duty of all who undertake the practical surgery of the eye, to qualify themselves for the efficient execution of those operations that are the most certain, and confer the most lasting benefits.

PREPARATION OF THE PATIENT.

Operations implicating the globe of the eye, demand for their success a state of health in which a wound can be inflicted on a delicate and sensitive organ with the greatest impunity. In the operation for extraction, unless union of the cornea be quickly effected by adhesion, success must always be more or less imperfect, and destruction of the organ will frequently ensue. A debilitated constitution requires to be improved to the highest standard that the idiosyncrasy of the person will allow.

Plethora should always be avoided. An accustomed eye soon detects the habit of body that is popularly called "rude health," and a person exhibiting it in a marked degree should be reduced by regulation of diet, exercise, and gentle purgation if necessary, till any excess disappears and the force of the circulation is rendered more natural.

Dr. Jacob, in his *brochure* on the operation for cataract with the fine needle, makes the following excellent remarks, which are not less practical than original :—

"The value of preparatory and after-treatment, as part of the surgeon's care in cataract operations, has been fully appreciated, and, in practice, amply made available ; but the value of a respectful consideration of all the functions of the animal economy upon which health depends has not been so well understood. It is assumed that a patient should be prepared for an operation by taking physic and abstaining from food ; yet a rational man, acquainted with the consecutive operation of each apparatus provided for the growth, repair, and preservation of the living being, may well doubt the correctness of such a view. The universal faith reposed in the practice of giving and taking physic has led practitioners not only to place too much reliance on that resource, but to resort to it sometimes to the injury of the patient; as I find in the case under consideration. In preparing a patient for operation, I do not act on the belief that empty bowels are essential to health, or that what are called *fæces* should not be found in the intestinal canal; on the contrary, I proceed on a conviction totally different. If a patient be in good health, notwithstanding an habitual retention of the contents of the bowels beyond the prescribed periods, I do not wish to risk an interruption of health by disturbing the natural functions of the stomach and bowels, and I therefore refrain from giving physic. But if the patient be not in good health, I of course endeavour to bring him into that condition by every means in my power, and resolutely resist every attempt to induce me to operate until I have accomplished that object. Above all things, the state of the digestive organs should be carefully studied, and if found defective, if possible, repaired. Nothing seems to require more attention than the condition of the tongue as indicative of the state of the stomach and bowels. If it be white, or coated with discoloured adhesive mucus, the functions of assimilation and nutrition are probably imperfectly performed, and a resulting tendency to destructive inflammation from local injury is engendered."

" It is usual in preparing for this and other operations to make great alterations in diet, substituting liquid for solid, and vegetable for animal aliments. This, however, must be done with caution, leading as it inevitably does to disturbance of the digestive function and interruption of the assimilating and nutritive processes, if suddenly or exclusively adopted. Without digestible nutritious food, good chyle and blood cannot be produced, and without good blood, local injuries are liable to suffer from destructive inflammation."

The whitish and rather coated tongue of the aged should not be mistaken for a symptom of unhealthiness. In them this organ is not so ready an index of the state of health as in early years; attention should therefore be paid to the urine, the deposition of uric acid, or of the urate of ammonia, being a sure indication of dyspepsia, or excess of nitrogenised food, or of fever; and that of phosphate of lime or the triple phosphate, of the opposite states of prostration and nervous depression. The abdominal evacuation should, with the least apparent necessity, be examined for evidence of the hepatic state, and for information respecting the digestion of food, particularly in those past the meridian of life, because it is then that these functions are mostly at fault, and all kinds of operations less successful. In the majority of persons far advanced in years, who have passed through operations under my hands, it has been necessary to increase, or, if I may so call it, force the circulation, by tonics and stimulants. Towards the limit of the natural term of life, we should not, without ample necessity, cut off the accustomed amount of daily nourishment or the usual stimuli.

The presence of active specific inflammation, as the strumous, gouty, syphilitic, or rheumatic, in any part of the body, would contra-indicate an operation; nor would it be prudent to operate on an eye that had recently been inflamed from any cause; a very long interval should be allowed to pass after the last trace of such disturbance.

 Organic disease in the chest is scarcely an impediment. While I was attending the practice of Mr. Tyrrell, he operated by extraction on the eye of a female, fifty-seven years old, who had valvular disease of the heart, ascites, and anasarca; the operation was quite successful, and the patient returned home on the eleventh day after its performance. Her heart had been diseased for five years.

Advanced age is not in itself an objection to operating, if nothing else forbid. The best attainable results have followed extraction after ninety, in the hands of Mr. Lawrence. The late Mr. Scott did the same operation successfully on a female between ninety and a hundred. I have several times performed it to my complete satisfaction after the eightieth year, and once as late as the eighty-sixth.

It is not yet generally agreed on by surgeons, when both eyes are equally affected, whether only one eye at a time should be operated on, or both at once. If extraction be the operation, my practice has been to do the one, and to let it recover before the other is touched. There is thereby less shock to the system; besides, at a first operation, there may be discovered some constitutional peculiarity of bad tendeney, which may in some measure be removed or reduced at the second. Patients almost invariably prefer single operation.

The season of the year most fitted for operating has also, and especially of late years, occupied attention. With reference to needle operations, I suspect it matters not; nor, perhaps, is any operation in our climate influenced by the mere degree of temperature, which is rarely in either extreme. In extracting in cold weather, I have the room to which the patient is confined kept at a uniform temperature, not lower than 60° Fahrenheit for the first few days. Many very excellent surgeons never extract in winter, and Mr. Tyrrell thought the best time for that operation to be between March and October. Where a choice is permitted, I should, as a rule, prefer that period, because regular exercise, prior to the operation, is less likely to be interfered with, from the greater certainty of settled weather; while the apartment can be better ventilated, and the patient will be able sooner to take out-door exercise, and recover his lost strength and spirits, the consequence of anxiety and confinement. Again, when the state of the eye is such as to render the success of the operation somewhat doubtful, I should prefer summer weather.

FIG. 121.

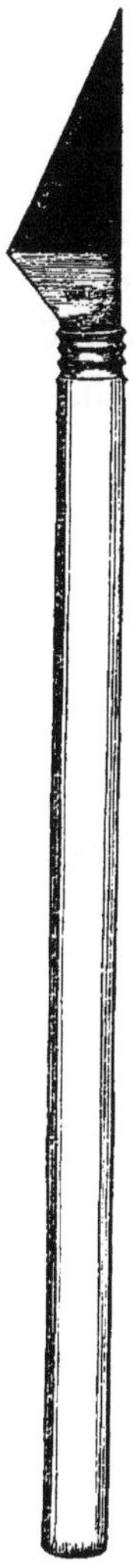

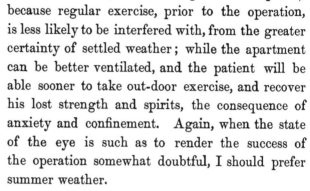

OPERATION FOR EXTRACTION.

CATARACT KNIFE.

Beer's Knife, more or less modified, is that which has obtained general approbation, the triangular blade fitting it for cutting a flap by one continuous movement. The form fig. 121 I employed for some years; but I found the breadth too great. I altered it to ten-twelfths of an inch, by seven-twentieths. I yet use this for a sunken eye, or where the eyeball cannot be well exposed.

FIG. 122.

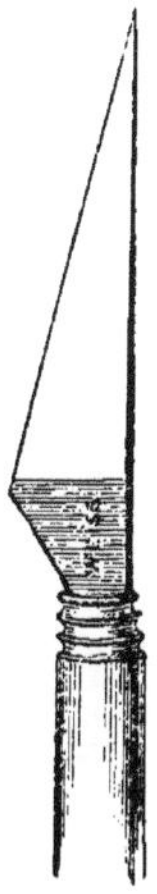

But I prefer the original Beer's, fig. 122, whenever it is applicable. If the angle be increased much beyond this, the cornea is less easily punctured, the aqueous humour is apt to escape prematurely, and the iris to fall on the edge of the instrument.

The following diagram, representing a cornea of full size, displays in the dotted lines the course the knife should take. Any breadth of blade greater than is required to accomplish

M M 2

such an incision, is superfluous.   The average diameter of the cornea is, in adults, about seventeen-fortieths of an inch; in old persons it is less.   In the very aged, it may be still more reduced.

FIG. 123.

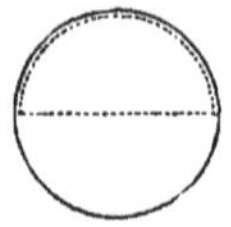

FIG. 124. 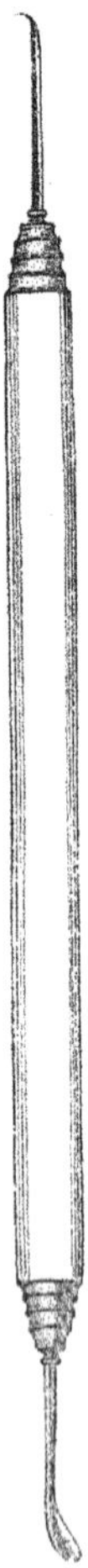   The thickness of the knife should be nicely regulated : there ought to be a slight increase from the point, which should be stiff, to the shoulder.   The back should neither be square nor obtusely rounded, but rolled off gradually from the middle of the blade, to an edge sufficiently thin, without being sharp.

CURETTE.

Both of the extremities of this instrument are considerably modified from the usual forms.   The spoon-like silver end peculiarly suits the purposes demanded of it ; the other, or needle limb, is curved only as much as is actually required, for the less the deviation from a straight line the greater is the facility in using it, and the less risk is there of injurious contact with the iris or the cornea.   A side view cannot, of course, convey an idea of the breadth, which is nearly that of the stem within a short distance of the point.   The very extremity only is sharp.

GUARDED CURETTE.

In one that I have had executed by Messrs. Weiss, the point is concealed by a little guard, so that when the instrument is closed it is dull, in consequence of which it can, with ease and safety, be carried to the required spot, where it is opened by pressure on the trigger in the handle, used, then allowed to close by remission of the pressure, and withdrawn.

FIG. 125.

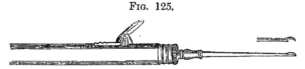

The larger figure (125) shows the instrument shut; the lesser FIG. 126. a little open. The ordinary curette of the shops is too large. Injury is apt to be in- FIG. 127. flicted on the iris in its passage, blood poured out, and its application to the capsule prevented, because of that part being obscured; or if these steps be well executed, mischief is often done in its withdrawal.

SECONDARY KNIFE.

I give the preference to one of this form (fig. 126). The point is rounded and blunt. A straight blade requires less force than a convex one, or concave, to direct it with effect; moreover, it is capable of receiving a keener edge, and these are advantages of higher importance here, because the occasion which calls for the secondary knife offers peculiar difficulties, owing to the flaccidity of the eye, the impractibility under the circumstances, of applying any pressure to keep it quite steady, and the necessity of cutting in a certain direction under unusually limited restrictions. When the instrument case contains one only, the blade should be longer.

SHARP HOOK.

This (fig. 127) is commonly called a lens hook. The point is sharp, yet the hook itself ought not to be very fine, for a very delicate extremity would not be sufficiently retained by the lens, and be more apt to become entangled in the parts over which it passes, or with which it comes in contact, and to scratch or otherwise injure them. It is an instrument very seldom needed, especially by a good operator.

Extraction is frequently referred to as one of the most difficult operations in surgery. While I fully admit that for accurate execution great nicety and tact are needed, and these are within the reach of most surgeons, I do not hesitate to assert that its difficulties are greatly exaggerated.

Putting aside those whose total want of manual tact, or great nervousness, disqualifies them for any manipulations in operative surgery requiring delicacy, I believe that with proper training and practice on the dead body, any surgeon may become a successful operator. Of course there have been, and ever will be, degrees of excellence, owing to the differences of natural aptitude, and of dexterity acquired by diligent study and practice. One of the best operators we have ever had in this kingdom was, in the first instance, so unsuccessful, that he was restrained from operating for two years at the institution to which he was attached; and during that time he was literally confined to the minor operations only. He had the good sense to submit with patience to this decree, and the issue was, that he became most dexterous. This valuable man was prematurely cut off, but he has left behind him for our example, his patience under temporary eclipse, his unwearied perseverance in overcoming his natural impediments, and his modesty and quiet dignity, when great and deserved success crowned his labours and his zeal.

My immediate preparation of a patient has been the administration of some mild laxative the day before operating, solely that the necessary quiet after the operation may not be disturbed for a day or two by the natural action of the bowels; for the probability is that they will not act for a few days after the effect of the medicine is over; but it is a practice that I do not insist on.

The state of the pupil, whether artificially dilated or not, can have little effect, either in placing the iris out of the reach of the knife, or throwing it in the way. It has been said, that if dilated, it is less manageable after the extraction, but this is very questionable indeed. I do not interfere with the natural state.

Whether a patient be sitting or lying down during the operation is of no particular moment, if he be quiet; but if likely to be restless, he ought to be placed on his back. In the earlier years of my practice, I adopted the former position. Now, I almost invariably use the couch.

The importance of a properly regulated light is evident; and an operator will, of course, choose that which, according to the arrangement of the room, suits best.

It is customay to bind up the eye not to be operated on if it have any sight; I object to the practice, because it possesses no advantage, and the formality tends to unnerve a patient.

It is well to have all the principal articles of clothing taken off, the patient prepared to go to bed, and a morning gown put on, to prevent the inconvenience of undressing afterwards.

I am in the habit of dividing the cornea in the upper part, preferring that section, as it possesses many advantages over the lower—such as the greater certainty in making it effectually, the less likelihood of the flap being interfered with by the eyelid, and the upper position of the pupil should the iris prolapse.

It is better to stand behind the patient in every instance, as it gives much greater command over the globe of the eye. But when the left eye is to be treated, if want of practice or deficiency of confidence disqualify the left hand, the operator must stand in front, or submit to the great disadvantage of resigning to another what he ought to do himself, as most important acts, and trust the retracting of the upper eyelid, and the steadying of the eyeball, to an assistant, while he uses the knife in the direction he prefers, upwards or downwards.

It is notorious that extraction in the left eye is much more frequently attended by failure than in the right, and the occur-

rence is of course attributable to the greater difficulty offered
by the position of this eye.

I shall now describe the operation. The preliminaries having
been arranged, an assistant gently draws down the lower eyelid,
resting his finger on the malar bone so that the eyeball be not
pressed. The operator stands behind the patient's head, which
is of course at a convenient height, places his hand on the
forehead, with the forefinger elevates and draws forward the
upper eyelid, locks it under the edge of the orbit, and with
the tip of the finger, which should be a little below the tarsus,
presses gently against the eyeball to prevent any upward
motion, while he places his middle finger on the inner side, to
counteract any movements · in an inward direction. Neither
finger encroaches on the cornea, but is kept away as far as
possible. He rests his other hand against the side of the face;

FIG. 128.

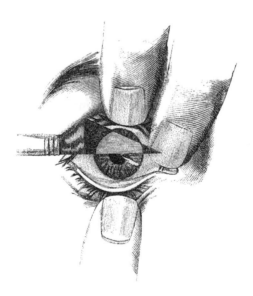

holds the knife lightly and unrestrained, by the thumb and
forefinger, or the second as well; enters it at the central and
external part of the cornea, a little less than half a line anterior

to the sclerotica, or just far enough to insure that the true corneal tissue is penetrated; passes it rapidly through the anterior chamber; and carries the point out on the inner side, at a spot as nearly as possible opposite to the entrance.

He thrusts the knife slowly along with the same continued movement, and takes care so to direct the edge in its entire course that it shall pass at a uniform distance from the sclerotica. As the incision advances, he remits the pressure, and discontinues before it is finished; prior to which, also, the assistant relaxes his hold. To prevent a jerk when finishing, he proceeds slowly, and allows the aqueous humour to escape by a slight twist, or the least withdrawal of the knife; places the end of the finger, or the back of the nail, against the remaining tag as a rest or support; and completes the cut by a sawing motion.

The preceding diagram delineates these several steps executed on the right eye.

Subsequently to a brief repose, he raises the eyelid sufficiently to expose the cornea, tells the patient to look towards his feet,

FIG. 129.

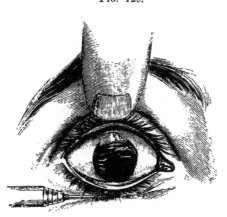

so that the eyeball may be directed downwards, introduces the curette beneath the corneal flap, and lacerates the capsule very freely across the entire area of the pupil. He now starts the cataract by pressing on the eyeball, above, through the medium of the eyelid, with the finger used as a wedge between it and the orbit, and below, with the curette, after the manner exemplified in fig. 129, or, as some prefer, applied against the sclerotica just below the cornea, increases it, and alternates it, till the opening of the lips of the cornea by the bulging of the iris indicates that the cataract has left its position, and steadily keeps it up till it has fairly protruded, when the elasticity of the cornea will suffice for the expulsion. The operation is now over, and if well done is generally bloodless.

My own practice is invariably to apply strips of court plaster, thoroughly wetted, to both eyes, even when only one has been operated on.

It matters not if the point of the knife be entered higher or lower than the centre of the cornea, provided that the counter-puncture correspond to it. It is a very common error for the operator to hold his knife in such a position that the edge, instead of the back, is in a line with the diameter of the cornea, which causes the instrument to take a wrong course, not including a sufficient portion of the cornea : from not being prac-tically aware of this fault, some surgeons frequently fail in extraction.

As the eyeball cannot always be kept motionless without an injurious amount of pressure, but may roll a little during the introduction and passage of the knife through the chamber, great nicety is required to adapt the hand to the yielding, for without this precaution a proper counter-puncture cannot be made. After the cornea is transfixed the eyeball is under the operator's control, and can then be correctly placed if it have rolled too much inwards.

A complication may arise by the iris falling in the way of the knife, an occurrence that may be produced by the prema-ture escape of the aqueous humour from undue pressure on the eyeball ; from not making a continuous onward movement with the knife, by which it is kept adapted to the incision ; or from what, in fact, amounts to the same thing, twisting it about, and causing the edges of the wound to gape. If the aqueous humour escape prior to the counter-puncture, the knife should be withdrawn, and the operation delayed. If, when the cornea be nearly divided, a considerable portion of the iris be in the way, the instrument should be taken out, and the section completed with the secondary knife, the blade of which must be passed completely under the remainder, and used in the most convenient direction. Every endeavour should be made not to cut the iris, because when wounded it almost always gets adherent to the cornea, and interferes with the healing of it, and the pupil is necessarily displaced. If a second pupil be made, the isthmus should at once be divided by the blunt-pointed iris scissors. It is recommended by several surgeons, always to attempt to free an entangled iris, by pressing it between the cornea and the knife; but I have seen many such efforts made without a single successful issue; however, I wish it to be understood, that I do not doubt the possibility of the iris being shaken off the edge of the knife, for the fact has been mentioned to me by surgeons who have done it. I feel perfectly sure that some of the rules laid down on this head by writers cannot, with safety to the eye, be reduced to practice.

The iris may or may not bleed when wounded, but the presence of blood in the chambers of the eye need not occasion any anxiety, as it is quickly absorbed.

If the cornea have been divided as I have directed, there will be ample room for the cataract to pass out; but in proportion as the incision is smaller, will there be difficulty in its exit; and when under a certain size, it cannot escape at all. A faulty section may arise from entering the knife too much above the transverse axis of the cornea, or too far from the sclerotica, or from running the point for some distance between the laminæ of the cornea; or with a good entrance, the counter-puncture may have been in the wrong place. Again, the cornea may be admirably transfixed; but instead, however, of the edge of the knife being kept parallel with the iris, it has been directed forwards and brought out too far from the sclerotica. All of these mistakes are equally bad; the most common, and therefore that to be most guarded against, is an imperfect counter-puncture, to obviate which very ingenious, but very useless, and even injurious instruments have been invented to fix the globe of the eye. It would be difficult to name a contrivance that has not been recommended. Certainly the most efficient and safe method when an operator needs such assistance, is for an assistant to lay hold of the conjunctiva at the lower part of the eyeball, with a pair of toothed forceps, as has been much recommended by Mr. France. But except there be actual necessity for any such help, it should not be employed, from the pain and annoyance it causes. I have heard patients speak of it as the worst part of the operation.

When the incision is inadequate, a fault which is always readily recognised by the cataract having partly passed through the pupil, and yet not escaping, the use of the secondary knife is the correct expedient, for any attempt at expulsion by squeezing would be fruitless, and likely to be fatal to the eye from the vitreous humour rushing out. The blade should be kept forwards with the extremity against the cornea, that the iris be not injured, and the cutting slowly executed by a succession of outward strokes on the outer extremity of the incision. A surgeon who operates even tolerably well will very seldom have to enlarge the incision—a proceeding which is certainly one of some danger; for according to my own experience, when it has been adopted, there has been a large average of failures, which is doubtless attributable to the cornea having been jagged, and the iris more or less bruised. Still, enlarging the wound is far preferable to forcing the cataract through a small aperture, for an easy exit is a very great essential to success. Some surgeons use scissors.

The importance of thoroughly lacerating the capsule, especially when it is thickened, is in general hardly sufficiently estimated, and the neglect of it is next in frequency to a defective corneal incision. Bulging of the iris, without the cataract commencing to escape, is the symptom of the laceration being effectual. The curette, introduced with the concavity upwards, should be run across from side to side, and from above to below, as far as the pupil will allow, and, unless this be done lightly, the cataract is in danger of being displaced. I have seen it used too freely, and the cataract, a softish one, actually broken up, so that only a part could be got out. On withdrawing the instrument, its direction should be reversed. Attention to these precautions will save the cornea and the iris from injury; but they are unnecessary when the guarded curette is used.

Pressing out the cataract should be a slow process. Sudden escape of it may paralyse the iris entirely or in part, and produce an irregular pupil. A cataract with a soft exterior comes out more easily than one in which there is not this degeneration, and less pressure is required.

Should the cataract not move forwards or evince some signs of displacement after the requisite degree of pressure, and should there be no impediment except that which may be attributed to encasement in a dense capsule, it must be removed with the lens hook. This little instrument being entered like the curette, is passed through the pupil and implanted in the cataract. Except in the hands of a most expert manipulator, this is certain to be attended with loss of the vitreous humour, from pressure in attempts to steady the eyeball, and only long practice in operating can give the delicacy of touch, the confidence, and the coolness that are required.

The vitreous humour may escape by the side of the cataract, in consequence of a faulty incision, too much pressure, dislocation with the curette, or undue fluidity. In the first instance, the section must be carefully enlarged. The lens hook must be brought into requisition and applied, if possible, to the back of the cataract. Should the cataract sink out of sight, it ought to be abandoned. Hæmorrhage may follow this lifting out of the cataract, but I have not myself met with an example, and I quote from Mr. Tyrrell, who informs us that in some cases where he has had to remove a cataract which had been displaced during the use of the curette, there has been subsequent hæmorrhage, without injury of the iris, to an extent that destroyed the eye, arising, as he supposed, from the central artery of the retina. In one case there was positive assurance that the iris was uninjured.

The cataract, if undergoing softening throughout, may fall

in pieces while emerging from the cornea, and some of the fragments remain in the anterior chamber. The spoon of the curette should be used to withdraw any of these that may interfere with the adaptation of the corneal flap, or perhaps lie between the iris and the cornea; but any that occupy the pupil may safely be left alone to the process of absorption.

If the circumference or soft part merely of the cataract remain, it should be left untouched, unless any portion occupy the incision of the cornea, for it is rapidly removed.

Sometimes the capsule of the lens occupies the pupil, or in some other way intrudes itself on our notice. It is dangerous to meddle with it, lest the hyaloid membrame be ruptured, and vitreous humour flow out. Except a portion of it should be in the corneal wound, all attempts at removal should be left for a future period.

The iris does not always recover itself and contract after the escape of the cataract, but may prolapse and be unmanageable. If after gently touching the eyeball a few times, or rubbing it through the closed eyelids, waiting a little, and again repeating the rubbing, the prolapsed portion be not removed, the guarded curette, or any appropriate appliance, must be called to our aid in replacing it. But this demands the most gentle manipulation, without which the hyaloid membrane will be ruptured. One attempt only should be made. There is always a chance of spontaneous return after all efforts have failed. Although the protruded part prevents rapid progress of the case, it may not materially interfere with success. The most troublesome prolapses are those complicated with escape of vitreous humour; and there is nothing that tries the young operator more than this condition. It is worse than useless to attempt the reduction of the iris. The best thing is to close the eye as quickly as possible over the gaping wound, lifting the upper eyelid over the eyeball, lest the corneal flap be further thrust down. With very much of the humour hanging out, it might be well to cut it through close to the iris, with the scissors. Of course the chances are greatly against success.

Loss of the vitreous humour, so often already alluded to, is perhaps the commonest untoward event in extraction. When it is dissolved, no operative skill can invariably prevent a partial escape. After operations that have been faultless, I have seen it trickle out like water. But the occurrence is generally due to accident from bad operating. It is a common thing with beginners for the cataract suddenly to burst out directly that the cornea is cut through. Spasmodic action of the muscles generally bears the blame. When the smallest part has been evacuated, the slightest pressure will occasion further discharge. All that need be said about the course to follow is expressed in the preceding paragraph. Some authors undertake to tell the effect that will be produced on vision according to the amount lost, and speak of a third, fourth, or fifth ; all this is mere conjecture : how is the quantity which has escaped to be decided on ? The abstraction of a very small quantity does not seem to be generally followed by a decidedly bad effect; but even when the amount is fortunately small, there are generally the accompanying disadvantages of prolapse of the iris, and prolonged healing, which is injurious in proportion as it is delayed, and may through this be fatal to the eye.

Adjustment of the flap of the cornea is the last particular of the operation requiring attention. In every instance it should be ascertained that there is adaptation and no eversion. With a prominent eye, the eyelid may displace it, turning it down. Instead of attempting replacement with the curette, which is always troublesome and not devoid of risk, the eye should be opened, the cilia taken hold of, and the eyelid raised, perhaps sometimes with the forceps, and lifted over. Inversion of the flap, which, it is said, may occur, would certainly require the curette, or some blunt instrument, to restore it.

A rare occurrence after extraction, but a most destructive one, is hæmorrhage. It never occurs, of course, except in diseased eyes; and in all but one of the cases that I have seen, there has been undue vascularity of the surface of the eyeball, than which there is no greater evidence of an unhealthy state of the vascular apparatus within. In the exceptional one there was merely darkness of the sclerotic coat. I operated on one of the eyes of the patient in whom this existed, removed the cataract with perfect satisfaction, and was about to close the eye, when bleeding commenced, and, continuing, forced out the vitreous humour, till the whole of it escaped; ultimately the retina was evacuated. A firm compress on the eye stopped further discharge. This was the first case of the kind I had seen associated with so little external change. I extracted the cataract from the other eye a few weeks afterwards, and precisely the same results ensued. In reviewing the several subjective symptoms throughout the entire duration of the cataract, there was nothing to indicate unhealthiness of the interior of the eye, beyond the rather frequent occurrence in the latter stage of small coloured spots. This, certainly more than the dusky hue of the surface of the eye, made me suspicious of some complication; and the expression of my opinion to that effect, together with some doubt about success, removed some of my responsibility, and saved no little annoyance.

My own views respecting the source of the bleeding in these instances, is given at page 326, in the chapter on "Staphyloma."

I saw a patient who was about to be operated on for cataract, with a degree of sclerotic vascularity which gave strong suspicions of such internal disease as would probably be followed by hæmorrhage. This did occur, and, as I have been told, the bleeding nearly cost the poor woman her life, by its continuance. Some so-called styptic was applied, and the case left to a nurse. A more competent surgeon who accidentally called, quickly applied a compress in a proper manner, and arrested it.

I took a note of a case that occurred in Mr. Tyrrell's practice, in which hæmorrhage appeared subsequent to extraction, and was not suppressed until after the cornea had healed, as the chambers of the eye were filled with blood, without there having been any escape of it. The blood was absorbed, and success ensued. I adduce this as a curious occurrence, rather than to illustrate what has gone before.

This is the proper place to notice those physical states of the eye, to which allusion has been made, that render extraction peculiarly difficult, and may require some modification of the ordinary operation.

Smallness of the anterior chamber is a common drawback to the safe execution of extraction. The dimensions may be so reduced that it cannot be done in the accustomed manner without considerable injury to the iris. The operator must decide when such limits are reached. I have seen one surgeon make the corneal section most successfully in a case which another had rejected. I have myself effected it in several instances, although at a first glance such a result seemed impossible. Much, therefore, is to be done by carefulness and lightness of touch. Tact also is demanded in the use of the knife, so as not to press it backwards against the eyeball, but, after the counter-puncture is made, rather to draw it forwards during the remainder of the cut. A healthy iris is not a perfect plane, but a little convex in front, at the centre. In any instance, therefore, in which there is a possibility of making a satisfactory counter-puncture, an operator need seldom fail in finishing the section as desired. Abnormal bulging of the iris may render it impossible to effect the counter-puncture safely, and therefore to operate with the triangular knife. But while such a state makes extraction more difficult, and I may say less certain, it does not forbid it. I have operated almost entirely, and successfully, with the secondary knife. I made an aperture with the triangular one, only just enough to admit the blunt extremity of the other, with which I effected an ample corneal flap, without wounding the iris. A careful assistant steadied the eyeball with a pair of forceps, so that there was scarcely any pressure exercised by the fingers. I should prefer this, as a rule, to displacing the cataract.

Smallness of the palpebral aperture offers an obstacle to steadying the eyeball with the fingers, without undue pressure, from actual want of space. Some mechanical means must be employed, and the use of the forceps is particularly indicated. Another disadvantage arising out of the same condition is, the

N N

encroachment of the eyelids so much on the cornea that there
is hardly room for the knife. The only thing I can recommend
for this is to use a smaller knife. I have seen a surgeon widen
the commissure by an incision at the outer angle: I thought the
proceeding to be unnecessary.

A small tag of adhesion between the iris and the capsule of
the lens can interfere but little, I suspect, if at all, with the
escape of the cataract. It would be different if the connexion were with the cataract itself. Should it be determined
on beforehand to cut through the adhesion, the position of it
must be well ascertained, or else it may not be readily made
out when the eye is flaccid. Probe-pointed scissors should be
employed.

Adhesion of the iris to the cornea is the last complication
I have to review. If merely an inconsiderable portion of the
pupil-margin were adherent, I should not hesitate to divide it
while making the section of the cornea, provided I could so
direct the knife that the remainder of the iris would escape
injury. When this is not practicable, the iris might perhaps
be separated by a preliminary operation.

Judicious after-treatment is no less essential to success than
careful preparation and good operating. I prefer sending my
patient to bed immediately that the operation is over, and keeping the eye closed for a certain period, with plaster, that the
adaptation of the cut surfaces may be maintained. I have
for some years discontinued the usually prescribed practice of
binding the eyes with a compress and bandage ; for any degree
of pressure on a wounded eye is injurious, and the heat and
discomfort inseparable from such coverings must often give a
disposition to, if it does not directly set up, inflammatory action.
Some surgeons put merely a fold of cloth over the eyes, and
support it with a bandage—but this has its disadvantages. The
aqueous humour, the lacrymal and conjunctival secretion, wet
the rag, cause it to adhere to the face, and produce discomfort
sufficient to disturb, or even prevent sleep. As a protection to
the eye from accident I employ a very large square stiff shade,

a little padded where it rests on the forehead, reaching from temple to temple and to the tip of the nose; and sustain it in position by elastic bands, one around, and two in a cross direction over the head; or some allied appliance—as a light wire frame covered with gauze. These guards have saved many eyes from destruction. They obviate the necessity and irksomeness of the patient keeping in one position, besides relieving his mind, as well as that of the operator, from much anxiety, simply because the eye cannot be accidentally struck. This renders unnecessary also the annoyance of fastening the hands, so that they cannot reach to the head. A celebrated ophthalmic surgeon of a past generation was operated on by his pupil and successor, and lost his eye by striking it while asleep.

Darkness of the apartment is a necessary condition well recognised, but it is too common to combine imperfect ventilation with it; the bed-curtains are drawn; every window is shut; the door is kept closed; and a foul atmosphere is generated. Absolute darkness is unnecessary: there may be a degree of light without being injurious, that will enable a person to move about the room; and ventilation should always be secured.

Special instructions must be given to the patient to endeavour to keep the eyeball quiet, and to repress any inclination to sneeze or to cough, and he should be apprised that there will be for a day or two an occasional gush of fluid from between the eyelids—aqueous humour, combined with lacrymal fluid,—or the unexpected occurrence will excite alarm.

A trustworthy and judicious nurse must be provided—one who will observe quiet, not talk unnecessarily with the patient, so as to excite him, although she may read to him; who will not communicate subjects likely to create anxiety or produce mental emotion, and who will obey to the letter, all orders respecting his diet.

If at the usual bed-time of the first day there be very decided restlessness and disinclination to sleep, I give an anodyne, usually hyoscyamus, unless I find that such is apt to disagree.

The nature of the aliment during the first few days is important : the usual practice is to prescribe slops, more under the idea, I believe, that actual chewing is hurtful to the eye than anything else. In man the action of the muscles of mastication cannot in any way influence the eyeball. The more I practise the more I am confirmed in the propriety of allowing, from the first, the usual diet at the usual times, only in rather less quantities. An old person who is confined and fed on slops is almost certain to have his digestive organs deranged, and if so, will most assuredly suffer from injurious prostration of strength, which may more or less interfere with success. I have had proof enough that starvation is no safeguard against inflammation, while it seems frequently to retard or to prevent the needed reparation. I am not aware that wholesome food, given in a state of system capable of assimilating it, will produce diseased action. I have had several opportunities of comparing the effects of a low and of a generous diet, and witnessing the advantages of the latter. Accustomed stimuli should not be absolutely prohibited ; in some cases they may be requisite at the beginning. Aged persons may have a degree of prostration directly after the operation, that demands alcoholic and other stimulants, followed by full diet.

From day to day the corners of the eye and the lower eyelid should be carefully cleaned with a bit of rag folded to form an angle, and wetted with warm water ; and the surfaces afterwards wiped dry. Unless the edges of the eyelids absolutely require cleansing, the quiet of the eye will be better secured by leaving them untouched. Should the plaster get hard, and so produce discomfort, I sop it thoroughly, remove it, and apply fresh pieces. The action of the bowels must be looked after, and if the third or fourth day arrive without an evacuation, a mild purgative, such as the compound rhubarb pill, a dose of castor oil, or any particular medicine known to agree, must be given, or an enema should be administered.

When seven clear days have been passed without unfavourable symptoms, success is pretty certain ; and after the edges of the eyelids have been thoroughly cleaned with warm water, the patient may be allowed to open the eye in a subdued light, to test the result of the operation. This would be too soon if any of the complications I have described have existed.

I have said nothing about the patient leaving his bed. I generally keep him there for the greater part of the week, or the whole, should there seem any necessity for it,—not always necessarily within the sheets. This is by some surgeons thought useless; but nowhere is he so secure from any accident to the eye. When it is remembered what is at stake, a few days passed in a recumbent posture should not be considered burdensome; but it is not generally thought so. I have found that when the bed is left, there is a risk of imprudent acts. After the second day I have no objection to allow the bed to be made.

The pernicious practice of opening the eye at an early period cannot be too strongly deprecated. An examination of this kind must be useless if the progress be favourable; if otherwise, it is certain to aggravate the mischief, and in no instance can it disclose symptoms for guidance more certain and more valuable than those of the patient's sensations, and the state of the eyelids, particularly of the upper. Without any valid reason there is often a desire to see the cornea; but as this cannot be exposed by the patient voluntarily, the upper eyelid, which is always very tender, is raised, pain is produced, and involuntary resistance follows, attended by spasmodic action of the orbital muscles. Several times I have observed the first bad symptoms immediately after this unhappy mistake. If nothing worse ensue, pain is sure to follow, which may last for hours or days. Should the cornea not be healed, prolapse of the iris by a gush of aqueous humour is most probable, and if already prolapsed there will almost certainly be an increase in the protrusion; but what is most to be feared is the accession of acute inflammation.

The admission of light to the eye must be carefully regulated, and a large shade should be worn for some weeks. Exercise should be taken directly that circumstances will admit.

The occasional rapidity with which the cornea may heal is astonishing.

A hospital patient, aged sixty-five, submitted to operation on the 22nd of the month, told me on the 25th that he had been trying his eye, and could see. The incision was united, and the chambers were filled with aqueous fluid, and on the 27th, contrary to my order, he left the house. A second patient, a female, aged eighty-two, finding on the third day, at which period the cornea had united, that she could see well, was with difficulty kept in the hospital a day longer. An elderly gentleman, a patient of mine, shaved himself before the glass on the fourth day. But these most imprudent acts would be the destruction of the large majority of eyes subjected to them; and every surgeon has seen the unfortunate issue of such foolhardiness.

Restoration to sight after extraction is very often effected without any inconvenience beyond the necessary confinement; indeed, pain rarely attends a successful case. Acute inflammation, as a direct consequence of the operation, is a cause of failure, but by no means so common as might be supposed. It usually appears early, within the first twenty-four hours. Almost suddenly, pain is felt in the eyeball, then in and around the orbit; the eyelids swell and inflame, and are soon of a bright red. Purulent discharge follows. The vascular and nervous systems become deranged. The worst result is the infiltration of the cornea with pus, and suppuration within the globe of the eye. The less severe effect is, adhesion of the capsule of the lens to the iris, or closure of the pupil, with some damage to the iris as well as to the retina. In every particular this state resembles that of acute inflammation consequent on accidental injury, the treatment of which, already fully given in Chapter IV., must be followed, with the exception of the use of antimony, as this drug may induce vomiting. Inflammation may appear some days after the operation when it is usually less severe: such an attack is generally considered to be iritis, because the most palpable effect is closure of the pupil, but it is in fact inflammation of the whole of the tunics.

Acute inflammation of the eyeball, of traumatic origin, very rapidly attains to that height which produces disorganization.

Even in a less intense degree, it so damages the eye that primary union of the cornea, a condition absolutely necessary for full success, is impossible. I must, therefore, strenuously warn the student not to expect to bring about by very active and heroic measures that which cannot be accomplished. It is but with full appreciation of this, which perhaps practice alone can give, that a surgeon can prevent himself from unnecessarily depleting his patient. Of late only has this common-sense view of the matter, drawn from the observation of facts, been received. There is really little scope for the exercise of art. But perhaps it would be more correct to say that the process which has been excited, in its inevitable stages, interferes with the quick repair of the wound. The practical discovery of this has induced many surgeons to doubt that treatment is at all beneficial, and so the effect of any saving influence is almost lost sight of. Except the eyeball at once pass into the suppurative stage, a very great deal may be done; and so much of it might be rescued from morbid changes, that ultimately useful vision may be secured. I would again refer my reader to Chapter IV., for much that is applicable here.

The student therefore should well understand the object of his treatment, and be aware of what it cannot effect, as well as what it might accomplish.

The only other remark that I will make respecting treatment is about mercury. It has been supposed on mere theoretical grounds that the administration will interfere with the healing of the cornea. As regards primary healing, all chance of this is gone before the use of it could be judiciously entertained; so that the question is disposed of on this score. That the mineral does not check the secondary healing process, or in any way suspend repair, if cautiously administered, is too well known to require proof here. It is an agent in which I have the fullest confidence. That it is capable of much abuse, I admit. My own rules for its administration have been fully given.

Sub-acute inflammation, which seems to be determined by the patient's low condition, is more common than the last, and is frequently mistaken for it. The attack comes on some days after the operation; the swollen eyelids have scarcely a flush of red, being rather of a darkish hue, and infiltrated with serum— the upper one exhibiting this the most. The cornea is gene- rally hazy, the wound not healed, and its edges thickened and creamy. The secretion is thin, and the conjunctiva, although chemosed, scarcely vascular. The external characters will generally offer sufficient guidance for treatment, and render it unnecessary to open the eye to see what are the changes within. The state of the system is the reverse of that in the acute attack : the circulation is feeble and languid, and the extremities often devoid of their natural warmth. I repeat here that the habitual hard pulse of the aged should not be allowed to deceive, when the condition of the eyelids and the feelings of the patient indicate that general power is required. The course of treatment is therefore apparent : it is, to support and to stimulate.

The well-marked extremes of the acute and sub-acute forms of inflammation do not, of course, always exist ; the local and general symptoms not in every instance affording sufficient criteria for the precise line of treatment; and it is here that blood-letting and purgatives to subdue pain may seal the fate of the eye. In all cases of doubt the rule should be to stimulate, rather than to attempt to depress. If a patient complain of more soreness and uneasiness about the eye than is generally inseparable from the operation, I order a full dose of hyoscy- amus, and wait the result. The feelings after taking food may in some measure furnish evidence of the condition of the system ; for example, in the case of a private patient, seventy years of age, who complained of pain in the eye two days after the operation, it was rather questionable what plan of treatment should be pursued, but all doubt was dispelled when he told me that the pain and the headache were for a time dissipated by food, and that this had occurred three times ; the hint was acted on, and the rather spare rations advantageously augmented. A better result was never seen. Cinchona is a valuable medicine in the sub-acute forms of inflammation with depression of the system, and the " Infusum cinchonæ spissatum " of the present London Pharmacopœia, is an excellent preparation, far superior to the preparations by Mr. Battley, which have been considerably over-estimated, and possess very much less virtue than they are reputed to have.

Occasionally, with the least possible evidence of an unfavourable state—that is, with only rather more discharge than usual, —the conjunctival secretion being in excess, it may be found on opening the eye that success is spoiled by the cornea being infiltrated with pus. I have seen this over and over, when there has not been the least swelling of the eyelid, or redness, and pain has not been complained of. It is most common in elderly persons. Severe symptoms, however, soon come on, and purulent discharge, with swelling of the eyelids, and pain, supervene. The eye is always severely damaged. This is an analagous state to deposition of pus in the cornea after injuries, already dwelt on.

A still more usually unfavourable condition than the last, but not comparable with it in bad effect, is non-union of the corneal wound. There may be mere suspension of the process; or the eye may be destroyed through chronic inflammation, consequent on the failure of it. It may be wholly without any accompanying symptom; the first intimation being when the eye is opened. Then it is discovered by the flatness of the cornea, in consequence of the aqueous humour not being retained, or the wound being a little open. With discharge of aqueous fluid from the eye rather longer than usual after the operation, I should suspect this state; but then the fluid may be the tears. Again there may be an absence of aqueous secretion. Generally, however, the patient tells you that he feels something in the eye,—it may be like a bit of grit, or an eyelash, or a small fly. This is produced by the iris protruding.

The treatment is, to close the eye with plaster, in the same manner as after the operation, and to continue this for several days. Nothing equals it in effect. Care, too, should be taken that there be no muscular effort, or any imprudent act, which is likely to cause the iris to be pushed out. The slightest indication of general feebleness should be attended to.

Prolapsus of the iris is the most frequent cause both of

temporary failure and imperfect success; and this whether the
prolapsus occur at the period of the operation, or subsequently.
The pupil is necessarily displaced, altered in form, and restricted
in motion; and the nearer it is dragged to the margin of the
cornea, and the smaller the opening that remains, the less perfect will vision be. It may be entirely destroyed; or, considerably enlarged. Among the causes of secondary protrusion,
are rough handling of the eye; opening it, or allowing the
patient to open it before the corneal section is healed; straining
efforts; pressure of any sort on the eyeball; sudden action of the
orbital muscles; sub-acute inflammation,—but it also happens
when there does not seem to be any reason for it. I suspect
that an imperfect corneal section, especially when in a bad
position, by being too anterior, favours the occurrence.

Tedious recovery is a sure consequence, owing to the delay of
the healing process, which will depend more on the position of
the prolapsed portion, and the degree to which the edges of the
cornea are thereby separated, than on the amount.

After watching very carefully, very many cases, both occurring after extraction and after accidents, in which the cornea has
been divided or ruptured; and after noticing the different kinds
of treatment that have been adopted by surgeons; I feel certain
that those in which there had been no additional irritation,
produced either by the use of nitrate of silver in substance or
solution, or by any other agent, made the best recoveries. I
have, therefore, left off all local applications. I keep the eye
closed till I find by the retained aqueous humour, that the parts
are healed. In these cases, as the iris may be pulled very much
forwards, the smallness of the space between it and the cornea
is no proof of the chamber being empty, although a sure
indication where there is no prolapse. I do not snip away any
of the protruding membrane, for whatever is not needed in the
formation of a proper cicatrix is sure to be efficiently and neatly
removed by a natural process, and with a better result than if
interfered with by art. The only occasion on which I venture to
assist nature is, when the iris bulges considerably by the pressure
of the aqueous fluid, and forms what is called staphyloma iridis;

then pricking the tumour occasionally, and giving vent to the fluid, will be advantageous in promoting contraction. In very aggravated cases, accompanied by considerable projection of the flap of the cornea, so effectual may be reparation in a few months, that all trace of the tumour has disappeared, a slight cicatrix only at the edge of the cornea testifying to the alteration.

Good vision is not incompatible with considerable prolapse ; the following figure, which shows very remarkable displacement, with much separation of the edges of the cornea, was taken from a patient in whom this is illustrated.

FIG. 130.

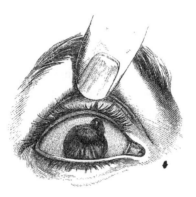

The subject was a lady who had been operated on by Mr. Tyrrell, about sixteen years prior to my having the sketch taken. She sees to read and write, notwithstanding that the greater part of the pupil is covered when the upper eyelid is free. The protruded iris, which is coated by a delicate white cicatrix, forms a boundary of the anterior chamber. The other eye was lost from sub-acute inflammation.

The adhesion of the cornea may give way, and prolapse ensue long after such an event seemed possible. I have known it occur so late as the seventh week.

Irregularity of the pupil sometimes occurs without prolapse of the iris, or adhesion of it to the cornea, in consequence of the injury sustained from stretching, during the escape of the cataract. The paralysed spot generally corresponds to the portion of iris over which the cataract has passed, just, in fact, where the greatest stretching has occurred, and is therefore in the direction of the incision of the cornea.

When persons begin to move about after the operation, to quit their rooms, and to get out, an attack of conjunctival inflammation is not very uncommon, especially if they are weak and the eye irritable, or they expose themselves imprudently to noxious influences, such as sudden atmospheric changes, damp, the heat of the fire, fatigue, excitement, and undue indulgence in drinking. Unless the symptoms be threatening, I generally rely on cold applications and the recumbent posture for a day or two. These slight paroxysms are often misunderstood, supposed to be the commencement of a violent attack, and the patient treated accordingly; but so long as pain is not the leading symptom there need not be any apprehension.

Inflammation of the entire eyeball may supervene long after such an occurrence is least expected. In one of my patients several weeks had passed, and up to the attack there had not been the least interruption to success. The inflammation was of a low type; pus was effused in the chambers of the eye; and the iris so affected that the pupil closed without any acute pain coming on, or much intolerance to light, or much surface vascularity.

Such occurrences point to the necessity of prudence and care on the part of patients, and watchfulness on the part of the surgeon.

An eye that has been operated on for cataract, however successfully, is never restored to the condition in which it was prior to the disease. No artificial compensation for the loss of the lens can enable it to exercise those rapid adaptations of focus from near to distant objects, beautifully provided for in the natural state. Glasses of two foci are always required, the one for reading, writing, or examining near objects, the other for looking at distant ones. These facts should always be pointed out to the patient or his friends; for the popular idea of cataract is that a scale or film grows over the eye, on the removal of which the organ may be as good as ever.

A surgeon should be cautious, even under the most favourable circumstances, never to overrate the chances of success of any operation for cataract, nor to allow it to be thought that any is infallible; and above all, when there is the slightest indication which would render the result questionable or imperfect, owing to individual peculiarity, or constitutional taint, hereditary or acquired, it is right as regards the patient, and a safe provision for himself, that all the particulars for and against operating should be stated clearly and intelligibly, without the least dissimulation.

The operation of extraction may be required under the less favourable condition of dislocation of the cataract; for certain changes in the eye, by which the vitreous humour is degenerated and the suspensory ligament is ruptured, may cause the opaque lens to fall into the anterior chamber or to rest on the iris, and produce a degree of irritation that demands removal. These are not common cases, but any one who sees large numbers of ophthalmic patients will occasionally meet with them. In an instance under my own care, of a female seventy years old, the cataract was partly detached, and swung by a lateral connexion; sometimes being just behind the pupil, sometimes nearly out of the field of vision. This state had probably existed three months before I saw her, and the eye now began to suffer from the occasional pressure of the cataract on the iris. There could be little doubt that in the other eye, about a year before, the cataract had dropped into the vitreous humour. The vision in each eye was tolerably good. I lost sight of my patient after a few visits.

If the displaced body be in the posterior chamber, I recommend an attempt to bring it forwards through the pupil; and the kind of needle with which this should be done, whether straight or curved, as well as the place of its introduction, whether through the cornea or sclerotica, must in a great measure depend on the circumstances of the case, and be left to the judgment of the operator : the anterior operation should be preferred when practicable. If in the anterior chamber, the opening in the cornea for its removal should, if possible, be made at a spot opposite to the site it occupies, and be ample ; the peculiar circumstances demanding a very easy exit for it.

Extraction may also be required for the removal of the nucleus of a lens, or of portions of it; and as this almost certainly requires the employment of the curette, a hook, or some similar instrument, an aperture in the cornea, larger than would be supposed, is needed.   Here, as in the ordinary extraction of a cataract, success depends mainly on the facility with which the body is removed.   If the lens have been displaced by violence, the hyaloid membrane will probably be ruptured.   The readiness, therefore, with which the vitreous humour will escape should be remembered.

The several steps of these operations, as not requiring modification according to the circumstances of each case, should be in strict accordance with the general rules.

The late Mr. Walker recommended the use of a grooved

FIG. 131.

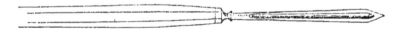

needle-knife for the extraction of a soft lens when dislocated into the posterior chamber ; and Mr. Wilde, in the " Dublin Journal" for 1847, speaks highly of it, and gives the following case of traumatic injury to the eye of a man aged thirty-two, in which he used it with success.   The iris was bulged forwards by the lens, which had been broken and softened, and partly protruded through the pupil, overlapping its edge so as to give it an irregular and deformed appearance.   The violence of the symptoms demanded the extraction of the lens, and the grooved needle was introduced at the under and outer side of the cornea, pushed through the centre of the lens, and the posterior capsule.

The effect was instantaneous. The aqueous fluid and the opaque and softened lens were immediately discharged along the groove in the knife. Great relief followed, and the report, twelve days after, states—"Sight nearly as good as ever, inflammation almost gone, no pain, nor any uneasiness; capsule disappearing."

FIG. 132.

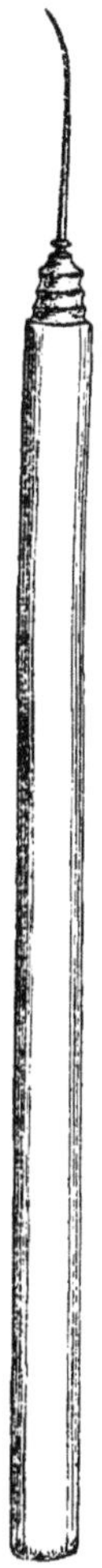

The preceding figure represents the needle now sold by Messrs. Weiss as Mr. Walker's, but it is smaller than that figured by Mr. Wilde, and the groove is very much narrower.

The irritability of the eye in these cases may induce an involuntary resistance that renders it impossible to operate with any chance of success, unless the patient be narcotized: the risk of injury to the eye from vomiting is not to be compared to the danger of operating without chloroform.

OPERATION FOR DISPLACEMENT.

NEEDLE FOR DISPLACEMENT.

It is obvious that a curved needle is better adapted to displace the lens into the vitreous humour below the level of the pupil, than a straight one: and were this the only circumstance to be regarded, the form of the curve would matter little; but the important condition in the operation—that the point of the needle be disengaged from the cataract when displaced, without further influencing its position,—establishes, I think, a ground of preference in favour of the instrument I here show (fig. 132). A gradually curved extremity, while it affords great facility for readily disengaging the point, allows the needle to enter the eye more easily, and renders it less dangerous to be used. The entire length need not exceed three-quarters of an inch, and the breadth of the broadest part the thirty-fifth of an inch. The point only should be sharp, the extremity wedge-shaped, and the body conical.

There are three ways of producing displacement : the oldest and now almost exploded method, " depression," is to press the cataract downwards till it disappears, as is meant to be shown in diagram 133.

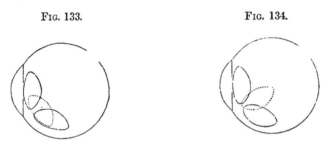

Fig. 133.   Fig. 134.

The second, " reclination," disposes of the cataract by tilting it backwards, and carrying the upper edge downwards, after the manner illustrated in the second sketch.

In the third, the cataract is pierced, and carried down in an oblique position, as represented in the following figure.

Fig. 135.

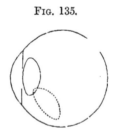

These diagrams must be regarded as demonstrating merely the theory of the several operations, for, in reality, the cataract does not pass through the many positions that are figured, so as ultimately to rest just at the desired situations ; there is the greatest uncertainty where it may actually go, especially in depression—an operation that I shall not describe, since, owing to the difficulty of pushing the cataract below the pupil, and getting it sufficiently covered by the vitreous humour without forcing it against the nervous coat of the eye, it is now superseded. Although the retina is very much less likely to be touched by a reclined than by a depressed cataract, the vitreous humour certainly suffers much more lesion, especially if it be healthy.

For the performance of reclination, of which I confess that I have but a very limited experience, the curved needle alone is required. It is indispensable that the pupil be fully dilated. An anterior operation through the cornea has been proposed and adopted, but is most inappropriate: it is only by passing the instrument through the sclerotica that sufficient command can be obtained for proper displacement. The position of the patient, that of the operator, and the manner of securing the eyelids and fixing the eye, are precisely the same as for extraction.

The needle, which should be held with the convexity upwards, and the handle a little depressed, to render the entrance of the curve more easy, is introduced exactly in the transverse axis of the eyeball, about the sixth of an inch behind the cornea, in which position injury will not be inflicted on the ciliary processes, retina, or long ciliary arteries, which vessels bifurcate posteriorly. It is directed inwards to the centre of the vitreous humour, the point carried forward, and made to appear between the upper part of the cataract and the

FIG. 136.

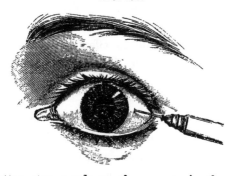

iris. The latter step needs much care, as in the natural state the circumference of the lens is in contact with the iris. It is then turned, and its concavity applied just above the centre of the cataract, which must first be tilted, and afterwards pressed backwards and downwards, as is shown in fig. 136, and made to assume a position as nearly as possible resembling the lowest of those in the diagram 134. The needle must be kept on the cataract for a few seconds, and then liberated by a slight rotatory motion, raised to the centre of the eye, and withdrawn. Each step of the process should be effected very slowly.

Should the cataract rise as soon as the needle is disengaged, the reclination must be repeated till it remain displaced. The reascension is certainly most often owing to the great elasticity of the vitreous humour, which must be in a healthy state to possess this.

Dr. Mackenzie advises that no attempt be made to dislocate the cataract till a sufficient opening has been effected in the posterior capsule. He says, except this be done, the resistance offered by the capsule and by the firm adhesion of the suspensory ligament of the lens to the ciliary body, will be impediments to the displacement. If the anterior part of the capsule be opaque, and have not been sufficiently torn in the first instance to allow of a clear pupil, the needle must be applied to it before being withdrawn. When of normal consistence, it is almost always ruptured. But the capsule may, if thickened, accompany the cataract, in spite of all our endeavours to the contrary. Should the cataract be accidentally projected into the anterior chamber, it must be extracted.

The cataract may fall in pieces under the pressure of the needle; it would be impossible to effect the depression of the fragments, and all that can be done is to leave them alone, unless they enter the anterior chamber, and produce irritation, when extraction is the proper course.

Complete pupillary adhesion renders displacement as inapplicable as extraction; for, independently of the pupil being so small that it would be impossible to see that the instrument is in its proper course, the iris must be considerably damaged before the needle could be made to appear in front of the cataract; and if the capsule were opaque and thickened, as in all probability it would be, it is more likely that the iris would separate from its ciliary attachments, than that the pupillary adhesions or the thickened capsule would give way under the pressure. It does not appear to me that one or two, or even more slight adhesions contra-indicate reclination, if the capsule of the lens be not much thickened. I should not attempt to break them down with the needle, as some surgeons have recommended.

The other operation for displacement requires the employment of a straight needle, such as that figured as a straight solution needle. This instrument is introduced through the sclerotica as far as in reclination ; but instead of being carried to the centre of the vitreous humour for the purpose of avoiding the cataract, it is intentionally passed by a rotatory motion into it, the lower part of which is then turned backwards, and in that oblique position carried downwards till the whole is just below the edge of the pupil, when the needle is to be most carefully withdrawn. This is supposed to be a modern operation, and is called the operation of Egerton, who practised it in Calcutta. I believe that the first notice of it in England was by Mr. Morgan in the " Guy's Hospital Reports " for April 1842. Whilst I attended the practice of the late Mr. Scott, in 1841, he used to adopt this method, a little modified and improved, and allusion is made to it in his work on Cataract, published in 1843. He thought it better not to transfix the cataract, on account of the danger of accidental dislocation, and the greater difficulty in subsequently detaching the needle ; and recommended instead that it should be pierced only to such a depth as will enable it to be carried backwards. According to him, if the needle can be introduced into two-thirds of the cataract, sufficient command will then be obtained for the displacement ; when it cannot be so used, the operation is not admissible.

The reputed advantages of Egerton's plan are, the less amount of injury to the hyaloid membrane, the greater facility with which the cataract can be placed in any position, the less probability of its rising, owing to the upper surface being covered by an unbroken part of the vitreous body, and the less chance of injury to the retina from any accidental mal-position of the cataract. It is better, it is said, to lacerate the anterior part of the capsule on an after occasion, through the cornea ; for otherwise there is risk of the cataract being touched and returned to its place.

These operations are likely to be followed by vomiting, and it is well to forewarn the patient of the probability of the occurrence.

Blood may be effused within the eye, but it is usually readily absorbed. A coagulum deposited under the conjunctiva at the spot where the needle entered the eye need not excite any fear; for it also readily disappears. Should a fungus be thrown out at the wound, and remain after sufficient time has been allowed for its spontaneous disappearance, it must be snipped off.

It is a grave objection to displacement, that in performing it the interior of a healthy eye must necessarily be considerably damaged. No condition of the vitreous humour can be said to be favourable to the operation. When from morbid change it yields readily to pressure, there is danger of the cataract gravitating, and resting on the retina; or floating about, and producing constant annoyance by temporarily interrupting vision; besides, it is then peculiarly liable to be dislocated through the pupil.

It is not surprising that acute inflammation of some, or of all the textures of the globe of the eye, with its destructive consequences, should often immediately follow displacement, and be as baneful as the most acute attack after extraction. But what is most imminent is a low, but certainly destructive, inflammation coming on at a later period; from pressure of the cataract on the iris, ciliary processes, or retina; from violence done to the structure of the vitreous humour; or from irritation occasioned by the unnatural position of the displaced body, in which case there will be all the symptoms that would occur if a foreign body were driven into the eye. The cataract may, in its new place, undergo partial or even entire absorption. For so long, therefore, as it is undissolved—and years may be required for the process—there is danger of this low inflammation.

Really there is no scope for successful treatment, should such symptoms arise. Dr. Mackenzie writes, "If the practitioner who has performed depression or reclination sees reason to suspect that the very means which he had adopted for restoring vision, threaten to destroy it, he ought not to hesitate about withdrawing the displaced lens from the eye entirely. Introducing a bent needle through the sclerotica, the cataract is to be raised into its former situation, pressed forward through the pupil, and kept in contact with the cornea till a section is made, a hook introduced, and the lens laid hold of, so that it may be extracted."

Moreover, from falls, blows on the head, or even without an apparent cause, the cataract may reascend in the track by which it was displaced, or pass into the anterior chamber, and require again to be thrust back, or extracted. Therefore, with all these contingencies, success can never be counted on. Neither repetition of the displacement, nor extraction, should, in my opinion, be hastily done when a cataract reascends, except in the very aged—in whom, from the greater density of the lens at that period of life, its solution is necessarily slowest,—or unless much irritation ensue; but the case should merely be watched, as experience justifies our giving a trial to the process of disintegration in an emergency like this.

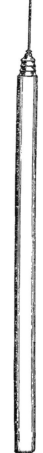

Fig. 137.

The after treatment is the same as that for extraction; quietude in bed is essential, for it is within the first week that there is the greatest likelihood of the cataract resuming its former place.

OPERATIONS FOR SOLUTION.

NEEDLES FOR SOLUTION.

STRAIGHT NEEDLE.

Solution needles cannot be too fine, provided they are strong enough to be guided with precision. The advantage of their delicacy was first strongly pointed out by Dr. Jacob, who, at an early period of his professional career, became strongly impressed with the injurious size of the needles in common use, and, being unable to procure what he desired, produced his well-known instrument, made out of an ordinary fine sewing-needle. Dr. Jacob's views on this subject, first published, I believe, in vol. iv. of the "Dublin Hospital Reports," have been made known through many channels. The latest account, however, is contained in a monograph on the operation for cataract with a fine sewing-needle through the cornea. In this, the difficulty of introducing the needle, from its roundness—and it is round throughout, even to the point,—and the risk of wounding or transfixing the iris, owing to the force necessary for its introduction, are fully described. These are certainly serious objections, but they are overcome by our present instrument-makers, who can produce a needle equalling Dr. Jacob's in size and strength, surpassing it in sharpness, and superior to it in shape. Such is the kind of needle shown at fig. 137 : the body is conical ; the largest part about the fortieth of an inch in thickness ; the extremity is wedge-shaped, and the point angular. The length, five-eighths of an inch, is as great as is consistent with sufficient stiffness, and ample for the use to which it is to be applied, as may be seen by reference to fig. 138, which is intended to show the size and position of the lens, and the distance required to be traversed by a needle, to reach the centre of that body.

Fig. 138.

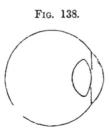

It is supposed that a cataract-needle may be made with cutting surfaces above its shoulders. Such an instrument would, however, be useless ; but it is impossible to put a keen knife-edge on the sides of a small needle. I speak on the authority of Mr. Weiss when I say that the needle which is sold and used under the impression of its being sharp above the shoulders, is merely thinned, or rolled off, but not sharp.

CURVED NEEDLE.

A curved needle, although neither so readily introduced, nor used with such precision as a straight one, is sometimes required, and should differ from the straight only in shape, and in the absence of shoulders, as in fig. 139. It is scarcely practicable, so say the instrument-makers, to make it with an angular point like the straight one.

FIG. 139.

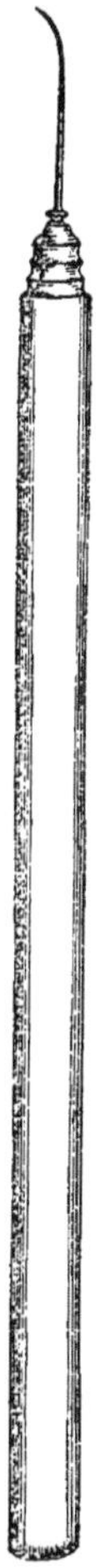

I find that many surgeons suppose a bent sewing-needle, as used by. Dr. Jacob, to possess peculiar appropriateness of temper. The idea is drawn from the circumstance that out of many papers of needles, each of which generally contains twenty-five, not one may take the bend when cold. I have known nearly two hundred broken before the curve could be obtained. This temper, only an accidental result in a few among masses prepared at a time, is just above what the needle-manufacturer desires, what in fact he avoids, but which can always be secured by the surgical instrument-maker. Jacob's needle is not less liable to break than an instrument forged by a good workman.

A cataract exhibiting the characteristics of softness is effectually removed through the process of absorption, by opening its capsule, and allowing the aqueous humour to be in contact with it.

There are two methods of operating, one through the cornea, another through the sclerotica; these are respectively designated anterior and posterior operations.

The anterior operation is more definite and simple; is less painful; inflicts less injury on the eye, for only one of its coats is punctured; can be done as effectually, and quicker than the other, the instrument never being out of view, and produces less irritation. It is moreover the easiest and safest of all operations for cataract, and is very generally applicable. I shall speak of it first.

The pupil should always be well dilated, not only to expose the cataract, but to place the iris out of the way of the needle. Whether the one or the other kind of needle shall be used, seems to be generally determined by the fancy of the operator: that either may do, is proved by the fact that each is exclusively used by different surgeons. There is, notwithstanding, a certain difference in their power which may be turned to decided advantage in particular cases. With the curved one a cataract can be more comminuted, and with less tearing of the capsule and less chance of dislocation of its nucleus, should there be one, than with the straight. The straight instrument is preferable, principally from being much easier to use.

The eye being steadied, and all the preliminaries arranged as for the other operations on cataract, the needle—the straight one—is introduced through the cornea near its circumference, the point carried to the centre of the cataract, as in the following sketch, and used according to the circumstances of the case. The curved needle is inserted with the concavity upwards, that

FIG. 140.

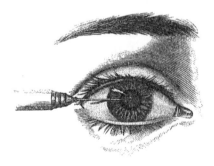

the stem may pass parallel to the iris, so as to avoid injuring it ; and when the pupil is reached, by a slight turn of the handle the point is brought on the cataract.

If the needle be kept well adapted to the wound in the cornea, the aqueous humour may not escape till the cataract has been pierced and the withdrawal is commenced. Should the humour have come away prematurely, the needle must be removed, and the operation delayed. Again, if the iris be wounded, and blood obscure the cataract, the operation must be deferred.

It should be a great principle in "solution" to procure absorption of the cataract in its natural position. The less that the lenticular matter is displaced, the less subject is the eye to irritation. The less, too, the capsule is torn in the early stage of the treatment, the less likely is it to contract adhesions to the iris, and therefore the more easy to be disposed of afterwards if it block up the pupil. At a first operation, on an ordinary soft lens, all that is desirable is to break the centre of the capsule, and to penetrate the cataract sufficiently to admit the aqueous humour to its texture; and this should be done gently, because rough usage will dislocate it.

I may say that dislocation is very readily effected, and is almost sure to ensue unless certain precautions are observed; the most important of these is, not to make a large aperture in the capsule so long as it retains its elasticity; for unless the breach be minute, there is great danger of an accidental increase in the opening by rupture, which will most likely allow the lens, or a portion of it, to escape. When the capsule is opaque, and consequently has lost much or all of its elasticity and liability to rupture, a large aperture will have the advantage of giving freer entrance to the aqueous humour, and, I may say, is necessary, to obviate the tendency of a wound in a capsule so altered, to unite. Not to carry the needle too deeply, nor to move it about too freely on the cataract, are further precautions against dislocation, to which must be added general delicacy of manipulation, in every step of the operation. The operator may be assured that the accident will occur, if he see the cataract move in the least degree.

Another reason against using the needle freely at first is, that the lens tissue swells very much when considerably broken, and pushes the capsule against the iris, when adhesion is inevitable. Indeed, these parts always adhere when in contact, during the process of absorption of the cataract,—a circumstance due, I suppose, to the capsule becoming inflamed. The first application of the needle will most likely cause opacity of the capsule, if it be not already opaque, and render the cataract still more cloudy. When the cataract has become very soft in its super- ficies, some of the degenerated matter may fall into the chambers of the eye, especially the anterior, and becoming flocculent, will soon be absorbed.

When there is fluid degeneration, the part so altered inevitably escapes on the capsule being punctured, and renders the aqueous fluid more or less turbid. Vomiting, attended with great pain in the eye, and sometimes around the orbit, is very frequently consequent on the escape of this ; but it may occur merely from the use of the needle, without lenticular matter of any kind having fallen into either of the chambers. The vomiting may be severe, and last even for days.

It has been supposed that the phenomena depend on the presence of some poisonous material, because if such a cataract be removed by extraction, in which case the capsule generally escapes entire, no such state follows. The treatment is, at once to evacuate the fluid material, by puncturing the cornea with one or other of the iris knives. The incision had better be made near the margin, and below. It may here be stated, too, that whenever there is escape of lenticular matter in any marked quantity, although not in a decidedly fluid state, the rule should be to evacuate it. The spoon of the curette may be needed to assist in the removal. The presence of any in- flammatory symptoms should not prevent this being done.

If the entire cataract should fall into the anterior chamber, or the nucleus of it accompany the soft superficies, extraction should be the rule. The most agonising pain, of a neuralgic character, in the eye, forehead, and head, is the usual accompa- niment. But the occupation of the anterior chamber is of little moment, compared with the disturbance that may ensue when the posterior chamber is the site of any portion of the lens material, principally, it would seem, from pressure on the iris. A cataract or its nucleus, when so situated, and producing irritation

likely to destroy the eye, must, if possible, be depressed, or·
brought into the anterior chamber by a needle, and extracted
—alternatives, I am happy to say, that have never been forced
on me.

The following quotation from Dr. Jacob's writings is valuable
in the consideration of this subject :—

" The surgeon who would succeed in restoring vision, by
exposing the lens to the contact of the aqueous humour, should
never forget that the most formidable impediment to his success
is, the inflammation which follows the operation; and that his
aim should therefore be to accomplish his object with the least
possible injury to the organ. He must also recollect that the
lens displaced, whether whole or in fragments, is equivalent to
a foreign body in the eye, and must therefore be so disposed that
it shall not press on the iris. A notion very generally prevails,
which I cannot but call a very mistaken one, that it is necessary
to place the fragments of the lens in the anterior chamber, to
accomplish their solution and absorption. The inexperienced
operator may rest assured that if he adopts such practice indiscriminately, he will have reason to repent of it.

" I have frequently had an opportunity of witnessing the
solution of cataract *in situ* after the capsule had been opened,
and I could with a magnifying glass observe from day to day
the change in form which occurred from the removal of particles
of cataract, until at last a portion has disappeared, and left a
passage for the light. In such a case I observed, three several
times, that when a small fragment fell out of the capsule into
the anterior chamber, pain and slight inflammation supervened,
and continued until the particle was absorbed."

In consequence of the softness of cataract in infancy, owing
to which there is so much less danger of the effects of inflammation from the lenticular substance being in the chambers of
the eye; as well as the little likelihood of inflammation consequent upon the operation itself, some surgeons have been induced
to recommend that the needle be very freely used to break it up,
and at the same time to eject the fragments from the capsule.
But even here the safer plan, and I am not sure of its not being

the quicker also, is, to endeavour to procure absorption with the cataract in its place.

The time required for absorption depends on circumstances connected with the nature of the cataract, as well as upon individual peculiarities. Under apparently the same conditions a cataract will resist the process of disintegration longer in some persons than in others. The presence of inflammation is said to suspend absorption. This is, in a measure, correct, but not altogether; it is only during intense inflammation that the absorption seems at a standstill, and not always, even then.

A single operation may suffice in many instances; and it certainly will when the lens has degenerated to fluidity. A repetition is generally made on the grounds that absorption has ceased, or is deviating in its rate, which is more frequently assumed than indicated; indeed, there is no positive proof of its cessation, and evidence goes to show that absorption, once begun, does not stop. However, it can be hastened. So long as I find, by examining the eye in profile, that lenticular matter yet projects from the capsule, I do nothing; but if, after the lapse of six or eight weeks, there is not evidence in the flattening of the capsule and the concavity of the iris, that the absorption is proceeding, the operation may be repeated. Much care is even necessary in using the needle subsequently; for, according to my observations, there is in after operations a greater tendency to inflammatory action; and hence the necessity for the greatest precautions to prevent dislocation of the nucleus of the cataract. On no account should there be a repetition when inflammation is present; nor do I think that anything can be gained by the renewed operation when the capsule is much opened, and the aqueous fluid is in free contact with the lenticular tissue.

If a sufficient interval be allowed, there are few cases that will not yield to two or three operations; and the fewer they are, the better the result. The most successful cases are those in which the pupil is normal, and without any adhesions to the capsule. For this there must have been great care in operating, and an absence of any inflammatory attack. But such results cannot be got with any attempt at quick absorption.

I have not said all that is necessary respecting the escape of any part of the cataract into the chambers of the eye. I have pointed out that fluid which may escape when the capsule is punctured, and which is always more or less coloured, should be let out. This applies also to any large amount of lenticular matter less disintegrated, dislocated at the time of the accident; and even the entire cataract, should it unfortunately be displaced. But when, during treatment, portions fall from the capsule into the anterior chamber, the proper course is to trust to the natural process of abruption, so long as no very decided irritation be excited. The same rule applies, too, to the displacement of the nucleus of the lens. I have watched large nuclei so situated, during the several weeks that were required for their dissipation, with scarcely any appreciable irritation.

The posterior operation for solution is performed precisely like that for "displacement," except that when the needle is brought in front of the cataract, it is used for laceration instead of reclination. This method is generally advocated solely on the score of affording greater facility for breaking up the cataract; hence it is recommended for infants, and some surgeons always practise it upon them. Mr. Tyrrell told me, shortly before his death, that he had operated on eight infants with congenital lenticular cataract, performing the posterior operation in one eye of each, and the anterior in the other; the result was that all did well, but those in which the posterior was performed, and the lens broken up and displaced, were cured the soonest. From this it is apparent that time only was saved by the posterior operation; a matter not of much importance, and the value of which cannot for a moment be insisted on here, from the want of precise evidence as to the subsequent power of vision in the respective eyes.

I give a very decided preference to the anterior operation, for the reasons already stated. By it the lens can be broken to any extent that is safe or necessary, if the curved needle be used, and with greater ease, I believe, than in the posterior operation. Mr. Saunders preferred it. The only reason why he ever performed the posterior was, from the supposed greater facility with which the lens could be comminuted. We are informed by Dr. Farre that "he finally attempted to diminish inflammation by performing his anterior instead of his posterior operation."

There is no surgeon living who has paid so much attention to needle operations as Dr. Jacob, of Dublin. The following quotation from his little work on the operation for cataract, before spoken of, expresses his opinion on the comparative value of these operations:—

"No anatomist, aware of the nature and number of the structures injured in the posterior operation, can for a moment assume that such injury does not cause more risk of destructive inflammation than the injury inflicted on the cornea in the anterior one; and no surgeon who has compared the effects and consequences of the two operations can for a moment maintain that the results of the puncture through the sclerotic are not more injurious than those following the puncture of the cornea. No man who knows what the penetrated structures are could venture to maintain that the conjunctiva, sclerotic, ciliary ligament and ciliary processes, could be traversed by an instrument with the same or less injury than is inflicted in traversing the cornea; and no man who has compared the dimensions and relations of the anterior and posterior chambers of the aqueous humour, could venture to maintain that the narrow space behind the iris affords a more accessible passage for the needle than the comparatively capacious chamber anterior to it. Neither can any man who has witnessed the sufferings caused by this posterior operation, or the destructive consequences of the inflammation which it produces, venture to assert that such mischief follows the anterior one. The truth in fact is, that this most valuable of all the methods devised for the removal of an opaque lens has been brought into discredit and almost into disuse by this bigoted preference of a method handed down to us from a remote antiquity, when surgery was in its infancy and anatomy not yet cultivated. I have every day to listen with wonder and no small vexation to the expressions of want of confidence in the operation for cataract, uttered, not only by patients, but by practitioners; and this I find is to be attributed to the experience people have had of the consequences of this bad method."

I understand that many continental surgeons abstain from the anterior operation, from the supposed liability of the cornea to inflammation, a dread participated in by many of our countrymen. On this question, the testimony of Dr. Jacob, to the following effect, is very valuable :—

"With respect to the objection made to this operation on the score of its endangering the cornea, and causing opacity of that structure, I can with safety state that there is nothing in it. I never yet saw vision impaired by any opacity caused by the wound of the needle, and very seldom indeed have I seen any opacity at all remain. In fact, as I have said elsewhere, I know no structure in the body which bears simple injury, such as a clean cut or puncture, better than the cornea. In the course of a long practice, I have met but one case in which suppurative inflammation took place in the puncture, and in that case the suppuration and subsequent ulceration were confined to a circle not an eighth of an inch in diameter, and left behind an opacity not larger than the head of a pin, at a distance from the pupil, and consequently not impairing sight. I have also met with cases, but very rarely indeed, in which the whole cornea suppurated, and the entire eye participated in the destructive inflammation, as sometimes happens from any operation for cataract; this, however, I have never considered a consequence of the peculiar nature of the puncture in this peculiar structure, but the result of constitutional derangement operating on local inflammation following injury. In fact, I looked upon it as of the same nature as the abscess of the cornea which follows very slight injury or irritable ulcer, and which takes place, not from the mere injury or ulcer, but from that state of the animal economy, whatever it may be, which is attended by these local destructive processes. But as I have said, this is a very unusual consequence of this operation; so much so, that I have often wondered that it does not occur

more frequently, seeing that it so often follows slight wounds
of the cornea by particles of stone or steel in stone-cutting or
metal turning. I repeat, therefore, emphatically that the surgeon need never be deterred from operating through the cornea
by any apprehension of the effects of injury on this more
than any other structure in the body he may be called upon
to divide."

During the treatment, the dilatation of the pupil should be
maintained till the capsule recedes, from the reduction in the
bulk of the cataract; or adhesion between its margin and the
torn capsule may ensue.

It has been supposed that expansion of the pupil may be
the cause of dislocating some of the contents of the capsule,
or even the entire cataract; but this is erroneous, as slight
reflection will show; on the contrary, dilatation may, besides
keeping the iris away from the capsule, be advantageous in
causing any portion of the cataract that might otherwise escape
into the posterior chamber, to fall into the anterior, where it is
by far less likely to be injurious.

Very slight irritation follows a well-executed operation on an
eye in which cataract is not complicated with some other
disease; and there is not the necessity for that strict observance
of quiet, so essential in the operations for extraction and displacement. However, the patient should remain in the house
for a few days, during which time the other eye should not be
used. Bright light should be excluded, and the diet carefully
regulated.

The pain which always follows the operation, but generally
very slight, must not be mistaken for the commencement of an
attack of acute inflammation. So long as the symptoms of
active inflammation are absent, narcotics and the application of
cold lotions alone need be employed.

By the mere contraction of the capsule, and its greater or
lesser separation from the suspensory ligament and hyaloid
membrane; or by retraction of its divided parts consequent on
absorption of the cataract, the pupil may be, and very often is,
sufficiently cleared. Should the aperture, from either of these

processes, not be ample enough, a special operation must be resorted to, which I shall describe under the head of capsular cataract.

Unless ill health forbid, congenital cataract should be operated on before the eyeball oscillates; and, as a rule, a child may be safely submitted to operation after the first month of life.

The operation for solution is certainly the safest of all for the removal of cataract, as regards any immediate danger to the eye. It would seem from the united testimony of surgeons, that congenital cataract, when operated on in infancy, or even rather later, during childhood, is that in which this operation is most eminently successful; and this is readily accounted for, since the soft cataract of later years often results from general disease in the eyeball, being merely a degeneration of the lens from mal-nutrition.

The late Mr. Gibson, so long ago as 1811, being dissatisfied with the result of solution, as then executed, used to extract soft cataracts. Having lacerated the capsule, some weeks later he opened the cornea and removed the cataract piecemeal with the curette. Mr. Travers also at one period advocated extraction, and has recorded his opinions concerning it in vol. v. of the "Medico-Chirurgical Transactions." But he changed his views after he learned what could be effected by the needle operation properly conducted. Of late there has been an attempt to introduce into English practice, a German novelty, and which is the old operation of Gibson, with this modification only, that there is no previous use of the needle.

It is called "Linear Extraction." The principle is to scoop out the lens through a small corneal incision. That it is possible for the eye to be more quickly restored to usefulness by this method than by absorption, no one can doubt; but it is more dangerous, almost beyond comparison. The majority of soft cataracts cannot be removed by extraction, even with a large corneal section, with safety to the eye. A considerable portion must be left behind, so that there is the immediate risk that attaches to extraction, while absorption must be relied on to remove what remains. That the difficulty is increased by a small channel of egress is obvious. I must utter my strong protest against it. The first case to which I saw the practice applied, was a most unfortunate one. With everything to give the strongest hope of success, so far as could be learnt from the state of the eyes, the worst result ensued. Both eyes were operated on at the same time. I was not present, and am unaware of the details. Six weeks after I was consulted by the young man with the hope of my conferring benefit. Both eyeballs were collapsed. The operator is a man of very decided skill. I have witnessed other distressing failures, besides seeing partial bad effects of this ill-chosen operation.

I have reserved till now to consider the complication of capsulo-lenticular cataract with entire pupillary adhesion, which is in many cases combined also with a deposit of lymph on the capsule. This state must be preceded by inflammatory action of an acute or chronic character. As it is for the most part a condition of early life, the lenticular cataract would necessarily be of the soft kind.

But, as observation of these cases shows, the lens quickly passes into destructive changes, that reduce its consistence; so that if the affection originate in adult age, or rather after that, in the middle period of life, the lens will scarcely remain of the density proper to those periods of life.

The operation for solution is peculiarly applicable. Even if the cataract be of the hard variety, there is no chance of mischief arising from its dislocation, or, at a later period, of fragments escaping into the chambers, because of the capsular thickness.

The operator must establish a sufficient aperture in the capsule to insure the entrance of the aqueous humour; and as the wound has a great tendency to unite quickly, this must be repeated, if necessary, at subsequent operations. As an unhealthy eye is being treated, the same cautious manipulating that I have pointed out as being necessary in all needle operations, must be observed.

The pupillary adhesions so far modify the case, that the progress of absorption is not easily watched, nor can it readily be said when the cataract is quite absorbed. The only positive proof of an empty capsule is concavity of the iris; and consequently increased size of the anterior chamber; but this is not always present, as the iris may be too much damaged to admit of it, and changes in the posterior part of the eye may certainly cause it to bulge. It may be only therefore, by two, three, or more operations, done at sufficient intervals, that there can be the required assurance of the cataract being removed.

Fig. 141.

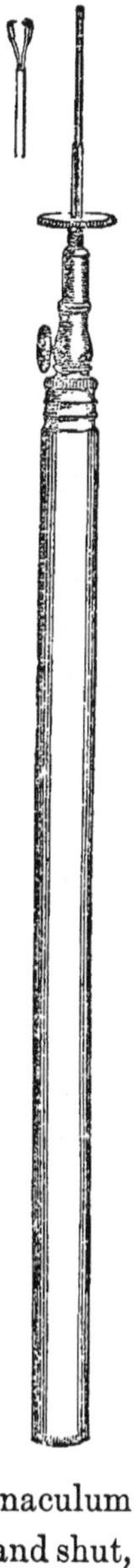

OPERATION FOR CAPSULAR CATARACT.

CAPSULE FORCEPS.

This modern instrument, for which we are indebted to the stimulus given to surgical instrument-makers by the Great Exhibition, combines delicacy of manufacture, simplicity, and remarkable ingenuity. The blades are brought into play by a canula, which encloses them; shutting when the canula is pushed forwards, and opening when it is withdrawn. Their expansion may be graduated by allowing more or less length for the canula to work over; an alteration which is provided for by the screw at the shoulder of the instrument that secures the stem of the blades. Much delicacy of workmanship is required in order that inequality shall not exist between the canula and the blades when the instrument is shut. Fig. 141 represents the forceps; the larger illustration showing them when closed, the smaller when open, and displays the tenaculum points. Fig. 142 portrays the sharp capsule forceps open and shut,

the mechanism of which is very beautiful. The larger and sharp
blade is perforated about the centre to receive the hooked end
of the lesser, and the surfaces where the two come into contact
are cross-cut, like common forceps. The object of these arrangements for taking secure hold of the capsule is at once apparent.
This, the more delicate instrument of the two, requires great
excellence of workmanship to perfect it. The sharp blade
should be sufficiently keen to enter the cornea readily, and the
lesser should have its edges so bevelled that there shall not be
any projecting angles, or any obtuseness to impede penetration.
It is an improvement for the canula to be worked with a

FIG. 142.

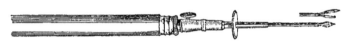

"trigger spring," which is arranged like that of the canula
scissors figured amongst the iris instruments. To the same
handle blades of different forms may be applied, and none
are more useful than curved ones.   Each time the instrument
is used, the canula should be removed, carefully wiped out
with threads drawn through by finely twisted wire, and the
other parts wiped and oiled.

When larger and more powerful forceps are required for
removing substances from within the eyeball, those with a
cross-spring answer the purpose best.   I introduce an effectual
pair with an excellent arrangement, fig. 143, made according
to my order by Messrs. Weiss.   One blade passes through the
other, as a security against any lateral movement, and this
adjustment enables a check to be placed against too great a
separation of them.   The extremities remain parallel at any
degree of opening.   The points are toothed.   The lesser
figure shows these magnified.

Fig. 144 represents a coarser and less expensive instrument
on the cross-spring principle, but one better adapted for seizing
a large body, and for penetrating deeper than the others.   The
smaller cut shows the actual size of the teeth.   Other forceps
for the same purpose are kept by the instrument-makers.

After the lens has been removed by extraction, solution, or displacement, the capsule may not roll up and contract out of the field of the pupil, in consequence of not having been sufficiently divided, or if divided, from its contractility being lost in consequence, perhaps, of being thickened; or, because

FIG. 143.

FIG. 144.

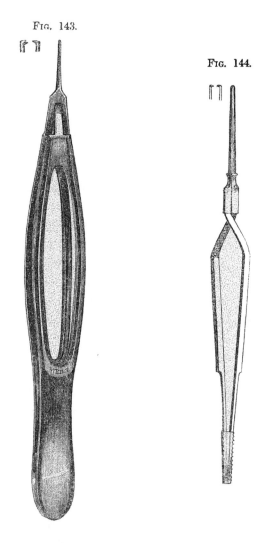

it is more or less adherent to the iris from inflammation. So far it is, therefore, surgically speaking, a secondary affection, and requires certain specific treatment.

Capsule is never absorbed; the bulk is diminished merely by rolling up, and this is always from without inwards—from circumference to centre: it must therefore be so disposed that contraction shall ensue; or it must be extracted.

No operation should be undertaken, except from necessity arising out of impediment to vision, and this ought to be well ascertained. There may be a sufficient aperture to afford excellent sight, while there is capsule within the area of the pupil. If therefore vision be as satisfactory as could be expected from the general state of the eye, and, above all, if it be not inferior to that which is capable of being restored by an operation for cataract, any portion of capsule that is visible had better be left alone. This may hold good, even although the centre of the pupil be not quite clear.

A very narrow strip of capsule passing across may not hinder the full and correct impressions of objects on the retina. This condition existed in the eye of a gentleman on whom I had performed the operation for solution. His sight was excellent. I did not readily determine whether I should, or should not, interfere. However, the following event settled the question of doing nothing. He went to the Derby, and on his return assured me that with his race-glass he watched the horses in the contest as well as before his eyes were diseased, and there was not any impediment to vision. The other eye was yet dark. There is therefore here some scope for judgment.

Irrespective of the impropriety of interfering when there is no need for it, it should never be lost sight of that the operation under consideration, with the rarest exceptions, must ever be under the unfavourable circumstances of being at a period when the eye has already been tired and weakened, sometimes severely so, and by so much the less able to resist injury. This finishing stroke consequently is not unfrequently very injurious, and even fatal.

The maxims for the student's guidance in operating are these:—To dilate the pupil. To exercise the utmost care and gentleness in manipulation, so that no unnecessary violence be inflicted, and no parts accidentally injured, especially the iris, and the vitreous humour, as they are most in danger of it. To endeavour to get the pupil clear in the centre, rather than in any other position. To avoid setting portions of the capsule free. To observe the same rules already propounded, in the description of the cataract operations, for the preliminary preparation of the patient, the steadying of the eyeball, and so forth. Not to puncture the cornea in a transparent part, when there is any opaque spot through which this may be done.

When a mere web of capsule interferes, probably it is so thin as readily to be torn through by a needle, and yet elastic enough to roll aside. The method of proceeding is too simple to be given in detail.

When a portion more dense, and probably adherent at a few points to the iris, is to be cleared, one needle probably will not suffice, and laceration must be done with two, as originally suggested by Mr. Bowman.

Two cataract needles are introduced through different parts of the cornea, and made to enter the capsule at the same spot, or as near as possible, and the mass is torn by the separation of their points. It must be obvious that by this measure also various manipulations may be exercised, according as circumstances demand.

The capsule may retain too slight an attachment to be attacked with one needle, or even two, or so lie on the surface of the vitreous humour, with one or more connexions stretching out from the circumference, that the needles are not applicable; it is one of the conditions necessary for their application that the membrane be free posteriorly. Or there may have been spontaneous absorption of the lens, in which case both hemispheres of the capsule will probably be opaque. Extraction then is required. While the incision in the cornea should be ample, it ought not much to exceed what is needed. The choice of instruments must mainly rest on the fancy of the operator: the smaller the volume of the capsule to be taken out, the more applicable will be the blunt canula-forceps. Extraction is not admissible when capsule is adherent to the iris.

A very troublesome disposition of the capsule is that of a large bar across the pupil. Although it is quite justifiable in some cases to make an attempt at rupture in the centre, there is the greatest uncertainty in the result. Attached, as it always is, to a larger portion at the circumference, a point often overlooked, it sinks under the pressure, and rises again by its own elasticity and that of the vitreous humour, directly that the force is remitted. The two needles might be satisfactorily used; or division effected with an iris knife, especially if there be adhesion to the iris. Or it might be extracted. The same applies when there are several bars.

The following representation conveys a very good idea of this last state. A soft cataract had been removed by solution. Several attempts had been made to break through the bands, without success, for under pressure they sank into the vitreous humour, from which they sprang unaltered to their former place; and the eye, unfortunately the only available one, remained with this impediment to vision.

FIG. 145.

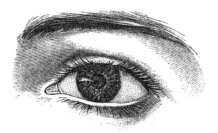

As the bars were very thin, and the capsule around very dense, and the iris free, I used the sharp forceps, and succeeded in twisting them off.

There are many advantages in being able to apply the sharp forceps, but the capsule must be capable of being drawn through the aperture that they make. As to the manner of execution, the instrument, held with the short limb anterior, is pushed through the cornea near its circumference, into the pupil; when it has arrived at the edge of the capsule, it is opened, the sharp blade passed behind, the short one in front, the opaque body seized, all pressure on the globe of the eye remitted, and the withdrawal commenced. A slightly twisting movement will facilitate detachment, and make the capsule clear the cornea more readily. It is essential that the aqueous humour be retained till the forceps are closed over the capsule—hence the necessity of the patient lying down : and should it have escaped prematurely, they must be withdrawn and the operation delayed. When possible, the blades should be made to pass on each side of the capsule, that effectual hold may be got by seizing both the surfaces ; but this cannot be done except the capsule be partially free, or has in some degree receded from its circumferential attachment ; otherwise the sharp blade must be carried through a part of it.

This second representation of capsular cataract is from the eye of an adult who had undergone the operation for solution, under the hands of a late distinguished surgeon. When the iris was in a natural state, the eye was nearly useless from the obscurity of the pupil.

FIG. 146.

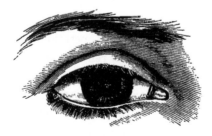

The great thickness of the central part of the capsule constituted an important difference between this and the above case, and it was a question whether the sharp forceps were applicable ; however, they were used, and successfully : the body of the mass came away, and the ring that remained was quite out of the way, when the pupil was undilated.

The only obstacle I know of to the use of these forceps, is extreme narrowness of the anterior chamber from adhesion of the iris to the cornea, which is usually conjoined with such close adaptation of parts, as to prevent the instrument being used except directly in front of the contracted pupil, where opacity of the cornea, which is so likely to ensue on a puncture from any large instrument, would be fatal to vision. Other attempts, therefore, must be made to dispose of the capsule; or other methods resorted to for restoring sight—artificial pupil, for instance.

Adhesion of the capsule to the iris is a serious complication. When the union is very limited, a preliminary operation with the curved needle may detach it, when extraction should follow. I have often done this, even when there has been extensive connexion, although the occurrence must be looked on as being very fortunate. More than once the capsule has separated in a mass, at the first endeavour to form a central aperture ; therefore it is quite allowable to attempt separation, which, however, should be abandoned after a careful, well-directed but inefficient trial. The iris, especially if altered in structure, will sometimes give way at the ciliary attachment, or tear at some part, rather than separate from what seems a slight attachment, and any rough attempt may be followed by paralysis.

Sometimes it is possible to detach the capsule at its circumference, when it rolls up against the iris, and a sufficiently clear space is left.

Inflammation often follows these operations, and, by uniting the divided edges of the capsule, renders abortive all that has been done. I was consulted by a lady who had during infancy been operated on by Mr. Saunders, in whom, in each eye, the capsule was united to the entire pupillary edge. One eye had been submitted to nine needle operations, and the other to eleven, to remove the cataract, and to make apertures in the capsule ; and in one only was there a sufficient opening.

In those most unfavourable cases, so constituted from the nature and extent of the adhesions of the capsule to the iris, the operator must rely on his judgment and his knowledge, to select and to apply that operation, or the combination of such operations, as may seem most desirable to effect his object. When the pupil has been so reduced that, even if tolerably cleared, there will scarcely be enough space for vision, the case is a proper one for an artificial pupil.

The toughness of capsule can scarcely be judged of from its appearance, when there is no deposit on, or in it; mere opacity affording no criterion of this quality.

Capsule detached, or torn through, may not readily roll up. I have seen instances in which it remained uninfluenced for two months, and even more, but then fully contracted.

Any loose bit of capsule that annoys, should be extracted if possible.

After an operation, the pupil should be kept dilated till all chance of adhesions has passed away.

CHAPTER XXIV.

CATARACT GLASSES.

SPECTACLES must not be worn until the eye has recovered from the action consequent on the several operations for cataract, and the light is not unpleasant, otherwise recovery may be considerably retarded, or the retina permanently injured; but after these requirements have been fulfilled, there can be no general reason for postponing their assistance. I have allowed them in three weeks, and I have been obliged to withhold them for nearly a year. At first they should be employed sparingly.

A choice must not be made without a very careful trial with many, the foci of which are closely graduated. A power of two-and-a-half inches' focus generally suffices for minute purposes, enabling ordinary print to be read at a convenient distance; that is, from six or eight to twelve, fourteen, or eighteen inches, and one of four inches' focus, for long ranges.

It is not uncommon for vision to improve some months after an operation; and when it is ascertained that the eye will take lower powers, a change should at once be effected.

As the lenses are necessarily heavy, the spectacle frames should be as light as is consistent with strength, steel being the metal most suited.

As cataract lenses are thick, project beyond the spectacle frame, and are therefore liable to be scratched or broken, pebble from its hardness is preferable to plate glass.

The rims of tortoiseshell which are usually placed between the frame and the lens, and designated " visuals," are totally useless, disfiguring to the wearer, and publishing to the world that he has had cataract.

A slight degree of intolerance to light may long remain after an operation; it may even be permanent. A tinted lens should then be used; and as pebble cannot be coloured, glass must be brought into requisition.

The frame should be nicely adjusted to the face, and be sufficiently wide that the centre of the lenses—and the lenses need not be circular—may be brought into correspondence with the optic axes. In order to save trouble, when only one eye is available, some persons have the near and the far-seeing lenses in the same frame, which obliges the bridge to be straight, so that they require to turn the spectacles merely. This is a foolish expedient, because there can never be proper adaptation for either side.

Mistakes in distances, especially in ascending or descending stairs, are common when spectacles are first worn, and the patient must be particularly warned that this may occur.

Many anecdotes are told about the wonderful compensative adjustment that has been witnessed in eyes that have lost their lenses when spectacles have been withheld, or only low powers used; and I have seen surprising examples, which all show that the eye should not be overtaxed, but judiciously assisted. This applies especially to children, and to young people. I always admonish my patients never to wear their spectacles except when they are actually wanted; and to use the eyes unassisted, whenever circumstances will admit, for all out-door pursuits.

It is almost incredible what trouble some patients give before they become satisfied with their spectacles and learn to use them. I make it a rule, which I follow whenever I can, to shift the burthen to the optician, as it is really his province. He must look after and attend to the endless details that are needed, as also the whims and fancies of restless and fickle people. For this reason, I have confined myself to a few general remarks that may be useful, and ought to be known by the surgeon.

From the power that the eye, unaided by spectacles, has sometimes acquired in children, it has been supposed that the crystalline lens may have been wholly or partially reproduced.

Its reproduction in some of the lower animals has been often proved. It is said by Mr. Wharton Jones that Textor has observed it in the human subject, and Valentin has discovered by the microscope that the regenerated substance possesses the same intimate structure as the lens. In a publication of the late Mr. Guthrie's, in 1834, on the certainty and safety with which the operation of extraction of cataract from the human eye may be performed, &c., p. 43, an instance is given of what the author considers to be regeneration of the lens. " Anne Wholly, aged twenty-three, came under my care nine years ago, when fourteen years old, having congenital cataracts of both eyes, on which I operated with success. Some circumstances induced her mother to go out of town suddenly, before the eyes were quite clear, and I did not see her again until the 11th of March last, when a small portion of capsule appeared to impede vision at the lower part of the pupil of the right eye, the left being quite free. Supposing that the removal of this portion of capsule would improve her sight, I proposed it to her, and on doing it, I found to my great surprise that the lens had been reproduced, and was quite transparent. It became, of course, opaque, and is now dissolving in the usual manner."

CHAPTER XXV.

ARTIFICIAL PUPIL.

CONDITIONS UNDER WHICH AN OPERATION MAY BE UNDERTAKEN, AND THOSE WHICH CONTRA-INDICATE IT—RELATIVE ADVANTAGES OF THE SEVERAL POSITIONS FOR A PUPIL — SIZE OF THE PUPIL — SHAPE OF THE PUPIL— CLASSIFICATION OF THE PRINCIPAL MORBID STATES OF THE EYE REQUIRING A FALSE PUPIL, WITH THE MOST APPROPRIATE OPERATIONS—CONCLUDING GENERAL REMARKS.

By artificial pupil is meant a passage opened in the iris for the admission of rays of light to the retina, when disease or accident has rendered the natural pupil inefficient.

When there is complete closure of the pupil by lymph, by the adhesion of its margin to an opaque capsule, or by prolapse of the iris; or when it is so eclipsed by an opacity of the cornea as not to admit of relief by artificial dilatation, there cannot be any doubt, abstractly, of the propriety of operating. When, however, there is but partial interruption to vision from any of these causes, it must frequently be a very nice practical question whether an operation should be undertaken, and the answer must be based on the degree of sight that exists, and the probability of being able to increase it by the means at our disposal.

The admissibility of making an artificial pupil when one eye is sound, or at least affords sufficient sight for the ordinary purposes of life, has been much discussed, and different conclusions have been arrived at. My own opinion is against operating, as a rule, so long as the one eye is efficient, except the pupil can be made in the centre of the iris; for, if the position do not correspond to the natural one, there will most probably be confusion of sight, double vision, or squint. The same applies to

making two pupils.   Even although the operation should not
altogether restore sight, and afford but a moderate amount of
vision, a person is much the gainer, especially in the lateral use
of the eye, and I have never had to regret making a false central
pupil, even when the crystalline lens has been absent.   I am
informed by Mr. S. Browne, of Belfast, whose knowledge of
ophthalmic surgery is very extensive, that he has frequently
operated while one eye was sound, to the great advantage of his
patients.

It would seem that confusion of vision does not, and is not
likely to, ensue, when there is perfect vision in the one eye.
This agrees with the fact that in coloboma iridis, on one side, no
confusion follows.   Again, persons with parallel eyes of different
refractive powers, and very dissimilar focal ranges, do not get
puzzled, and would not, so far as I can learn, like the less useful
eye to be obscured.   Even the slight addition of the improvement to the countenance by a restored pupil, is an advantage not
to be thrown away.

A dissimilarity in the position of the pupils is generally, but
not always, followed by disturbance of vision—why only occasionally I am not able to say ; I only know the fact that, under
apparently the same circumstances, when the pupils disagree,
sometimes there will be this derangement, sometimes not any. .

The morbid states of the eyeball that forbid an operation are
generally very palpable, and are declared in altered states of the
cornea, the iris, and the retina.

When the true tissue of the cornea has been lost, and its
place supplied by a cicatrix, an operation is contra-indicated,
although there may be a part of the cicatrix nearly or quite
transparent, for the iris is necessarily incorporated with the new
material.   If at a loss to detect the cicatrix, touch the part with
the point of an instrument, and the palpable thinness will decide
the presence of the abnormal material.

An operation is also contra-indicated when the iris is adherent to the corneal tissue, as an aperture could not be made in
the portion so adhering, for it is an indispensable condition that
these parts be distinct, however closely they may lie ; although

actual apposition renders operating very difficult. It is not, therefore, esssential, as I shall show, that an anterior chamber should exist.

An iris that has lost its characteristic fibrous appearance and lustre, and bulges, affords but a doubtful prospect of success, from the tendency there is for the breach that is made in it to close by adhesive inflammation; and, moreover, the eye in general is certainly, for the most part, so disorganized as to render the application of an operation questionable; still, no structural change in the iris, taken alone, imperatively forbids a trial at a false pupil.

To determine whether the retina has entirely lost its function is certainly not difficult. A moderate light may be intercepted by closure of the pupil, combined with capsulo-lenticular cataraet; but bright rays would always reach it. The sclerotica and the choroid are not impenetrable to light. When, however, the retina is feeble—and it frequently is in the class of cases under consideration,—the propriety of operating cannot always be readily decided, for although yet sensitive, it may be practically spoiled; but the rule of affording every chance for restoring some vision, assists us out of the difficulty, justifying an attempt under discouraging conditions. It must, therefore, occasionally happen, that a well-made pupil proves unavailing. After severe purulent ophthalmia, the eyeball is generally too much damaged to admit of this relief. With a disorganized retina, and a fluid vitreous humour, the external appearances of the eye may be most encouraging.

The several morbid states of the ocular appendages mentioned at page 523, as being more or less obnoxious to the operations for cataract, apply also here, although less forcibly, and should be, as far as possible, removed or reduced, prior to operating.

There are certain conditions, local and general, that are essential to ensure the success of the operation.

The local condition is, freedom of the eyeball from active or chronic inflammation. A long interval should be allowed to elapse after the cessation of the disease which has occasioned the loss of the pupil. When inflammation of the entire globe of the eye has been the cause, the disappearance of preternatural surface vascularity proves the cessation of the more active state ; the absence of the subjective symptoms of flashes, coruscations, and intolerance of light, and the decrease in the size, the number, or the blackness of muscæ, are the criteria of the more chronic condition having subsided.

In certain traumatic cases, closure of the pupil is the only trace of the mischief which the eye has sustained ; but when the closure results from inflammatory causes, especially of long duration, the eyeball rarely becomes freed from an unnatural vascularity, or varicosity, which, in most cases, must be regarded as an irrecoverable state of the blood-vessels, rather than as evidence of the persistence of the morbid condition. If the original disease have long passed away, and a fair trial have been given to means calculated to subdue inflammation,—if the health be good, and the eye be free from irritability,—and if there be much encouragement from the soundness of the retina,—I consider such varicose condition of no importance, and do not hesitate to operate.

The general condition includes the absence, in an active form, of any virus or taint that may have induced the ophthalmic affection. When syphilis, gout, rheumatism, or struma, are yet predominant, it is dangerous to operate, owing to the great probability of re-establishing severe local disease. It has been said that when loss of the pupil in childhood has arisen from any scrofulous affection, an operation should not be performed under puberty. I really think that this should be discretional, as the disadvantages of keeping a child blind are most assuredly very great.

An eye that has seemed to be in an almost hopeless con- dition directly after the subsidence of the disease that has rendered its pupil useless, may, on the restoration of the general health, improve considerably, and be brought into a proper state for a successful operation. Thus it is that an iris which had been for several months apparently permanently spoiled, will lose much of its dulness, and even recover some of its colour ; and a cornea that has been densely opaque, will clear to an extent incredible to those unaccustomed to observe eye-diseases : indeed, so great may be its restoration, especially in children, that an operation for an artificial pupil should never be attempted on account of such opacity, until every suitable means have been tried for its removal, and a considerable time allowed for their operation, as well as for that of the restorative power of nature. The importunity of patients to be relieved from blindness, and the anxiety of surgeons lest they should appear to be negligent, are not unfrequent causes of premature operations.

That a central position for an artificial pupil is superior to a lateral one is most obvious, and is indicated by the natural arrangement of the eye, the configuration of the cornea, the lens, the vitreous body, and even the retina, the most sensitive part of which is opposite the pupil. This has no doubt been recognised ever since the general introduction of the operation for the false aperture, though, perhaps, it has not always been acted upon. The imperfections of a lateral aperture, arising from the interception of the light by the intervention of the ciliary processes, have been long pointed out, especially by Scarpa ; the indistinctness of the image formed by the circumference of the lens, and the disadvantage of its falling on a part of the retina not the most sensitive, are facts which the elements of physiology teach us, and the details of practice confirm. As a natural effort to obviate these defects, when the pupil is external, the eye generally squints inwards. It has often been a matter of surprise to me how slightly vision has been interfered with by central opacities of the cornea, so long as the pupil was natural, and its margin extended a little beyond the opaque part ; and also, where there has been general, although slight, loss of corneal transparency, with a perfect state of pupil. As a rule, therefore, I have ever preferred forming a pupil centrally, even though it should be by the side of a dense opacity of the cornea, or be somewhat shaded, to choosing the circumference of the iris, though there the cornea may be transparent.

There is much diversity of opinion regarding the most

advantageous spot to be selected, when a pupil cannot be made
centrally, supposing all parts of the iris circumference to be available. This discrepancy arises from the real difficulty that invests
the subject, inasmuch as we are almost without the assistance of
practical deductions ; for it is seldom that the results of lateral
pupils can be compared with each other, owing to the very
different states of the eye, and the variation in the sizes and in
the shapes of the pupils in different individuals. I will state
the opinions of some of our most distinguished ophthalmic
surgeons on the matter ; and first, that of the late Mr.
Guthrie :—

  "When an artificial pupil cannot be made in the centre of
the iris (from whatever cause), the other parts of it are eligible
in the following order :—1st, The inferior part of the iris
inclining inwards ; 2nd, The internal, a little below the transverse diameter of the eye ; 3rd, The inferior and external : the
upper part being the least eligible, from the eyelid covering
that portion of the cornea in the natural state of the eye. The
lower and inferior parts of the iris are to be preferred, for the
following reasons : because the line of vision being through that
part, the eye is less removed from its natural axis, and consequently less squinting is occasioned than when vision is acquired
in any other direction ; and if both eyes are operated upon, the
axes of vision are made more nearly parallel. A decided preference of a position not higher than the centre of the iris is
founded upon the natural position of by far the greater number
of objects of vision which it is essential for a person to see
being viewed forwards or downwards."

  Mr. Lawrence writes,—"When a lateral opening is to be
made, in consequence of the circumference of the cornea only
remaining transparent, the nasal side of the iris should be
chosen on the level of the natural pupil ; then comes the
temporal side. The normal place of the opening is nearer
to the nasal than to the temporal edge of the cornea ; the
axis of vision, therefore, with a pupil in the former situation,
coincides more nearly with that of the perfect eye than when
it occupies the latter place. The next best situation is the

lower and outer part of the iris, after which comes the lower; but the optic axis then deviates widely from its natural direction. The least favourable position is above; for a pupil is not of much use here, as the upper eyelid interferes with it, so that the eye must be turned downwards, and even then sight is imperfect."

Dr. Mackenzie prefers the nasal edge of the cornea, and gives as one of his reasons, the deformity which is caused by a pupil at the temporal edge; a consideration that I think ought scarcely to have any weight in the question. He thinks, besides, that when the pupil is behind the temporal edge of the cornea, a person finds it difficult to turn the eye so as to bring the pupil into the necessary direction to embrace the usual range of objects.

Mr. Tyrrell directs that when the position and extent of opacity of the cornea does not forbid, the pupil should always be brought downwards and outwards; and when that cannot be effected, it should be directed downwards, and never, unless compelled by circumstances, should it be drawn upwards. He does not make any mention of an internal position.

M. Desmarres, the most recent French writer on ophthalmic surgery, advises a choice in the following order : first the internal side, then the lower, next the external inferior.

My own opinion is in favour of an aperture at the inferior margin of the iris, as next best to the centre, because I think that position possesses the greatest advantages, and it is that which I should adopt whenever it can be easily executed; but where retraction of the eyeball, or a prominent cheek, at all interfered with the ready use of instruments, I would make it downwards and outwards.

When circumstances oblige us to place the pupil laterally, we should endeavour, if opacity of the cornea do not interfere, to make it ample enough, without extending the aperture to the very margin of the iris, for the reasons above stated.

It is well to have some principle by which we may regulate the size of an artificial pupil, when the physical peculiarities of

the case do not limit its dimensions. The multiplicity of the
conditions to be taken into account, especially when the crystalline lens has been lost, renders it difficult to solve the pro-
blem on purely theoretical grounds, and experience must be
our guide. When the aperture is to be central, we should
endeavour to make it of a size corresponding to the pupil in a
state between dilatation and contraction. In the middle of the
iris, however, size seems of less importance than when the aperture is lateral; for then, except it be of a certain capacity,
sufficient light will not enter, and if very large, too much will
be admitted, and confusion of vision must ensue. For the side
pupil, the simple slit, or still better, the pear-shape, with the
apex outwards, are to be preferred.

The form of the new pupil is seldom entirely under our
control; practical surgeons well know this. Therefore, in
general, an operator should not be dissatisfied if he can effect
an aperture of any figure at the spot he desires, provided it be
ample. At the time of operating it is for the most part
impossible to say what will be the outline, or even the size of
the future pupil; a small slit in a flaccid iris may, when the
chambers of the eye are filled with the aqueous fluid, expand
beyond expectation, and the excision of an apparently insufficient
portion may form an opening well shaped, and equal to that
required.

IRIS SCISSORS.

In the scissors represented at fig. 147, one blade is probe-pointed, and longer and broader than its fellow, which is sharp. When the two are closed, the lesser blade is completely shielded by the greater, the instrument being then blunt, as is shown in

FIG. 147.   FIG. 148.

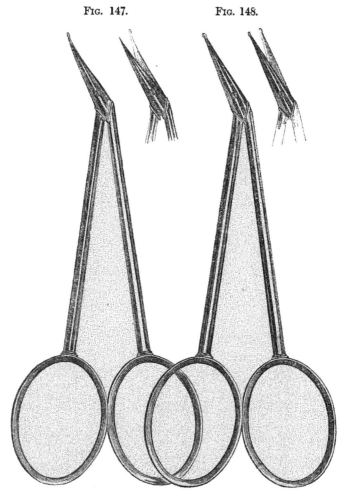

the larger wood-cut. Great nicety of workmanship is required for the sharp limb to be fine enough to penetrate the iris readily, and to have also a cutting edge to the very extremity.

The scissors, fig. 148, are merely blunt-pointed.

IRIS KNIVES

These instruments should be sufficiently thin to penetrate the cornea and the iris readily. They need not be sharp beyond

FIG. 149.　　FIG. 150.　　FIG. 151.

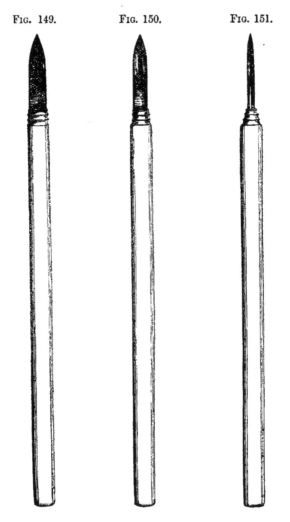

the shoulder. Different sizes are necessary in order that the incision of the cornea may not exceed that required for the iris. The smallest, called a broad needle, is generally useful.

IRIS HOOKS.

The first, fig. 152, known as Tyrrell's, owes its efficiency to its long and narrow recess, within which the iris can be securely retained.   As a precaution against the capsule of the lens being

FIG. 152.   FIG. 153.   FIG. 154.

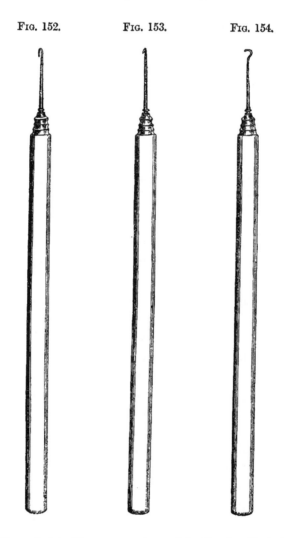

injured, the point is blunt, smooth, and inclined a little inwards. I also use one with a shorter bend and more interspace, when I require to draw out a smaller bit of the iris.

Fig. 153 is like a lady's crochet needle, but has a blunter and more prominent barb. I have found it useful on certain occasions when it has been necessary to disengage the instrument readily from the iris. Fig. 154 illustrates a hook that I have often used in the necessarily varied manipulations required in the formation of an artificial pupil.

IRIS CANULA SCISSORS.

The mechanism of this instrument resembles that of the capsule forceps described among the cataract instruments, except

FIG. 155.

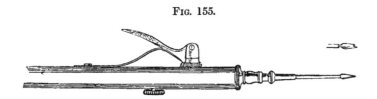

that the canula is worked by a spring, and this is necessary here, because it is required to be moved backwards and forwards repeatedly.

The lesser figure, representing the instrument partly open, shows the form of the blades, one of which is blunt. There are blades of different sizes, some with both extremities sharp, others, for particular occasions, with both dull.

The supposed value of these scissors is that they can be used without previously incising the cornea, which allows the aqueous humour to escape; but unless the blades be thin enough, and so wrought that they may penetrate readily, they will not only be ineffectual, but are very likely to inflict severe injury on the cornea and the iris.

To Mr. Wilde, of Dublin, is due the credit of this addition to our ophthalmic instrument case. His announcement of the invention is in the " Medical Times" for December, 1850.

Perhaps the simplest, and at the same time the most practical and concise manner of treating the operative part of this subjcet is, to classify the principal states of the eye admitting of an artificial pupil, and to annex to each its generally appropriate operation.

1. CLOSURE OF THE PUPIL, FROM INFLAMMATION OR PROLAPSE OF THE IRIS; THE CRYSTALLINE LENS ABSENT, THE CORNEA CLEAR, OR IF PARTIALLY OPAQUE, THE OPACITY NOT INTER-FERING WITH THE FORMATION OF A CENTRAL APERTURE IN THE IRIS.

Incision.—Incision with Extension.—Incision with Excision.

When inflammation has destroyed the pupil, the iris does not necessarily alter its position; it does not bulge from the loss of communication between the chambers of the eye, provided its tonicity is preserved, and then the size of the anterior chamber is not only undiminished, a matter of importance in operating, but may be actually increased by the falling back of parts in consequence of the loss of the lens. There may be but a mere trace of the remains of the pupil; or the aperture, very much contracted, may be closed by lymph or capsule.

When prolapse of the iris through the cornea has shut up the pupil, there must always be a reduction in the size of the anterior chamber, the diminution depending on the position through which the iris has escaped. Both these states may be combined; the pupil may be closed from inflammation, and the iris may be prolapsed.

The operation of "incision," with the knife, is the most appropriate when the iris retains enough of its physical properties to gape on being divided, and the less it has suffered from the effects of inflammation the more certain will be the result. "We need not hesitate to assert," writes Dr. Mackenzie, "that in every case in which the substance of the iris is not greatly altered by inflammation, we may con-fidently expect a successful issue to the operation by incision, in whatever direction, or in whatever part of the iris the incision is made, above or below, or in the line of the natural pupil, and whether it is a mere pin-hole or extends to two-thirds of the diameter of the iris."

Independently of the superiority of a central pupil, it must certainly be an advantage, as tending to produce a more perfectly formed aperture, to divide the iris in its centre, that the circumferential or dilating portion may act equally on the divided part. Perhaps, too, there may be some practical advantage in cutting through those fibres in the centre of the iris, by the interlacing of which a sort of sphincter muscle is provided; besides, it is in these pupillary fibres, if I may so call them, that there is generally the greatest agglutination from inflammation.

I invariably operate through the cornea. The following manner of steadying the eye, is applicable to all these operations. An assistant draws down the lower eyelid, resting his finger on the malar bone. I raise the upper eyelid with my forefinger, and with the tip of it, and that of the middle finger, steady the eyeball, after the manner indicated by this diagram,

Fig. 156.

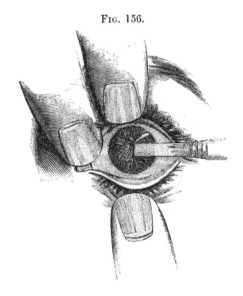

which represents an operation on the left eye. If in any case the steadying of the eyeball, by holding the conjunctiva with a pair of forceps, be serviceable, it should be adopted.

With the first or second-sized iris knife, according to the circumstances of the case, I divide the cornea as near to the circumference as practicable, and penetrate the iris as centrally as possible, thrusting the blade up to the shoulder. In the above figure, the second knife is introduced, but for most cases the largest is required.

The aperture thus made is about the third of the diameter of the iris, elliptical and vertical.

A great deal of stress is usually laid on the special fitness of "incision" in cases where the iris is on the stretch from prolapsus. Without going into the question of the greater elasticity or contractility of the part under such circumstances, but giving it as my opinion, that this property is much overrated, I would suggest that the choice of the operation, so far as the state of the iris can be taken as a guide, should be made to depend on its actual structural condition; because any advantage that the mere stretching could afford, might be lost by slight interstitial change, and inflammation of the eyeball is often a cause of the prolapse.

The annexed sketch of a pupil closed by prolapse of the iris is from a man seventy years of age, who applied to me after having

Fig. 157.

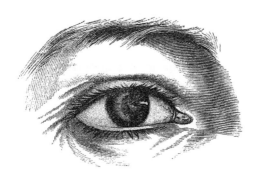

undergone the operation for extraction. The broad white line on the outer side of the cornea indicates the cicatrix of the faulty incision, to the entire extent of which the iris was adherent. I suspect that a large portion of the iris, including a part of the pupillary margin, had been cut off in making the section of the cornea. The pupil, reduced to a minute aperture, was nearly useless. The other eye was quite lost in the attempt to extract. With the second-sized knife I divided the iris obliquely upwards and inwards, endeavouring to make the incision divaricate from the upper end of the narrow slit that existed. My object was accomplished. Not the slightest untoward symptom ensued, and in a week the man left the hospital with good vision.

This second sketch of the eye was taken several months afterwards, and exhibits the form of the new pupil. The

FIG. 158.

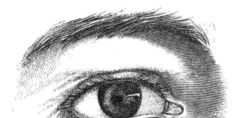

artist has shown the reduction in the opacity of the cornea, the consequence of the natural process of repair.

Perhaps this may be the most appropriate place to describe that inefficient state of the pupil which so frequently exists after the operation for solution when the iris is adherent to the capsulo-lenticular cataract, and which may be due to the smallness of the aperture in the capsule, or the lymph that has been effused, or to the diminutiveness of the pupil, even although it may be quite clear, and to which "incision" is suited when the iris will retract.

J. Browne, twenty-one years old, an inmate of the St. Pancras Workhouse, had been operated on at some institution in London. When he came to me, at the Ophthalmic Hospital, I found that the lenticular cataract had been absorbed, and that the capsule, though partly detached, yet blocked up the pupil, which was too much contracted to be of much use if cleared, and I therefore determined to make an artificial one. The figure 159 represents the state of the eye.

FIG. 159.

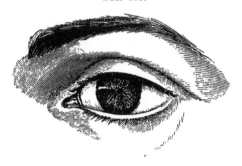

The operation of "incision" with the knife was performed, and an ample pupil resulted. The capsule separated from the iris during the operation, but retained a part of its natural attachment, and, moving backwards and forwards, occasionally produced much inconvenience by temporarily interrupting vision. After the lapse of a few months I attempted to remove it. I incised the cornea with the second-sized iris knife, and with the blunt canula capsule forceps withdrew the greater part.

FIG. 160.

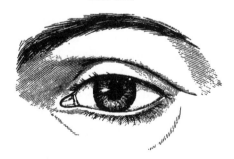

The portion that remained, being behind the iris at the inner side of the eye, did not interfere with vision, which was excellent. Fig. 160 shows the after state of the pupil.

It was by "incision" performed through the sclerotica that Cheselden, the well-known originator of artificial pupil, used to operate; his method fell into disrepute and was almost abandoned, when Sir W. Adams revived it. From Adams' account of himself he was very successful, and he attributed this to making a more free incision in the iris than his predecessor, and using a long and very narrow scalpel, known as Adams' iris knife, which is still to be found among most sets of ophthalmic instruments. While in his last book, "Adams on the Eye," he speaks in the most laudatory terms of his operation, as he was wont to call it, he does not omit to tell of the difficulty of making a sufficient aperture, and the risk in the attempt, of detaching the iris at its circumference; the cause of both of which, namely, operating through the sclerotica, seems to have escaped his notice. Irrespective of these objections, however, is the very serious one of the great violence necessarily inflicted on the eye by operating posteriorly.

The great advantages of the operation I advocate are, its being executed through the cornea; the certainty of being able to make the pupil at the desired spot; the division of the iris before the aqueous humour is lost, and therefore while it is tense, by an incision, which, owing to the form of the knife, is effected with such slight pressure that there is no risk of detachment from its natural connexions.

The reasons that I have advanced in the chapter on Cataract for the superiority of the anterior operation for solution over the posterior, as respects injuring fewer textures of the eye, apply here also, and with greater force, because of the larger wound inflicted; but, more than this, in the old posterior operation, there is generally much bleeding within the eye, and the blood may proceed from many sources, whereas in the anterior, the iris is the only part from which it can issue, and very frequently it does not bleed when cut.

To render "incision" with the knife more generally applicable, by adapting it to cases in which the iris has not sufficient tone to contract when merely incised; or when it is more or less tied or fixed, by being prolapsed, or adherent to capsule; I proposed, some years ago, a modification of the above operation; namely, to divide the iris, and with the hook ($_{fig.}$ 154) to draw outwards the outer lip of the wound, till a sufficient gap is made. An aperture is thus effected, by tearing, by stretching, and by the folding inwards of the flap of iris. This may be denominated "incision with extension."

The following sketch shows two pupils I made after this

FIG. 161.

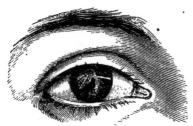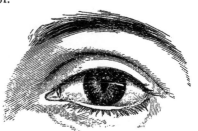

method. The man had been operated on for cataract, by "extraction." Mr. Tyrrell performed on the right eye; the remains of the natural pupil, displaced by prolapse of the iris, and closed by lymph, are seen above the artificial one. I extracted on the left side. The pupil was closed by inflammation.

I have done this operation very often.

It not unfrequently happens that a dense layer of lymph or thickened capsule blocks up the pupil, and forms an impediment to "incision" with the knife, at least to the formation of a central aperture by it; perhaps, too, the iris is not healthy enough to retract when cut; but with the aid of another mode of operating, "excision," the details of which are given in Section 2, we are enabled to make the pupil towards the centre of the iris, and to secure for it a better shape than by any other means. The following case will explain this. I performed the operation for "solution" on a youth eighteen years of age, whose iris was adherent to the capsulo-lenticular cataract, but could not, by any endeavour, make a patent opening in the

R R

dense capsule, and the lymph on it, nor detach the mass from the pupil. Having divided the iris close to the capsule, with the largest iris knife, I seized the outer portion with the hook (fig. 154), drew it without the cornea, and cut off a piece. Fig. 162 represents the eye after the operation. A portion of

FIG. 162.

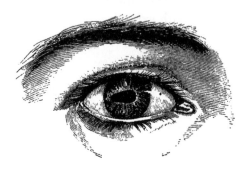

the capsule is seen at the inner side of the pupil; the remainder of it lay rolled up behind. The two black dots at the margin of the cornea indicate two very minute portions of the iris that prolapsed. This patient recovered sufficient vision to enable him to get his living as an errand lad. The other eye was quite disorganized. By making the incision a little internal to the centre of the iris, when practicable, the pupil will be still more central.

When capsule alone blocks up the pupil, the process of tearing it through with two needles, as given at page 583, might be applicable, and should be considered. I have not myself, however, found it as well adapted here, as when applied to capsule that is merely in the field of vision and does not adhere to the iris, or at least is but partially adherent, so that there is pupillary movement.

Janin's operation improved by Maunoir is usually recommended in these cases, and especially when the unhealthy condition of the iris renders " incision " alone inapplicable. The principle of it is, to form a flap of a portion of the iris, by the shrivelling of which an aperture may result.

The cornea is divided towards its margin to about a fourth of

its circumference, and the scissors (fig. 147), introduced sideways till they reach the desired spot, then turned, opened, the
iris pierced with the sharp limb, and the instrument carried on
till sufficiently advanced, as indicated by the blunt limb that
traverses the anterior chamber, when the cutting is effected.
A second incision is then to be made at an acute angle with
the first.   The two should be as nearly as possible in correspondence with the diverging lines in the following diagram :—:

FIG. 163.

The line at the margin represents the incision of the cornea.
Mr. Tyrrell advised that the flap of the iris should be depressed
towards the vitreous body by the scissors, on account of its
liability to unite.   He writes :—" I formerly used to take out
a piece of the iris, but I afterwards found the above modification of the operation to answer exceedingly well."

This is a complicated operation, and according to my experience a most uncertain one.

2. PARTIAL OPACITY OF THE CORNEA, OBSCURING THE PUPIL ;
THE IRIS UNADHERENT ; THE LENS AND ITS CAPSULE TRANS-
PARENT.

Excision.—Iriddesis.

'Excision,' which is of very old date, is the operation adapted
for this condition, and that which I have generally executed.

The cornea should be incised to about a fourth of its circumference, close to its margin, and in that direction which may
seem most desirable for a lateral pupil.   Should the iris prolapse—an occurrence not unusual,—it is seized with a pair of
forceps, drawn out sufficiently, and the required portion, including the pupil-edge, cut off with the scissors.   As there is
danger of making the pupil too large, the operator must be
cautious.   If the iris bulge, it is safer to make the corneal

incision with the cataract knife, because it is less likely to be penetrated, and the lens is less exposed to danger.

When the iris does not prolapse, the wound may be opened with the spoon of the curette, or a short Tyrrell's hook may be employed, the ordinary one being apt to draw out too much in these cases, the pupillary margin caught, and the retraction made. There may be some embarrassment in withdrawing the hook, on account of its catching the edge of the cornea, to avoid which it should be half rotated when it arrives at that part. The capsule of the lens may be touched with impunity by a blunt and smooth instrument. Some operators employ the forceps.

The opacity of the cornea may so obscure the pupil that the hook cannot be readily applied to its margin; in such a case the iris must be withdrawn with a pair of forceps. I object to an attempt to cause its protrusion by pressing on the eye, from the attendant danger of dislocating the lens.

It is a matter of nicety to decide how much of the iris should be excised; and nothing but actual practice can ever teach this. However, I may state that too much is likely to be removed rather than too little. The nearer the scissors are applied to the hook, the smaller will be the pupil. The operation is finished by endeavouring to return within the eye any part of the iris that yet protrudes. When it is returned, the healing is more quickly effected.

Mr. Tyrrell improved on this by incising the cornea to a very limited extent with the " broad needle," seizing the iris with his hook, and retaining it in the wound,—strangulating it, as the process is generally called. A channel so made is pear-shaped, the apex at the margin of the cornea,—and this is a good form for a lateral pupil. But the process of strangulation is so uncertain, from the frequent spontaneous extrication of the iris from the wound,—an occurrence of great likelihood when it is healthy and has not any adhesions,—that I do not trust to it, but perform the older operation.

A method of operating in this condition has been introduced

by Mr. Critchett, and, according to his description of the operation,—" Iriddesis," as he calls it, in the first volume of the "Ophthalmic Hospital Reports," p. 220,—it is here particularly applicable. It is the simplest class of case to which it is suitable; namely, a central defined opacity of the cornea, in which it is only required that the natural pupil should be slightly moved to one side, and brought opposite a transparent part.

The patient, if at all restless, being placed under the influence of chloroform, the wire speculum is inserted, and the eye is fixed by seizing a small fold of conjunctiva with a pair of forceps. A small opening is then made with a broad needle into the anterior chamber; it should be close to the sclerotic, and just large enough to admit the canula forceps, with which the iris is caught near, but not close to, its ciliary attachment, and drawn out until the pupil is sufficiently displaced; the small piece thus made to prolapse is secured and strangulated in a loop of floss silk, previously slipped over the canula forceps, and, at the proper time, brought down and drawn tight, by holding each end in a pair of ordinary forceps; the ends of the silk are then cut off, and the operation is complete. The prolapsed iris soon shrinks, and the ligature may generally be removed on the second day.

The advantages are, that the circular fibres of the iris are not lacerated, and the natural margin of the pupil remains uninjured; while its size, form, and direction can be exactly regulated according to the exigencies of the case, and the natural motory power in some measure retained.

This is certainly a valuable addition to ophthalmic surgery. I speak from frequent personal use of it. I have at times deviated from the above manner of operating, as regards the details, such as not holding the eyeball with the forceps, and the manner of applying the noose. Like all the other operations for artificial pupil, it must be adapted to the fitting cases. It does not entirely supersede " excision,"—for example, when there is a mere crescent of transparent cornea at the circumference.

3. CLOSURE OF THE PUPIL BY LYMPH, THE LENS AND ITS
CAPSULE TRANSPARENT OR OPAQUE.

Tearing away a bit of the iris.—Excision.—Operation for "solution."—Laceration of capsule.—Incision.—Excision.—Operation for "extraction."—Division of iris adhesions.

Until within a very recent period, in England at least, it was generally supposed that the lens and capsule become entirely opaque when a deposit of lymph completely closes the pupil, a condition in which the iris is necessarily adherent to the capsule of the lens. Dr. Mackenzie certainly alludes to transparency of the lens and capsule in connexion with closure of the pupil by lymph; but then he does not admit that the lymph is adherent to the capsule of the lens. "Closure of the pupil from inflammation of the iris, without any opacity of the capsule, or any adhesion between it and the iris, is certainly a very rare occurrence, and, from the appearance presented, is exceedingly liable to be taken for a case of closure of the pupil with adhesion to an opaque capsule." With due deference to such authority, I must record my disbelief that such a state can exist: I think that the lymph must bind the iris to the capsule of the lens. Even so great a pathologist as the late Mr. Dalrymple maintained the prevalent opinion that the lens and capsule are always rendered opaque, as I had an opportunity of knowing from himself, in a consultation very shortly before his death. I understand that the German surgeons first showed the fallacy of the opinion, and taught, that while the centre of the capsule just under a deposit of lymph may be opaque, the rest of it, and the whole lens, may be transparent. With this knowledge we now avoid the destruction of the lens, and proceed to make a pupil in a manner that shall not injure it or the capsule. Of course we cannot determine beforehand, with certainty, whether they are transparent: the history of the case, and the perception of light which the patient may possess, will afford us some guide; but we ought, whenever there is a probability of the absence of opacity of these parts, to proceed on the assumption of their integrity. Prior to Mr. Tyrrell's time, when the formation of an artificial pupil was undertaken, this state of the eye was a sad puzzle to surgeons, the chief difficulty being how to dispose of the lens. Mr. Tyrrell, by introducing "drilling," which is merely the operation for "solution," was supposed to have overcome the difficulty.

When the lens and its capsule are transparent, there seem to be only two appropriate operations; for in any by which the iris is transfixed, or cut, these parts can hardly escape injury. One of them is very modern and very simple. The cornea is punctured, the blunt canula forceps introduced, a portion of the iris close to the pupil is seized, and a piece gradually torn away, drawn out, and cut off.

The other operation that is applicable, "excision," has been already sufficiently described in Section 2; and all that need be said here is, that if the iris do not prolapse when the cornea is opened, as in such a case it probably may not, or cannot, a part of it must be seized with a pair of forceps, withdrawn, and excised. It does not appear in any of the cases related by Gibson, who was a great authority on "excision," that he executed it when the iris was adherent to the capsule of the lens by means of lymph. He restricted it, as most operators have since his time, to those cases in which the pupil was lost by the iris adhering to the cornea, or was obscured by corneal opacity, or in which both of these states existed. Indeed, the operation has by some been erroneously deemed impracticable, unless the pupil be in part free, so as to admit of a portion of the iris being readily drawn out.

A young woman, twenty-one years old, applied at the Central London Ophthalmic Hospital, with trichiasis. An artificial pupil in that eye quickly attracted my notice. It was the most efficient I had ever seen at the side of the iris; for, with the naked eye, small print could be read, but she was short-sighted, seeing distant objects better through a concave glass. The lens was present. The accompanying figure is a representation of the eye after the trichiasis was removed.

FIG. 164.

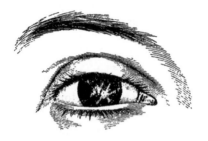

The iris had lost its fibrous appearance, and the remains of the pupil in its centre, closed by lymph, was just perceptible. The girl could not tell who was the operator; she knew only from her mother's account, that when a child, she was taken to a gentleman in London, who operated, and restored sight, which had been lost in infancy, from a severe attack of inflammation. She suspected that the late Mr. Alexander operated.

When a portion of the circumference of the iris cannot be withdrawn, excision is inapplicable, and a piece must be torn away.

When the pupil is adherent to a capsulo-lenticular cataract, the age of the patient is my chief guide to the course I shall adopt. In early life, and before the fortieth year, I should first operate on the lenticular cataract for "solution;" and after a full and sufficient time had been allowed for absorption—and I beg to refer to this in the chapter on Cataract—I should make the pupil, either by tearing through the capsule, by "incision," or otherwise, as may seem most necessary. I would adopt the same plan in old age, if I had any proof, or strong suspicion of the degeneration of the lens; no uncommon change in this state.

When, however, there is the hard cataract of age, my plan is to extract the cataract, and to make the pupil at the same time. This was first practised and made public by the late Mr. Travers. He cut the cornea as for "extraction," raised the centre of the iris with a pair of forceps, cut off a piece, and then removed the cataract. When there is too small an anterior chamber to allow the corneal section to be made in the ordinary way, I have used the secondary knife, as described in the cataract operation. I have besides, with excellent success, extracted the cataract, partly by tearing through the capsule and the exudation on it, and partly by snipping the iris with the scissors. On one occasion, with the curette alone, I separated the pupillary adhesions enough to admit of the escape of the cataract, and with the best results.

4. PARTIAL CLOSURE OF THE PUPIL BY LYMPH, THE LENS AND ITS CAPSULE TRANSPARENT.

Excision.—Iriddesis.

This state differs from the last described merely in the pupil not being entirely lost. "Excision" is chiefly applicable here. The cornea should be punctured near the margin with the smallest iris knife, the hook most suitable introduced, the point carefully inserted into the opening of the pupil, which would necessarily be very small, and an endeavour made to tear out a piece of the iris. Sometimes a thin strip is brought away, which may or may not be snipped off, according to the length of the piece; sometimes only a fissure is made; the result depending very much on the condition of the iris, whether it be considerably altered in structure or not; if much damaged, the hook readily tears out. It may, therefore, be necessary, at a future period, to enlarge the fissure. Of course this should not be attempted till it has been well ascertained that the pupil so made is insufficient; for a linear pupil, apparently too narrow, may afford good sight. After it has been determined in which direction the enlargement shall be made, the cornea is punctured on the corresponding side, the hook introduced, the margin of the fissure seized, withdrawn, and cut off or strangulated, according to circumstances. A triangular-shaped opening will be made.

The hook is more in contact with the capsule of the lens in this, than in any other operation for artificial pupil; yet if properly made, and carefully used, it will not inflict any injury.

It matters not, as far as the performance of the operation is concerned, at which side of the eye the free portion of the pupil be situated, for the stem of the hook may be so bent as to allow the instrument to be used in any direction; but I would suggest that it might be better, when the iris is unadherent in a direction not the best suited for the manipulation, to employ the canula forceps, and make an aperture in the most advantageous situation.

To obviate the inconvenience arising from the loss of the aqueous humour in the preliminary incision with the knife, and which consists chiefly in the alterations that take place in the relative position of the iris and the lens, several surgeons have suggested the use of a sharp hook that may be pushed through the cornea, and applied to the iris while the anterior chamber is yet filled.

FIG. 165.

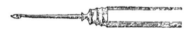

I have given the instrument a fair trial; the difficulty, however, in withdrawing it is a fatal objection. Besides, the liability of wounding the lens, and the impossibility of re-application on the same occasion, are strong objections against any general employment of it, and much narrow its applicability.

With particular care in reference to preventing the escape of the aqueous humour, by not pressing on the eyeball, but steadying it by having the conjunctiva held with forceps, employing the spring-wire eyelid retractor, by making the incision in the cornea with care, and withdrawing the knife gently, and exactly as it was introduced, without twisting, that the wound may not gape, so little of this fluid will generally ooze out, that the loss may be practically unimportant.

The operation "Iriddesis," described in Section 2, is also applicable here, if not by one tying, by two, at a few lines apart, whereby a triangular aperture is made. It must be mentioned that the iris may be too rotten to be tied.

5. DIMINUTION OR CLOSURE OF THE PUPIL FROM PROLAPSE OF THE IRIS, OR ADHESION OF IT TO THE CORNEA IN CONSEQUENCE OF A WOUND, A PENETRATING ULCER, A SLOUGH, OR SUPPURATION OF THE CORNEA ; THE CORNEA MORE OR LESS OPAQUE, THE LENS AND ITS CAPSULE TRANSPARENT, OR OPAQUE, OR THE LENS LOST.

Cutting or tearing through the adhesions.—Excision.—
Incision.—Iriddesis.—Separation.

Under this head occur the greater number of cases requiring an artificial pupil ; and of these, the majority arise from ulceration of the cornea and prolapse of a part of the iris ; but as, in a surgical point of view, it is the same whether the pupil be lost by prolapse, or by mere adhesion of the iris to the cornea, I shall not practically recognise any difference.

When a small part of the margin of the pupil is prolapsed, the aperture being merely diminished, and the opacity of the cornea is limited, or if extensive, not so dense as to obstruct light, the practice should be to detach the iris from the cornea, without injuring the capsule of the lens, and thus to make the pupil central. A slight tag of the iris may be readily divided with the smallest iris knife, and the operation is simple. The cornea is punctured at the spot where the adhesion can be most readily reached, subject only to the rule of avoiding that part under which the pupil will fall ; the knife is directed between the iris and the cornea with great care, as the anterior chamber is necessarily small, and applied at once to the part to be severed. If it be carried too far, and then withdrawn, the aqueous humour will escape, and the operation probably fail. I have torn away the connexion with the blunt hook.

When a large portion of the pupil is adherent—in which case no inconsiderable part of the body of the iris is generally tied to the cornea,—it is scarcely possible to operate in the above manner; for in attempting to divide the iris the aqueous humour escapes, and then the operation must be abandoned, or the capsule of the lens will be wounded and rendered opaque. I have witnessed many marked failures of this kind.

I have frequently incised the cornea, and divided some of the connexions with the blunt iris scissors, and established useful pupils. In a few instances I have used the scissors to the utmost, and torn the remainder through with one or other of the blunt hooks; but I do not recommend it, on account of the tediousness of the proceeding, and the violence it inflicts.

" Excision " is often well adapted. I have made some excellent pupils by it.

It is supposed that the canula scissors are well suited to this class of cases, but I find that they are not generally applicable; and when they may be used with freedom, the iris knife may also be employed, and I think with greater safety. There is not generally space enough for them to be worked in, without their inflicting injury to the back of the cornea, or to the capsule of the lens. A very great objection to them is the lacerated wound they inflict when pushed through the cornea, especially in an unhealthy cornea. Their withdrawal is not easy. However, that they may be used when the pupil is much deranged, there can be no doubt, and I have applied them myself, although not latterly. The following example of their employment in Mr. Bowman's practice, I take from the " Medical Times." The case, too, serves to illustrate very extensive adhesions of the iris :—

The patient, thirty-six years old, had lost the left eye by a blow. The right was rendered useless by a severe inflammation, which ended in sloughing of the cornea. A dense leucoma occupied the greater part of the cornea, nearly concealing the lower portion of the iris, and obscuring the pupil. When the eye was shaded so as to dilate the pupil, it rose a little above the leucoma, and his sight was considerably improved. Still, the cornea was slightly hazy above the leucoma, to nearly its upper margin. The lens appeared to be *in sitû*, and perfectly clear. The lower edge of the pupil adhered to the leucoma.

The scissors were introduced at the outer side of the cornea, where it was very nebulous, and pushed on as far as the existing pupil, where it lay almost, but not quite, obscured by the leucoma, for atropine had been applied. The shorter, blunt-pointed blade was then passed behind the upper border of the pupil, and the long sharp-pointed one in front of the iris, and the upper margin of the pupil cut to the extent of about 1-16th of an inch. Vision was improved. The man returned home. He came back for inspection. He stated that he saw more distinctly when the eye was shaded; and as it was found that the pupil enlarged slightly upwards when that took place, the operation was repeated and the iris incised at the same point, but to a greater extent, so as to place the pupil permanently in the condition in which it was found to serve most efficiently the purposes of vision. A minute strip of iris remained between the two cuts.

FIG. 166.

No inflammation followed; nor did the capsule of the lens become opaque, although it was, as the report says, "evidently touched with the scissors, and that, too, not slightly." This was, therefore, a fortunate escape.

The first diagram shows the size of the pupil before operation. The oblique line indicates the course of incision by the scissors. The line at the margin points out the position at which the cornea was divided. The second diagram represents the pupil after the first operation.

My own practice here has been to make a linear pupil with the hook after the manner given in Section 3.

" Iriddesis " also is applicable.

When the pupil is quite closed, the choice of an operation must depend chiefly on the extent of the corneal opacity, and the supposed state of the lens. In the following instance I adopted double " incision." A girl, nine years old, whose right eye had been quite destroyed by an attack of purulent ophthalmia in infancy, was placed under my care by Mr. Harding, of Percy Street, for the purpose of having an artificial pupil made in the left. The central lower part of the cornea was occupied by a dense cicatrix (fig. 167) to the entire extent of

FIG. 167. .

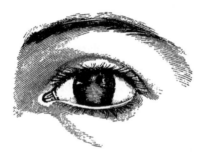

which the iris was adherent, the pupil being of course lost ; and the rest of the cornea was more or less opaque. Acting on the supposition that the lens had escaped, or having become opaque was absorbed, my opinion being founded on what I had observed in parallel cases, I incised the iris at the outer and upper part with the second-sized iris knife, but its texture was too much damaged for a gap to ensue. However, the incision did not close, and a few weeks afterwards I divided the cornea on the outer side, near its margin, and with the iris scissors (fig. 147) cut the iris transversely at each extremity of the incision ; and a good-sized, well-shaped, and well-placed pupil resulted, as the sketch shows.

Scarcely any inflammation followed either operation. The

lens was absent. Very little benefit ensued, for the retina was, it appeared, too much damaged to admit of useful sight. This loss of power is a very common effect of purulent ophthalmia. The general damage of the eye is always more than would be suspected, except by those who have experience in the matter.

In parallel cases it must be left to the judgment of the operator, whether "incision," combined with extension or with "excision," as described in Section 1, page 603, should be done.

When the lens is present, and supposed to be not opaque, the question is, whether a portion of the iris should be torn away with the capsule-forceps, as described at page 615; or Mr. Tyrrell's operation adopted, namely, that of incising the iris close to the cornea, with the smallest iris knife, and with the blunt hook withdrawing a portion of it, as in the operation for enlarging a pupil, pages 612 and 617. The latter is the more hazardous of the two to the capsule of the lens.

When, with extensive adhesion, only just the circumference of the cornea is transparent, "separation," or the tearing away of the iris from its natural attachment, is the only resource; for then it would be most imprudent to incise that part of the cornea for the execution of any of the other operations, lest opacity of it should ensue. When the transparent portion is at the upper or the inner side, even although it be not so very limited, "separation" may be required, from the impediments to the performance of other operations in such situations. But it should be restricted to these cases, and these only, as it is an operation that inflicts much injury, and, according to my own experience, is less successful than any of the methods of making a false pupil that I have described. Besides this, it may be stated in general, that eyes requiring it are most unfavourable for an operation, as they are usually the wrecks of disease, and fall only just within the compass of operative surgery. The cornea, besides having dense opacities from slough or penetrating ulceration, is frequently staphylomatous; and adhesions of the iris to it diminish, or even destroy, the anterior chamber, whereby the operation is rendered very difficult. It need not be done as a rule, except there be the absolute necessity of incising the cornea through an opaque spot. I have often found space enough for "incision," when at first " separation " seemed the only alternative.

To execute "separation" the cornea should be divided obliquely with the second-sized iris knife, opposite, or as nearly as possible opposite, the portion of the iris to be detached, and so far only from its margin that, when enough of the iris is torn away, it shall readily reach the incision, so as to allow of a part of it being cut off or strangulated. If the incision be very far, too much will be separated. The next step is the important one of extracting the piece of iris. The canula-forceps are very applicable, and I have used them with perfect satisfaction. They are far preferable to the hook, because they more certainly retain the tissue of a diseased iris, and are less likely to injure the capsule of the lens, and are easier withdrawn. The hook that I have employed is the ordinary "lens hook" figured among the cataract instruments. Dr. Mackenzie, in his review of the last edition of this work, in the " British and Foreign Medico-Chirurgical Review," vol. ix., in speaking of this hook says, that from its liability to let the iris loose after the separation has begun, and to tear through the iris when the membrane is unbound, it is inferior to Schlagintweit's hook, or even the hook forceps of Reisinger. Also, that the withdrawal of the simple hook, with the portion of separated iris, is more difficult than that of the guarded hook of Schlagintweit. As I have never used either of the hooks, I introduce these remarks.

Whichever be the instrument selected, it should be carried in front of the iris to its margin, where it is implanted, separation effected, and a portion of the iris withdrawn and cut off. It must be kept close to the cornea while being withdrawn, lest the capsule of the lens be injured. The circumference of the iris being a little behind the sclerotica, the extremity must pass out of sight to seize it. The withdrawal of the hook through the cornea requires adroitness, and unless the aperture be ample, the iris will probably be shaken off; the size should therefore bear some relation to that of the hook, being of course always much larger. When the operation is successful, the form of pupil that usually results resembles that shown in the annexed sketch,

FIG. 168.

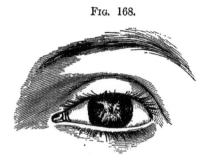

which was taken from a person I met with, on whom I did not operate; and I may observe that in this instance the operation had been badly chosen, and the pupil badly placed, and that vision was very defective.

There is, I believe, greater uncertainty in the execution of "separation" than any of the foregoing operations; it is, more-ever, attended with great pain. Instead of a portion of iris of the required size separating, a mere strip of it may give way, or, what is more common in a diseased state, the instrument may tear out without effecting any separation. Sometimes, directly that the detachment is commenced, blood is poured out, and the subsequent steps of the operation obscured.

A male, twenty-two years of age, applied to me at the Central London Ophthalmic Hospital, to know if his right eye could be submitted to an operation similar to one which had been performed on his left, by Mr. Wilde, of Dublin—namely, "separation." I have never seen an instance to which this form of operation was more adapted, or a better example of its execution. Fig. 170 is a sketch of the eye. A severe attack of purulent ophthalmia, which had completely destroyed the right eye, had also rendered opaque the cornea of the left, with the exception of a strip at the outer and upper edge, which was hazy.

The iris had entirely lost its fibrous appearance, and was, as far as I could judge, in actual contact with the cornea. The remainder of it was adherent to the leucoma. There was sufficient sight to read very large print, such as the titles of books, without glasses; to do which, however, the eyelids were

FIG. 169.

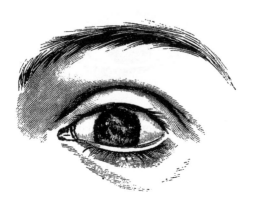

almost closed, to diminish the aperture and reduce the rays of light. I did not ascertain whether the lens was present. In an answer from Mr. Wilde, to whom I wrote about this person, I learn that in the majority of cases in Ireland requiring artificial pupil, purulent ophthalmia has so damaged the eye, that " separation " is the operation most suitable, and that for the most part he strangulates the iris in the wound in the cornea, though he sometimes cuts it off, and then the pupil is less triangular. In this instance he thinks that the latter must have been practised.

The following case combined morbid alterations in the crystalline lens, its capsule, the iris, and the cornea. The patient was submitted to my treatment by Mr. E. A. Lloyd, of Bedford Row. He had been injured by an explosion of gunpowder. The right eye was quite lost. The cornea of the other was densely opaque in the central portion, and some black dots showed where grains of the powder had entered. The pupil, so far as could be made out, was adherent to an opaque capsule, from which bands of adhesion, apparently of lymph, passed to the opaque part of the cornea. The iris was discoloured, but not bulging. I suspected that the lens was absent; that, as some years had elapsed since the accident, it had been removed by absorption. I cut through the cornea at the lower and outer edge of the cicatrix, and incised the iris, but an attack of inflammation frustrated my operation. Some months afterwards I divided the cornea near the circumference, again 'incised' the iris, and attempted to draw out the external portion with a blunt hook; but as this was not readily effected I desisted, lest there should be an escape of the vitreous humour, which was supposed to be degenerated. When the eye was opened a week after, a small and irregular, but useful pupil was discovered, and in a few days the man was able to walk alone in the streets. Mr. R. Taylor took the following sketch of the eye.

FIG. 170.

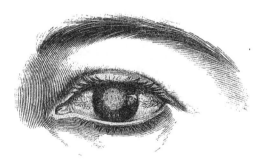

The pupil will be observed at the outer and lower part of the corneal opacity; the vessels at each corner of the eye were the remains of the very active inflammation that had existed; such probably will be always present. The lens was absorbed, and the capsule had contracted towards the centre, and was quite away from the position of the pupil; very likely the iris knife had torn it from its external attachments.

When a pupil, diminished from prolapse of the iris through a more or less opaque cornea, is associated with capsulo-lenticular cataract, a troublesome complication exists. A careful survey of all the circumstances must be taken before it can be well decided whether it be proper and advisable to treat the cataract first, as for 'solution;' to make the pupil first, and to treat the cataract after; or, to form the pupil, and to 'extract' the cataract at the same time, as described in Section 3.

According to the arrangement of my subject, I include in this section that displacement, and generally, too, that diminution of the pupil which is apt to occur after the operation for 'extraction,' and which is nearly always produced by prolapse of the iris. When the aperture is very small, and the iris therefore tense, I have enlarged it by simple "incision" with the knife. When, although perhaps large enough, it has been too much displaced to be of full benefit—that is, by being concealed under the upper eyelid—"incision" with the knife is not generally applicable, but it may be done with the scissors. Divide the cornea to the required extent with the cataract knife, and with the scissors make a snip in the centre of the free edge.

I have had occasion to adopt "excision."

"Iriddesis" may be applied.

When a much reduced pupil is associated with adherent capsule, more than one attempt may be needed to get the required opening. The method I have most generally adopted is "incision," and I have combined with it "extension" or "excision," according to the state of the iris, whether more or less healthy, or diseased.

The above sections include all the individual alterations in the eye that admit of the formation of an artificial pupil; and the operations described are the most fitting according to my knowledge, and they comprise all that are practised in this department by modern surgeons. Some other methods have been suggested by a recent continental writer, but their inapplicability is so self-evident, that I shall not speak of them. To describe those that have been superseded and are now obsolete, would not be compatible with the character of this work, which is professedly practical.

The classification I have made has been solely for the sake

of perspicuity and brevity, and I hope it has been made suffi-ciently clear, that the choice of any particular operation must be based on a careful examination and analysis of all the particulars of the case. The peculiarity in each instance must be the guide to the method most suited.

The after treatment is the same as when the operation for 'extraction' has been performed; the most important points being the quiet of the patient, perfect rest to the eye, opiates, and cold to subdue pain.

Blood poured out into the chambers of the eye need not cause any apprehension. I am not aware that it is attended with any disadvantage, it is soon absorbed, and does not require any special treatment; but I have considered this subject in detail in connexion with injuries, in a previous chapter.

It is possible that atropine may be beneficial after operating, by keeping the edges of the pupil more apart; it should always be used, except when a part of the iris has been left stran-gulated.

The advantage of having a patient chloroformed during these operations is very great, and should never be foregone, except for cogent reasons.

When the crystalline lens has been lost, particular spectacles will of course be requisite; for rules respecting their use I beg to refer to the chapter on Cataract Glasses. However, I may state that when the pupil is away from the centre of the iris, it may be requisite to adapt this appliance accordingly. Here much ingenuity is required, but an optician who has had practice in such cases readily sees what is needed. Similar contrivances are sometimes necessary when, without loss of the lens, glasses are wanted.

Certain mechanical contrivances may be of advantage when the pupil is too large, such as a diaphragm in a spectacle frame, with a hole or a slit to look through. I have found that several patients with lateral pupils have seen better when the side light has been shut out by a sort of goggle.

CHAPTER XXVI.

Iridectomia, or Iridectomy, as it is expressed in English, is the term originally introduced to express the operation for the formation of an artificial pupil, by removing a bit of the iris. More commonly, however, we say, "artificial pupil by excision." Iridectomy, which has been performed of late years to cure certain states of the eye attended with considerable structural lesion, is therefore nothing novel, but, on the contrary, an old operation directed to a modern purpose. The new application has been much discussed, as well as disputed, and very opposite opinions are held. It is yet so fresh in the professional mind, and such is the desire to get information, that I suspect no other subject in this volume will be so quickly referred to, or so frequently.

For my own sake, and not less for that of truth, I shall most carefully abstain from any expressions that may possibly lead to controversy; and partizanship I am not likely to fall into. At the same time I shall, inoffensively, freely give my own opinion and conviction, founded on what I have seen, and withal endeavour to be concise.

Iridectomy was first performed by Professor Graefe, of Berlin, and quickly taken up in England, in consequence of certain circumstances, which it is unnecessary to narrate. But, strange to tell, Graefe's writings on the subject are by no means generally known, even by some surgeons who practise the operation. His original papers, extending to a great length, appeared in the "Archiv für Ophthalmologie," in the years

1856, -7, and -8. They have been translated by Mr. Windsor, in the Sydenham Society's volume for 1859, from which I make these short abstracts.

FIRST MEMOIR.—Graefe's attention was first drawn to the efficacy of the treatment in internal inflammations of the eyeball, by observing the results of the operation for artificial pupil by excision after irido-choroiditis, with closed pupil. In such cases he ascertained by experiment, "that the increased power of vision was in no way dependent on re-absorption of the pupillary exudations, but was entirely to be ascribed to an improvement in the choroidal complications." The whole condition of the eyeball was improved, and liability to relapses prevented.

Encouraged by success, he proceeded to operate on cases in which, after previous iritis with pupillary exclusion, there had resulted atrophy of the globe of the eye, from secondary choroiditis. He treated by repeated iridectomy many cases in which the globe had become very soft, and much flattened by the action of the recti muscles, and it was ultimately perfectly refilled. He relates the case of a man to whom he had formerly given a certificate of incurable blindness, on account of atrophy of both globes; vision was limited to a dull quantitative sensation of light. At the time of writing, the operation having been performed six times, the patient could count fingers at the distance of some feet, and distinguish letters of the largest print, and the vision was weekly improving.

Atrophy of the globe he considers as the result of "choroidal stasis." When the choroidal circulation stagnates, or is vitiated by inflammation, the nutrition of the vitreous body fails, and its volume diminishes. When atrophy has exceeded a certain extent, the eye cannot recover its previous volume.

In irido-choroiditis with adhesions, the synechiæ act injuriously on the iris by keeping it tense, and thus there is a constant tendency to recurrence of the inflammation.

Iridectomy may act in two ways. First, the muscular tension is materially reduced, and thus the adhesions no longer cause disease ; and second, the size of the iris being diminished, its vessels will have relatively to secrete more aqueous humour, and will thus be constantly relieved to a greater extent.

I beg to observe that this explanation is based on the supposition that the aqueous humour is secreted by the vessels of the iris, a theory which is not generally admitted by physiologists of this country.

Glaucoma is not here alluded to.

SECOND MEMOIR.—In this Graefe considers iridectomy as applied to glaucoma, which he divides into three heads: 1. Acute glaucoma; 2. Chronic glaucoma; 3. Amaurosis with excavation of the optic nerve.

In acute glaucoma there is generally a premonitory stage, characterised by increasing presbyopia, coloured spectra round the flame of a lamp or candle, intercurrent obscurations, everything appearing grey and misty during the attack; sometimes slight contraction of the field of vision. Gradually the obscurations become more frequent and more intense, the pupil large and sluggish, and generally neuralgic pain is felt in the brow and temples; and this stage lasts for an indefinite period—months, or years—and is succeeded by the outbreak, generally sudden, of the acute stage, of which the symptoms are: intense pain of the eye, forehead, temples, and side of the nose, injection of the sub-conjunctival vessels, with or without chemosis, anterior chamber hazy, cornea dull, pupil irregularly dilated, iris of a dirty hue and pressed forwards, vision entirely gone, or much diminished, photopsia, chromopsia.

As the attack recedes, sight may remain as it was, or it may be partially or nearly entirely restored, but the pupil remains sluggish, and the field of vision often contracted. Successive attacks may occur, progressively destroying the function of the retina; or without fresh inflammatory symptoms, the visual field gradually contracts and becomes eccentric, the iris assumes a greyish hue, the pupil is dilated and fixed, the globe becomes harder and harder, and the cornea perfectly anæsthetic. Should the humours become clear, as they frequently do, there are seen round spots of retinal ecchymosis, and frequently larger choroidal extravasations; also constantly progressively increasing excavation of the optic nerve, with arterial pulsation, either spontaneous or appearing on the slightest compression with the finger.

Extensive retinal ecchymoses diminish to some extent the acuteness of vision, but do not by any means explain the blindness of glaucoma. [He is arguing against the retina being the seat of the disease.]

" I have ascertained, in a number of cases, that most (perhaps all?) of the retinal ecchymoses do not occur until after iridectomy, and yet that, at the time of observation, there is very great improvement of vision."

These ecchymoses differ in form from those of apoplectic retinitis, which are striped, following the course of the fibres. In glaucoma they are round and regular, seated exclusively on the veins, for the most part where the larger trunks unite. He traces such ruptures not to disease of the vessels, but to the sudden removal, by paracentesis or iridectomy, of mechanical pressure.

Choroidal ecchymoses disappear far more rapidly than retinal. The latter usually continue two or three weeks after iridectomy, sometimes considerably longer.

Besides performing iridectomy in chronic and recurrent iritis, and in various forms of irido-choroiditis, Graefe found it especially useful in ulcerations and infiltrations of the cornea, in partial staphyloma of the cornea, and in staphyloma of the sclerotica.

After a very minute consideration of the exact pathology of the disease, he concludes thus :—

" I consider acute glaucoma to be a choroiditis (or irido-choroiditis), with diffuse imbibition of the vitreous body (and aqueous humour), and in which increase of the intra-ocular pressure, compression of the retina, and the well-known series of secondary symptoms, are produced by the increased volume of the vitreous humour."

In chronic glaucoma there is an absence of distinct and periodically recurring inflammation. The pupil gradually dilates, the iris becomes discoloured, the globe becomes tenser, the sub-conjunctival veins dilated, the visual field contracted, the vision diminished in acuteness. Ciliary neurosis is seldom absent, but the attacks are seldom violent. There is haziness of the aqueous humour, which may appear and disappear many times in the course of the day. The cornea gradually loses its sensibility. At a relatively early period of the disease the ophthalmoscope shows progressive excavation of the optic nerve, with arterial pulsation. The background of the eye always appears somewhat indistinct—whether from vitreous or aqueous turbidity, it is difficult to determine. There may be choroidal ecchymoses in the equatorial region.

Amaurosis with excavation of optic nerve. These cases ought to be distinguished from chronic glaucoma, the pathogenesis being different. Exactly the same form of lesion as in glaucoma occurs in the optic nerve, but the glaucomatous habitus is altogether absent in the external parts of the eye. As a rule, arterial pulsation does not occur spontaneously, but it is excited by slight pressure. The chromopsiæ are not so prominent. The essential character is gradual limitation of the field of vision, generally spreading from one side. These cases do not, as asserted by some, ultimately assume the appearance of glaucoma. No other transformations than those of atrophy of the optic nerve and retina have been seen. The disease is not accompanied by irido-choroiditis. There is a twofold method by which lesions of the optic nerve take place : first, by pressure on the surface of the papilla (glaucoma) ; second, by traction from within the trunk of the nerve.

" In the present state of our knowledge, the lesion of the optic nerve alone is no longer to be considered as defining glaucoma, because in a series of cases it has a pathogenesis quite foreign to glaucoma."

Attributing the blindness in glaucoma, and its intractability to treatment, to intra-ocular pressure, Graefe sought some method of permanently relieving this pressure. The results of iridectomy in chronic iritis and various forms of irido-choroiditis induced him to try it also in glaucoma—first, in the premonitory stage; second, in the acute period; third, in the later period of inflammatory glaucoma; fourth, in chronic glaucoma; fifth, in amaurosis with excavation of the optic nerve.

1. In the premonitory stage the operation was satisfactory. The ciliary neuroses and chromopsiæ ceased. The obscurations did not reappear.

2. In acute glaucoma the results are very striking. "Vision was *perfectly restored* in all cases in which the operation was performed before the termination of two weeks from the occurrence of inflammation." The ciliary neuroses generally cease immediately after the operation. The improvement of vision is most striking during the first two weeks, but continues for at least six weeks. Iridectomy has no influence over the second eye, which may be attacked with glaucoma shortly after a successful operation on the first.

3. In the later period of acute glaucoma, a duration of many weeks, even of many months, does not absolutely exclude complete restoration. The prognosis depends on the circumstances of individual cases. It is favourable when the field of vision and the optic disc have been normal in the remission preceding the last attack; more and more unfavourable in proportion as the field of vision is contracted, and the papilla excavated. Still, great improvement takes place in many cases; and even where vision is permanently lost, iridectomy prevents the recurrence of inflammation and ciliary neurosis.

4. In chronic glaucoma the prognosis depends, as in the last, on the state of the field of vision and of the optic papilla. Great improvement in some cases, in others slight. At all events, it is a better mode of treatment than any other.

5. Amaurosis, with excavation of the optic nerve. No improvement.

In performing the operation, the iris must be removed quite up to its ciliary attachment. "The excised piece must be as large as possible," and the more intense the symptoms, the larger must be the piece excised.

THIRD MEMOIR.—The third memoir is chiefly confirmatory of the former two. He strongly recommends the performance of iridectomy in the premonitory stage, as affording complete and permanent relief. " The ultimate result is still more perfect than when it is performed in the inflammatory stage, soon after the disease has broken out."

In acute glaucoma, the more immediately the operation is performed the better. In two cases, where one eye was operated on the first or second day of the attack, and the other from the fourth to the seventh, there was a marked superiority in those in which the early operation had been performed.

In the advanced stage of acute glaucoma, the result is very various, and depends, as previously shown, on the amount of lesion the eye has undergone. In proportion as the impairment of vision depends on pressure or opacities of the refractive media, the greater improvement may be expected; the more it depends on lesion of the optic nerve, the less improvement is to be expected.

" The uncertainty of the result in the later stages of glaucoma, especially as regards duration, is so directly opposed to its completeness and durability in the acute period, that the advice *to operate immediately and without hesitation* cannot be too urgent. I must most decidedly reject the recommendation to try first paracentesis—advice which has been urged from unfounded ideas of caution. Three years' extensive experience has taught me that the results of paracentesis are, in the infinite majority of cases, temporary only." " My clinic presents a considerable number of cases where one eye has been treated by paracentesis in former years, the other by iridectomy. Only a glance at the fate of these different eyes is needed, *to induce the abandonment of all other treatment in glaucoma than that of the immediate performance of iridectomy.*"

In chronic glaucoma the operation " is indicated so long as any considerable amount of vision remains, though in many cases negative results, and in others only temporary ones, will be obtained."

He finds his theory (of pressure) supported by the observation he has frequently made, that immediately after iridectomy the excavation of the optic entrance is much diminished: the papilla becomes flatter. Another proof is the condition of increased refraction. In two cases on which he had operated, the patients " saw with a convex (+ 6) glass large print many inches farther off before the operation than after, although the vision had been rendered very much better by the treatment." It is probable that the presbyopia in glaucoma is caused by the flattening of the cornea, and its diminution after treatment, by increased curvature of the same part.

The amount of success depends intimately on the period at which it is performed.

In the premonitory period, when the intercurrent obscurations, contraction of the visual field, and ciliary pain, are marked and progressing, it ought to be done, and will be entirely successful.

In acute glaucoma, Graefe "predicts complete restoration of vision where moderate quantitative perception of light exists, and the operation is performed before the expiration of a fortnight from the date of the first inflammatory attack." In older cases the amount of improvement depends on the extent of atrophy of the optic nerve and retina.

The full extent of improvement is not attained till several weeks or months after the operation, though it may commence in a few hours. The ophthalmoscope shows a gradual disappearance of the retinal hæmorrhages, and absence of pulsation. The eye regains its normal tension, the iris becomes bright, and usually remains motionless.

In chronic glaucoma the disease is arrested, and the existing amount of sight preserved. More rarely the improvement is temporary; atrophy progresses, but pain does not recur.

Before making any remarks, I shall give a partial abstract of a paper on Glaucoma, by Mr. Hulke, published in the " Medico-Chirurgical Transactions," vol. xliii., because the appearances of the eye during life are very carefully noted, and there are several records of minute dissections, performed during the early stages of the disease, which are particularly valuable, since opportunities for such investigations must become more rare as any sure method of treating the affection is discovered.

Mr. Hulke's general description of acute and chronic glaucoma does not differ in any respect from that of other authors. But he calls particular attention to the flattening of the cornea —the result, as has been shown experimentally, of excessive distension.

Respecting the ophthalmoscopic signs, "excavation of the optic nerve-entrance, and pulsation of the central artery of the retina, are considered pathognomonic of glaucoma." Frequently there are seen small dotted hæmorrhage in the retina and filmy clots in the vitreous humour. The excavation is indicated by a bluish-grey colour of the periphery of the optic disc, and a peculiar arrangement of its vessels. When slight, these undergo a sudden diminution at the margin ; when the hollow is deep, they are abruptly bent, or their continuity apparently interrupted at the margin. It is partly due to compression, but mainly secondary to it, and owing to atrophy. In extreme excavation the bottom of the hollow lies outside the level of the choroidal foramen. He has dissected an eyeball where the lamina cribrosa itself was pushed outwards. The retinal hæmorrhages come from ruptured capillaries which have become varicose and saculated from over-distension.

The vitreous humour, both in acute and chronic glaucoma, continues for a long time much firmer than natural. He has been much struck with this in several eyes which he has dissected at an early period of the disease, and has verified the same fact in the living eye, by puncturing the sclerotic, and endeavouring in vain to squeeze out some of the vitreous humour. It is only in old cases, where all the other tissues are involved in a common atrophy, that it becomes diffluent. In a recent dissection of acute glaucoma, he found a thin stratum of yellow serum between the hyaloid and the membrana limitans of the retina. In a very typical case, he observed also, on dissection, the hollow of a large sclerotic staphyloma, wholly filled with very firm vitreous humour, in no way differing from the remainder.

The subjective symptoms of glaucoma are, he thinks, one and all due to excessive intra-ocular pressure; and this through an increase of the vitreous humour, both in quantity and firmness. As the humour is nourished by the vascular tunics, this increase must be owing to disturbance of the process of nutrition. There is good reason for believing that a congested or inflammatory state of the choroid is the first step. He agrees with Graefe, that acute glaucoma is a *serous choroiditis*. He has ascertained by actual measurement that a considerable dilatation of the larger veins exists, and of the choroidal capillaries. The retina is probably only passively concerned. The calibre of its arteries is scarcely enlarged. The arterial walls become hypertrophied. This, and the venous hyperæmia, seem to be due to obstruction to the efflux of blood at the optic nerve-entrance.

He has failed to connect glaucoma with gout, atheroma of the vascular system, albuminuria, or diabetes. A certain period of life—enfeebled constitution—broken rest—mental anxiety—predispose to it; also some injuries, and diseases of the eye, especially penetrating wounds of the ciliary region, injuring the lens—and advanced sclerotico-choroidal staphyloma, and chronic irido-choroiditis.

The whole pathology, then, of the disease of glaucoma, according to the above observers, is that, in the first instance, the choroid circulation gets deranged, hypertrophy of the vitreous humour ensues by endosmosis, as a consequence, and the retina is acted on secondarily by pressure.

Respecting the theory of the treatment, it is hardly necessary to point out that Graefe removes a portion of the iris, because, as he supposes, this diaphragm is the source of the aqueous secretion, and that by reducing it, less fluid is poured out, less pressure is therefore produced, and accordingly as the operation is done, as to time, so is the retina completely arrested from injury—rescued from complete destruction. No allusion is made to any influence exerted on the part which is stated to be the original seat of the disease—the choroid; nor to the progress of the affection, nor to the enlarged vitreous humour. That strong objections may be raised against the hypothesis must be apparent; but I leave the reader to ponder over it, and shall remark only, that even if it be granted that the iris is the sole source of the aqueous secretion, after the removal of an eighth of it, or even a sixth, enough is left, I consider, for an abundant supply. Indeed, if the aqueous fluid produce an injurious or disorganizing pressure, so long as the chambers of the eye are filled by it,—no matter if the secretion proceed from a mere speck of secreting surface,—the deleterious effect must be exerted. It also appears to me, that for Graefe's theory to be correct, the fluid should be reduced to a definite amount, actually less than the space that exists for its reception. But this difficulty occurs,—what would stop the vitreous humour from becoming more hypertrophied?

I suspect one of the physiological properties of the aqueous humour to be accommodation to the varying size of the chambers of the eye during the several periods of life: that the quantity is regulated by the space destined to be filled. I think, too, that this is not altogether lost in diseased states: for instance, when there is a large staphyloma of the cornea, the amount is more abundant; when the chambers are reduced— either from pressure posteriorly, so that the lens is near the cornea, or touches it, or from mechanical injury to the cornea— it is less.

There is no more marked characteristic of glaucoma than the smallness of the chambers from the lens being thrust forwards, and, consequently, the paucity of aqueous fluid.

I would observe with respect to the idea of the retina not being originally diseased, that lesion of it may exist, inscrutable alike by the ophthalmoscope and the microscope.

But it must not be supposed that I am writing against iridectomy with a spirit of opposition,—most certainly I am doing nothing of the kind; I am merely giving my views on the *rationale* that has been advanced.

There is just one more point connected with excision of the iris which I should like to notice. In the first memoir, that in which Graefe treats of irido-choroiditis, he attributes a large portion of the success to the reduction of the muscular tension of the iris. However this may hold good when the iris is entirely adherent to the capsule of the lens, and all communication between the chambers of the eye is cut off, it cannot, I suspect, at all apply when it is free. I am not aware that Graefe states anything to the contrary. Another surgeon has advanced a very remarkable as well as novel theory. It is his opinion, that by it a more direct communication is opened between the vitreous and aqueous regions of the eye, which facilitates the play of currents between them, and thus allows any excess of fluid behind to come forward to the corneal surface, through which exosmosis is much easier than through the posterior coats—the sclerotica, choroid, and retina. As applied to a condition in which there is a communication between the fluid in the chambers of the eye, it is to me unintelligible. The exosmosis, too, is equally obscure.

The operation differs in no essential particular from that for artificial pupil by excision when the pupil is free. It is merely on a more extended scale. More iris is to be taken away, and the cornea must therefore be incised to a greater extent. Graefe says that there is a direct relation between the amount of iris lost and the effect on the disease; but that not so much as a third, nor even a fourth, need be excised. He operates with a lance-shaped knife, introduced half a line behind the junction of the cornea and sclerotica, and directed so that its point may pass into the anterior chamber exactly at the point of union. To prevent hæmorrhage he recommends slight compression for dalf an hour, or an hour, and to be gradually relaxed.

But the general condition of the eye makes the proceeding less easy than establishing a false pupil. The strip of iris is to be excised to the very circumference. The cornea therefore must be cut through at the extreme margin, or the incision planned according to the method of Graefe. As the iris bulges, being sometimes in actual contact with the cornea, it is apt to be penetrated; indeed, it is sure to be, without great care. With such an accident, the lens, which is almost always thrust forwards, will in all probability be wounded. Bleeding, too, is likely to ensue and obscure the other steps of the operation, or render it imprudent to proceed. Even if the iris escape being touched, the lens is still somewhat exposed to injury, because of its anterior position, and the wide area of the pupil.

Bleeding from the iris is a very common occurrence during and after the excision, and some operators endeavour to evacuate as much blood as they can, by pressing along the cornea with the curette, or by opening the corneal incision with the same instrument.

I proceed now to speak of the result of iridectomy in glaucoma. That the operation has been recklessly performed by being applied to cases to which it is wholly inapplicable, according even to its propounder's theory, I have had frequent proof. It is useless to give particulars. Graefe, as I must remind my reader, lays great stress on the curative results, according to the stages of the disease.

I am sorry to say I have seen several instances in which iridectomy has been applied where there was no glaucoma, and to the injury of the patient. In most of these it has been done, as the modern phrase goes, "in anticipation of the disease." I have saved many patients from being subjected to it, in whom there was very slight defective sight from haziness of the vitreous humour, or whose eyes were affected merely with sclerotic inflammation. I have had the satisfaction in ascertaining by actual inspection, that some of these—all that I have been able to watch—have completely recovered.

But all those things tell nothing against iridectomy, if it be a valuable operation. Certainly not; they only show the abuse of the measure. The same indiscretions may, and do, attend our most valuable operations. A man may operate for stone where there is none in the bladder; or proceed to relieve a strangulated hernia, where there is no rupture. But in the present instance, with the existence of great difference of opinion about the utility of the procedure, and when men are seeking for evidence from facts, the exposure of such error and malpractice is of value, because it shows that there may be conclusions from very insufficient, as well as wrong data.

It remains for me to give the result of my experience from what I have seen of the operation in glaucomatous eyes, in the practice of others, and from my own. Respecting the first, the cases have been, with but few exceptions, of the chronic form of the disease. In some of them there was certainly a slight improvement of vision for a few days, but in none has this been more than temporary. Pain has also been relieved, and in a few has been so long absent, that it has been supposed to be for ever removed, when with sad disappointment it has returned. Some of these had been published as most successful cases. Of the acute kind I can give no better report.

My own operations have not been numerous. Having been disappointed in the result in some well-selected cases of acute glaucoma (and these have been few, for with no small field of observation I do not find such cases common), I could not make that strong recommendation to patients, which they required respecting the success of an operation, or the possibility of success, to induce all to submit to it.

While I wish it most fully to be understood that I do not condemn iridectomy, I must express my own conviction that I attribute all the good effect which may follow to the mere tapping of the aqueous humour. I have found as much benefit to sight and reduction of pain from this, as I have been able to trace to the other measure. In a private patient of mine, seen by several other medical men, there was sub-acute glaucoma in one eye of nine months' standing. This lady had coruscations, and much pain. She could read nothing. The iris bulged, and the pupil was slightly dilated. Two days after the first tapping she could manage to read a part of one of the articles in the "Times." The pain was relieved, and the coruscations lessened. Vision then got as bad as before, and a slight attack of acute inflammation supervened. Several tappings at intervals of a week enabled her to read large type, but not with clear vision. The pain quite left her, and the coruscations almost disappeared. This improved state lasted five months, as long as I attended her; during which time there was no accession of inflammation. The vitreous humour was always too hazy to afford a satisfactory examination of the fundus of the eye.

I do not by any means infer, or wish it to be understood, that I believe tapping the aqueous humour to be a remedy for glaucoma. That it is capable, occasionally, of affording relief I am sure; but as I have not yet practised it, either as extensively as I wish, nor with that degree of accurate observation which is necessary to establish facts, I would rather say no more about it.

There is quite authority enough, even from some of our English surgeons, to warrant any inquiring student to undertake iridectomy. If a man, whose opinion in surgical matters is considered to be of a superior kind, more especially in ophthalmic subjects, speaks of it as a sure and certain remedy in glaucoma, and as arresting the disease and restoring sight in a marvellous manner, surely it ought not to be left untried. I will merely suggest that, if the trial be made, fitting cases should be selected; and that full and well-authenticated reports, extending over a sufficient period, be given by the operator to the public; and withal, that the facts be attested by others. The anonymous reports in the medical journals, on most operations, are as a rule of less value, when accuracy is needed, than is supposed; and in the present case, those that have been published are not exempt from this charge.

I will mention, digressively, that I have found removal of the lens, and some of the vitreous humour, to produce relief from suffering that nothing seemed to influence; I have done it only when there has been no sight. The first case made so great an impression on me, that I published it in the "Medical Times and Gazette" for July 26th, 1859, with remarks; the following is an abstract of it:—

A female, of middle age, was sent to me in private by Mr. Wall, of Paddington, with acute glaucoma of the left eye, which was very tense, and much injected. The pupil was dilated, and the iris pressed forwards by the semi-opaque lens. Vision was quite lost. I was consulted solely on account of the severe suffering, sometimes lasting for several consecutive hours, but more generally in paroxysms, which nothing had been able to subdue. The extreme vascularity of the eyeball, and the general plethora, induced me to order cupping to the temple, and purgatives. Not the slightest benefit ensued. Opiates, both locally and generally, were then tried, with no more effect than securing better nights' rest than hitherto; but as the general health was deranged by the narcotics, they were discontinued. Other drugs were administered in vain. Thus, after a period of five months, the patient got no material benefit either from myself or from any other surgeon by whom she had been treated, and she had applied to several. She expressed her desire to submit to any operation likely to afford relief, and she was the more anxious as the right eye was certainly sympathetically affected, as manifested by intolerance to light and lacrymation. Rather than extirpate the eyeball, a practice that had been recommended to my patient, I determined to try the experiment of extracting the opaque lens, and evacuating some of the vitreous humour. I effected this without wounding the iris. The vitreous humour was apparently quite normal ; and compress and bandage were applied to prevent hæmorrhage, and with success.

The acute pain ceased. There was less uneasiness during the healing process, which was quickly effected, than is often experienced in operations for the extraction of cataract, complicated with loss of any of the vitreous body. Five weeks after the operation there had been no recurrence of pain, nor was there any other abnormal appearance about the eye, except that the pupil was irregular, a part of it being adherent to the corneal wound, but without prolapse. The right eye lost the sympathetic irritation.

There are two subjects that I desire to notice before closing this part of my subject—the condition of vision after iridectomy, and the unfavourable effects of the operation.

The state of the pupil after a fully-performed iridectomy, one in which as much iris has been removed as is said to be sufficient for the intended purpose—for " small iridectomy " is declared to be useless—is such, that were the glaucomatous state to be entirely removed, and the most perfect condition of the retina established, vision could not, I think, be restored, but must be confused and inaccurate. Yet we are told of " perfect recovery of sight," of a patient " seeing well" with both eyes, and " can read pearl type without the aid of glasses,'' &c. This is difficult to comprehend. We know that when the pupil is dislocated, after the operation for the extraction of cataract, and in other instances of like displacement, there may be an amount of sight that is, under the circumstances, rather surprising; but the cases are not parallel, because that, in the latter, the pupil is mostly small, and drawn aside. After iridectomy, a very large area is added to the existing, and often much expanded pupil. Any circumstance, either iridectomy or otherwise, which leaves such a space in the iris, must, according to all that I have learned, impair the vision.

A gentleman, who had been submitted to iridectomy in one eye, applied to me. Both eyes, it appeared, had been the subject of some disease that produced mistiness of vision, but he would allow only one to be operated on. The disease disappeared, and the eye that was untouched quite recovered. The other, so far as I could tell from my examination, was defective only to the extent occasioned by the loss of the iris.

I attended a private patient for three attacks of severe rheumatic inflammation of the eyeball. When I saw her first, the iris was already more or less adherent to the capsule of the lens, and the retina almost insensible; the last accession of inflammation completed the adhesion of any portion of the pupil that had been free, and destroyed all sight. The lens was not opaque. She was in course of attendance on me when she was induced, by a physician, to consult another surgeon for this eye; and it so happened, that the morning on which she called the other eye, as she expressed it, was rather red, and felt a little weak; but sight was not in the least impaired. Iridectomy was proposed, and the advantages so forcibly placed before her, and so admirably contrasted with the inevitable blindness that would follow were it neglected, that the terms were accepted. The operation was immediately executed on both eyes. I saw the lady four months afterwards. The disorganized eye was of course no better. The other was rendered so very imperfect by the operation,—that is, by the excision of so large a portion of the iris,—that she could not read the largest type, nor do any kind of plain or worsted-work, nor see anything distinctly. How far the use of a pair of goggles, with a small hole in a black diaphragm, may relieve these particular cases, I cannot say.

The unfavourable results of iridectomy have not been fully published. Little or nothing is said about the dangers, and still less about the possible bad results. There are no statistics on this head. We have had only a few hints about the escape of the vitreous humour, and hæmorrhage within the eyeball. I am told that some eyes have been lost by both occurrences. That .the lens may become opaque without being wounded, but simply and directly as the consequence of the operation, I can testify, as it has happened in my own practice; and I have seen it occur to another surgeon.

Having gone so far into this interesting subject, I am sure that I cannot close it better than with this quotation, which I take from the second edition of Mr. Dixon's " Practical Study of the Diseases of the Eye."

" The facility with which the operation of ' Iridectomy,' as it has been called, can be performed, has led to its being practised in an immense number of cases ; and were we contented with the array of so-called cures which have resulted, we should, indeed, believe that glaucoma, hitherto so helpless a disease, had been brought as much under control as cataract itself. But a careful criticism will convince us that many of the ' cases of acute glaucoma cured by operation,' were simply cases of acute inflammation of the sclerotic, implicating to a slight extent the iris and cornea, and attended with severe neuralgia and impairment of vision,—cases which would have yielded to judicious treatment if no *iridectomy* had been performed. A few cases, supposed to be chronic glaucoma, were probably nuclear cataract in an early stage ; and the removal of a portion of iris, by exposing the still transparent periphery of the lens, improved (of course only temporarily) the patient's sight. Of other instances which have come under my own observation, where the operation has been unsuitably performed or proposed, I forbear to speak. There remains a mass of cases of glaucoma, diagnosed by careful and competent surgeons, and skilfully operated upon by them, sufficiently numerous to enable them to draw their own conclusions as to the real value of the 'new operation.' For myself, I may state that, although I could not recognise as sound the theory upon which the operation was brought forward as a cure for glaucoma, I tried it in a series of carefully-selected and well-marked cases of the following forms of disease:—'Amaurosis with excavated optic nerve'—as Graefe has termed a peculiar morbid condition; chronic glaucoma, where the lens had not yet lost its transparency; and in cases of acute glaucoma, characterised by sudden impairment of sight, rapidly followed by inflammation of the eyeball, dilated and fixed pupil, severe neuralgia, and total loss of vision.

"In neither of the first two classes did I find—nor had I expected to find—any improvement to result. Nor in the third class was sight restored; but the inflammation seemed to be arrested, and the neuralgia was either very much lessened or it wholly ceased. I cannot, however, attribute this result to the removal of a portion of iris, but mainly to the evacuation of the aqueous humour through the large corneal wound."

Other operations have been devised for glaucoma, and I proceed to notice them in abstract. The first that I shall give is by Mr. Hancock, whose writings on the subject are in the "Lancet" for February 11th, 1860. He says:—

"I believe that glaucoma, whether acute or chronic, is essentially a disease of the blood and blood-vessels, and that the effusion or infusion, as may be described, is the result of this condition, which, if not arrested, sooner or later, destroys sight."

He observed that, "in acute glaucoma, the eyeball is constricted, and marked by a circular depression at the point corresponding to the ciliary muscle, whilst the vessels round this point are gorged to a great degree. The eyeball is elongated in its antero-posterior diameter, and the cornea lessened in all its diameters, and rendered more conical than natural: whilst, when the patient turns his eyeball sideways, irregular bulging of the sclerotica (staphyloma) is exposed to view."

"All these considerations," he continues, "led me to suspect that the ophthalmoscopic and pathological appearances of the blood-vessels were greatly enhanced by, if not, in some instances, entirely due to, the obstruction of the circulation, caused by the undue and excessive constriction exerted on them by the spasmodic, or extreme contraction of the ciliary muscle, analogous to the spasm so often observed in the muscular fibres of the urethra, as well as in the sphincter ani muscle in certain affections of those parts."

To obviate the injurious effects of this spasm, he determined to divide the ciliary muscle. He says that the practice has been attended with the best results.

His mode of operating is thus given:—"I introduce a Beer's cataract knife at the outer and lower margin of the cornea, where it joins the sclerotica. The point of the knife is pushed obliquely backwards and downwards until the fibres of the sclerotica are divided obliquely for rather more than one-eighth of an inch; by this incision the ciliary muscle is divided, whilst the accumulated fluid flows by the edge of the knife."

The alleged advantages are:—1, It obviates the objections to iridectomy; 2, It relieves pain by the removal of the constriction of the eyeball, and the consequent pressure upon the nerves, from the undue contraction of the ciliary muscle; 3, By it the accumulation of fluid is evacuated, and the impediment to the circulation through the blood-vessels being got rid of, they are placed in a favourable condition to recover their normal state; and a probability of a recurrence of the effusion is greatly diminished; 4, By the situation and oblique direction of the incision, a free drainage of the fluid is provided for; 5, The iris is but slightly wounded, and the pupil is preserved of its original size and shape, and in its normal situation ; 6, The danger of wounding the lens is avoided.

Mr. Hancock is opposed by every other observer when he says that the cornea becomes conical in glaucoma—flattening is one of the most characteristic symptoms.

It is not probable, I think, that such a muscle as the ciliary could contract with sufficient force to groove the hard and stony eyeball of glaucoma ; still less likely is it that such spasm could be continuous.

I ought to mention that Mr. Hulke says, he has several times verified by dissection the co-existence of a hard painful glauco-matous state of the eyeball, with advanced atrophy and fatty degeneration of the muscle.

Mr. Solomon has devised a method of dividing the ciliary muscle in glaucoma, which he terms "intra-ocular myotomy." It is performed " by entering a Beer's cataract knife at the corneo-sclerotic union, and then pushing it through the pillars of the iris into the muscle ; the flat surfaces of the blade being opposed on the one side to the sclerotic, and on the other to the rim of the lens." He limits the incision in the muscle to two lines—$\frac{1}{6}$th of an inch. "The intra-ocular incision cuts across a bundle of the radial fibres of the ciliary muscle, branches of the ciliary nerves of the third pair, and perhaps of the fifth."

The anterior chamber is generally penetrated, and the posterior put in communication with the wound. By this operation, " the circulation in the choroid is regulated, and the stony hardness of the eyeball in glaucoma, and the extreme tension in cases of acute choroido-iritis, sub-acute syphilitic iritis, with recent pupillary occlusion, hydrophthalmia, with the ciliary neurosis which attends these disorders, are either cured or much relieved."

He has performed the operation successfully in cases of acute and chronic glaucoma, choroiditis, conical cornea, myopia, presbyopia, asthenopia, &c. &c.   " Medical Times and Gazette," May 19th, 1861.

I conclude this chapter with Mr. Nunneley's operation. His papers are contained in the "Lancet" for January 19th and 26th, 1861.

He believes, from report and from experience, that cures more or less complete have followed the performance of iridee- tomy, but considers the reasoning by which such results are attempted to be explained, as unsatisfactory. "When it was first proclaimed that the removal of a large portion—the more the better—of what had hitherto been supposed to be an impor- tant, nay, essential tissue for satisfactory vision, and the injury of which in a much less degree would, in the great majority of cases, render a sound eye useless, would be found to be a perfect cure for an eye already almost hopelessly diseased, it appeared so astounding that, like many others, I waited before doing it until the reports of some of those who had more faith than I had, gave the result as so uniformly successful, that doubt gave way before recorded facts, and though unconvinced by the reasoning, longer resistance to them appeared like obstinacy."

He thinks that "all that iridectomy accomplishes in the cure of acute glaucoma and glaucomatous diseases is in the greater degree and more permanent manner in which it affords relief to intra-ocular pressure than paracentesis, as performed previous to its introduction, did." The removal of the iris he considers as an evil to be avoided : "The good accompanying its removal does not, in my judgment, result from the loss of the iris itself, but from allowing a greater yielding of the eyeball—in all probability owing to a greater division of its curve being made when a large portion of the iris is taken away, than when none of it is removed—and thus permanently lessening its tension, as well as affording a longer continued drain of the aqueous humour." If this be the case, it is desirable to operate effectually for the relief of tension without injuring the iris, as he demurs to the idea that removal of part of this muscle diminishes the secretion of the aqueous humour. He continues,—"Observing that the eyeball is often distended to the utmost limit which the comparatively unyielding sclerotica and cornea will allow, and that the pain and acutely distressing symptoms in the ball and about the orbit commonly occur in proportion to the rapidity with which the distension takes place,' whether the disease be glaucoma, iritis, or choroido-iritis,—and knowing that the most unyielding portion of the globe is the point of junction of the sclerotic, cornea, iris, and ciliary muscle, which may not unfrequently, in very decided cases of hydrophthalmia, be observed as a depressed ring between the bulging sclerotic and cornea,—it occurred to me that division of this part would afford the desired relief, and that not improbably the good gained in Von Graefe's operation in reality depends upon the removal of the resistance of this part, and not upon the ablation of the iris."

The operation which, in accordance with these views, he devised, he describes as follows :—

" The manner in which I have operated is to puncture the sclerotic coat with the point of a sharp thin knife—a small cataract knife, or very narrow, short bistoury answers very well —not less than one-eighth of an inch behind its junction with the cornea, and carry it on to about the same extent through the cornea, making altogether an incision about one-third of an inch long. Care must be taken to pass the knife sufficiently deep to completely divide those textures, and yet not so deep as to touch the lens, which I once did, owing to the patient starting at the moment the incison was made. Care also must be taken not to make the incision too long. A larger incision in the sclerotic, besides unnecessarily wounding important tissues, is useless, and if carried too far towards the centre of the cornea, though allowing this afterwards to yield more, is bad, for it may allow the lens to be displaced into the aqueous chamber ; and if the iris should adhere to the whole extent of the corneal section, as it is likely to do, particularly if a portion of its whole breadth has been removed, not only will there be dragging of it, but the section becomes opaque, and hence the field of vision is lessened. In making the section, if the point of the knife has been well kept in, the outer margin of the iris will be divided. Sometimes the iris bulges through the section. I have tried the effect of simply leaving the prolapsed iris in the wound, of cutting it off, and also of pulling out a larger portion, and cutting off a strip through the entire width. In this latter plan the operation more nearly assimilates with Von Graefe's iridectomy, only that the section through the unyielding tissues is made directly across their junction, instead of into or parallel with it, whereby a greater expansion in it is allowed, and not nearly so much of the iris is removed. If none of the iris be cut off or tied, the pupil usually recovers its circular form; if some be excised, it remains oval and attached to the corneal cicatrix, in proportion to the size of the piece removed, but in a much less degree than would be *à priori* anticipated. The degree of deformity is very slight indeed."

As to the situation of the incision, Mr. Nunneley prefers "the centre of the lower corneal curvature" as most generally convenient.

At the time of writing, he had performed the operation in about twenty cases, and prefers it to that of Von Graefe. " It has, so far as I can judge, afforded all the relief that the more serious proceeding has done, and appears to be free from its inconveniences." His experience had extended over a period of eighteen months.

CHAPTER XXVII.

THE OPHTHALMOSCOPE.

I MUST remind my reader that, in accordance with the title of the book, he must not expect to find more in connexion with this subject than is needed for what I undertake to teach. While I shall be explicit enough for this, and even sufficiently comprehensive to enable the student to learn how to use the instrument,—besides in general pointing out what is healthy appearance and what is not,—I shall abstain from entering into the treatment of the internal diseases of the eye.

It seems to be generally agreed, and I believe with correct- ness, that the source of this discovery, which has revolution- ized ophthalmic nosology, and rendered obsolete nearly every- thing that has been written or taught on the deep-seated diseases of the eye, is to be traced to a communication in the twenty- ninth volume of the "Medico-Chirurgical Transactions," by William Cumming, Esq., formerly House-Surgeon to the London Hospital. The title of the paper is, "On a Luminous Appear- ance of the Human Eye, and its Application to the Detection of Disease of the Retina and Posterior Part of the Eye."

It would appear that Mr. Cumming's attention was attracted to the subject from the description of cat's-eye amaurosis by several authors; the name being used to infer that the appearance was like the luminous glare of the eyes of some animals by the reflection of the light from a brilliant tapetum. What was seen, they thought to be the condition of disease; and Mr. Cumming started with his investigations under that supposition. None of the writers, he says, mention a reflection from the posterior part of the perfectly-formed healthy eye of the human subject, nor had he heard of any one else who described such a condition; and he undertakes to show that the healthy human eye is equally luminous, or nearly equally, with the eye of the cat, or dog, or other animal, when observed under favourable circumstances. It was not long before he discovered that the cat's-eye amaurosis about which he found the statement of writers to be at variance on all points, was a matter of imagination. He found that "it existed in all eyes when the pupil was dilated." With our superior knowledge, we may justly infer that the mass of recorded cases of amaurosis were not diseases of the nervous apparatus of the eye.

"Most of the cases," he continues, "appear, then, to have been nought but the observance of the natural luminosity, and that it should be seen in amaurosis only is nowise strange: the more minute examination bestowed upon cases of this kind, and the probably dilated state of the pupil, are reasons why it should have been seen in it alone."

His simple process of examination is this :—"Let the person under examination sit or stand eight or ten feet from a gaslight, looking a little to the side; standing near the gas-light, we have only to approach as near as possible to the direct line between it and the eye to be viewed, at once to see the reflection. Or, in a dark room, a candle being placed four or five feet from the eye, if we approach the direct line between them, we shall be able at once to see it in many cases. If solar light be admitted through a newly-closed shutter into a dark room, the luminosity may be seen when the pupil is tolerably dilated, the patient standing five or six feet from the aperture, and the observer occupying the position before indicated."

" These, then," he continues, " are the circumstances necessary for seeing the luminosity. That the eye must be at some
distance from the source of light, the distance being greater in
proportion to the intensity; that the rays of light diffused
around the patient, and sometimes around the eye itself, should
be excluded ; that the observer should occupy a position as near
as possible to the direct line between the source of light and the
eye examined : hence it is sometimes necessary for the observer
to stand obliquely, that his eye may approach nearer to the
direct line.

" The appearance of the reflection itself not only varies much
in colour and intensity in different persons, but also from
the circumstances under which it is seen ; viz., the greater or
less intensity of light, the position of the eye examined, and
the distance at which it is viewed."   Many other similar modes
are given.

Among the physiological conditions of the eye enunciated by
Mr. Cumming, are these : that the choroid is the principal
reflecting structure, the light returned from the retina and
concavity of the hyaloid body doubtlessly increasing the effect ;
that the brilliancy is considerably augmented from the concen-
trating influence of the concave shape of the retina, and the
focal distance of the lens; that the luminosity of the healthy
eye appears to be in proportion to the light colour of the pigment. The reflection from the albino is evident in ordinary
daylight. He further observes :—

" In persons of fair complexion and blue or gray irides, it is
generally more brilliant and more readily seen than in those of
dark skin and irides. In the mulatto it is also dusky ; but in
them, as in persons of swarthy complexion, a silvery reflection
is sometimes seen, and is most probably a reflection from the
retina. In the albino this reflection, produced by the vascular
choroid, is most brilliant, and lightest in tint. In proportion to
the darkness of the pigment, its lustre is diminished and the
colour becomes more dusky."

Perhaps there appears a contradiction here, but there is really
no discrepancy. The choroid is found to reflect most where

the pigment is wanting. The pigment has nothing to do with the reflection : on the contrary, it interferes with it, and therefore lessens the illuminating power. In man, the pigment is less abundant and less intense in colour than in many of the lower animals; it is brown, rather than black.

It was, then, the first grand principle, the comprehensive idea, that Mr. Cumming gave us. He did not see the optic disc, nor the retinal vessels. The perfecting of the discovery and the practical application, involving, as they did, the difficulty of inventing an instrument and the working out of much detail, were reserved for other labourers. These were found in Germany. It would be fruitless to trace the instrument through its stages of development. I will merely give the names of its several improvers, as far as I can ascertain, in the order of time : they are, Helmholtz, Ruete, Coccius, and Anagnostakis.

The ophthalmoscope at present in use is a portable little concave mirror, made of silvered glass, having a hole of sufficient dimensions in the centre, with a handle of about four inches. The hole is usually too small: it should be of sufficient size to admit of distinct vision when the instrument is held with the requisite obliquity; the edges should be smooth and free from splinters.

A double convex lens, of from two and a half to three inches' focus, is needed as an appendage; but the power should be regulated by the requirements of the observer. It should be set in a frame with a stem of three or four inches long, which renders it more readily used. I know that mirrors of different curve, and lenses of varying power, compose the apparatus of some surgeons. That these varieties can be brought into requisition according to one's fancy, is undoubted; but I believe that they possess no utility, no decided practical advantage.

The ophthalmoscope demands an artificial light. Under an emergency, I have employed a candle, and, with its faint illumination, have gathered some, although an imperfect, idea of the interior of the eye. A steady lamp-flame is needed for the full effect. I employ a gas-lamp much used by the artizans of the watchmaking district of Clerkenwell, and sold at a lamp-shop in Clerkenwell-green. A very light-blue chimney whitens the light, and the eye is then seen more naturally.

The examination should be made in a dark room.

As a rule, the eye should be prepared by having the pupil dilated by belladonna, or some of its salts. Now and then persons are met with, especially when fair and young, whose naturally expanded pupils enable us to dispense with the artificial enlargement, particularly if it be not more than a mere glance within the eye that is needed; and above all, near-sighted eyes may be so examined. But generally, in adult age, and still more in old age, with its discoloured lens, and in all cases where a thorough survey is called for, the natural pupil will not suffice. Vain discussions have been wasted on this question, which may be resolved into this common-sense view, that if the desired object can be accomplished without interfering with the pupil, all the better, as the sequel will show; if it cannot, dilatation must be resorted to.

The pupil is generally more contracted by the light of day than by the light of the ophthalmoscope. Often when it has appeared too small to allow of any serviceable examination, it has dilated sufficiently on the room being darkened, and remained of such capacity as to afford all that was desired.

Unnecessary dilatation should always be avoided, because this unnatural state produces positive discomfort, from indistinct vision, the degree and duration of which, from days to weeks, is proportionate to the dilatation and the healthiness of the eye. Patients frequently leave the surgeon on account of this effect, even when they have been forewarned. In spite of all assurance to the contrary, they are likely to attribute the temporary annoyance to the use of the ophthalmoscope, and to declare how detrimental it has been to them. Any increase of disease is often set down to the same cause.

It is not generally known, indeed I have not seen it mentioned, that, when a strong solution of atropine is used to the one eye, the vision of the other is apt to be impaired for one, two, three, or even more days, and that without any apparent alteration in the pupil. The power of adjustment seems to suffer particularly. I shall not stop to discuss the physiology of this. It is quite sufficient for all practical purposes to mention the fact. These are reasons why such powerful applications should be avoided ; and weak ones answer our purpose well. Half a grain of the sulphate of atropia to an ounce of water is what I ordinarily employ. A single drop, put on the conjunctiva, suffices. I depress the lower eyelid, and with a brush, my finger, or any convenient thing, apply the drop. Dilatation is much slower with the weak form, but it passes away quickly, and the disagreeables incidental to the stronger do not appear. Dr. Garrod has shown by his experiments that dilatation may be obtained by a grain in several ounces of water ; but it must be remembered that healthy eyes are easier influenced than diseased ones.

It has been asserted that the retina is likely to become congested by the atropine. I have not been able to confirm this ; and it is difficult to reconcile such a statement with the observation of my colleague, Mr. Taylor,—that the eye is more tolerant to the ophthalmoscopic examination when atropine is used, than otherwise.

But indiscriminate dilatation is required by the learner. I must confess to have gained much information in the earlier parts of my studies from the examination of the healthy eye as well as the diseased ; and I have found that sometimes an appearance which I would have set down as morbid, in consequence of coexisting symptoms, should not be so esteemed, as the same condition might be seen in the perfectly healthy organ.

This is the manner of conducting an examination. The patient sits by the side of a convenient table. The lamp is placed close to his head ; the flame put on a level with the eye, from which it is screened by a little metal plate fixed to the burner. Or his hand may be used as a screen. The observer takes his position directly in front, and sits slightly elevated, holding the ophthalmoscope close to his own eye, in an oblique position, to receive the light from the lamp, and at about eighteen or twenty inches from the patient's eye, on which he throws the reflection. Looking through the central aperture, he moves the instrument forwards, and endeavours to get the focus. A diffused reddish glare shows that the interior of the eye is illuminated. With a little adjusting, the retinal vessels or the optic disc may be seen. The exact focus is now obtained. If, however, it should be desired to illuminate the eye still more for examination, or to magnify the parts at the fundus, the lens is now used. This is held before the eye at its focal range, and the ophthalmoscope and it, manœuvred till the desired definition is acquired.

The following figure is intended to illustrate the directions that I have given.

Fig. 171.

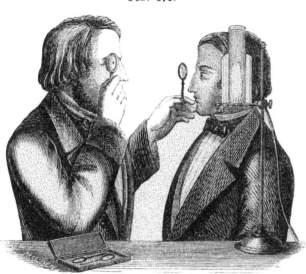

The student must be prepared to meet with different degrees of illumination, and different shades of light—reddish, orange-red, orange, yellow, or buff. It is no easy matter to get a tolerably practical knowledge of the healthy state; much investigation and abundant opportunities are needed, and withal, remarkable patience. It is only by familiarity with the variations of the healthy or physiological states, that we can ever detect morbid changes, and especially slight structural alterations. Here is the chief difficulty of the process; it has been the stumbling-block of many, and caused no few aspirants to depreciate the discovery.

The annexed diagram is a magnified view of the fundus of the left eye, and gives an idea of the optic disc and the vessels diverging from it. It expresses all that a woodcut can convey.

FIG. 172.

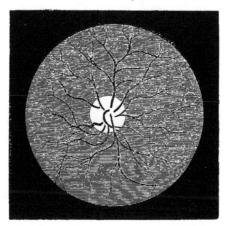

As might naturally be expected, ingenuity has been exercised in endeavouring to devise an easier way of getting the focus, and of maintaining it when found; for, in truth, the method in ordinary use is like making a microscopic examination with the lenses held in our hands.

I have seen and used many instruments devised for this purpose, yet I have met with but one that has answered—Liebreich's, of German invention. It consists of the mirror and the lens set in a tube, to each of which is attached an adjustment: the whole is clamped to a table. The patient's head is fixed, partly by resting on the edge of the table, and partly by a chin-support.

Nothing can be more satisfactory than an examination in this way, when the focus is got; it is just the thing for the uninitiated, after an experienced observer has made the arrangement.

Such an instrument greatly facilitates ophthalmoscopic drawings; but it possesses, as far as I know, no other practical use, and its machinery renders it somewhat cumbrous for ordinary application. Besides this, it is not so generally applicable for inspecting diseased eyes. The simple instrument, once learned, is enough for our purpose.

It must be remembered, in using the ordinary ophthalmoscope,—the perforated concave mirror, with a convex lens,—that the parts at the fundus of the eye are not seen in their natural position, but in an inverted one. The macula lutea would, therefore, appear as if on the nasal side, instead of on the temporal, and so also as regards the retinal vessels. All, in fact, seem to the observer in the same relative positions as the objects under examination by a microscopist are seen to him, when working with a compound microscope.

When the convex lens is not used, the objects are not reversed; but for them to be well seen, the mirror must be held inconveniently close to the patient's eye.

The principle of the ophthalmoscope is not self-evident. If the question be asked why a reflector is necessary, and why the eye cannot be illuminated by the very lamp from which the light is borrowed, the answer may not be readily found. A stream of light thrown into the pupil is reflected back by the retina and choroid, as before shown. This ensues whenever a luminous body, a lamp or candle, is held before the eye; but, except under the circumstances detailed, we see no reflection. It is because our eye is not in the focus, the flame is in the direct line of reflection, and it cannot be seen through. This is overcome by using the mirror, which receives the light and represents the flame; and, by means of the hole, the eye can be placed in the focus.

To those who would investigate the matter scientifically, I recommend a most valuable and accurate work of sixty-six pages, involving high calculations, " On the Theory of the Ophthalmoscope," by George Rainy, M.D., Glasgow.

Physical peculiarities, apart from disease, render inspection of the eye more or less easy, or difficult. Sometimes the exploration is quickly made, at others it is tediously obtained; the unsteadiness, too, of a patient has its influence.

An examination should not be uselessly or unreasonably long. It would be unpleasant to any one, to say the least of it, to have a concentrated light on his retina for the greater part of an hour, and this persons seem to forget when they are learning to use the ophthalmoscope. We know that it is not very uncommon for the fundus of the eye to become preternaturally red during an ordinary inspection—a fact always to be remembered, and to be guarded against by avoiding a lengthened sitting, or by resting the eye for a few seconds when the process is necessarily prolonged. No surgeon with any common sense would employ the ophthalmoscope when it would give pain or cause any uneasiness. It is just in such cases that the internal examination of the eye is not needed; there is enough indication to direct our treatment. The intolerance to light is a significant symptom; and, if it be associated with any surface-redness, there is evidence of inflammation of the eyeball.

On occasions where there is slight sensitiveness to light—so slight as to warrant a careful and brief examination,—I reduce the lamp-flame, and illuminate less: toleration will then embolden us to employ more light, should it be required.

The examiner is likely to fatigue his own eye by the consecutive inspection of several subjects. I have known indistinctness of vision to be produced, and to last for days. The prevention is, to avoid continuous work, or to use the eyes alternately.

NORMAL CONDITIONS.

OPTIC DISC.—By this is meant the termination of the optic nerve, before it expands into the retina. It is of a pinkish-white colour, in health, set, as it were, in a field of red. Its normal form is circular, but it varies, being frequently oval, vertically, rarely horizontally. Sometimes it is more or less angular, according to the encroachments of the choroid on its margin. A perfectly pearly white optic disc is an abnormal appearance, and is generally associated with some intra-cranial lesion. It becomes white in advanced atrophy of the optic nerve.

Hyperæmia of the optic disc is not necessarily a diseased state, although generally bordering thereon. It is astonishing what an amount of vascularity may exist without impairing the function of the retina. This is especially the case among those persons whose eyes are continually at work on minute objects, under all kinds of adverse circumstances—hot rooms, bright lights, &c. It is only from a just appreciation of the state of the whole interior of the eye which practice alone can give, that a correct diagnosis can be formed.

As the prolonged axis of the optic nerve would strike the cornea near its outer edge, in order to bring the optic disc central to the dilated pupil, it is necessary to direct the patient to turn his eye somewhat inwards, or towards the tip of the observer's ear on the side furthest from the eye examined. Should the disc not be readily found, a large vessel will generally be seen on focussing, which, if followed, will lead to it.

Anatomy shows that the centre of the optic nerve, as it enters the eye, and is about to form the retina, is slightly depressed. As the fibres expand, radiating over the fundus of the eye, the edge of the disc is a little elevated, forming what is called the " colliculus," thus giving to the centre a comparatively depressed appearance. According to the thickness of this colliculus, or of the more superficial layers of the retina at this part, or according as the dark choroid encroaches on the contracted portion of the optic nerve at the scleral aperture, so will there be a more or less shaded ring around the disc; but this state must not be set down as morbid, for it is frequently found, and is quite compatible with healthy vision.

The subject of the various changes which take place in the optic disc, both in health and disease, is of the highest interest to the anatomist and pathologist. It hardly falls within the

scope of this work to enter into much detail on the microscopical investigations, which render the foreign, more especially
the German publications, of such value. One paper is of
high interest in reference to these changes. I allude to that
by H. Müller, published in the "Archiv. für Ophthalmologie,"
Band IV., Abth. 2, s. 1, 1858, and entitled "Ueber Niveau-
Veränderungen an der Eintritts stelle des sehnerven," which is
accompanied by diagramatic woodcuts.

THE CENTRAL ARTERY OF THE RETINA perforates the optic
disc about the middle; it generally divides into two branches,
the directions of which are upwards and downwards. These
soon divide into pairs, which may be traced dividing dichotomously towards the periphery of the retina; their ultimate
capillaries are, of course, not singly visible: they pass over each
other, or interlace.

The artery is smaller than the vein, and is of a brighter red;
it has a sharper outline, and a more direct course. There are
frequently one or two small arterial branches, which perforate
the disc independently, and radiate outwards, but not quite to
the macula lutea.

The veins are of a darker red; the thinner coats enable
their contents to be more readily seen; usually the branches
pass out of the eye through two or three apertures, and unite
in the optic nerve. They are of a larger diameter than the
arteries, their outline more dusky, and their course more tortuous.
A beginner will not, at first, make out these differences so
readily. Slight pressure on the eyeball produces a venous
pulse, alternating with that of the wrist. Increased pressure
will produce an arterial pulse, synchronous with it. The arterial
pulse is evident in diseased states of the interior of eyeball,
accompanied, it is supposed, by intra-ocular pressure. Excessive
pressure empties both artery and vein, and arrests the pulse in
both.

THE RETINA, in health, is chiefly recognised by its vessels;
for, ordinarily, its transparency prevents any other mode of

detection. It is best examined in those who have dark eyes, when it may be detected as a faint-bluish haze, overspreading the choroid. The vessels usually stand out clear. It must be remembered that they ramify chiefly in the fibrous lamina. They are therefore most superficially situated to the observer.

The retina is said by Coccius to be more transparent in delicate, young, brown-eyed individuals, than in those older and more robust. It is more transparent towards the periphery than in the neighbourhood of the optic disc, because the fibrous lamina is thinner as we approach the ora serrata.

The retinal arteries have sometimes a peculiar appearance, as though the centre of the canal was transparent, and the blood coursed along the sides of its wall. In retinitis, apoplexy of the retina, and other morbid states, they give way, and clots are effused, the small coagula taking the course of the vessels.

THE PUNCTUM CENTRALE RETINÆ, or macula lutea, is with great difficulty to be found, as it so slightly differs in structure from the rest of the retina. It is situated external to the optic disc, directly in the axis of the eye. It is not discernible under ordinary conditions, but its position may be noted by the retinal vessels passing above and below it, and not across. The parts about it appear to possess a deeper shade of colour. In young presbyopic persons, it may be seen as an indistinct spot, the greyish haze of the retina being absent.

THE CHOROID, more than the retina, gives the red colour to the interior of the eye; and although the vessels, which are parallel rather than arborescent, are larger than those of the retina, they are not visible ordinarily. When the pigment which intervenes between them and the retina is scanty, as in old persons among white people, they are more discernible. In these states the reflection is of a more orange-red colour. In the albino, where the pigment is absent, they are still more visible.

Donders has observed pulsation in the choroidal veins in white rabbits, and it is said to have been seen in man, in eyes deficient in pigment, being produced by slight pressure.

In certain states of disease, where the pigment is removed, the vessels are quite apparent. In the dark races, in whom the pigment abounds, there is no trace of them, and the light is but faintly reflected.

In the negro the pigment is so abundant, and its presence produces so marked an effect, that the fundus of the eye can scarcely be illuminated, and it reflects a brown colour, especially where there is an anæmic choroid.

Among Europeans, we trace the larger vessels by the irregular markings or mottlings of a dusky colour, which are in contrast to the vascular interspaces which contain more pigment, and are therefore darker.

Patches of brilliant white reflection from the fundus of the eye are due to atrophy of the choroid in those parts, by which the sclerotic is seen shining through. The edges of these patches often assume a circular form, as though a piece had been stamped out with a punch.

The Cornea, the Crystalline Lens, and the Humours of the Eye in the healthy state are, of course, perfectly transparent. In the examination of these media, only a modified light should be used, and for the more anterior parts the convex lens is not required, for strong glare would render slight opacities almost transparent. It is advantageous for the patient to turn his eye in different directions, from one side to the other, towards the ceiling, &c. &c., because by an oblique investigation opacities and other changes may be detected which otherwise would escape observation. For example:

On the cornea—opacities from various causes, disturbance of its epithelial layer, incipient conical cornea.

On the capsule—opacities, pigmental deposit.

On the lens—striæ of commencing cataract, or the slight haziness of the nuclear form of the disease.

In the vitreous humour—floating flocculi, &c. &c.

Few surgeons have long been engaged in active duty, without being aware of the difficulty attendant on the diagnosis of incipient cataract. Indeed, till the ophthalmoscope appeared, we were necessarily often in difficulty; and no one felt this more than myself, as the means at our disposal—the catoptric test and the concentrated light—were not enough. It was especially so in old age, when the natural coloration of the lens, the amber hue, existed, and particularly when it was unusually developed, for then posterior streaks of opacity of this body, or general haziness, were easily overlooked. The coloration itself was liable to be mistaken for disease, when there coexisted impaired vision from any cause. Whenever, therefore, there is a suspicion of cataract, an ophthalmoscopic investigation should be instituted. With very high illumination, as already hinted, opacities may even be less apparent than without the ophthalmoscope. It is on this account, too, that the eye should be examined at first with the reflector alone. A source of fallacy must here be guarded against. The dots of pigment that are so often seen on the capsule of the lens, as the result of inflammatory attacks, by which the iris and the capsule have been brought into apposition, as also cicatrices or spots on the cornea, must not be mistaken for cataract opacities. It is enough to direct attention to this point to prevent a mistake. Positively, cataract may now be detected before a person is himself aware of it. I have several times discovered one or more slight streaks of opacity, when, as yet, a person has been unaware of any defective sight. When I am applied to by a patient with cataract in one eye, I often inspect the other with the ophthalmoscope, and thus it is that I have acquired this knowledge.

The pupil should be fully dilated, that the circumference of the lens, as well as the centre, may be thoroughly examined.

Linear opacities appear like black lines on the red field of the fundus.

When the entire lens is affected, and the opacity, but yet slight, there is not a general haze merely, but distinct, although irregular, marking of more opaque parts.

By this investigation the absence of the lens may be detected, by small shrunken portions of the capsule around the periphery of the posterior chamber.

It requires some practice to recognise the different depths of the vitreous humour in which floating particles occur. For the complete examination of this body, it is necessary to have the pupil fully dilated, and even then it must be borne in mind, that that portion of it in the neighbourhood of the ciliary bodies, is necessarily hidden from an investigation. It should be inspected with and without the convex lens; carefully attended to, and modifications of the intensity of the light must be carefully focussed. Besides this, the patient should be directed to move his eye quickly to the right and left, upwards and downwards. Deposits are thereby often thus rendered visible, when otherwise they would escape by sinking below the field of vision. When the humour is preternaturally fluid—no uncommon event,—any morbid products in it are readily set in motion.

It may be well to mention that the portion of the fundus of the eye which is subjected to ophthalmoscopic examination is much smaller than may be generally imagined. Probably, if it be stated that about two or three times the diameter of the optic disc in all directions is the full amount of surface available for examination, a tolerably correct estimate is given.

PATHOLOGICAL CONDITIONS.

The pathological changes which take place in the optic disc are naturally very intimately associated with those that are seen in the retina; thus, anæmia, hyperæmia, apoplexies, extravasations, and pigmental changes, which affect the one, are more or less developed in the other. Still there are some abnormal appearances in the disc itself, which are peculiar to its structure, and should be fully appreciated, especially as it is the first part examined in an ophthalmoscopic investigation. Two of the most important of these are present in atrophy of the optic nerve and in glaucoma.

In atrophy of the nerve, its fibres degenerate, and the nerve itself gradually changes into a mere cord of fibro-cellular tissue; the diameter of the disc is consequently somewhat diminished, and in advanced cases it becomes what is called "cupped." From its ordinary pinkish tinge it gradually assumes a bluish-grey appearance, the scleral ring, however, showing more distinct and broader than usual. The meshes of the lamina cribrosa may be distinguished, but this gradually disappears, and the disc eventually assumes a dead-white tendinous appearance. The vessels, at first, appear less in number, and gradually become finer and finer. As a matter of course, with this form of atrophy and degeneration of the nerve, the retina and its elements suffer as well; a gradually increasing amblyopia, amaurosis, in its most literal sense, being the final result. It is the most complete and irremediable form of blindness. It is most common in old persons.

In glaucoma, the optic disc presents a "cupped" appearance as well; but here this is supposed to be dependent, to a considerable extent, upon excessive intra-ocular pressure. The surface of the disc seems pressed backwards, and the cupping is generally associated with the other ophthalmoscopic signs of the disease, viz.—pulsation of the vessels, capillary hæmorrhages, &c. This cupped appearance may readily be made out in the early stages of the affection, before the humours of the eye have become turbid. At one time, this aspect of the disc was considered to depend upon a projection of the extremity of the nerve, which gives it, as it were, a "bossed" resemblance. However, this turned out to be merely an optical illusion arising from the effect of the light, in consequence of the disc being examined in an inverted position. Dr. Mackenzie has so clearly explained the cause of this illusion in No. XI., page 255, of the "London Ophthalmic Hospital Reports," that I shall quote his lucid explanation. "We judge that an object, viewed with a single eye, is convex or concave, solely by the manner in which light is reflected from the body under examination. The light which falls obliquely on a convex surface illuminates that side which is nearer to the source of light; the side further from it is in shade. The light which falls obliquely on a concave surface illuminates that side which is further from the source of light; the side nearer it is in shade. Let the source of light remain in the same position, but invert the image of the object illuminated, so that the light which falls on the furthest side of it may seem to be on the near side—which is the case when we look through the compound microscope—at the hollow in a bit of paper, or when we examine the optic papilla through the compound microscope formed for the occasion by the patient's eye, plus the convex lens held in front of it; and both the dimple in the paper and the papilla, although they are actually cupped or concave, will then appear convex and prominent.

" If, on the other hand, we turn the convex side of the dimple in the paper uppermost, and view it with the compound microscope, it appears concave. The inversion of its image causes the light which falls on its near side to appear as if it fell on its further side, and thus the eye is subjected to a deception—the reverse of the former, and from which it cannot free itself. If there be cases, then, in which the end of the optic nerve within the eye actually projects in a convex form, they will offer, when examined in the direct method, the appearance of a cup or depression."

The disposition of the vessels of the disc is remarkable, and also decisive of its excavated or depressed condition. If we trace them from the periphery towards the centre, we shall find that, as they approach the edge of the disc, they seem suddenly to stop short, and resume their course on the disc at another point; the fact being that the vessels have turned over the edge, formed a sort of curve, and consequently appear on the disc itself at another place, deeper. It is in the bend of the vessels, that pulsation is most readily seen.

To estimate rightly the pathological changes which take place in the complex and delicate structure of the retina, the following important points should be borne in mind:—The natural transparency of the membrane when in a healthy state, which allows of the retinal vessels being seen sharply defined. The arteries, containing their bright-red contents, chiefly ramifying in the fibrous layer of the retina, dividing more or less dichotomously, and running their direct course towards the ora serrata. The veins not quite so sharply defined, having a more tortuous course, thicker in diameter, with darker contents, and often turgid, especially as they leave the eye through the optic disc. The close connexion of the capillaries of the choroid coat with the outer layers of the retina. These facts, together with the subjective symptoms, should be duly weighed in diagnosing simple hyperæmia from a more advanced state of inflammation.

When hyperæmia of the retina has passed into inflammation, there is increased redness, which may either be generally diffused or partially, over its surface, and is owing to an increased development of the capillaries. The optic disc becomes more injected in very acute cases; its white surface invisible from over-injection, and only to be traced by the main trunks springing from its centre. After a time ecchymoses appear, in the form of small punctiform spots on the surface of the retina; and as the disease progresses, hæmorrhages, from rupture of the walls of the retinal vessels. The turgescence of the veins is much increased, and according to Liebreich they show pulsation; are much augumented in diameter and tortuosity, and exhibit a hazy outline.

The retina now becomes dimmed, owing to exudation on its surface; or the vitreous humour turbid, rendering a clear view of the fundus impossible. I have generally found these exudations take place in that more chronic form of retinitis which occurs in feeble suckling women, "retinitis lactantium;" and it is at this period of the complaint at which the majority of hospital patients seek advice, the sight having become seriously impaired.

Retinitis may terminate favourably, the prognosis being much more favourable when the disease is early diagnosed and treated, and before exudations and hæmorrhages have materially damaged the structure of the organ. It may terminate in inflammatory softening. In fatty degeneration, recognised by white projecting spots of a peculiar opalescent transparency and of variable size. Extravasation; and what is called apoplexy of the retina is, doubtless, frequently preceded by the degeneration; and this state is intimately associated with heart and kidney disease.

An interesting case, illustrating the form of retinitis associated with "Bright's disease," is given by Dr. R. Liebreich in the "Archiv. für Ophthalmologie," Band V., Abth. 2, s. 265, 1859, with a coloured illustration. The following is an abstract of it:—

"The disease develops itself as follows:—At first, retinal hyperæmia, the veins fuller and more tortuous as they rise and fall in their course, becoming dark-red, and sharply outlined, or covered with the slightly dulled retina. Blood, sometimes in the form of radiating streaks, is deposited between the nerve-fibres, sometimes as oval or round spots, which increases the dimness, so that the vessels can hardly be found in the dark-red fundus. The optic disc is ill defined, appearing faintly, and streaky and opaque. Small white round elevated spots are seen in different parts of the fundus oculi; these increase in number, and surround the optic disc: there is, however, a greyish part of the retina left, of a tolerably round form, and of about three or four times the diameter of the disc. From its periphery a thick milk-white layer of granule cells elevates itself, the outer irregular, but sharp contour, of which is continued along the course of the larger vessels. Later, changes take place in the retina on the edge of the layer; the granule cells do not appear as large white spots which coalesce, but as groups of small white ones, which arrange themselves peculiarly in the form of rays, while the middle of the macula lutea, in contrast to the clear white surrounding part, appears dark-red. Small white spots also show themselves in the periphery. In the normal parts of the retina small ecchymoses soon take place, and more extensive extravasations, which cover a great part of this layer of fat, which transforms it into a dark-red surface; or, sometimes the retina becomes detached in its normal part. In some cases, there is a gradual disappearance of these changes, and there only remains the signs of slight retinal atrophy; viz., a white optic disc, and fine retinal vessels."

The opaque white spots appear to be of the nature of fatty degeneration; they are so considered by Heymann, although they have been set down by Virchow as enlargements of the ganglia cells. Further microscopic research is certainly wanted on this subject. The occurrence of these retinal extravasations should always lead the surgeon to investigate the state of the heart and kidneys. When of small extent, they do not much interfere with vision. Even when they are numerous, so long as they avoid the macula lutea, the sight is but partially impaired.

The retinitis pigmentosa of Donders applies to a form of chronic inflammation leading to atrophy of the organ, commencing in its periphery, and extending backwards to the disc. It is characterised by irregular pigmentary deposits over the fundus. I have no experience of this form of disease.

Atrophy of the retina is a consequence of chronic inflammations. It sometimes occurs as a congenital defect.

The retina may be atrophied in parts, as the results of lymph effusions from choroiditis. When this is associated with atrophy of the optic nerve, a cupping of the disc is observed. A progressive diminution of the field of vision from the periphery towards the centre, together with diminution of defining power, is the usual course of this irremediable form of degeneration: it is frequently the cause of slow progressive blindness in old people. Strong convex glasses generally assist the sight in these patients for a time.

Detachment of the retina from the choroid may be the result of accident—for instance, blows on the eyeball, or about the orbit; but the majority of patients who apply to me attribute it to other causes. It has been discovered after rising suddenly from a stooping posture. In some cases, the separation has, doubtless, existed unobserved for some time. Such patients assign no particular cause for the defect. Almost invariably the eye itself shows no external evidence of the internal changes.

The causes of those detachments are, fluid effusions of various natures, chiefly, however, serous; sub-retinal dropsy, hydrophthalmia posterior; or, firm, solid deposits.

The subjective symptoms generally are hemiopia; sometimes a dark cloud moves before the eye.

The objective symptoms are not generally very manifest; for although occasionally with a fully dilated pupil, in a young person, a bluish moving shred may be seen, the ophthalmoscope is needed to discover the cause of impaired vision. The instrument should be first used alone, and by a dull light; afterwards the lens must be employed for minute investigation, because the recognition of the retinal vessels is important as a diagnostic sign.

The displacement may be limited; or the whole retina detached, in a funnel-shaped form, in which case the optic nerve is more or less hidden by its folds.

Loss of transparency, and ultimately complete opacity, are the consequences of the separation; but when these effects occur is uncertain.

The vitreous humour is frequently more fluid than usual, perhaps from its dilution with effused serum.

It is but of slight practical moment as to which part of the retina is most frequently, or originally detached; but the extent to which the loss of connexion takes place, is of the highest importance as regards vision. A fair amount of sight is retained as long as that around the macula lutea is sound, and this even when the optic disc is encroached on by any bulging part. The vessels continue their course, following the folds into which the membrane is thrown,—now appearing in high relief, and now vanishing out of focus. They vary much in colour; often they appear like fine black lines in the edge of the folds: this is dependent, according to Liebreich, on the nature of the effusion—the darker they are, the more opaque the substance beneath.

Detachments of the retina and choroid from the sclerotica are very rare, and the two coats are thrust forward into the vitreous humour, in the form of a roundish tumour. The retinal vessels may be clearly distinguished, leaving the fundus, and coming forwards. Sometimes, according to Liebreich, the choroidal vessels may be seen.

The vitreous humour, generally unhealthy, is probably partly absorbed.

The diagnosis between this and simple detachment of the retina, consists in the absence of the retinal folds and the floating of the membrane.

Lesions of this kind are generally caused by blood effused between the sclerotica and choroid; or by tubercle, or growths of a malignant nature.

It will be easily understood, that from the peculiar structure of the choroid—almost entirely composed of vascular tissues, together with a richly furnished pigmental layer,—alterations in this membrane are of frequent occurrence, and I believe that the majority of pathological changes which take place in the interior of the eye may be referred originally to chronic inflammation of this coat.

Alteration in the deposition of the pigment is one of the most striking of the morbid alterations. The pigment cells are frequently amassed together in some parts of the fundus; whilst in others the white, and somewhat circular spaces, caused by the sclerotic shining through the atrophied choroid, show their disappearance. Dissection discovers that the retina and the other layers of the choroid are perfect over these white spots, but that the hexagonal pigment epithelium is absent. The choroidal vessels, which at first are rendered more evident, finally disappear, and a more complete atrophy is the result. A very good representation of the effects of long continued chronic choroiditis, the result of a blow five years before, is given in my colleagues', Messrs. Taylor and Hulme's Illustrations of the Use of the Ophthalmoscope, fig. 4, plate 1, vol. ii., "Archives of Medicine." The deficiency of the pigment in some parts, with the orange-red choroidal vessels showing on the white sclerotica, and the irregular deposition of it about the fundus, and especially around the rim of the optic disc, are very well shown, and give that peculiar appearance to the eye which Desmarres has called the "choroide tigrée." The patient complained of considerable confusion of vision; but she could see to discern objects when brought opposite to the healthy portion of the choroid.

Irregular pigmental deposits must not always be considered as abnormal, as they frequently occur in healthy eyes.

Colloid degeneration of the choroid is a disease of rare occurrence; the elucidation of which is due to Professor Donders, of Utrecht, and a full account has been published by him in the "Archiv. für Ophthalmologie," Band I., Abth. 2, s. 107, 1854-5. It occurs in young children as well as in adults. The ophthalmoscopic appearances are, small round pearly deposits, diffused more or less over the fundus of the eye. Producing pressure on the choroidal epithelium, they cause its absorption, and the shining appearance of the colloid globules may then be made out. Vision is but slightly affected in the early stages, but sooner or later, as the disease extends, it proportionally diminishes. Donders considers the disease to be first developed in the nuclei of the pigment cells; Müller, that the elastic lamina of the choroid is the seat of the growths. I am inclined to believe in the latter; and in the dissection of an eye shown to me by Mr. Hulme, the colloid globule seemed clearly to originate in a thickening of this membrane.

Among the important effects of choroiditis are, fluid effusion, either in the membrane itself, between it and the sclerotica, or it and the retina. Also, effusions of blood, varying in extent, either from traumatic or constitutional causes. Semi-fluid exudations on its surface, and even a solid deposit—as tubercle, cancer, &c.,—have been seen.

Hyperæmia of the choroid is one of those early stages of ophthalmic changes for the recognition of which we are almost entirely indebted to the ophthalmoscope. It is diagnosed by a scarlet injection of its capillaries, which gives to it the red velvety appearance peculiar to this state. The capillary layer is that chiefly involved, and the pressure of the injected vessels on the retina naturally results in considerable confusion of vision.

The pigmentary arborizations more or less disappear ; but due consideration must be made in valuing this symptom, as to the complexion of the patient.   It is this state which, if unchecked by treatment, leads on to exudations, hæmorrhages, and other pigmental changes called by the Germans, " pigment maceration."

Hyperæmia of the choroid sometimes merely occurs in circumscribed patches; and it may be as well to remind the reader that, from the disposition of the vascular system of the choroid, a variable degree of thickness of the membrane is present in different parts of the fundus.

Choroidal exudations, especially if they be of a plastic nature, are easily diagnosed.   The amount of discomfort to vision will depend upon the nature and density of the effusion, and the duration of time before absorption is complete will depend also upon the same cause.   Unfortunately, when of lymph, they are apt to remain stationary, and by their position and pressure often cause absorption and atrophy of the choroid, with more or less detriment to the retinal outer coats.   They may also become the seat of other morbid degenerations.   They are generally of a greyish colour, and the retinal vessels may often be traced running over their surface, which is for the most part slightly elevated.

Injuries to the choroid from traumatic causes, as blows, &c., are of frequent occurrence, and more or less damaging to vision. When caused by direct injury, the impairment of vision will be dated from the accident, and it will be in proportion generally to the amount of extravasation.   Small isolated vessels may be ruptured, but much more generally the effusion of blood is extensive, and the clot may be observed occupying a considerable and important extent of the field of vision, either behind an uninjured retina, or else rupturing the latter, and projecting through it into the vitreous humour.   That such is sometimes the case is revealed by time ; the cicatrices left after the absorption of the blood showing the nature of the injury.

I have seen extravasation in which I have had but little doubt that the larger choroidal vessels had been ruptured.

Professor Esmarch, of Kiel (Archiv. für Ophthalmologie; Band IV., Abth. 1, s. 350, 1858), gives an interesting case of perforation of the retina by choroidal hæmorrhage, which he had the opportunity of watching for some time. The Professor states his opinion, to the effect that small perforations of the retina may cicatrize without a mark; but extensive openings generally leave a visible scar, with proportionate defect in vision. The case is illustrated diagrammatically, showing the progressive absorption of the clot.

An instance of choroidal hæmorrhage, without rupture of the retina, is given also by Messrs. Taylor and Hulme (Archives of Medicine, vol. ii., pl. 1, fig. 3). The retinal vessels could be made out, passing uninjured over the effused clot underneath; as the clot absorbed, it assumed a rounded, discoid shape, with a white centre. Probably blood effusion may be the origin of those brownish discoid spots often seen, and which differ in marked respect from the irregular pigmental deposits.

Smaller choroidal extravasations are met with in various stages of absorption. I believe they are always associated with changes in the pigmentary layer. Granular disease of the kidney may have the same influence on the vessels of this membrane as I have shown may take place in those of the retina.

A few words may be said about an abnormal condition of the eye, frequently found in myopic persons, which, as it depends upon a posterior bulging of the sclerotica with thinning, near the entrance of the optic nerve, and consequent elongation of the antero-posterior axis of the eye, has been designated "posterior staphyloma." It has been considered as a result of chronic inflammation of that part of the two outer tunics of the eye, "Sclero-choroiditis posterior."

To Professor Von Graefe is due the credit of first interpreting this affection. It is diagnosed at once by the ophthalmoscope as a white crescentic figure, of which the concave border is in connexion with the edge of the optic disc, while the convex is directed outwards towards the macula lutea. It varies in size; generally its horns embrace about half of the disc; but when it increases, which it sometimes does very sensibly, it is by extension of the extremities, and sometimes they surround the disc completely. It is then generally of a whiter colour than the disc itself, the border of which is recognised by a slight pink or grey shade. It rarely commences on the inner side of the eye.

The choroid is present over the crescent, as the larger vessels may be seen dipping into the cavity, but they lose their outline by being out of focus. The pigment epithelium appears to be absent, and probably also the capillaris, thus rendering the sclerotica apparent. Pigment is frequently deposited at the edge of the disc. The retina would seem to be normal, as sometimes small retinal vessels pass outwards, and can be traced sharply defined over the white sclerotic background.

With this condition the eyeball does not maintain its sphericity. There is either a tendency to a thinning of the sclerotica at the ciliary margin, or a slight departure from the perfect form between the insertions of the muscles. I have not had an opportunity of examining, microscopically, an eye thus affected, but I should imagine some degeneration of the sclerotic texture would be found.

Although this crescent is so frequently present in myopic eyes, it can hardly be said to be perfectly diagnostic of this condition, as I have examined the eyes of many genuine cases of myopia, without finding the least trace of such alteration.

FINIS.

INDEX.

Reed and Pardon, Printers, Paternoster-row, London.

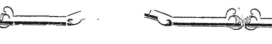

London, New Burlington Street,
May, 1866.

MESSRS. CHURCHILL & SONS'

Publications,

IN

MEDICINE

AND THE VARIOUS BRANCHES OF

NATURAL SCIENCE.

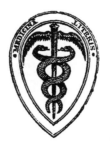

"It would be unjust to conclude this notice without saying a few words in favour of Mr. Churchill, from whom the profession is receiving, it may be truly said, the most beautiful series of Illustrated Medical Works which has ever been published."—*Lancet.*

"All the publications of Mr. Churchill are prepared with so much taste and neatness, that it is superfluous to speak of them in terms of commendation."—*Edinburgh Medical and Surgical Journal.*

"No one is more distinguished for the elegance and *recherché* style of his publications than Mr. Churchill."—*Provincial Medical Journal.*

"Mr. Churchill's publications are very handsomely got up: the engravings are remarkably well executed."—*Dublin Medical Press.*

"The typography, illustrations, and getting up are, in all Mr. Churchill's publications, most beautiful."—*Monthly Journal of Medical Science.*

"Mr. Churchill's illustrated works are among the best that emanate from the Medical Press."—*Medical Times.*

"We have before called the attention of both students and practitioners to the great advantage which Mr. Churchill has conferred on the profession, in the issue, at such a moderate cost, of works so highly creditable in point of artistic execution and scientific merit."—*Dublin Quarterly Journal.*

A CLASSIFIED INDEX

TO

MESSRS. CHURCHILL & SONS' CATALOGUE.

CLASSIFIED INDEX.

MR. F. A. ABEL, F.R.S., & MR. C. L. BLOXAM.

HANDBOOK OF CHEMISTRY: THEORETICAL, PRACTICAL, AND TECHNICAL. Second Edition. 8vo. cloth, 15s.

MR. ACTON, M.R.C.S.

I.

A PRACTICAL TREATISE ON DISEASES OF THE URINARY AND GENERATIVE ORGANS IN BOTH SEXES. Third Edition. 8vo. cloth, £1. 1s. With Plates, £1. 11s. 6d. The Plates alone, limp cloth, 10s. 6d.

II.

THE FUNCTIONS AND DISORDERS OF THE REPRODUC-TIVE ORGANS IN CHILDHOOD, YOUTH, ADULT AGE, AND ADVANCED LIFE, considered in their Physiological, Social, and Moral Relations. Fourth Edition. 8vo. cloth, 10s. 6d. III.

PROSTITUTION: Considered in its Moral, Social, and Sanitary Bearings, with a View to its Amelioration and Regulation. 8vo. cloth, 10s. 6d.

DR. ADAMS, A.M.

A TREATISE ON RHEUMATIC GOUT; OR, CHRONIC RHEUMATIC ARTHRITIS. 8vo. cloth, with a Quarto Atlas of Plates, 21s.

MR. WILLIAM ADAMS, F.R.C.S.

I.

ON THE PATHOLOGY AND TREATMENT OF LATERAL AND OTHER FORMS OF CURVATURE OF THE SPINE. With Plates. 8vo. cloth, 10s. 6d. II.

ON THE REPARATIVE PROCESS IN HUMAN TENDONS AFTER SUBCUTANEOUS DIVISION FOR THE CURE OF DEFORMITIES. With Plates. 8vo. cloth, 6s. III.

SKETCH OF THE PRINCIPLES AND PRACTICE OF SUBCUTANEOUS SURGERY. 8vo. cloth, 2s. 6d.

DR. WILLIAM ADDISON, F.R.S.

I.

CELL THERAPEUTICS. 8vo. cloth, 4s.

II.

ON HEALTHY AND DISEASED STRUCTURE, AND THE TRUE PRINCIPLES OF TREATMENT FOR THE CURE OF DISEASE, ESPECIALLY CONSUMPTION AND SCROFULA, founded on MICROSCOPICAL ANALYSIS. 8vo. cloth, 12s.

DR. ALDIS.

AN INTRODUCTION TO HOSPITAL PRACTICE IN VARIOUS COMPLAINTS; with Remarks on their Pathology and Treatment. 8vo. cloth, 5s. 6d.

DR. SOMERVILLE SCOTT ALISON, M.D.EDIN., F.R.C.P.

THE PHYSICAL EXAMINATION OF THE CHEST IN PUL-MONARY CONSUMPTION, AND ITS INTERCURRENT DISEASES. With Engravings. 8vo. cloth, 12s.

THE ANATOMICAL REMEMBRANCER; OR, COMPLETE POCKET ANATOMIST. Sixth Edition, carefully Revised. 32mo. cloth, 3s. 6d.

DR. MCCALL ANDERSON, M.D.

I.

PARASITIC AFFECTIONS OF THE SKIN. With Engravings. 8vo. cloth, 5s. II.

ECZEMA. 8vo. cloth, 5s.

III.

PSORIASIS AND LEPRA. With Chromo-lithograph. 8vo. cloth, 5s.

DR. ANDREW ANDERSON, M.D.

TEN LECTURES INTRODUCTORY TO THE STUDY OF FEVER.

Post 8vo. cloth, 5s.

DR. THOMAS ANDERSON, M.D.

HANDBOOK FOR YELLOW FEVER: ITS PATHOLOGY AND

TREATMENT. To which is added a brief History of Cholera, and a method of Cure. Fcap. 8vo. cloth, 3s.

DR. ARLIDGE.

ON THE STATE OF LUNACY AND THE LEGAL PROVISION

FOR THE INSANE; with Observations on the Construction and Organisation of Asylums. 8vo. cloth, 7s.

DR. ALEXANDER ARMSTRONG, R.N.

OBSERVATIONS ON NAVAL HYGIENE AND SCURVY.

More particularly as the latter appeared during a Polar Voyage. 8vo. cloth, 5s.

MR. T. J. ASHTON.

I.

ON THE DISEASES, INJURIES, AND MALFORMATIONS

OF THE RECTUM AND ANUS. Fourth Edition. 8vo. cloth, 8s.

I.

PROLAPSUS, FISTULA IN ANO, AND HÆMORRHOIDAL

AFFECTIONS; their Pathology and Treatment. Second Edition. Post 8vo. cloth, 2s. 6d.

MR. W. B. ASPINALL.

SAN REMO AS A WINTER RESIDENCE. With Coloured Plates.

Foolscap 8vo. cloth, 4s. 6d.

MR. THOS. J. AUSTIN, M.R.C.S.ENG.

A PRACTICAL ACCOUNT OF GENERAL PARALYSIS:

Its Mental and Physical Symptoms, Statistics, Causes, Seat, and Treatment. 8vo. cloth, 6s.

DR. THOMAS BALLARD, M.D.

A NEW AND RATIONAL EXPLANATION OF THE DIS-

EASES PECULIAR TO INFANTS AND MOTHERS; with obvious Suggestions for their Prevention and Cure. Post 8vo. cloth, 4s. 6d.

DR. BARCLAY.

I.

A MANUAL OF MEDICAL DIAGNOSIS. Second Edition.

Foolscap 8vo. cloth, 8s. 6d.   II.

MEDICAL ERRORS.—Fallacies connected with the Application of the

Inductive Method of Reasoning to the Science of Medicine. Post 8vo. cloth, 5s.

DR. T. HERBERT BARKER, M.D., F.R.S, & MR. ERNEST EDWARDS, B.A.

PHOTOGRAPHS OF EMINENT MEDICAL MEN, with brief

Analytical Notices of their Works. Nos. I. to VI., price 3s. each.

DR. BARLOW.

A MANUAL OF THE PRACTICE OF MEDICINE. Second

Edition. Fcap. 8vo. cloth, 12s. 6d.

DR. BARNES.

THE PHYSIOLOGY AND TREATMENT OF PLACENTA

PRÆVIA; being the Lettsomian Lectures on Midwifery for 1857. Post 8vo. cloth, 6s.

DR. BASCOME.

A HISTORY OF EPIDEMIC PESTILENCES, FROM THE
EARLIEST AGES. 8vo. cloth, 8s.

DR. BASHAM.

ON DROPSY, AND ITS CONNECTION WITH DISEASES OF
THE KIDNEYS, HEART, LUNGS AND LIVER. With 16 Plates. Third Edition. 8vo. cloth, 12s. 6d.

MR. H. F. BAXTER, M.R.C.S.L.

ON ORGANIC POLARITY; showing a Connexion to exist between
Organic Forces and Ordinary Polar Forces. Crown 8vo. cloth, 5s.

MR. BATEMAN.

MAGNACOPIA: A Practical Library of Profitable Knowledge, commu-
nicating the general Minutiæ of Chemical and Pharmaceutic Routine, together with the generality of Secret Forms of Preparations. Third Edition. 18mo. 6s.

MR. LIONEL J. BEALE, M.R.C.S.

I.

THE LAWS OF HEALTH IN THEIR RELATIONS TO MIND
AND BODY. A Series of Letters from an Old Practitioner to a Patient. Post 8vo. cloth, 7s. 6d.

II.

HEALTH AND DISEASE, IN CONNECTION WITH THE
GENERAL PRINCIPLES OF HYGIENE. Fcap. 8vo., 2s. 6d.

DR. BEALE, F.R.S.

I.

URINE, URINARY DEPOSITS, AND CALCULI: and on the
Treatment of Urinary Diseases. Numerous Engravings. Second Edition, much Enlarged. Post 8vo. cloth, 8s. 6d.

II.

THE MICROSCOPE, IN ITS APPLICATION TO PRACTICAL
MEDICINE. With a Coloured Plate, and 270 Woodcuts. Second Edition. 8vo. cloth, 14s.

III.

ILLUSTRATIONS OF THE SALTS OF URINE, URINARY
DEPOSITS, and CALCULI. 37 Plates, containing upwards of 170 Figures copied from Nature, with descriptive Letterpress. 8vo. cloth, 9s. 6d.

MR. BEASLEY.

I.

THE BOOK OF PRESCRIPTIONS; containing 3000 Prescriptions.
Collected from the Practice of the most eminent Physicians and Surgeons, English and Foreign. Third Edition. 18mo. cloth, 6s.

II.

THE DRUGGIST'S GENERAL RECEIPT-BOOK: comprising a
copious Veterinary Formulary and Table of Veterinary Materia Medica; Patent and Proprietary Medicines, Druggists' Nostrums, &c.; Perfumery, Skin Cosmetics, Hair Cosmetics, and Teeth Cosmetics; Beverages, Dietetic Articles, and Condiments; Trade Chemicals, Miscellaneous Preparations and Compounds used in the Arts, &c.; with useful Memoranda and Tables. Sixth Edition. 18mo. cloth, 6s.

III.

THE POCKET FORMULARY AND SYNOPSIS OF THE
BRITISH AND FOREIGN PHARMACOPŒIAS; comprising standard and approved Formulæ for the Preparations and Compounds employed in Medical Practice. Eighth Edition, corrected and enlarged. 18mo. cloth, 6s.

DR. HENRY BENNET.

I.

A PRACTICAL TREATISE ON INFLAMMATION AND OTHER DISEASES OF THE UTERUS. Fourth Edition, revised, with Additions. 8vo. cloth, 16s.

II.

A REVIEW OF THE PRESENT STATE OF UTERINE PATHOLOGY. 8vo. cloth, 4s.

III.

NUTRITION IN HEALTH AND DISEASE. Post 8vo. cloth, 5s.

IV.

WINTER IN THE SOUTH OF EUROPE; OR, MENTONE, THE RIVIERA, CORSICA, SICILY, AND BIARRITZ, AS WINTER CLIMATES. Third Edition, with numerous Plates, Maps, and Wood Engravings. Post 8vo. cloth, 10s. 6d.

PROFESSOR BENTLEY, F.L.S.

A MANUAL OF BOTANY. With nearly 1,200 Engravings on Wood. Fcap. 8vo. cloth, 12s. 6d.

DR. BERNAYS.

NOTES FOR STUDENTS IN CHEMISTRY; being a Syllabus compiled from the Manuals of Miller, Fownes, Berzelius, Gerhardt, Gorup-Besanez, &c. Fourth Edition. Fscap. 8vo. cloth, 3s.

MR. HENRY HEATHER BIGG.

ORTHOPRAXY: the Mechanical Treatment of Deformities, Debilities, and Deficiencies of the Human Frame. With Engravings. Post 8vo. cloth, 10s.

DR. BILLING, F.R.S.

ON DISEASES OF THE LUNGS AND HEART. 8vo. cloth, 6s.

DR. S. B. BIRCH, M.D.

CONSTIPATED BOWELS: the Various Causes and the Rational Means of Cure. Second Edition. Post 8vo. cloth, 3s. 6d.

DR. GOLDING BIRD, F.R.S.

I.

URINARY DEPOSITS; THEIR DIAGNOSIS, PATHOLOGY, AND THERAPEUTICAL INDICATIONS. With Engravings. Fifth Edition. Edited by E. LLOYD BIRKETT, M.D. Post 8vo. cloth, 10s. 6d.

II.

ELEMENTS OF NATURAL PHILOSOPHY; being an Experimental Introduction to the Study of the Physical Sciences. With numerous Engravings. Fifth Edition. Edited by CHARLES BROOKE, M.B. Cantab., F.R.S. Fcap. 8vo. cloth, 12s. 6d.

MR. BISHOP, F.R.S.

I.

ON DEFORMITIES OF THE HUMAN BODY, their Pathology and Treatment. With Engravings on Wood. 8vo. cloth, 10s.

I.

ON ARTICULATE SOUNDS, AND ON THE CAUSES AND CURE OF IMPEDIMENTS OF SPEECH. 8vo. cloth, 4s.

MR. P. HINCKES BIRD, F.R.C.S.

PRACTICAL TREATISE ON THE DISEASES OF CHILDREN AND INFANTS AT THE BREAST. Translated from the French of M. BOUCHUT, with Notes and Additions. 8vo. cloth. 20s.

MR. BLAINE.

OUTLINES OF THE VETERINARY ART; OR, A TREATISE
ON THE ANATOMY, PHYSIOLOGY, AND DISEASES OF THE HORSE, NEAT CATTLE, AND SHEEP. Seventh Edition. By Charles Steel, M.R.C.V.S.L. With Plates. 8vo. cloth, 18s.

DR. BOURGUIGNON.

ON THE CATTLE PLAGUE; OR, CONTAGIOUS TYPHUS IN
HORNED CATTLE: its History, Origin, Description, and Treatment. Post 8vo. 5s.

MR. JOHN E. BOWMAN, & MR. C. L. BLOXAM.

I.

PRACTICAL CHEMISTRY, including Analysis. With numerous Illustrations on Wood. Fifth Edition. Foolscap 8vo. cloth, 6s. 6d.

II.

MEDICAL CHEMISTRY; with Illustrations on Wood. Fourth Edition,
carefully revised. Fcap. 8vo. cloth, 6s. 6d.

DR. JAMES BRIGHT.

ON DISEASES OF THE HEART, LUNGS, & AIR PASSAGES;
with a Review of the several Climates recommended in these Affections. Third Edition. Post 8vo. cloth, 9s.

DR. BRINTON, F.R.S.

I.

THE DISEASES OF THE STOMACH, with an Introduction on its
Anatomy and Physiology; being Lectures delivered at St. Thomas's Hospital. Second Edition. 8vo. cloth, 10s. 6d.

II.

THE SYMPTOMS, PATHOLOGY, AND TREATMENT OF
ULCER OF THE STOMACH. Post 8vo. cloth, 5s.

MR. BERNARD E. BRODHURST, F.R.C.S.

I.

CURVATURES OF THE SPINE: their Causes, Symptoms, Pathology,
and Treatment. Second Edition. Roy. 8vo. cloth, with Engravings, 7s. 6d.

II.

ON THE NATURE AND TREATMENT OF CLUBFOOT AND
ANALOGOUS DISTORTIONS involving the TIBIO-TARSAL ARTICULATION. With Engravings on Wood. 8vo. cloth, 4s. 6d.

III.

PRACTICAL OBSERVATIONS ON THE DISEASES OF THE
JOINTS INVOLVING ANCHYLOSIS, and on the TREATMENT for the RESTORATION of MOTION. Third Edition, much enlarged, 8vo. cloth, 4s. 6d.

MR. THOMAS BRYANT, F.R.C.S.

I.

ON THE DISEASES AND INJURIES OF THE JOINTS.
CLINICAL AND PATHOLOGICAL OBSERVATIONS. Post 8vo. cloth, 7s. 6d.

II.

THE SURGICAL DISEASES OF CHILDREN. The Lettsomian
Lectures, delivered March, 1863. Post 8vo. cloth, 5s.

DR. BRYCE.

ENGLAND AND FRANCE BEFORE SEBASTOPOL, looked at
from a Medical Point of View. 8vo. cloth, 6s.

DR. BUCKLE, M.D., L.R.C.P.LOND.

VITAL AND ECONOMICAL STATISTICS OF THE HOSPITALS,
INFIRMARIES, &c., OF ENGLAND AND WALES. Royal 8vo. 5s.

DR. BUDD, F.R.S.
I.
ON DISEASES OF THE LIVER.
Illustrated with Coloured Plates and Engravings on Wood. Third Edition. 8vo. cloth, 16s.

II.
ON THE ORGANIC DISEASES AND FUNCTIONAL DIS-
ORDERS OF THE STOMACH. 8vo. cloth, 9s.

DR. JOHN CHARLES BUCKNILL, & DR. DANIEL H. TUKE.
A MANUAL OF PSYCHOLOGICAL MEDICINE: containing
the History, Nosology, Description, Statistics, Diagnosis, Pathology, and Treatment of
Insanity. Second Edition. 8vo. cloth, 15s.

MR. CALLENDER, F.R.C.S.
FEMORAL RUPTURE: Anatomy of the Parts concerned. With Plates.
8vo. cloth, 4s.

DR. JOHN M. CAMPLIN, F.L.S.
ON DIABETES, AND ITS SUCCESSFUL TREATMENT.
Third Edition, by Dr. Glover. Fcap. 8vo. cloth, 3s. 6d.

MR. ROBERT B. CARTER, M.R.C.S.
I.
ON THE INFLUENCE OF EDUCATION AND TRAINING
IN PREVENTING DISEASES OF THE NERVOUS SYSTEM. Fcap. 8vo., 6s.

II.
THE PATHOLOGY AND TREATMENT OF HYSTERIA. Post
8vo. cloth, 4s. 6d.

DR. CARPENTER, F.R.S.
I.
PRINCIPLES OF HUMAN PHYSIOLOGY. With numerous Illus-
trations on Steel and Wood. Sixth Edition. Edited by Mr. HENRY POWER. 8vo.
cloth, 26s.

II.
A MANUAL OF PHYSIOLOGY. With 252 Illustrations on Steel
and Wood. Fourth Edition. Fcap. 8vo. cloth, 12s. 6d.

III.
THE MICROSCOPE AND ITS REVELATIONS. With nume-
rous Engravings on Steel and Wood. Third Edition. Fcap. 8vo. cloth, 12s. 6d.

DR. CHAMBERS.
I.
LECTURES, CHIEFLY CLINICAL. Fourth Edition. 8vo. cloth, 14s.

II.
DIGESTION AND ITS DERANGEMENTS. Post 8vo. cloth, 10s. 6d.

III.
SOME OF THE EFFECTS OF THE CLIMATE OF ITALY.
Crown 8vo. cloth, 4s. 6d.

DR. CHANCE, M.B.
VIRCHOW'S CELLULAR PATHOLOGY, AS BASED UPON
PHYSIOLOGICAL AND PATHOLOGICAL HISTOLOGY. With 144 Engravings on Wood. 8vo. cloth, 16s.

MR. H. T. CHAPMAN, F.R.C.S.
I.
THE TREATMENT OF OBSTINATE ULCERS AND CUTA-
NEOUS ERUPTIONS OF THE LEG WITHOUT CONFINEMENT. Third
Edition. Post 8vo. cloth, 3s. 6d.

II.
VARICOSE VEINS: their Nature, Consequences, and Treatment, Pallia-
tive and Curative. Second Edition. Post 8vo. cloth, 3s. 6d.

MR. PYE HENRY CHAVASSE, F.R.C.S.

I.

ADVICE TO A MOTHER ON THE MANAGEMENT OF
HER CHILDREN. Eighth Edition. Foolscap 8vo., 2s. 6d.

II.

ADVICE TO A WIFE ON THE MANAGEMENT OF HER
OWN HEALTH. With an Introductory Chapter, especially addressed to a Young Wife. Seventh Edition. Fcap. 8vo., 2s. 6d.

MR. LE GROS CLARK, F.R.C.S.

OUTLINES OF SURGERY ; being an Epitome of the Lectures on the
Principles and the Practice of Surgery, delivered at St. Thomas's Hospital. Fcap. 8vo. cloth, 5s.

MR. JOHN CLAY, M.R.C.S.

KIWISCH ON DISEASES OF THE OVARIES: Translated, by
permission, from the last German Edition of his Clinical Lectures on the Special Pathology and Treatment of the Diseases of Women. With Notes, and an Appendix on the Operation of Ovariotomy. Royal 12mo. cloth, 16s.

DR. COCKLE, M.D.

ON INTRA-THORACIC CANCER. 8vo. 6s. 6d.

MR. COLLIS, M.B.DUB., F.R.C.S.I.

THE DIAGNOSIS AND TREATMENT OF CANCER AND
THE TUMOURS ANALOGOUS TO IT. With coloured Plates. 8vo. cloth, 14s.

DR. CONOLLY.

THE CONSTRUCTION AND GOVERNMENT OF LUNATIC
ASYLUMS AND HOSPITALS FOR THE INSANE. With Plans. Post 8vo. cloth, 6s.

MR. COOLEY.

COMPREHENSIVE SUPPLEMENT TO THE PHARMACOPŒIAS.

THE CYCLOPÆDIA OF PRACTICAL RECEIPTS, PRO-
CESSES, AND COLLATERAL INFORMATION IN THE ARTS, MANU-FACTURES, PROFESSIONS, AND TRADES, INCLUDING MEDICINE, PHARMACY, AND DOMESTIC ECONOMY; designed as a General Book of Reference for the Manufacturer, Tradesman, Amateur, and Heads of Families. Fourth and greatly enlarged Edition, 8vo. cloth, 28s.

MR. W. WHITE COOPER.

ON WOUNDS AND INJURIES OF THE EYE. Illustrated by
17 Coloured Figures and 41 Woodcuts. 8vo. cloth, 12s.

II.

ON NEAR SIGHT, AGED SIGHT, IMPAIRED VISION,
AND THE MEANS OF ASSISTING SIGHT. With 31 Illustrations on Wood. Second Edition. Fcap. 8vo. cloth, 7s. 6d.

SIR ASTLEY COOPER, BART., F.R.S.

ON THE STRUCTURE AND DISEASES OF THE TESTIS.
With 24 Plates. Second Edition. Royal 4to., 20s.

MR. COOPER.

A DICTIONARY OF PRACTICAL SURGERY AND ENCYCLO-
PÆDIA OF SURGICAL SCIENCE. New Edition, brought down to the present time. By SAMUEL A. LANE, F.R.C.S., assisted by various eminent Surgeons. Vol. I., 8vo. cloth, £1. 5s.

MR. HOLMES COOTE, F.R.C.S.

A REPORT ON SOME IMPORTANT POINTS IN THE
TREATMENT OF SYPHILIS. 8vo. cloth, 5s.

DR. COTTON.

I.

ON CONSUMPTION : Its Nature, Symptoms, and Treatment. To
which Essay was awarded the Fothergillian Gold Medal of the Medical Society of
London. Second Edition. 8vo. cloth, 8s.

II.

PHTHISIS AND THE STETHOSCOPE; OR, THE PHYSICAL
SIGNS OF CONSUMPTION. Third Edition. Foolscap 8vo. cloth, 3s.

MR. COULSON.

I.

ON DISEASES OF THE BLADDER AND PROSTATE GLAND.
New Edition, revised. *In Preparation.*

II.

ON LITHOTRITY AND LITHOTOMY; with Engravings on Wood.
8vo. cloth, 8s.

MR. WILLIAM CRAIG, L.F.P.S., GLASGOW.

ON THE INFLUENCE OF VARIATIONS OF ELECTRIC
TENSION AS THE REMOTE CAUSE OF EPIDEMIC AND OTHER
DISEASES. 8vo. cloth, 10s.

MR. CURLING, F.R.S.

OBSERVATIONS ON DISEASES OF THE RECTUM. Third
Edition. 8vo. cloth, 7s. 6d.

II.

A PRACTICAL TREATISE ON DISEASES OF THE TESTIS,
SPERMATIC CORD, AND SCROTUM. Third Edition, with Engravings. 8vo.
cloth, 16s.

DR. DALRYMPLE, M.R.C.P., F.R.C.S.

THE CLIMATE OF EGYPT: METEOROLOGICAL AND MEDI-
CAL OBSERVATIONS, with Practical Hints for Invalid Travellers. Post 8vo. cloth, 4s.

MR. JOHN DALRYMPLE, F.R.S., F.R.C.S.

PATHOLOGY OF THE HUMAN EYE. Complete in Nine Fasciculi:
imperial 4to., 20s. each; half-bound morocco, gilt tops, 9l. 15s.

DR. HERBERT DAVIES.

ON THE PHYSICAL DIAGNOSIS OF DISEASES OF THE
LUNGS AND HEART. Second Edition. Post 8vo. cloth, 8s.

DR. DAVEY.

I.

THE GANGLIONIC NERVOUS SYSTEM: its Structure, Functions,
and Diseases. 8vo. cloth, 9s.

II.

ON THE NATURE AND PROXIMATE CAUSE OF IN-
SANITY. Post 8vo. cloth, 3s.

MR. DIXON.

A GUIDE TO THE PRACTICAL STUDY OF DISEASES OF
THE EYE. Third Edition. Post 8vo. cloth, 9s.

DR. DOBELL.

I.

DEMONSTRATIONS OF DISEASES IN THE CHEST, AND

THEIR PHYSICAL DIAGNOSIS. With Coloured Plates. 8vo. cloth, 12s. 6d.

II.

LECTURES ON THE GERMS AND VESTIGES OF DISEASE,

and on the Prevention of the Invasion and Fatality of Disease by Periodical Examinations.
8vo. cloth, 6s. 6d.

III.

A MANUAL OF DIET AND REGIMEN FOR PHYSICIAN

AND PATIENT. Third Edition (for the year 1865). Crown 8vo. cloth, 1s. 6d.

IV.

ON TUBERCULOSIS: ITS NATURE, CAUSE, AND TREAT-

MENT; with Notes on Pancreatic Juice. Second Edition. Crown 8vo. cloth, 3s. 6d.

V.

ON WINTER COUGH (CATARRH, BRONCHITIS, EMPHY-

SEMA, ASTHMA); with an Appendix on some Principles of Diet in Disease—
Lectures delivered at the Royal Infirmary for Diseases of the Chest. Post 8vo. cloth,
5s. 6d.

DR. TOOGOOD DOWNING.

NEURALGIA: its various Forms, Pathology, and Treatment. THE

JACKSONIAN PRIZE ESSAY FOR 1850. 8vo. cloth, 10s. 6d.

DR. DRUITT, F.R.C.S.

THE SURGEON'S VADE-MECUM; with numerous Engravings on

Wood. Ninth Edition. Foolscap 8vo. cloth, 12s. 6d.

MR. DUNN, F.R.C.S.

AN ESSAY ON PHYSIOLOGICAL PSYCHOLOGY. 8vo. cloth, 4s.

SIR JAMES EYRE, M.D.

I.

THE STOMACH AND ITS DIFFICULTIES. Fifth Edition.

Fcap. 8vo. cloth, 2s. 6d.

II.

PRACTICAL REMARKS ON SOME EXHAUSTING DIS-

EASES. Second Edition. Post 8vo. cloth, 4s. 6d.

DR. FENWICK.

ON SCROFULA AND CONSUMPTION. Clergyman's Sore Throat,

Catarrh, Croup, Bronchitis, Asthma. Fcap. 8vo., 2s. 6d.

SIR WILLIAM FERGUSSON, BART., F.R.S.

A SYSTEM OF PRACTICAL SURGERY; with numerous Illus-

trations on Wood. Fourth Edition. Fcap. 8vo. cloth, 12s. 6d.

SIR JOHN FIFE, F.R.C.S. AND MR. URQUHART.

MANUAL OF THE TURKISH BATH. Heat a Mode of Cure and

a Source of Strength for Men and Animals. With Engravings. Post 8vo. cloth, 5s.

MR. FLOWER, F.R.C.S.

DIAGRAMS OF THE NERVES OF THE HUMAN BODY,

exhibiting their Origin, Divisions, and Connexions, with their Distribution to the various
Regions of the Cutaneous Surface, and to all the Muscles. Folio, containing Six
Plates, 14s.

MR. FOWNES, PH.D., F.R.S.

I.

A MANUAL OF CHEMISTRY; with 187 Illustrations on Wood.
Ninth Edition. Fcap. 8vo. cloth, 12s. 6d.
Edited by H. BENCE JONES, M.D., F.R.S., and A. W. HOFMANN, PH.D., F.R.S.

II.

CHEMISTRY, AS EXEMPLIFYING THE WISDOM AND
BENEFICENCE OF GOD. Second Edition. Fcap. 8vo. cloth, 4s. 6d.

III.

INTRODUCTION TO QUALITATIVE ANALYSIS. Post 8vo. cloth, 2s.

DR. D. J. T. FRANCIS.

CHANGE OF CLIMATE; considered as a Remedy in Dyspeptic, Pul-
monary, and other Chronic Affections; with an Account of the most Eligible Places of
Residence for Invalids, at different Seasons of the Year. Post 8vo. cloth, 8s. 6d.

DR. W. FRAZER.

ELEMENTS OF MATERIA MEDICA; containing the Chemistry
and Natural History of Drugs—their Effects, Doses, and Adulterations. Second Edition.
8vo. cloth, 10s. 6d.

MR. J. G. FRENCH, F.R.C.S.

THE NATURE OF CHOLERA INVESTIGATED. Second
Edition. 8vo. cloth, 4s.

C. REMIGIUS FRESENIUS.

A SYSTEM OF INSTRUCTION IN CHEMICAL ANALYSIS,
Edited by LLOYD BULLOCK, F.C.S.
QUALITATIVE. Sixth Edition, with Coloured Plate illustrating Spectrum Analysis. 8vo.
cloth, 10s. 6d.——QUANTITATIVE. Fourth Edition. 8vo. cloth, 18s.

DR. FULLER.

ON DISEASES OF THE CHEST, including Diseases of the Heart
and Great Vessels. With Engravings. 8vo. cloth, 12s. 6d.

II.

ON DISEASES OF THE HEART AND GREAT VESSELS.
8vo. cloth, 7s. 6d.   III.

ON RHEUMATISM, RHEUMATIC GOUT, AND SCIATICA:
their Pathology, Symptoms, and Treatment. Third Edition. 8vo. cloth, 12s. 6d.

DR. GAIRDNER.

ON GOUT; its History, its Causes, and its Cure. Fourth Edition. Post
8vo. cloth, 8s. 6d.

MR. GALLOWAY.

I.

THE FIRST STEP IN CHEMISTRY. Third Edition. Fcap. 8vo.
cloth, 5s.   II.

THE SECOND STEP IN CHEMISTRY; or, the Student's Guide to
the Higher Branches of the Science. With Engravings. 8vo. cloth, 10s.

III.

A MANUAL OF QUALITATIVE ANALYSIS. Fourth Edition.
Post 8vo. cloth, 6s. 6d.   IV.

CHEMICAL TABLES. On Five Large Sheets, for School and Lecture
Rooms. Second Edition. 4s. 6d.

MR. J. SAMPSON GAMGEE.

HISTORY OF A SUCCESSFUL CASE OF AMPUTATION AT
THE HIP-JOINT (the limb 48-in. in circumference, 99 pounds weight). With 4
Photographs. 4to cloth, 10s. 6d.

MR. F. J. GANT, F.R.C.S.

I.

THE PRINCIPLES OF SURGERY : Clinical, Medical, and Operative. With Engravings. 8vo. cloth, 18s.

II.

THE IRRITABLE BLADDER : its Causes and Curative Treatment. Post 8vo. cloth, 4s. 6d.

DR. GIBB, M.R.C.P.

ON DISEASES OF THE THROAT AND WINDPIPE, as reflected by the Laryngoscope. Second Edition. With 116 Engravings. Post 8vo. cloth, 10s. 6d.

MRS. GODFREY.

ON THE NATURE, PREVENTION, TREATMENT, AND CURE OF SPINAL CURVATURES and DEFORMITIES of the CHEST and LIMBS, without ARTIFICIAL SUPPORTS or any MECHANICAL APPLIANCES. Third Edition, Revised and Enlarged. 8vo. cloth, 5s.

DR. GORDON, M.D., C.B.

CHINA, FROM A MEDICAL POINT OF VIEW, IN 1860 AND 1861; With a Chapter on Nagasaki as a Sanatarium. With Plans. 8vo. cloth, 10s. 6d.

DR. GRANVILLE, F.R.S.

I.

THE MINERAL SPRINGS OF VICHY : their Efficacy in the Treatment of Gout, Indigestion, Gravel, &c. 8vo. cloth, 3s.

II.

ON SUDDEN DEATH. Post 8vo., 2s. 6d.

DR. GRAVES, M.D., F.R.S.

STUDIES IN PHYSIOLOGY AND MEDICINE. Edited by Dr. Stokes. With Portrait and Memoir. 8vo. cloth, 14s.

DR. S. C. GRIFFITH, M.D.

ON DERMATOLOGY AND THE TREATMENT OF SKIN DISEASES BY MEANS OF HERBS, IN PLACE OF ARSENIC AND MERCURY. Fcap. 8vo. cloth, 3s.

MR. GRIFFITHS.

CHEMISTRY OF THE FOUR SEASONS — Spring, Summer, Autumn, Winter. Illustrated with Engravings on Wood. Second Edition. Foolscap 8vo. cloth, 7s. 6d.

DR. GULLY.

THE SIMPLE TREATMENT OF DISEASE; deduced from the Methods of Expectancy and Revulsion. 18mo. cloth, 4s.

DR. GUY AND DR. JOHN HARLEY.

HOOPER'S PHYSICIAN'S VADE-MECUM; OR, MANUAL OF THE PRINCIPLES AND PRACTICE OF PHYSIC. Seventh Edition, considerably enlarged, and rewritten. Foolscap 8vo. cloth, 12s. 6d.

GUY'S HOSPITAL REPORTS. Third Series. Vols. I. to XI., 8vo., 7s. 6d. each.

DR. HABERSHON, F.R.C.P.

I.

PATHOLOGICAL AND PRACTICAL OBSERVATIONS ON DISEASES OF THE ABDOMEN, comprising those of the Stomach and other Parts of the Alimentary Canal, Œsophagus, Stomach, Cæcum, Intestines, and Peritoneum. Second Edition, with Plates. 8vo. cloth, 14s.   II.

ON THE INJURIOUS EFFECTS OF MERCURY IN THE TREATMENT OF DISEASE. Post 8vo. cloth, 3s. 6d.

DR. C. RADCLYFFE HALL.

TORQUAY IN ITS MEDICAL ASPECT AS A RESORT FOR
PULMONARY INVALIDS. Post 8vo. cloth, 5s.

DR. MARSHALL HALL, F.R.S.

PRONE AND POSTURAL RESPIRATION IN DROWNING
AND OTHER FORMS OF APNŒA OR SUSPENDED RESPIRATION.
Post 8vo. cloth. 5s.   II.

PRACTICAL OBSERVATIONS AND SUGGESTIONS IN MEDI-
CINE. Second Series. Post 8vo. cloth, 8s. 6d.

MR. HARDWICH.

A MANUAL OF PHOTOGRAPHIC CHEMISTRY. With
Engravings. Seventh Edition. Foolscap 8vo. cloth, 7s. 6d.

DR. J. BOWER HARRISON, M.D., M.R.C.P.
I.

LETTERS TO A YOUNG PRACTITIONER ON THE DIS-
EASES OF CHILDREN. Foolscap 8vo. cloth, 3s.

II.

ON THE CONTAMINATION OF WATER BY THE POISON
OF LEAD, and its Effects on the Human Body. Foolscap 8vo. cloth, 3s. 6d.

DR. HARTWIG.
I.

ON SEA BATHING AND SEA AIR. Second Edition. Fcap.
8vo., 2s. 6d.   II.

ON THE PHYSICAL EDUCATION OF CHILDREN. Fcap.
8vo., 2s. 6d.

DR. A. H. HASSALL.
I.

THE URINE, IN HEALTH AND DISEASE; being an Ex-
planation of the Composition of the Urine, and of the Pathology and Treatment of
Urinary and Renal Disorders. Second Edition. With 79 Engravings (23 Coloured).
Post 8vo. cloth, 12s. 6d.   II.

THE MICROSCOPIC ANATOMY OF THE HUMAN BODY,
IN HEALTH AND DISEASE. Illustrated with Several Hundred Drawings in
Colour. Two vols. 8vo. cloth, £1. 10s.

MR. ALFRED HAVILAND, M.R.C.S.

CLIMATE, WEATHER, AND DISEASE; being a Sketch of the
Opinions of the most celebrated Ancient and Modern Writers with regard to the Influence
of Climate and Weather in producing Disease. With Four coloured Engravings. 8vo.
cloth, 7s.

DR. HEADLAND.

ON THE ACTION OF MEDICINES IN THE SYSTEM.
Being the Prize Essay to which the Medical Society of London awarded the Fothergillian Gold Medal for 1852. Third Edition. 8vo. cloth, 12s. 6d.

DR. HEALE.
I.

A TREATISE ON THE PHYSIOLOGICAL ANATOMY OF
THE LUNGS. With Engravings. 8vo. cloth, 8s.

II.

A TREATISE ON VITAL CAUSES. 8vo. cloth, 9s.

MR. CHRISTOPHER HEATH, F.R.C.S.

I.
PRACTICAL ANATOMY: a Manual of Dissections. With numerous Engravings. Fcap. 8vo. cloth, 10s. 6d.

II.
A MANUAL OF MINOR SURGERY AND BANDAGING, FOR THE USE OF HOUSE-SURGEONS, DRESSERS, AND JUNIOR PRACTITIONERS. With Illustrations. Third Edition. Fcap. 8vo. cloth, 5s.

MR. HIGGINBOTTOM, F.R.S., F.R.C.S.E.

A PRACTICAL ESSAY ON THE USE OF THE NITRATE OF SILVER IN THE TREATMENT OF INFLAMMATION, WOUNDS, AND ULCERS. Third Edition, 8vo. cloth, 6s.

DR. HINDS.

THE HARMONIES OF PHYSICAL SCIENCE IN RELATION TO THE HIGHER SENTIMENTS; with Observations on Medical Studies, and on the Moral and Scientific Relations of Medical Life. Post 8vo. cloth, 4s.

MR. J. A. HINGESTON, M.R.C.S.

TOPICS OF THE DAY, MEDICAL, SOCIAL, AND SCIENTIFIC. Crown 8vo. cloth, 7s. 6d.

DR. HODGES.

THE NATURE, PATHOLOGY, AND TREATMENT OF PUERPERAL CONVULSIONS. Crown 8vo. cloth, 3s.

DR. DECIMUS HODGSON.

THE PROSTATE GLAND, AND ITS ENLARGEMENT IN OLD AGE. With 12 Plates. Royal 8vo. cloth, 6s.

MR. JABEZ HOGG.

A MANUAL OF OPHTHALMOSCOPIC SURGERY; being a Practical Treatise on the Use of the Ophthalmoscope in Diseases of the Eye. Third Edition. With Coloured Plates. 8vo. cloth, 10s. 6d.

MR. LUTHER HOLDEN, F.R.C.S.

I.
HUMAN OSTEOLOGY: with Plates, showing the Attachments of the Muscles. Third Edition. 8vo. cloth, 16s.

II.
A MANUAL OF THE DISSECTION OF THE HUMAN BODY. With Engravings on Wood. Second Edition. 8vo. cloth, 16s.

MR BARNARD HOLT, F.R.C.S.

ON THE IMMEDIATE TREATMENT OF STRICTURE OF THE URETHRA. Second Edition, Enlarged. 8vo. cloth, 3s.

DR. W. CHARLES HOOD.

SUGGESTIONS FOR THE FUTURE PROVISION OF CRIMINAL LUNATICS. 8vo. cloth, 5s. 6d.

DR. P. HOOD.

THE SUCCESSFUL TREATMENT OF SCARLET FEVER;
also, OBSERVATIONS ON THE PATHOLOGY AND TREATMENT OF CROWING INSPIRATIONS OF INFANTS. Post 8vo. cloth, 5s.

MR. JOHN HORSLEY.

A CATECHISM OF CHEMICAL PHILOSOPHY; being a Familiar
Exposition of the Principles of Chemistry and Physics. With Engravings on Wood. Designed for the Use of Schools and Private Teachers. Post 8vo. cloth, 6s. 6d.

MR. LUKE HOWARD, F.R.S.

ESSAY ON THE MODIFICATIONS OF CLOUDS. Third Edition,
by W. D. and E. HOWARD. With 6 Lithographic Plates, from Pictures by Kenyon. 4to. cloth, 10s. 6d.

DR. HAMILTON HOWE, M.D.

A THEORETICAL INQUIRY INTO THE PHYSICAL CAUSE
OF EPIDEMIC DISEASES. Accompanied with Tables. 8vo. cloth, 7s.

DR. HUFELAND.

THE ART OF PROLONGING LIFE. Second Edition. Edited
by ERASMUS WILSON, F.R.S. Foolscap 8vo., 2s. 6d.

MR. W. CURTIS HUGMAN, F.R.C.S.

ON HIP-JOINT DISEASE; with reference especially to Treatment
by Mechanical Means for the Relief of Contraction and Deformity of the Affected Limb. With Plates. Re-issue, enlarged. 8vo. cloth, 3s. 6d.

MR. HULKE, F.R.C.S.

A PRACTICAL TREATISE ON THE USE OF THE
OPHTHALMOSCOPE. Being the Jacksonian Prize Essay for 1859. Royal 8vo. cloth, 8s.

DR. HENRY HUNT.

ON HEARTBURN AND INDIGESTION. 8vo. cloth, 5s.

PROFESSOR HUXLEY, F.R.S.

LECTURES ON THE ELEMENTS OF COMPARATIVE
ANATOMY.—ON CLASSIFICATON AND THE SKULL. With 111 Illus. trations. 8vo. cloth, 10s. 6d.

MR. JONATHAN HUTCHINSON, F.R.C.S.

A CLINICAL MEMOIR ON CERTAIN DISEASES OF THE
EYE AND EAR, CONSEQUENT ON INHERITED SYPHILIS; with an appended Chapter of Commentaries on the Transmission of Syphilis from Parent to Offspring, and its more remote Consequences. With Plates and Woodcuts, 8vo. cloth, 9s.

DR. INMAN, M.R.C.P.

I.

ON MYALGIA: ITS NATURE, CAUSES, AND TREATMENT;
being a Treatise on Painful and other Affections of the Muscular System. Second Edition. 8vo. cloth, 9s.

II.

FOUNDATION FOR A NEW THEORY AND PRACTICE
OF MEDICINE. Second Edition. Crown 8vo. cloth, 10s.

DR. ARTHUR JACOB, F.R.C.S.

A TREATISE ON THE INFLAMMATIONS OF THE EYE-BALL.
Foolscap 8vo. cloth, 5s.

DR. JAGO, M.D.OXON, A.B.CANTAB.

ENTOPTICS, WITH ITS USES IN PHYSIOLOGY AND
MEDICINE. With 54 Engravings. Crown 8vo. cloth, 5s.

MR. J. H. JAMES, F.R.C.S.

PRACTICAL OBSERVATIONS ON THE OPERATIONS FOR
STRANGULATED HERNIA. 8vo. cloth, 5s.

DR. PROSSER JAMES, M.D.

SORE-THROAT: ITS NATURE, VARIETIES, AND TREAT-
MENT; including the Use of the LARYNGOSCOPE as an Aid to Diagnosis. Post
8vo. cloth, 4s. 6d.

DR. HANDFIELD JONES, M.B., F.R.C.P.

CLINICAL OBSERVATIONS ON FUNCTIONAL NERVOUS
DISORDERS. Post 8vo. cloth, 10s. 6d.

DR. HANDFIELD JONES, F.R.S., & DR. EDWARD H. SIEVEKING.

A MANUAL OF PATHOLOGICAL ANATOMY. Illustrated with
numerous Engravings on Wood. Foolscap 8vo. cloth, 12s. 6d.

DR. JAMES JONES, M.D., M.R.C.P.

ON THE USE OF PERCHLORIDE OF IRON AND OTHER
CHALYBEATE SALTS IN THE TREATMENT OF CONSUMPTION. Crown
8vo. cloth, 3s. 6d.

MR. WHARTON JONES, F.R.S.
I.

A MANUAL OF THE PRINCIPLES AND PRACTICE OF
OPHTHALMIC MEDICINE AND SURGERY; with Nine Coloured Plates and
173 Wood Engravings. Third Edition, thoroughly revised. Foolscap 8vo. cloth, 12s. 6d.

II.

THE WISDOM AND BENEFICENCE OF THE ALMIGHTY,
AS DISPLAYED IN THE SENSE OF VISION; being the Actonian Prize Essay
for 1851. With Illustrations on Steel and Wood. Foolscap 8vo. cloth, 4s. 6d.

III.

DEFECTS OF SIGHT: their Nature, Causes, Prevention, and General
Management. Second Edition. Fcap. 8vo. 2s. 6d.

A CATECHISM OF THE MEDICINE AND SURGERY OF
THE EYE AND EAR. For the Clinical Use of Hospital Students. Fcap. 8vo. 2s. 6d.

V.

A CATECHISM OF THE PHYSIOLOGY AND PHILOSOPHY
OF BODY, SENSE, AND MIND. For Use in Schools and Colleges. Fcap. 8vo.,
2s. 6d.

MR. FURNEAUX JORDAN, M.R.C.S.

AN INTRODUCTION TO CLINICAL SURGERY; WITH A
Method of Investigating and Reporting Surgical Cases. Fcap. 8vo. cloth, 5s.

MR. JUDD.

A PRACTICAL TREATISE ON URETHRITIS AND SYPHI-
LIS: including Observations on the Power of the Menstruous Fluid, and of the Dis-
charge from Leucorrhœa and Sores to produce Urethritis: with a variety of Examples,
Experiments, Remedies, and Cures. 8vo. cloth, £1. 5s.

DR. LAENNEC.

A MANUAL OF AUSCULTATION AND PERCUSSION. Trans-
lated and Edited by J. B. SHARPE, M.R.C.S. 3s.

DR. LANE, M.A.

HYDROPATHY; OR, HYGIENIC MEDICINE. An Explanatory
Essay. Second Edition. Post 8vo. cloth, 5s.

MR. LAWRENCE, F.R.S.

I.

LECTURES ON SURGERY. 8vo. cloth, 16s.

II.

A TREATISE ON RUPTURES. The Fifth Edition, considerably
enlarged. 8vo. cloth, 16s.

DR. LEARED, M.R.C.P.

IMPERFECT DIGESTION: ITS CAUSES AND TREATMENT.
Fourth Edition. Foolscap 8vo. cloth, 4s.

DR. EDWIN LEE.

I.

THE EFFECT OF CLIMATE ON TUBERCULOUS DISEASE,
with Notices of the chief Foreign Places of Winter Resort. Small 8vo. cloth, 4s. 6d.

II.

THE WATERING PLACES OF ENGLAND, CONSIDERED
with Reference to their Medical Topography. Fourth Edition. Fcap. 8vo. cloth, 7s. 6d.

III.

THE BATHS OF GERMANY. Fourth Edition. Post 8vo. cloth, 7s.

IV.

THE BATHS OF SWITZERLAND. 12mo. cloth, 3s. 6d.

V.

HOMŒOPATHY AND HYDROPATHY IMPARTIALLY AP-
PRECIATED. With Notes illustrative of the Influence of the Mind over the Body.
Fourth Edition. Post 8vo. cloth, 3s. 6d.

MR. HENRY LEE, F.R.C.S.

I.

ON SYPHILIS. Second Edition. With Coloured Plates. 8vo. cloth, 10s.

II.

ON DISEASES OF THE VEINS, HÆMORRHOIDAL TUMOURS,
AND OTHER AFFECTIONS OF THE RECTUM. Second Edition. 8vo. cloth, 8s.

DR. ROBERT LEE, F.R.S.

I.

CONSULTATIONS IN MIDWIFERY. Foolscap 8vo. cloth, 4s. 6d.

II.

A TREATISE ON THE SPECULUM; with Three Hundred Cases.
8vo. cloth, 4s. 6d.

III.

CLINICAL REPORTS OF OVARIAN AND UTERINE DIS-
EASES, with Commentaries. Foolscap 8vo. cloth, 6s. 6d.

IV.

CLINICAL MIDWIFERY: comprising the Histories of 545 Cases of
Difficult, Preternatural, and Complicated Labour, with Commentaries. Second Edition.
Foolscap 8vo. cloth, 5s.

DR LEISHMAN, M.D., F.F.P.S.

THE MECHANISM OF PARTURITION: An Essay, Historical and
Critical. With Engravings. 8vo. cloth, 5s.

MR. LISTON, F.R.S.

PRACTICAL SURGERY. Fourth Edition. 8vo. cloth, 22s.

MR. H. W. LOBB, L.S.A., M.R.C.S.E.

ON SOME OF THE MORE OBSCURE FORMS OF NERVOUS AFFECTIONS, THEIR PATHOLOGY AND TREATMENT. Re-issue, with the Chapter on Galvanism entirely Re-written. With Engravings. 8vo. cloth, 8s.

DR. LOGAN, M.D., M.R.C.P.LOND.

ON OBSTINATE DISEASES OF THE SKIN. Foolscap 8vo. cloth, 2s. 6d.

LONDON HOSPITAL.

CLINICAL LECTURES AND REPORTS BY THE MEDICAL AND SURGICAL STAFF. With Illustrations. Vols. I. and II. 8vo. cloth, 7s. 6d.

LONDON MEDICAL SOCIETY OF OBSERVATION.

WHAT TO OBSERVE AT THE BED-SIDE, AND AFTER DEATH. Published by Authority. Second Edition. Foolscap 8vo. cloth, 4s. 6d.

DR. MACKENZIE, M.D., M.R.C.P.

THE PATHOLOGY AND TREATMENT OF PHLEGMASIA DOLENS, as deduced from Clinical and Physiological Researches. Lettsomian Lectures on Midwifery. 8vo. cloth, 6s.

MR. M'CLELLAND, F.L.S., F.G.S.

THE MEDICAL TOPOGRAPHY, OR CLIMATE AND SOILS, OF BENGAL AND THE N. W. PROVINCES. Post 8vo. cloth, 4s. 6d.

DR. MACLACHLAN, M.D., F.R.C.P.L.

THE DISEASES AND INFIRMITIES OF ADVANCED LIFE. 8vo. cloth, 16s.

DR. GEORGE H. B. MACLEOD, F.R.C.S.E.

I.

OUTLINES OF SURGICAL DIAGNOSIS. 8vo. cloth, 12s. 6d.

II.

NOTES ON THE SURGERY OF THE CRIMEAN WAR; with REMARKS on GUN-SHOT WOUNDS. 8vo. cloth, 10s. 6d.

MR. JOSEPH MACLISE, F.R.C.S.

I.

SURGICAL ANATOMY. A Series of Dissections, illustrating the Principal Regions of the Human Body.
The Second Edition, imperial folio, cloth, £3. 12s.; half-morocco, £4. 4s.

II.

ON DISLOCATIONS AND FRACTURES. This Work is Uniform with the Author's "Surgical Anatomy;" each Fasciculus contains Four beautifully executed Lithographic Drawings. Imperial folio, cloth, £2. 10s.; half-morocco, £2. 17s.

DR. McNICOLL, M.R.C.P.

A HAND-BOOK FOR SOUTHPORT, MEDICAL & GENERAL; with Copious Notices of the Natural History of the District. Second Edition. Post 8vo. cloth, 3s. 6d.

DR. J. MACPHERSON, M.D.

CHOLERA IN ITS HOME; with a Sketch of the Pathology and Treatment of the Disease. Crown 8vo. cloth, 5s.

DR. MARCET, F.R.S.

I.

ON THE COMPOSITION OF FOOD, AND HOW IT IS ADULTERATED; with Practical Directions for its Analysis. 8vo. cloth, 6s. 6d.

II.

ON CHRONIC ALCOHOLIC INTOXICATION; with an INQUIRY INTO THE INFLUENCE OF THE ABUSE OF ALCOHOL AS A PRE-DISPOSING CAUSE OF DISEASE. Second Edition, much enlarged. Foolscap 8vo. cloth, 4s. 6d.

DR. MARKHAM.

I.

DISEASES OF THE HEART: THEIR PATHOLOGY, DIAG-

NOSIS, AND TREATMENT. Second Edition. Post 8vo. cloth, 6s.

II.

SKODA ON AUSCULTATION AND PERCUSSION. Post 8vo.

cloth, 6s.

SIR RANALD MARTIN, K.C.B., F.R.S.

INFLUENCE OF TROPICAL CLIMATES IN PRODUCING

THE ACUTE ENDEMIC DISEASES OF EUROPEANS; including Practical Observations on their Chronic Sequelæ under the Influences of the Climate of Europe. Second Edition, much enlarged. 8vo. cloth, 20s.

DR. MASSY.

ON THE EXAMINATION OF RECRUITS; intended for the Use of

Young Medical Officers on Entering the Army. 8vo. cloth, 5s.

MR. C. F. MAUNDER, F.R.C.S.

OPERATIVE SURGERY. With 158 Engravings. Post 8vo. 6s.

DR. MAYNE.

I.

AN EXPOSITORY LEXICON OF THE TERMS, ANCIENT

AND MODERN, IN MEDICAL AND GENERAL SCIENCE, including a complete MEDICAL AND MEDICO-LEGAL VOCABULARY. Complete in 10 Parts, price 5s. each. The entire work, cloth, £2. 10s.

II.

A MEDICAL VOCABULARY; or, an Explanation of all Names,

Synonymes, Terms, and Phrases used in Medicine and the relative branches of Medical Science, intended specially as a Book of Reference for the Young Student. Second Edition. Fcap. 8vo. cloth, 8s. 6d.

DR. MERYON, M.D., F.R.C.P.

PATHOLOGICAL AND PRACTICAL RESEARCHES ON THE

VARIOUS FORMS OF PARALYSIS. 8vo. cloth, 6s.

DR. MILLINGEN.

ON THE TREATMENT AND MANAGEMENT OF THE IN-

SANE; with Considerations on Public and Private Lunatic Asylums. 18mo. cloth, 4s. 6d.

DR. W. J. MOORE, M.D.

I.

HEALTH IN THE TROPICS; or, Sanitary Art applied to Europeans

in India. 8vo. cloth, 9s.

II.

A MANUAL OF THE DISEASES OF INDIA. Fcap. 8vo. cloth, 5s.

PROFESSOR MULDER, UTRECHT.

THE CHEMISTRY OF WINE. Edited by H. BENCE JONES, M.D.,

F.R.S. Fcap. 8vo. cloth, 6s.

DR. BIRKBECK NEVINS.

THE PRESCRIBER'S ANALYSIS OF THE BRITISH PHAR-

MACOPEIA. Third Edition, enlarged to 295 pp. 32mo. cloth, 3s. 6d.

DR. NOBLE.

THE HUMAN MIND IN ITS RELATIONS WITH THE BRAIN AND NERVOUS SYSTEM. Post 8vo. cloth, 4s. 6d.

MR. NUNNELEY, F.R.C.S.E.

I.

ON THE ORGANS OF VISION: THEIR ANATOMY AND PHYSIOLOGY. With Plates, 8vo. cloth, 15s.

II.

A TREATISE ON THE NATURE, CAUSES, AND TREATMENT OF ERYSIPELAS. 8vo. cloth, 10s. 6d.

DR. O'REILLY.

THE PLACENTA, THE ORGANIC NERVOUS SYSTEM, THE BLOOD, THE OXYGEN, AND THE ANIMAL NERVOUS SYSTEM, PHYSIOLOGICALLY EXAMINED. With Engravings. 8vo. cloth, 5s.

MR. LANGSTON PARKER.

THE MODERN TREATMENT OF SYPHILITIC DISEASES, both Primary and Secondary; comprising the Treatment of Constitutional and Confirmed Syphilis, by a safe and successful Method. Fourth Edition, 8vo. cloth, 10s.

DR. PARKES, F.R.S., F.R.C.P.

I.

A MANUAL OF PRACTICAL HYGIENE; intended especially for the Medical Officers of the Army. With Plates and Woodcuts. 2nd Edition, 8vo. cloth, 16s.

II.

THE URINE: ITS COMPOSITION IN HEALTH AND DISEASE, AND UNDER THE ACTION OF REMEDIES. 8vo. cloth, 12s.

DR. PARKIN, M.D., F.R.C.S.

THE CAUSATION AND PREVENTION OF DISEASE; with the Laws regulating the Extrication of Malaria from the Surface, and its Diffusion in the surrounding Air. 8vo. cloth, 5s.

MR. JAMES PART, F.R.C.S.

THE MEDICAL AND SURGICAL POCKET CASE BOOK, for the Registration of important Cases in Private Practice, and to assist the Student of Hospital Practice. Second Edition. 2s. 6d.

DR. PAVY, M.D., F.R.S., F.R.C.P.

DIABETES : RESEARCHES ON ITS NATURE AND TREATMENT. 8vo. cloth, 8s. 6d.

DR. PEACOCK, M.D., F.R.C.P.

ON SOME OF THE CAUSES AND EFFECTS OF VALVULAR DISEASE OF THE HEART. With Engravings. 8vo. cloth, 5s.

DR. PEET, M.D., F.R.C.P.

THE PRINCIPLES AND PRACTICE OF MEDICINE; Designed chiefly for Students of Indian Medical Colleges. 8vo. cloth, 16s.

DR. PEREIRA, F.R.S.

SELECTA E PRÆSCRIPTIS. Fourteenth Edition. 24mo. cloth, 5s.

DR. PICKFORD.

HYGIENE; or, Health as Depending upon the Conditions of the Atmosphere, Food and Drinks, Motion and Rest, Sleep and Wakefulness, Secretions, Excretions, and Retentions, Mental Emotions, Clothing, Bathing, &c. Vol. I. 8vo. cloth, 9s.

MR. PIRRIE, F.R.S.E.

THE PRINCIPLES AND PRACTICE OF SURGERY. With
numerous Engravings on Wood. Second Edition. 8vo. cloth, 24s.

**PHARMACOPŒIA COLLEGII REGALIS MEDICORUM LON-
DINENSIS.** 8vo. cloth, 9s.; or 24mo. 5s.
IMPRIMATUR.
Hic liber, cui titulus, PHARMACOPŒIA COLLEGII REGALIS MEDICORUM LONDINENSIS.
Datum ex Ædibus Collegii in comitiis censoriis, Novembris Mensis 14to 1850.
                  JOHANNES AYRTON PARIS. *Præses.*

PROFESSORS PLATTNER & MUSPRATT.

THE USE OF THE BLOWPIPE IN THE EXAMINATION OF
MINERALS, ORES, AND OTHER METALLIC COMBINATIONS. Illustrated
by numerous Engravings on Wood. Third Edition. 8vo. cloth, 10s. 6d.

DR. HENRY F. A. PRATT, M.D., M.R.C.P.
I.

THE GENEALOGY OF CREATION, newly Translated from the
Unpointed Hebrew Text of the Book of Genesis, showing the General Scientific Accuracy
of the Cosmogony of Moses and the Philosophy of Creation. 8vo. cloth, 14s.
II.

ON ECCENTRIC AND CENTRIC FORCE: A New Theory of
Projection. With Engravings. 8vo. cloth, 10s.
III.

ON ORBITAL MOTION: The Outlines of a System of Physical
Astronomy. With Diagrams. 8vo. cloth, 7s. 6d.
IV.

ASTRONOMICAL INVESTIGATIONS. The Cosmical Relations of
the Revolution of the Lunar Apsides. Oceanic Tides. With Engravings. 8vo. cloth, 5s.
V.

THE ORACLES OF GOD: An Attempt at a Re-interpretation. Part I.
The Revealed Cosmos. 8vo. cloth, 10s.

THE PRESCRIBER'S PHARMACOPŒIA; containing all the Medi-
cines in the British Pharmacopœia, arranged in Classes according to their Action, with
their Composition and Doses. By a Practising Physician. Fifth Edition. 32mo.
cloth, 2s. 6d.; roan tuck (for the pocket), 3s. 6d.

DR. JOHN ROWLISON PRETTY.

AIDS DURING LABOUR, including the Administration of Chloroform,
the Management of Placenta and Post-partum Hæmorrhage. Fcap. 8vo. cloth, 4s. 6d.

MR. LAKE PRICE.

PHOTOGRAPHIC MANIPULATION; Treating of the Practice of
the Art, and its various appliances to Nature. With Fifty Engravings on Wood. Post
8vo. cloth, 6s. 6d.

MR. P. C. PRICE, F.R.C.S.

AN ESSAY ON EXCISION OF THE KNEE-JOINT. With
Coloured Plates. With Memoir of the Author and Notes by Henry Smith, F.R.C.S.
Royal 8vo. cloth, 14s.

DR. PRIESTLEY.

**LECTURES ON THE DEVELOPMENT OF THE GRAVID
UTERUS.** 8vo. cloth, 5s. 6d.

DR. RADCLIFFE, F.R.C.P.L.

LECTURES ON EPILEPSY, PAIN, PARALYSIS, AND
CERTAIN OTHER DISORDERS OF THE NERVOUS SYSTEM, delivered at
the Royal College of Physicians in London. Post 8vo. cloth, 7s. 6d.

MR. RAINEY.

ON THE MODE OF FORMATION OF SHELLS OF ANIM

OF BONE, AND OF SEVERAL OTHER STRUCTURES, by a Proce
Molecular Coalescence, Demonstrable in certain Artificially-formed Products. Fcap
cloth, 4s. 6d.

DR. F. H. RAMSBOTHAM.

THE PRINCIPLES AND PRACTICE OF OBSTETRIC M

CINE AND SURGERY. Illustrated with One Hundred and Twenty Plates on
and Wood; forming one thick handsome volume. Fourth Edition. 8vo. cloth, 22

DR. RAMSBOTHAM.

PRACTICAL OBSERVATIONS ON MIDWIFERY, with a Sele

of Cases. Second Edition. 8vo. cloth, 12s.

PROFESSOR REDWOOD, PH.D.

A SUPPLEMENT TO THE PHARMACOPŒIA: A concis

comprehensive Dispensatory, and Manual of Facts and Formulæ, for the use of
tioners in Medicine and Pharmacy. Third Edition. 8vo. cloth, 22s.

DR. DU BOIS REYMOND.

ANIMAL ELECTRICITY; Edited by H. Bence Jones, M.D., F

With Fifty Engravings on Wood. Foolscap 8vo. cloth, 6s.

DR. REYNOLDS, M.D LOND.

I.

EPILEPSY: ITS SYMPTOMS, TREATMENT, AND RELAT

TO OTHER CHRONIC CONVULSIVE DISEASES. 8vo. cloth, 10s.

II.

THE DIAGNOSIS OF DISEASES OF THE BRAIN, SPI

CORD, AND THEIR APPENDAGES. 8vo. cloth, 8s.

DR. B. W. RICHARDSON.

I.

ON THE CAUSE OF THE COAGULATION OF THE BL

Being the Astley Cooper Prize Essay for 1856. With a Practical App
8vo. cloth, 16s.

II.

THE HYGIENIC TREATMENT OF PULMONARY CONSU

TION. 8vo. cloth, 5s. 6d.

III.

THE ASCLEPIAD. Vol. I., Clinical Essays. 8vo. cloth, 6s. 6d.

DR. RITCHIE, M.D.

ON OVARIAN PHYSIOLOGY AND PATHOLOGY.

Engravings. 8vo. cloth, 6s.

DR. WILLIAM ROBERTS, M.D., F.R.C.P.

AN ESSAY ON WASTING PALSY; being a Systematic Treatis

the Disease hitherto described as ATROPHIE MUSCULAIRE PROGRESS
With Four Plates. 8vo. cloth, 5s.

DR. ROUTH.

INFANT FEEDING, AND ITS INFLUENCE ON LI

Or, the Causes and Prevention of Infant Mortality. Second Edition. Fcap. 8vo. clot

DR. W. H. ROBERTSON.

I.

THE NATURE AND TREATMENT OF GOUT. 8vo. cloth, 10s. 6d.

II.

A TREATISE ON DIET AND REGIMEN. Fourth Edition. 2 vols. 12s. post 8vo. cloth.

DR. ROWE.

NERVOUS DISEASES, LIVER AND STOMACH COM-PLAINTS, LOW SPIRITS, INDIGESTION, GOUT, ASTHMA, AND DIS-ORDERS PRODUCED BY TROPICAL CLIMATES. With Cases. Sixteenth Edition. Fcap. 8vo. 2s. 6d.

DR. ROYLE, F.R.S., AND DR. HEADLAND, M.D.

A MANUAL OF MATERIA MEDICA AND THERAPEUTICS. With numerous Engravings on Wood. Fourth Edition. Fcap. 8vo. cloth, 12s. 6d.

DR. RYAN, M.D.

INFANTICIDE: ITS LAW, PREVALENCE, PREVENTION, AND HISTORY. 8vo. cloth, 5s.

ST. BARTHOLOMEW'S HOSPITAL.

A DESCRIPTIVE CATALOGUE OF THE ANATOMICAL MUSEUM. Vol. I. (1846), Vol. II. (1851), Vol. III. (1862), 8vo. cloth, 5s. each.

MR. T. P. SALT, BIRMINGHAM.

A PRACTICAL TREATISE ON RUPTURE: ITS CAUSES, MANAGEMENT, AND CURE. And the various Mechanical Contrivances employed for its Relief. With Engravings. Post 8vo. cloth, 3s.

DR. SALTER, F.R.S.

ON ASTHMA: its Pathology, Causes, Consequences, and Treatment. 8vo. cloth, 10s.

DR. SANKEY, M.D.LOND.

LECTURES ON MENTAL DISEASES. 8vo. cloth, 8s.

DR. SANSOM, M.B.LOND.

CHLOROFORM: ITS ACTION AND ADMINISTRATION. A Hand-book. With Engravings. Crown 8vo. cloth, 5s.

MR. SAVORY.

A COMPENDIUM OF DOMESTIC MEDICINE, AND COMPA-NION TO THE MEDICINE CHEST; intended as a Source of Easy Reference for Clergymen, and for Families residing at a Distance from Professional Assistance. Seventh Edition. 12mo. cloth, 5s.

DR. SCHACHT.

THE MICROSCOPE, AND ITS APPLICATION TO VEGETABLE ANATOMY AND PHYSIOLOGY. Edited by Frederick Currey, M.A. Fcap. 8vo. cloth, 6s.

DR. SCORESBY-JACKSON, M.D., F.R.S.E.

MEDICAL CLIMATOLOGY; or, a Topographical and Meteorological Description of the Localities resorted to in Winter and Summer by Invalids of various classes both at Home and Abroad. With an Isothermal Chart. Post 8vo. cloth, 12s.

DR. SEMPLE.

ON COUGH: its Causes, Varieties, and Treatment. With some practical Remarks on the Use of the Stethoscope as an aid to Diagnosis. Post 8vo. cloth, 4s. 6d.

DR. SEYMOUR.

I.

ILLUSTRATIONS OF SOME OF THE PRINCIPAL DIS-
EASES OF THE OVARIA: their Symptoms and Treatment; to which are prefixed
Observations on the Structure and Functions of those parts in the Human Being and in
Animals. With 14 folio plates, 12s.

II.

THE NATURE AND TREATMENT OF DROPSY; considered
especially in reference to the Diseases of the Internal Organs of the Body, which most
commonly produce it. 8vo. 5s.

DR. SHAPTER, M.D., F.R.C.P.

THE CLIMATE OF THE SOUTH OF DEVON, AND ITS
INFLUENCE UPON HEALTH. Second Edition, with Maps. 8vo. cloth, 10s. 6d.

MR. SHAW, M.R.C.S.

THE MEDICAL REMEMBRANCER; OR, BOOK OF EMER-
GENCIES: in which are concisely pointed out the Immediate Remedies to be adopted
in the First Moments of Danger from Drowning, Poisoning, Apoplexy, Burns, and other
Accidents; with the Tests for the Principal Poisons, and other useful Information.
Fourth Edition. Edited, with Additions, by JONATHAN HUTCHINSON, F.R.C.S. 32mo.
cloth, 2s. 6d.

DR. SHEA, M.D., B.A.

A MANUAL OF ANIMAL PHYSIOLOGY. With an Appendix of
Questions for the B.A. London and other Examinations. With Engravings. Foolscap
8vo. cloth, 5s. 6d.

DR. SIBSON, F.R.S.

MEDICAL ANATOMY. With coloured Plates. Imperial folio. Fasci-
culi I. to VI. 5s. each.

DR. E. H. SIEVEKING.

ON EPILEPSY AND EPILEPTIFORM SEIZURES: their
Causes, Pathology, and Treatment. Second Edition. Post 8vo. cloth, 10s. 6d.

MR. SINCLAIR AND DR. JOHNSTON.

PRACTICAL MIDWIFERY: Comprising an Account of 13,748 Deli-
veries, which occurred in the Dublin Lying-in Hospital, during a period of Seven Years.
8vo. cloth, 15s.

DR. SIORDET, M.B.LOND., M.R.C.P.

MENTONE IN ITS MEDICAL ASPECT. Foolscap 8vo. cloth, 2s. 6d.

MR. ALFRED SMEE, FRS.

GENERAL DEBILITY AND DEFECTIVE NUTRITION; their
Causes, Consequences, and Treatment. Second Edition. Fcap. 8vo. cloth, 3s. 6d.

DR. SMELLIE.

OBSTETRIC PLATES: being a Selection from the more Important and
Practical Illustrations contained in the Original Work. With Anatomical and Practical
Directions. 8vo. cloth, 5s.

MR. HENRY SMITH, F.R.C.S.

I.

ON STRICTURE OF THE URETHRA. 8vo. cloth, 7s. 6d.

II.

HÆMORRHOIDS AND PROLAPSUS OF THE RECTUM:
Their Pathology and Treatment, with especial reference to the use of Nitric Acid. Third
Edition. Fcap. 8vo. cloth, 3s.

III.

THE SURGERY OF THE RECTUM. Lettsomian Lectures. Fcap.
8vo. 2s. 6d.

DR. J. SMITH, M.D., F.R.C.S.EDIN.

HANDBOOK OF DENTAL ANATOMY AND SURGERY, FOR
THE USE OF STUDENTS AND PRACTITIONERS. Fcap. 3vo. cloth, 3s. 6d.

DR. W. TYLER SMITH.
I.

A MANUAL OF OBSTETRICS, THEORETICAL AND PRAC-
TICAL. Illustrated with 186 Engravings. Fcap. 8vo. cloth, 12s. 6d.
II.

THE PATHOLOGY AND TREATMENT OF LEUCORRHŒA.
With Engravings on Wood. 8vo. cloth, 7s.

DR. SNOW.

ON CHLOROFORM AND OTHER ANÆSTHETICS: THEIR
ACTION AND ADMINISTRATION. Edited, with a Memoir of the Author, by
Benjamin W. Richardson, M.D. 8vo. cloth, 10s. 6d.

MR. J. VOSE SOLOMON, F.R.C.S.

TENSION OF THE EYEBALL; GLAUCOMA: some Account of
the Operations practised in the 19th Century. 8vo. cloth, 4s.

DR. STANHOPE TEMPLEMAN SPEER.

PATHOLOGICAL CHEMISTRY, IN ITS APPLICATION TO
THE PRACTICE OF MEDICINE. Translated from the French of MM. BECQUEREL
and RODIER. 8vo. cloth, reduced to 8s.

MR. PETER SQUIRE.
I.

A COMPANION TO THE BRITISH PHARMACOPÆIA.
Third Edition. 8vo. cloth, 8s. 6d.
II.

THE PHARMACOPÆIAS OF THIRTEEN OF THE LONDON
HOSPITALS, arranged in Groups for easy Reference and Comparison. 18mo. cloth,
3s. 6d.

DR. STEGGALL.
STUDENTS' BOOKS FOR EXAMINATION.
I.

A MEDICAL MANUAL FOR APOTHECARIES' HALL AND OTHER MEDICAL
BOARDS. Twelfth Edition. 12mo. cloth, 10s.
II.

A MANUAL FOR THE COLLEGE OF SURGEONS; intended for the Use
of Candidates for Examination and Practitioners. Second Edition. 12mo. cloth, 10s.
III.

GREGORY'S CONSPECTUS MEDICINÆ THEORETICÆ. The First Part, con-
taining the Original Text, with an Ordo Verborum, and Literal Translation. 12mo.
cloth, 10s.
IV.

THE FIRST FOUR BOOKS OF CELSUS; containing the Text, Ordo Verb-
orum, and Translation. Second Edition. 12mo. cloth, 8s.
V.

FIRST LINES FOR CHEMISTS AND DRUGGISTS PREPARING FOR EX-
AMINATION AT THE PHARMACEUTICAL SOCIETY. Second Edition.
18mo. cloth, 3s. 6d.

MR. STOWE, M.R.C.S.

A TOXICOLOGICAL CHART, exhibiting at one view the Symptoms, Treatment, and Mode of Detecting the various Poisons, Mineral, Vegetable, and Animal. To which are added, concise Directions for the Treatment of Suspended Animation. Twelfth Edition, revised. On Sheet, 2s.; mounted on Roller, 5s.

MR. FRANCIS SUTTON, F.C.S.

A SYSTEMATIC HANDBOOK OF VOLUMETRIC ANALYSIS; or, the Quantitative Estimation of Chemical Substances by Measure. With Engravings. Post 8vo. cloth, 7s. 6d.

DR. SWAYNE.

OBSTETRIC APHORISMS FOR THE USE OF STUDENTS COMMENCING MIDWIFERY PRACTICE. With Engravings on Wood. Third Edition. Fcap. 8vo. cloth, 3s. 6d.

MR. TAMPLIN, F.R.C.S.E.

LATERAL CURVATURE OF THE SPINE: its Causes, Nature, and Treatment. 8vo. cloth, 4s.

DR. ALEXANDER TAYLOR, F.R.S.E.

THE CLIMATE OF PAU; with a Description of the Watering Places of the Pyrenees, and of the Virtues of their respective Mineral Sources in Disease. Third Edition. Post 8vo. cloth, 7s.

DR. ALFRED S. TAYLOR, F.R.S.

I.

THE PRINCIPLES AND PRACTICE OF MEDICAL JURIS-PRUDENCE. With 176 Wood Engravings. 8vo. cloth, 28s.

II.

A MANUAL OF MEDICAL JURISPRUDENCE. Eighth Edition. With Engravings. Fcap. 8vo. cloth, 12s. 6d.

III.

ON POISONS, in relation to MEDICAL JURISPRUDENCE AND MEDICINE. Second Edition. Fcap. 8vo. cloth, 12s. 6d.

MR. TEALE.

ON AMPUTATION BY A LONG AND A SHORT RECTAN-GULAR FLAP. With Engravings on Wood. 8vo. cloth, 5s.

DR. THEOPHILUS THOMPSON, F.R.S.

CLINICAL LECTURES ON PULMONARY CONSUMPTION; with additional Chapters by E. SYMES THOMPSON, M.D. With Plates. 8vo. cloth, 7s. 6d.

DR. THOMAS.

THE MODERN PRACTICE OF PHYSIC; exhibiting the Symptoms, Causes, Morbid Appearances, and Treatment of the Diseases of all Climates. Eleventh Edition. Revised by ALGERNON FRAMPTON, M.D. 2 vols. 8vo. cloth, 28s.

MR. HENRY THOMPSON, F.R.C.S.

I.

STRICTURE OF THE URETHRA; its Pathology and Treatment. The Jacksonian Prize Essay for 1852. With Plates. Second Edition. 8vo. cloth, 10s.

II.

THE DISEASES OF THE PROSTATE; their Pathology and Treatment. Comprising a Dissertation "On the Healthy and Morbid Anatomy of the Prostate Gland;" being the Jacksonian Prize Essay for 1860. With Plates. Second Edition. 8vo. cloth, 10s.

III.

PRACTICAL LITHOTOMY AND LITHOTRITY; or, An Inquiry into the best Modes of removing Stone from the Bladder. With numerous Engravings, 8vo. cloth, 9s.

DR. THUDICHUM.

I.

A TREATISE ON THE PATHOLOGY OF THE URINE,

Including a complete Guide to its Analysis. With Plates, 8vo. cloth, 14s.

II.

A TREATISE ON GALL STONES: their Chemistry, Pathology,

and Treatment. With Coloured Plates. 8vo. cloth, 10s.

DR. TILT.

I.

ON UTERINE AND OVARIAN INFLAMMATION, AND ON

THE PHYSIOLOGY AND DISEASES OF MENSTRUATION. Third Edition.
8vo. cloth, 12s.

II.

A HANDBOOK OF UTERINE THERAPEUTICS, AND OF

MODERN PATHOLOGY OF DISEASES OF WOMEN. Second Edition.
Post 8vo. cloth, 6s.

III.

THE CHANGE OF LIFE IN HEALTH AND DISEASE: a

Practical Treatise on the Nervous and other Affections incidental to Women at the Decline
of Life. Second Edition. 8vo. cloth, 6s.

DR. GODWIN TIMMS.

CONSUMPTION: its True Nature and Successful Treatment. Crown

8vo. cloth, 10s.

DR. ROBERT B. TODD, F.R.S.

I.

CLINICAL LECTURES ON THE PRACTICE OF MEDICINE.

New Edition, in one Volume, Edited by DR. BEALE, *8vo. cloth,* 18s.

II.

ON CERTAIN DISEASES OF THE URINARY ORGANS, AND

ON DROPSIES. Fcap. 8vo. cloth, 6s.

MR. TOMES, F.R.S.

A MANUAL OF DENTAL SURGERY. With 208 Engravings on

Wood. Fcap. 8vo. cloth, 12s. 6d.

MR. JOSEPH TOYNBEE, F.R.S., F.R.C.S.

THE DISEASES OF THE EAR: THEIR NATURE, DIAG-

NOSIS, AND TREATMENT. Illustrated with numerous Engravings on Wood.
8vo. cloth, 15s.

DR. TUNSTALL, M.D., M.R.C.P.

THE BATH WATERS: their Uses and Effects in the Cure and Relief

of various Chronic Diseases. Third Edition. 8vo. cloth, 2s. 6d.

DR. TURNBULL.

I.

AN INQUIRY INTO THE CURABILITY OF CONSUMPTION,

ITS PREVENTION, AND THE PROGRESS OF IMPROVEMENT IN THE
TREATMENT. Third Edition. 8vo. cloth, 6s.

II.

A PRACTICAL TREATISE ON DISORDERS OF THE STOMACH

with FERMENTATION; and on the Causes and Treatment of Indigestion, &c. 8vo.
cloth, 6s.

DR. TWEEDIE, F.R.S.

CONTINUED FEVERS: THEIR DISTINCTIVE CHARACTERS,
PATHOLOGY, AND TREATMENT. With Coloured Plates. 8vo. cloth, 12s.

VESTIGES OF THE NATURAL HISTORY OF CREATION.
Eleventh Edition. Illustrated with 106 Engravings on Wood. 8vo. cloth, 7s. 6d.

DR. UNDERWOOD.

TREATISE ON THE DISEASES OF CHILDREN. Tenth Edition,
with Additions and Corrections by HENRY DAVIES, M.D. 8vo. cloth, 15s.

DR. UNGER.

BOTANICAL LETTERS. Translated by Dr. B. PAUL. Numerous
Woodcuts. Post 8vo., 2s. 6d.

MR. WADE, F.R.C.S.

STRICTURE OF THE URETHRA, ITS COMPLICATIONS
AND EFFECTS; a Practical Treatise on the Nature and Treatment of those
Affections. Fourth Edition. 8vo. cloth, 7s. 6d.

DR. WALKER, M.B.LOND.

ON DIPHTHERIA AND DIPHTHERITIC DISEASES. Fcap.
8vo. cloth, 3s.

DR. WALLER.

ELEMENTS OF PRACTICAL MIDWIFERY; or, Companion to
the Lying-in Room. Fourth Edition, with Plates. Fcap. cloth, 4s. 6d.

MR. HAYNES WALTON, F.R.C.S.

SURGICAL DISEASES OF THE EYE. With Engravings on
Wood. Second Edition. 8vo. cloth, 14s.

DR. WARING, M.D., F.L.S.

A MANUAL OF PRACTICAL THERAPEUTICS. Second Edition,
Revised and Enlarged. Fcap. 8vo. cloth, 12s. 6d.

DR. WATERS, M.R.C.P.
I.

THE ANATOMY OF THE HUMAN LUNG. The Prize Essay
to which the Fothergillian Gold Medal was awarded by the Medical Society of London.
Post 8vo. cloth, 6s. 6d.
II.

RESEARCHES ON THE NATURE, PATHOLOGY, AND
TREATMENT OF EMPHYSEMA OF THE LUNGS, AND ITS RELA-
TIONS WITH OTHER DISEASES OF THE CHEST. With Engravings. 8vo.
cloth, 5s.

DR. ALLAN WEBB, F.R.C.S.L.

THE SURGEON'S READY RULES FOR OPERATIONS IN
SURGERY. Royal 8vo. cloth, 10s. 6d.

DR. WEBER.

A CLINICAL HAND-BOOK OF AUSCULTATION AND PER-
CUSSION. Translated by JOHN COCKLE, M.D. 5s.

MR. SOELBERG WELLS, M.D., M.R.C.S.

ON LONG, SHORT, AND WEAK SIGHT, and their Treatment by the Scientific Use of Spectacles. Second Edition. With Plates. 8vo. cloth, 6s.

MR. T. SPENCER WELLS, F.R.C.S.

I.

DISEASES OF THE OVARIES: THEIR DIAGNOSIS AND TREATMENT. Vol. I. 8vo. cloth, 9s.

II.

SCALE OF MEDICINES WITH WHICH MERCHANT VES-SELS ARE TO BE FURNISHED, by command of the Privy Council for Trade; With Observations on the Means of Preserving the Health of Seamen, &c. &c. Seventh Thousand. Fcap. 8vo. cloth, 3s. 6d.

DR. WEST.

LECTURES ON THE DISEASES OF WOMEN. Third Edition. 8vo. cloth, 16s.

DR. UVEDALE WEST.

ILLUSTRATIONS OF PUERPERAL DISEASES. Second Edition, enlarged. Post 8vo. cloth, 5s.

MR. WHEELER.

HAND-BOOK OF ANATOMY FOR STUDENTS OF TH FINE ARTS. With Engravings on Wood. Fcap. 8vo., 2s. 6d.

DR. WHITEHEAD, F.R.C.S.

ON THE TRANSMISSION FROM PARENT TO OFFSPRING OF SOME FORMS OF DISEASE, AND OF MORBID TAINTS AN TENDENCIES. Second Edition. 8vo. cloth, 10s. 6d.

DR. WILLIAMS, F.R.S.

PRINCIPLES OF MEDICINE : An Elementary View of the Causes, Nature, Treatment, Diagnosis, and Prognosis, of Disease. With brief Remarks or Hygienics, or the Preservation of Health. The Third Edition. 8vo. cloth, 15s.

THE WIFE'S DOMAIN : the YOUNG COUPLE—the MOTHER—the NURSE —the NURSLING. Post 8vo. cloth, 3s. 6d.

DR. J. HUME WILLIAMS.

UNSOUNDNESS OF MIND, IN ITS MEDICAL AND LEGAL CONSIDERATIONS. 8vo. cloth, 7s. 6d.

DR. WILLIAMSON, SURGEON-MAJOR, 64TH REGIMENT.

I.

MILITARY SURGERY. With Plates. 8vo. cloth, 12s.

II.

NOTES ON THE WOUNDED FROM THE MUTINY IN INDIA: with a Description of the Preparations of Gunshot Injuries contained in the Museum at Fort Pitt. With Lithographic Plates. 8vo. cloth, 12s.

MR. ERASMUS WILSON, F.R.S.

I.
THE ANATOMIST'S VADE-MECUM: A SYSTEM OF HUMAN ANATOMY. With numerous Illustrations on Wood. Eighth Edition. Foolscap 8vo. cloth, 12s. 6d.

II.
DISEASES OF THE SKIN: A Practical and Theoretical Treatise on the DIAGNOSIS, PATHOLOGY, and TREATMENT OF CUTANEOUS DISEASES. Fifth Edition. 8vo. cloth, 16s.

THE SAME WORK; illustrated with finely executed Engravings on Steel, accurately coloured. 8vo. cloth, 34s.

III.
HEALTHY SKIN: A Treatise on the Management of the Skin and Hair in relation to Health. Seventh Edition. Foolscap 8vo. 2s. 6d.

IV.
PORTRAITS OF DISEASES OF THE SKIN. Folio. Fasciculi I. to XII., completing the Work. 20s. each. The Entire Work, half morocco, £13.

V.
THE STUDENT'S BOOK OF CUTANEOUS MEDICINE AND DISEASES OF THE SKIN. Post 8vo. cloth, 8s. 6d.

VI.
ON SYPHILIS, CONSTITUTIONAL AND HEREDITARY; AND ON SYPHILITIC ERUPTIONS. With Four Coloured Plates. 8vo. cloth, 16s.

VII.
A THREE WEEKS' SCAMPER THROUGH THE SPAS OF GERMANY AND BELGIUM, with an Appendix on the Nature and Uses of Mineral Waters. Post 8vo. cloth, 6s. 6d.

VIII.
THE EASTERN OR TURKISH BATH: its History, Revival in Britain, and Application to the Purposes of Health. Foolscap 8vo., 2s.

DR. G. C. WITTSTEIN.

PRACTICAL PHARMACEUTICAL CHEMISTRY: An Explanation of Chemical and Pharmaceutical Processes, with the Methods of Testing the Purity of the Preparations, deduced from Original Experiments. Translated from the Second German Edition, by STEPHEN DARBY. 18mo. cloth, 6s.

DR. HENRY G. WRIGHT.

HEADACHES; their Causes and their Cure. Fourth Edition. Fcap. 8vo. 2s. 6d.

DR. YEARSLEY, M.D., M.R.C.S.

I.
DEAFNESS PRACTICALLY ILLUSTRATED; being an Exposition as to the Causes and Treatment of Diseases of the Ear. Sixth Edition. 8vo. cloth, 6s.

II.
ON THE ENLARGED TONSIL AND ELONGATED UVULA, and other Morbid Conditions of the Throat. Seventh Edition. 8vo. cloth, 5s.

CHURCHILL'S SERIES OF MANUALS.

Fcap. 8vo. cloth, 12s. 6d. each.

"We here give Mr. Churchill public thanks for the positive benefit conferred on the Medical Profession, by the series of beautiful and cheap Manuals which bear his imprint."— *British and Foreign Medical Review.*

AGGREGATE SALE, 141,000 COPIES.

ANATOMY. With numerous Engravings. Eighth Edition. By ERASMUS WILSON, F.R.C.S., F.R.S.

BOTANY. With numerous Engravings. By ROBERT BENTLEY, F.L.S., Professor of Botany, King's College. and to the Pharmaceutical Society.

CHEMISTRY. With numerous Engravings. Ninth Edition. By GEORGE FOWNES, F.R.S., H. BENCE JONES, M.D., F.R.S., and A. W. HOFMANN, F.R.S.

DENTAL SURGERY. With numerous Engravings. By JOHN TOMES, F.R.S.

MATERIA MEDICA. With numerous Engravings. Fourth Edition. By J. FORBES ROYLE, M.D., F.R.S., and FREDERICK W. HEADLAND, M.D., F.L.S.

MEDICAL JURISPRUDENCE. With numerous Engravings. Eighth Edition. By ALFRED SWAINE TAYLOR, M.D., F.R.S.

PRACTICE OF MEDICINE. Second Edition. By G. HILARO BARLOW, M.D., M.A.

The MICROSCOPE and its REVELATIONS. With numerous Plates and Engravings. Third Edition. By W. B. CARPENTER, M.D., F.R.S.

NATURAL PHILOSOPHY. With numerous Engravings. Fifth Edition. By GOLDING BIRD, M.D., M.A., F.R.S., and CHARLES BROOKE, M.B., M.A., F.R.S.

OBSTETRICS. With numerous Engravings. By W. TYLER SMITH, M.D., F.R.C.P.

OPHTHALMIC MEDICINE and SURGERY. With coloured Plates and Engravings on Wood. Third Edition. By T. WHARTON JONES, F.R.C.S., F.R.S.

PATHOLOGICAL ANATOMY. With numerous Engravings. By C. HANDFIELD JONES, M.B., F.R.C.P., and E. H. SIEVEKING, M.D., F.R.C.P.

PHYSIOLOGY. With numerous Engravings. Fourth Edition. By WILLIAM B. CARPENTER, M.D., F.R.S.

POISONS. Second Edition. By ALFRED SWAINE TAYLOR, M.D., F.R.S.

PRACTICAL ANATOMY. With numerous Engravings. (10s. 6d.) By CHRISTOPHER HEATH, F.R.C.S.

PRACTICAL SURGERY. With numerous Engravings. Fourth Edition. By Sir WILLIAM FERGUSSON, Bart., F.R.C.S.

THERAPEUTICS. Second Edition. By E. J. Waring, M.D., F.L.S.

Printed by W. BLANCHARD & SONS, 62, Millbank Street, Westminster.

9 781330 586389